PHYSICAL THERAPY CASE FILES®
Acute Care

Erin E. Jobst, PT, PhD
Associate Professor
School of Physical Therapy
College of Health Professions
Pacific University
Hillsboro, Oregon

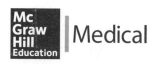

McGraw-Hill Education | Medical

New York   Chicago   San Francisco   Lisbon   London   Madrid   Mexico City
Milan   New Delhi   San Juan   Seoul   Singapore   Sydney   Toronto

Physical Therapy Case Files®: Acute Care

1 2 3 4 5 6 7 8 9 0   DOC/DOC   18 17 16 15 14 13

ISBN 978-0-07-176380-6
MHID 0-07-176380-5

Notice

Medicine is an ever-changing science. As new research and clinical experience broaden our knowledge, changes in treatment and drug therapy are required. The authors and the publisher of this work have checked with sources believed to be reliable in their efforts to provide information that is complete and generally in accord with the standard accepted at the time of publication. However, in view of the possibility of human error or changes in medical sciences, neither the editors nor the publisher nor any other party who has been involved in the preparation or publication of this work warrants that the information contained herein is in every respect accurate or complete, and they disclaim all responsibility for any errors or omissions or for the results obtained from use of the information contained in this work. Readers are encouraged to confirm the information contained herein with other sources. For example and in particular, readers are advised to check the product information sheet included in the package of each drug they plan to administer to be certain that the information contained in this work is accurate and that changes have not been made in the recommended dose or in the contraindications for administration. This recommendation is of particular importance in connection with new or infrequently used drugs.

This book was set in Goudy by Cenveo® Publisher Services.
The editors were Catherine A. Johnson and Christina M. Thomas.
The production supervisor was Catherine H. Saggese.
Project management was provided by Yashmita Hota, Cenveo Publisher Services.
The designer was Janice Bielawa.
RR Donnelley was the printer and binder.

Library of Congress Cataloging-in-Publication Data

Jobst, Erin E.
    Physical therapy case files : acute care / Erin E. Jobst.
        p. ; cm.
    Includes bibliographical references and index.
    ISBN 978-0-07-176380-6 (pbk.) — ISBN 0-07-176380-5 (pbk.)
    I. Title.
    [DNLM: 1. Physical Therapy Modalities—Case Reports.   2. Needs Assessment—Case Reports.   WB 460]
    615.8′2—dc23   2012027971

CONTENTS

Heather Dillon Anderson, PT, DPT, NCS
Assistant Professor
Physical Therapy Program
Neumann University
Aston, Pennsylvania

Scott M. Arnold, PT
Supervisor, Rehabilitative Services
Mayo Clinic Florida
Instructor
Physical Medicine and Rehabilitation
Mayo College of Medicine
Jacksonville, Florida

Ronald De Vera Barredo, PT, DPT, EdD, GCS
Associate Professor and Department Head
Department of Physical Therapy
Tennessee State University
Nashville, Tennessee

Christina N. Brown, PT, DPT
Physical Therapist
Community Memorial Hospital
Hamilton, NY
Adjunct Faculty
Utica College
Utica, New York

Paz Susan Cabanero-Johnson, PT, DScPT, MA
Health Care Education Specialist/Project Manager
Department of Veterans Affairs
VA Medical Center Perry Point Campus
Perry Point, Maryland

Lawrence P. Cahalin, PhD, PT, CCS
Professor
University of Miami
Leonard M. Miller School of Medicine
Department of Physical Therapy
Coral Gables, Florida

Joyce M. Campbell, PT, PhD
Professor
Department of Physical Therapy
College of Health and Human Services
California State University, Long Beach
Long Beach, California

Doris Y. Chong, PT, DScPT, MSc, NCS
Clinical Associate
Department of Rehabilitation Sciences
The Hong Kong Polytechnic University
Hong Kong

Alisa L. Curry, PT, DPT
PT Clinical Coordinator
Program Manager - Center for Joint Replacement
Washington Hospital Healthcare System
Fremont, California

CPT Jeremy Fletcher, PT, DPT, CSCS
4th Infantry Brigade Combat Team, Third Infantry Division
Fort Stewart, Georgia

Judith R. Gale, PT, DPT, MPH, OCS
Associate Professor
Department of Physical Therapy
Creighton University
Omaha, Nebraska

Anne K. Galgon, PT, PhD, NCS
Assistant Professor
Department of Physical Therapy
Temple University
Philadelphia, Pennsylvania

Leslie B. Glickman, PT, PhD
Department of Physical Therapy and Rehabilitation Science
University of Maryland, School of Medicine
Baltimore, Maryland

Sharon L. Gorman, PT, DPTSc, GCS
Associate Professor
Department of Physical Therapy
Samuel Merritt University
Oakland, California

Rose Hamm, DPT, CWS
Assistant Professor of Clinical Physical Therapy
University of Southern California
Los Angeles, California

Jeff Hartman PT, DPT, MPH
Physical Therapist
Methodist Hospital
Emergency Medicine and Trauma Center
Indianapolis, Indiana

Larisa Reed Hoffman, PT, PhD
Assistant Professor
School of Physical Therapy
Rueckert-Hartman College for Health Professions
Regis University
Denver, Colorado

Erin E. Jobst, PT, PhD
Associate Professor
School of Physical Therapy
College of Health Professions
Pacific University
Hillsboro, Oregon

Karen Kemmis, PT, DPT, MS, GCS, CDE, CEEAA
Physical Therapist
Physical Medicine & Rehabilitation and Joslin Diabetes Center
 & University Endocrinologists
SUNY Upstate Medical University
Syracuse, New York

David John Lorello, PT, DPT
Physical Therapist
Maricopa Integrated Health System
Arizona Burn Center
Phoenix, Arizona

John D. Lowman, PT, PhD, CCS
Assistant Professor
Department of Physical Therapy
School of Health Professions
University of Alabama at Birmingham
Birmingham, Alabama

David W. Mandel, PhD, PT
Assistant Clinical Professor
Department of Physical Therapy
University of Miami Miller School of Medicine
Coral Gables, Florida

Jo-Anne Marcuz, MScPT, BSc
Physical Therapist
Department of Rehabilitation Services and Division of Rheumatology
The Hospital for Sick Children
Toronto, Ontario
Canada

Margaret L. McNeely, MSc PT, PhD
Assistant Professor
Department of Physical Therapy & Department of Oncology
University of Alberta
Rehabilitation Medicine Department
Cross Cancer Institute
University of Alberta
Edmonton, Alberta
Canada

Lindsey M. Montana, PT, DPT, CCS
Senior Physical Therapist
Department of Rehabilitation Services
Memorial Sloan-Kettering Cancer Center
New York, New York

Karen Mueller, PT, DPT, PhD
Professor
Program in Physical Therapy
Northern Arizona University
Flagstaff, Arizona

Barbara E. Nicholson, PT, MSPT, CLT-LANA
Providence St. Vincent's Medical Center
Portland, Oregon

Jaime C. Paz PT, DPT, MS
Associate Chair
Clinical Professor
Division of Physical Therapy
Walsh University
North Canton, Ohio

Brooke B. Pettyjohn, SPT
Doctor of Physical Therapy Program
Lynchburg College of Virginia
Lynchburg, Virginia

Amanda Stoltz, PT, DPT
Physical Therapist
Shriners Hospital for Children
Portland, Oregon

Mary Swiggum, PT, PhD, PCS
Assistant Professor
Doctor of Physical Therapy Program
Lynchburg College of Virginia
Lynchburg, Virginia

Anne K. Swisher PT, PhD, CCS
Associate Professor
Division of Physical Therapy
West Virginia University
Morgantown, West Virginia

Nicholas S. Testa, SPT
Doctorate of Physical Therapy Candidate
Utica College
Utica, New York

Laura White, PT, DScPT, GCS
Director of Clinical Education
University of South Alabama
Physical Therapy Department
Mobile, Alabama

Kristi Whitney-Mahoney PT, MSc, BScPT
Physical Therapist, Practitioner in Rheumatology ACPAC (C)
Division of Rheumatology
The Hospital for Sick Children
University of Toronto
Toronto, Ontario
Canada

ACKNOWLEDGMENTS

The original idea for these textbooks is that of Eugene C. Toy, the series editor of the Case Files™ for many years. The original Case Files™ books are designed to teach medical students and residents through patient case scenarios. I would like to thank Joseph Morita, my original editor from McGraw-Hill, who chose me to bring this vision of Dr. Toy's case-based learning to the field of physical therapy. Without his faith and persistent encouragement, I never could have done this project. I am also indebted to Catherine Johnson and Christina Thomas at McGraw-Hill for guiding me through the role of a Series Editor.

These books certainly would not exist without the contributors. I am so greatly indebted to each contributor of these cases. Thank you for sharing your academic knowledge, clinical expertise, time, and patience with my many editorial questions and comments.

I would especially like to thank every physical therapy student who I have had the pleasure of teaching. You are the reason I strive to share knowledge and bring evidence-based practice into the daily practice of physical therapy. I hope these cases help bring the evidence into action!

Finally, I would like to thank my fabulous husband Ken for not only supporting me at every step of my career and life, but also for making it so much fun.

Erin E. Jobst, PT, PhD

As the physical therapy profession continues to evolve and advance as a doctoring profession, so does the rigor of entry-level physical therapist education. Students must master fundamental foundation courses while integrating an understanding of new research in all areas of physical therapy. Evidence-based practice is the use of current best evidence in conjunction with the expertise of the clinician and the specific values and circumstances of the patient in making decisions regarding assessment and treatment. Evidence-based practice is a major emphasis in physical therapy education and in clinical practice. However, the most challenging task for students is making the transition from didactic classroom-based knowledge to its application in developing a physical therapy diagnosis and implementing appropriate evidence-based interventions. Ideally, instructors who are experienced and knowledgeable in every diagnosis and treatment approach could guide students at the 'bedside' and students would supplement this training by self-directed independent reading. While there is certainly no substitute for clinical education, it is rare for clinical rotations to cover the scope of each physical therapy setting. In addition, it is not always possible for clinical instructors to be able to take the time necessary to guide students through the application of evidence-based tests and measures and interventions. Perhaps an effective alternative approach is teaching by using clinical case studies designed with a structured clinical approach to diagnosis and treatment. At the time of writing the *Physical Therapy Case Files* series, there were no physical therapy textbooks that contain case studies that utilize and reference current literature to support an illustrated examination or treatment. In my own teaching, I have designed case scenarios based on personal patient care experiences, those experiences shared with me by my colleagues, and searches through dozens of textbooks and websites to find a case study illustrating a particular concept. There are two problems with this approach. First, neither my own nor my colleagues' experiences cover the vast diversity of patient diagnoses, examinations, and interventions. Second, designing a case scenario that is not based on personal patient care experience or expertise takes an overwhelming amount of time. In my experience, detailed case studies that incorporate application of the best evidence are difficult to design "on the fly" in the classroom. The two-fold goal of the *Physical Therapy Case Files* series is to provide resources that contain multiple real-life case studies within an individual physical therapy practice area that will minimize the need for physical therapy educators to create their own scenarios and maximize the students' ability to implement evidence into the care of individual patients.

The cases within each book in the *Physical Therapy Case Files* series are organized for the reader to either read the book from "front to back" or to randomly select scenarios based on current interest. A list of cases by case number and by alphabetical listing by health condition is included in Section III to enable the reader to review his or her knowledge in a specific area. Sometimes a case scenario may include a more abbreviated explanation of a specific health condition or clinical test than was provided in another case. In this situation, the reader will be referred to the case with the more thorough explanation.

Every case follows an organized and well thought-out format using familiar language from both the World Health Organization's International Classification of Functioning, Disability, and Health (ICF) framework[1] and the American Physical Therapy Association's *Guide to Physical Therapist Practice*.[2] To limit redundancy and length of each case, we intentionally did not present the ICF framework or the *Guide's* Preferred Practice Patterns within each case. However, the section titles and the language used throughout each case were chosen to guide the reader through the evaluation, goal-setting, and intervention process and how clinical reasoning can be used to enhance an individual's activities and participation.

The front page of each case begins with a patient encounter followed by a series of open-ended questions. The discussion following the case is organized into seven sections:

1. **Key Definitions** provide terminology pertinent to the reader's understanding of the case. **Objectives** list the instructional and/or terminal behavioral objectives that summarize the knowledge, skills, or attitudes the reader should be able to demonstrate after reading the case. **PT considerations** provides a summary of the physical therapy plan of care, goals, interventions, precautions, and potential complications for the physical therapy management of the individual presented in the case.

2. **Understanding the Health Condition** presents an abbreviated explanation of the medical diagnosis. The intent of this section is *not* to be comprehensive. The etiology, pathogenesis, risk factors, epidemiology, and medical management of the condition are presented in enough detail to provide background and context for the reader.

3. **Physical Therapy Patient/Client Management** provides a summary of the role of the physical therapist in the patient's care. This section may elaborate on how the physical therapist's role augments and/or overlaps with those of other healthcare practitioners involved in the patient's care, as well as any referrals to additional healthcare practitioners that the physical therapist should provide.

4. **Examination, Evaluation, and Diagnosis** guides the reader how to: organize and interpret information gathered from the chart review (in inpatient cases), appreciate adverse drug reactions that may affect patient presentation, and structure the subjective evaluation and physical examination. Not every assessment tool and special test that could possibly be done with the patient is included. For each outcome measure or special test presented, available reliability, validity, sensitivity, and specificity are discussed. When available, a minimal clinically important difference (MCID) for an outcome measure is presented because it helps the clinician to determine the 'the minimal level of change required in response to an intervention before the outcome would be considered worthwhile in terms of a patient/client's function or quality of life.'[3]

5. **Plan of Care and Interventions** elaborates on a few physical therapy interventions for the patient's condition. The advantage of this section and the previous section is that each case does *not* exhaustively present every outcome measure, special test, or therapeutic intervention that *could be* performed. Rather, only selected outcome measures or examination techniques and interventions

are chosen. This is done to simulate a real-life patient interaction in which the physical therapist uses his or her clinical reasoning to determine the *most appropriate* tests and interventions to utilize with that patient during that episode of care. For each intervention that is chosen, the evidence to support its use with individuals with the same diagnosis (or similar diagnosis, if no evidence exists to support its use in that particular patient population) is presented. To reduce redundancy, standard guidelines for aerobic and resistance exercise have not been included. Instead, the reader is referred to guidelines published by the American College of Sports Medicine[4], Goodman and Fuller[5], and Paz and West.[6] For particular case scenarios in which standard guidelines are deviated from, specific guidelines are included.

6. **Evidence-Based Clinical Recommendations** includes a minimum of three clinical recommendations for diagnostic tools and/or treatment interventions for the patient's condition. To improve the quality of each recommendation beyond the personal clinical experience of the contributing author, each recommendation is graded using the Strength of Recommendation Taxonomy (SORT).[7] There are over one hundred evidence-grading systems used to rate the quality of individual studies and the strength of recommendations based on a body of evidence.[8] The SORT system has been used by several medical journals including *American Family Physician*, *Journal of the American Board of Family Practice*, *Journal of Family Practice*, and *Sports Health*. The SORT system has been chosen for two reasons: it is simple and its rankings are based on patient-oriented outcomes. The SORT system has only three levels of evidence: A, B, and C. Grade A recommendations are based on consistent, good-quality patient-oriented evidence (*e.g.*, systematic reviews, meta-analysis of high-quality studies, high-quality randomized controlled trials, high-quality diagnostic cohort studies). Grade B recommendations are based on inconsistent or limited-quality patient-oriented evidence (*e.g.*, systematic review or meta-analysis of lower-quality studies or studies with inconsistent findings). Grade C recommendations are based on consensus, disease-oriented evidence, usual practice, expert opinion, or case series (*e.g.*, consensus guidelines, disease-oriented evidence using only intermediate or physiologic outcomes). The contributing author of each case provided a grade based on the SORT guidelines for each recommendation or conclusion. The grade for each statement was reviewed and sometimes altered by the editors. Key phrases from each clinical recommendation are bolded within the case to enable the reader to easily locate where the cited evidence was presented.

7. **Comprehension Questions and Answers** include two to four multiple-choice questions that reinforce the content or elaborate and introduce new, but related concepts to the patient's case. When appropriate, detailed explanations about why alternative choices would not be the best choice are also provided.

My hope is that these real-life case studies will be a new resource to facilitate the incorporation of evidence into everyday physical therapy practice in various settings and patient populations. With the persistent push for evidence-based healthcare to promote quality and effectiveness[9] and the advent of evidence-based reimbursement guidelines, case scenarios with evidence-based recommendations will be an added benefit as physical therapists continually face the threat of decreased reimbursement rates for their services and will need to demonstrate evidence supporting their services. I hope physical therapy educators, entry-level physical therapy students, practicing physical therapists, and professionals preparing for Board Certification in clinical specialty areas will find these books helpful to translate classroom-based knowledge to evidence-based assessments and interventions.

1. World Health Organization. International Classification of Functioning, Disability and Health (ICF). Available from: http://www.who.int/classifications/icf/en/. Accessed August 7, 2012.

2. American Physical Therapy Association. *Guide to Physical Therapist Practice (Guide)*. Alexandria, VA: APTA; 1999.

3. Jewell DV. *Guide to Evidence-Based Physical Therapy Practice*. Sudbury, MA: Jones and Barlett; 2008.

4. *ACSM's Guidelines for Exercise Testing and Prescription*, 8th ed. Wolters Kluwer/Lippincott Williams & Wilkins; 2010.

5. Goodman CC, Fuller KS. *Pathology: Implications for the Physical Therapist*. 3rd ed. Philadelphia, PA: W.B. Saunders Company; 2009.

6. Paz JC, West MP. *Acute Care Handbook for Physical Therapists*. 3rd ed. St. Louis, MO: Saunders Elsevier; 2009.

7. Ebell MH, Siwek J, Weiss BD, et al. Strength of Recommendation Taxonomy (SORT): a patient-centered approach to grading evidence in the medical literature. *Am Fam Physician*. 2004;69:548-556.

8. Systems to rate the strength of scientific evidence. Summary, evidence report/technology assessment: number 47. AHRQ publication no. 02-E015, March 2002. Available from: http://www.ahrq.gov/clinic/epcsums/strengthsum.htm. Accessed August 7, 2012.

9. Agency for Healthcare Research and Quality. Available from: www.ahrq.gov/clinic/epc/. Accessed August 7, 2012.

Introduction

When I first started working with patients in the hospital setting in the mid-1990s, the physical therapist's role was somewhat limited both in the type of patients we worked with and the extent of our assessments and interventions. Now, acute care physical therapy is in the process of ongoing evolution and physical therapists in the acute care setting must understand increasingly medically complex patients to provide individualized assessments, education, therapeutic exercise programs, assistive device training, and positioning programs that are supported by the best evidence currently available. There is accumulating evidence supporting the effectiveness of early mobilization in improving quality of life, function, prevention of complications of inactivity, and even in reducing length of hospital stay in critically ill patients. As a result, current practitioners, faculty, and students need to stay abreast of the most recent information available. In the absence of understanding medically complex patients and the appropriate and safe application of outcome measures and interventions in this population, the acute care setting can unfortunately seem either overwhelming in its scope and pace or possibly just a setting to be a technician in order to "get the patients up and walk them."

This text contains 31 cases contributed by some of the preeminent physical therapy researchers, educators, and master therapists in the acute care setting. Cases include a spectrum of diagnoses involving neurologic, orthopaedic, cardiac, pulmonary, infectious, inflammatory, integumentary, oncological, and postsurgical conditions affecting individuals across the lifespan (26 adult cases and 5 pediatric cases). Each case presents practice patterns supported by the strongest available research. Several cases are more unusual and highlight the expanding roles of the acute care physical therapist. For example, Jeff Hartman illustrates how physical therapists are utilized in emergency departments of several hospitals in his case of a patient presenting with low back pain. Anne Galgon and Heather Anderson describe the clinical decision-making process for differentiating between causes of dizziness in what initially appears as a "straightforward" patient after an elective total hip arthroplasty. Karen Mueller eloquently elaborates on the basis by which an acute care physical therapist would support the recommendation of a hospice evaluation for a patient and the role of the physical therapist in the hospice setting.

These cases are designed to inspire reflections on current clinical practice and to incite students and therapists to apply the ever-growing evidence in the management of fragile patients in the fast-paced and interprofessional hospital environment. It is my hope that these cases also "bring to life" the excitement of working in the challenging acute care environment in which uniquely trained physical therapists provide the best evidence-based care for acutely ill patients. As physical therapists expand and apply the evidence base supporting physical therapy management of patients in the acute care setting, the recognition of acute care physical therapy as a specialty area of practice within physical therapy may soon follow.

Thirty-One Case Scenarios

Cerebrovascular Accident

Sharon L. Gorman

CASE 1

A 69-year-old male presented to the emergency department (ED) after awakening this morning with aphasia and right hemiparesis. His wife phoned emergency medical services immediately and the patient arrived at the ED with the acute stroke team in attendance 30 minutes after the patient awoke with these signs. The patient's wife stated that the patient went to bed at approximately 10:30 p.m. the evening before without these complaints. The patient's prior medical history includes type 2 diabetes managed with metformin (Glucophage XR0) and hypertension controlled with atenolol (Tenormin). A computed tomography (CT) scan upon arrival to the ED showed evidence of a left middle cerebral artery (MCA) ischemic stroke with no evidence of hemorrhage. The acute stroke team determined that the patient was not a candidate for thrombolytic therapy, and they subsequently admitted him to the hospital. Physician admission referrals include "evaluate and treat by physical and occupational therapy" and "speech therapy for videofluoroscopy and aphasia treatment." It is currently 1:30 p.m. on the day of admission and the patient has just arrived on the Neurosciences floor of the hospital. The unit's case manager has approached the physical therapist to ask when the evaluation will be performed so she can begin working on his discharge to an acute rehabilitation unit, if indicated.

▶ Based on his health condition, what do you anticipate will be the contributors to activity limitations and impairments?
▶ What are the examination priorities?
▶ What are the most appropriate physical therapy interventions?
▶ What precautions should be taken during physical therapy interventions?
▶ What are possible complications interfering with physical therapy?

KEY DEFINITIONS

APHASIA: Inability to read, write, and/or speak due to damage to language centers of the brain

COMPUTED TOMOGRAPHY (CT): Diagnostic imaging procedure that uses radiography and computers to produce cross-sectional images of the body

DYSPHAGIA: Difficulty swallowing

HEMIPARESIS: Inability to move one side of the body

HYPERTENSION: Increased blood pressure, defined as $\geq$ 140/90 mm Hg most of the time[1]

ISCHEMIC STROKE: Disruption of cerebral circulation caused by a blocked artery due to either an embolus or thrombus

SUBLUXED SHOULDER: Glenohumeral joint instability often seen after stroke due to muscle imbalances caused by hemiplegia and/or abnormal muscle tone

TISSUE PLASMINOGEN ACTIVATOR (tPA): Thrombolytic drug used to break up and dissolve clots that cause heart attacks or strokes

TYPE 2 DIABETES: Disease in which blood glucose levels are persistently elevated due to the body's inability to make or use insulin appropriately

VIDEOFLUOROSCOPY: Examination of swallowing using a series of radiographs of patient swallowing radiopaque dye in various food consistencies (thin liquid, thick liquid, solid, etc.)

Objectives

1. Describe indications for use of tPA.
2. Identify the medical purpose for maintaining hypertension post-stroke.
3. Describe signs and symptoms consistent with hemorrhagic conversion and increased intracranial pressure.
4. Prescribe appropriate early mobility in an individual post-stroke, including management of common post-stroke complications.

Physical Therapy Considerations

PT considerations during management of the individual immediately after ischemic stroke:

▶ **General physical therapy plan of care/goals:** Increase activity and participation; increase strength and/or normalize muscle tone on involved side; prevent or minimize loss of range of motion (ROM), strength, and aerobic functional capacity; improve quality of life

▶ **Physical therapy interventions:** Neuromuscular re-education; functional training; pre-gait and gait training; patient/family education and training on positioning and ROM exercises; coordination of care with interprofessional team; prescription of supportive devices; provision of discharge recommendations taking into account the appropriate location and level of rehabilitation services the patient requires and can tolerate (*e.g.*, skilled nursing vs. acute rehabilitation), ability of spouse and/or family to assist, patient safety, environmental and contextual issues at home

▶ **Precautions during physical therapy:** Monitor vital signs, pain management in coordination with medical team, abnormal lab values, progressive weightbearing on hemiplegic side, protection of joints on hemiplegic side, protection of skin in insensate areas

▶ **Complications interfering with physical therapy:** Post-stroke complications such as deep vein thrombosis, aspiration pneumonia, and/or urinary tract infection; extension of stroke during initial few days after stroke, hemorrhagic conversion; edema on hemiplegic side; shoulder subluxation on hemiplegic side

Understanding the Health Condition

A stroke, also referred to as cerebrovascular accident (CVA) or brain attack, is an acute brain disorder of vascular origin accompanied by neurologic dysfunction persisting more than 24 hours.[2] In the United States, there are more than 750,000 people who have a stroke each year.[3] Stroke is the third leading cause of death in the country, and represents more serious long-term disability than any other disease.[3] Nearly 75% of all strokes happen in persons over the age of 65 years, and one's risk of stroke doubles with each decade after 55 years of age.[3] African Americans as a group have more strokes and more mortality due to stroke than any other ethnic or racial group in the United States.[3] The risk factors, both modifiable and nonmodifiable, are listed in Table 1-1.

Strokes are classified according to their primary cause, either ischemic or hemorrhagic. Ischemic strokes, caused by thrombi or emboli, account for 80% to 88% of all strokes.[4] Hemorrhagic strokes, presenting either as intracerebral or subarachnoid hemorrhages, represent the remaining 12% to 20% of CVAs.[4] The incidence of strokes has remained relatively stable since the mid-1980s, but mortality has

Table 1-1 RISK FACTORS FOR STROKE[4-6]	
Nonmodifiable	Older age[a] African American race Male sex[a]
Modifiable	Hypertension[a] Cigarette smoking Heart disease Diabetes[a] Transient ischemic attack

[a]The patient in this case has four risk factors present.

declined, suggesting a declining mortality rate among people after stroke.[6] Even with these declines, approximately 25% of people die in the year following their stroke.[6] Individuals who survive greater than 6 months after their stroke have substantial morbidity including hemiparesis (48%), inability to ambulate (22%), complete or partial dependence for activities of daily living (ADLs; 24%-53%), aphasia (12%-18%), and depression (32%).[6]

With ischemic stroke, neuronal tissue is directly damaged by loss of blood flow and subsequent hypoxia. In addition to the directly damaged brain tissue, additional *secondary* damage occurs near the directly affected area. After cerebral artery occlusion, it is hypothesized that thromboemboli begin to form at the distal portions of the artery. The surrounding neurons may become hypoxic due to microvessel occlusion secondary to astrocyte swelling.[4] Fibrin formation in surrounding gray matter also contributes to surrounding occlusion and secondary damage. These perfusion and inflammation cascade changes in the surrounding neuronal tissue cause secondary neuronal damage referred to as ischemic penumbra.[4] If this region can have blood flow normalized soon after stroke, additional irreversible damage can be avoided. Metabolic changes throughout the brain after ischemic stroke can also lead to additional cerebral damage. Uncoupled oxygen consumption, excitotoxic neurotransmitter cascades, and changes in perfusion pressure after hypoxia are all mechanisms thought to extend tissue damage beyond the area of direct vascular blockage.[4]

Deficits seen after ischemic stroke are directly related to the region of the brain affected, making knowledge of cerebral circulation useful in anticipating potential deficits seen in patients after stroke. Figure 1-1 shows the arterial supply of the

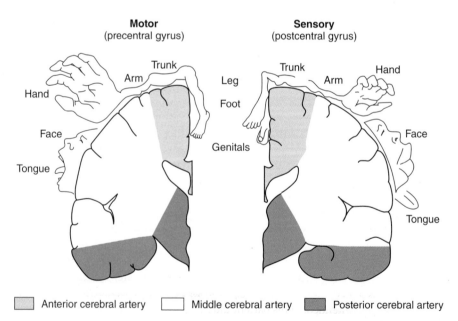

Figure 1-1. Arterial supply of the primary motor and sensory cortex (coronal view). (Reproduced with permission from Greenberg DA, Simon RP. *Clinical Neurology*. 7th ed. New York: McGraw-Hill; 2009. Figure 9-9.)

primary and sensory cortices. A large MCA infarction secondary to a total or near total occlusion commonly presents as hemiplegia and hemianesthesia on the contralateral side of the body. Global aphasia, involving both expressive and receptive aphasia, may be present if the involved hemisphere is the dominant hemisphere.[4] With more distally located infarctions, variations in clinical presentation commonly include hemiplegia and hemianesthesia greater in the face and upper body, expressive aphasia, Wernicke's aphasia, and spatial agnosia.[4] This patient had a large infarction and presented to the ED with dense, nearly complete hemiplegia and hemianesthesia on the right side of his body. He was also experiencing global aphasia.

Thrombolytic therapy for treatment of acute ischemic stroke has received regulatory approval in many countries throughout the world, including the United States. In 1995, the National Institute of Neurological Disorders and Stroke (NINDS) reported that treatment of acute ischemic stroke with injected tPA within 3 hours of stroke symptoms yielded substantial benefit.[7] Patients receiving tPA have increased survival rates and less dependency on measures of functional status in multiple studies.[7,8] However, there are many logistical challenges to health systems that can limit widespread tPA use in clinical practice. Acute stroke care systems have been re-engineered to try to limit obstacles to using tPA in the treatment of acute ischemic stroke. Most of these issues are related to time factors such as early presentation to the ED immediately after the onset of symptoms, "door-to-needle time" for tPA administration being less than 60 minutes, and the need for fast imaging studies upon presentation to the ED.[8,9] Inclusion and exclusion criteria for the administration of tPA post-acute ischemic stroke are described in Table 1-2.

For patients who meet inclusion and exclusion criteria, the recommendations are for intravenous (IV) administration of tPA to be given as quickly as possible within the 3-hour time limit from the onset of stroke signs and symptoms.[8] Because the effectiveness of tPA diminishes rapidly over time, recommendations suggest that physicians do not use IV tPA in patients whose stroke onset was between 3 and 4.5 hours prior to presentation to the hospital; however, the recommendations *do not directly recommend against* its use.[8] After 4.5 hours from stroke onset, the recommendation is *against* using tPA.[8] Streptokinase is no longer recommended as a thrombolytic agent for ischemic stroke due to trial and meta-analyses showing increased early mortality and symptomatic intracranial hemorrhage (ICH).[8] Intra-arterial (IA) tPA administration is recommended under specific guidelines for patients with MCA occlusion at medical centers with "appropriate neurologic and interventional expertise."[8] This includes patients with angiographically visualized MCA occlusion without major early infarction signs on baseline CT or MRI scan who can be treated within 6 hours of symptom onset.[8] Bleeding problems are the most common complication after tPA administration. Symptomatic ICH is the most severe complication seen in 6% to 7% of those receiving tPA, increasing as high as 15.7% in those patients who did not meet inclusion/exclusion criteria.[8] In patients who are not tPA candidates after acute ischemic stroke, the use of early aspirin therapy, if not otherwise contraindicated, is recommended.[8] This patient did not meet the time requirement for tPA therapy. Calculation of the time since onset of stroke uses the last time the patient was seen functioning normally. Since this patient's stroke likely occurred sometime during the night while he was asleep, the time his wife saw him when he went to bed

Table 1-2 ACCP EVIDENCE-BASED CLINICAL PRACTICE GUIDELINES FOR tPA ADMINISTRATION[8]	
Inclusion criteria	• Age ≥ 18 years • Clinical diagnosis of stroke with clinically meaningful neurologic deficit • Clearly defined time of onset of < 180 minutes before treatment • Baseline CT showing no evidence of ICH
Exclusion criteria	• Minor or rapidly improving symptoms or signs • CT signs of ICH • Seizure at stroke onset • Stroke or serious head injury within 3 months • Major surgery or serious trauma within 2 weeks • GI or urinary tract hemorrhage within 3 weeks • Systolic BP > 185 mm Hg • Diastolic BP > 110 mm Hg • Aggressive treatment required to lower BP • Glucose < 50 mg/dL or > 400 mg/dL • Symptoms of subarachnoid hemorrhage • Arterial puncture at a noncompatible site or lumbar puncture within 1 week • Platelet count < 100,000/mm^3 • Heparin therapy within 48 hours associated with elevated aPTT • Clinical presentation suggesting post-myocardial infarction pericarditis • Pregnant women • Anticoagulation due to oral anticoagulants (INR > 1.7)

Abbreviations: ACCP, American Academy of Chest Physicians; aPTT, activated partial thromboplastin time; BP, blood pressure; CT, computerized tomography; GI, gastrointestinal; ICH, intracranial hemorrhage; INR, international normalized ratio.

was used. While this patient did have an MCA infarct and his CT scan was without hemorrhage, it showed a large left MCA infarction on his initial CT scan, but he presented to the ED longer than 6 hours after symptom onset, placing him outside of the tPA protocol. The patient's CT scan with infarction to the left MCA is shown in Fig. 1-2. His thrombolytic intervention consisted of 200 mg per day of aspirin, which was started in the ED.

Newer modalities to treat ischemic stroke include mechanical neurothrombectomy devices for clot retrieval or to speed clot lysis. The MERCI Retriever System (Concentric Medical, Mountain View, CA) and Penumbra System (Penumbra, Alameda, CA) are the two FDA-approved devices that may be an option for patients ineligible for traditional tPA therapy.[10] Recanalization (i.e., resolution of the arterial occlusion) rates after mechanical neurothrombectomy vary significantly from 43% to 100%. The most common complications are symptomatic harm (0%-10%), asymptomatic ICH (1%-43%), and vessel perforation or dissection (0%-7%).[10] Predictors of harm with neurothrombectomy devices include older age, prior history of stroke, and higher baseline stroke severity scores.[10] Currently, neurothrombectomy devices have limited use due to the cost and technical expertise required to use the devices. More clinical outcome data are required before more substantial recommendations about their use can be formulated.[8,10] The hospital in which this patient was admitted had a MERCI Retriever System, but the patient's admission

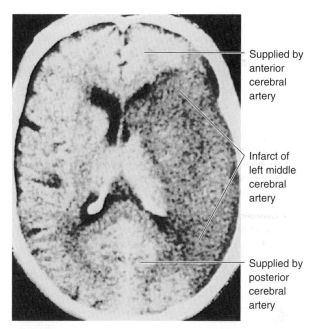

Supplied by
anterior
cerebral
artery

Infarct of
left middle
cerebral
artery

Supplied by
posterior
cerebral
artery

Figure 1-2. Computed tomography image of a horizontal section of the head showing an infarct caused by middle cerebral artery occlusion. (Reproduced with permission from Waxman SG, ed. *Clinical Neuroanatomy.* 26th ed. New York: McGraw-Hill; 2010. Figure 12-14.)

stroke severity score was low enough and the acute stroke team did not think he would be a suitable candidate for neurothrombectomy.

Hemorrhagic conversion (or hemorrhagic transformation) is a complication seen after ischemic stroke. With hemorrhagic conversion, reperfusion into the initial ischemically damaged vessels can result in hemorrhage through the damaged blood–brain barrier.[4] Two forms of hemorrhagic conversion may occur: hemorrhagic infarction (HI) or the less prevalent parenchymatous infarction (PH). Both of these types can be seen on CT scans. HI occurs regularly as a natural evolution of acute embolic strokes usually within the first 48 hours after stroke and primarily in the zone of the original infarction.[11] Incidence varies from 51% to 71% in autopsy studies, 26% to 43% in CT studies of noncoagulated patients, and 20% of cardioembolic strokes.[11] Most HIs are asymptomatic and are seen on CT scans of patients who are exhibiting stable or improving medical status. PH is less common than HI and is associated primarily with anticoagulation therapy. A low incidence of PH (2%-9%) is seen post-CVA in noncoagulated patients.[11] Although most HIs do not influence clinical presentation, PH is often associated with clinical deterioration due to development of a mass effect and extension of the damage beyond the original infarct territory. Proposed mechanisms of hemorrhagic conversion include blood pressure rises in the immediate post-stroke period and untreated hyperglycemia, but more research is needed to better understand the role of hypertension and elevated blood glucose on the development of hemorrhagic conversion.[11]

Because of the risk of hemorrhagic conversion and cerebral edema, the medical team has traditionally tried to **manage blood pressure post-CVA**. After acute stroke, blood pressure spontaneously increases in as many as 75% to 80% of patients, but usually decreases spontaneously during the first few days.[12] A recent double-blinded, placebo-controlled trial ($n = 2029$) investigating whether routine use of blood pressure–lowering medication in the acute post-CVA period improved mortality and functional outcomes found *no* beneficial effect on functional outcomes and a nonsignificant increased risk for worse functional outcomes at 6 months post-stroke.[13] Recent medical management has recognized that lowering blood pressure after acute ischemic stroke may actually decrease cerebral perfusion; thus, current recommendations are that physicians should not in routine practice prescribe blood pressure–lowering drugs within the first week of acute stroke.[12,14]

Early mobility for persons post-stroke has been shown to decrease morbidity and mortality, reduce disability after stroke, and reduce the number of patients requiring nursing home care.[15-18] In the United States, early mobility programs and clinical pathways have been incorporated into best practices internationally. These are required for a facility to attain certification as a **Primary Stroke Center**.[15,18] The AVERT (A Very Early Rehabilitation Trial) study was a large, multicenter randomized controlled trial out of Australia designed to investigate the safety, outcomes, and cost-effectiveness of early mobility rehabilitation programs in persons after acute stroke ($n = 56$).[15,16] The study protocol was designed for wide generalizability; inclusion and exclusion criteria and a basic outline of the interventions are listed in Table 1-3.

In 2008, the results of the safety portion of the AVERT trial were published showing that standard care plus early mobility did not increase the number of deaths and had similar outcomes on other safety measures such as falls, early neurologic deterioration, physiological monitoring compliance, and patient fatigue after interventions.[16] Nearly all deaths were in the most severe stroke participants regardless of whether they received standard care or standard care plus early mobility. In 2011, phase II of the AVERT trial reported on walking outcomes in persons in the standard care plus early mobility group ($n = 71$), indicating that early mobility participation led to a faster return to walking and was highly associated with good functional outcomes.[17] Specifically, Barthel Index scores were higher at 3 months post-CVA and Rivermead Motor Assessment scores were improved at both 3 and 12 months post-CVA, indicating improved functional outcomes in those who received early mobility interventions. This patient was admitted to a hospital with a Primary Stroke Center certification using early mobility protocols for appropriate patients.

Physical Therapy Patient/Client Management

Assessments and interventions during the immediate acute post-stroke period should include: determination of patient endurance (a key consideration for acute rehabilitation discharge recommendations); prevention of complications such as skin breakdown, edema in hemiplegic limbs, shoulder subluxation, and/or loss of ROM and minimization of poor postural or movement patterns such as contraversive pushing, improper mobility sequencing, and/or maladaptive static postures. Techniques

Table 1-3 PROTOCOL USED IN AVERT RANDOMIZED CONTROLLED TRIALS[15-17]	
Inclusion criteria	• Patients >18 years with first or recurrent stroke admitted within 24 hours of symptom onset • React to verbal commands (but not necessarily fully alert) • Systolic BP between 120 and 220 mm Hg • Oxygen saturation > 92% (with or without supplementation) • HR between 40 and 100 bpm • Temperature < 38.5°C
Exclusion criteria	• Premorbid (retrospective) modified Rankin Scale score >3 • Deterioration within the first hour of admission to the stroke unit or direct admission to intensive care • Concurrent progressive neurologic disorder • Acute coronary syndrome • Severe heart failure • Confirmed or suspected lower limb fracture preventing mobilization • Requiring palliative care
Interventions	• Receive usual standard care on stroke unit, and in addition: • Physiological monitoring of BP, HR, oxygen saturation, and temperature before each mobilization attempt within the first 3 days of stroke • Emphasis to assist patient to be upright and out of bed (sitting or standing as able) at least twice per day • Intervention delivered 6 days per week

Abbreviations: BP, blood pressure; HR, heart rate; bpm, beats per minute.

to normalize muscle tone and improve body awareness should be augmented with functional mobility tasks to reinforce familiar movement patterns while regaining activity-level movements using a task-oriented approach.[19] The primary focus during the immediate post-stroke phase is determining the most appropriate discharge destination and continued rehabilitation needs of the patient.[20-22] Constant monitoring for severe complications such as extension of the CVA, hemorrhagic conversion, or altered intracranial pressure is ongoing, since these signs and symptoms may be most readily recognized during therapy sessions. Signs of increased intracranial pressure include: altered consciousness, headache, seizure, sluggish ipsilateral papillary response to light, blurred or double vision, increased blood pressure and bradycardia (late signs), contralateral paresis, abnormal posturing (late sign), and vomiting.[23]

Examination, Evaluation, and Diagnosis

Prior to seeing this patient, a full chart review should be completed, with particular attention to physician orders such as post-stroke blood pressure parameters and other referrals for rehabilitation services (*i.e.*, occupational therapy, speech/language pathology). Imaging reports need to be reviewed because the type and location of the CVA can give important functional and prognostic information. Emergency medical services and/or ED notes should be reviewed for a clear picture of the initial presentation of the patient, history leading to presentation to the ED, and time since the onset of symptoms. Social work or case management notes (if available this early in the patient's hospitalization) could provide valuable insight into the home environment and situation as well as any third-party payer issues that may affect discharge planning. Review of the medical and/or surgical interventions and time given/started is important because these factors may help determine when physical therapy should be initiated and at what intensity.

The facility where this patient was admitted is certified as a Primary Stroke Center and uses an early mobility protocol for initiation of rehabilitation therapies, as indicated by the referrals written on admission for physical therapy, occupational therapy, and speech/language pathology. However, consideration of the patient's admission, medical treatment, and stroke severity all impact the therapist's decision about *when* therapy can safely be initiated. All decisions about when to initiate rehabilitation are aimed at reducing risk and harm and maximizing early mobility opportunities. Persons with hemorrhagic CVAs are managed with the following considerations: any neurosurgical procedures, cerebral vasospasm protocols, serial cerebral imaging to detect increased shifts or mass effect, and monitoring of mean arterial pressure, intracranial pressure, and cerebral perfusion pressure. For patients with ischemic CVAs, like this patient, the administration of tPA including route of administration (IV vs. IA) and the performance of mechanical neurothrombectomy are additional factors to consider prior to initiation of physical therapy. Table 1-4 summarizes considerations and current evidence-based recommendations for early mobility in persons with acute ischemic CVA.

The patient in this case did not receive either tPA or mechanical neurothrombectomy. His head CT was negative for hemorrhage, so early mobilization could be initiated based on his physiologic tolerance for increasing activity and ongoing

Table 1-4 EARLY MOBILITY CONSIDERATIONS POST-ACUTE ISCHEMIC CVA[16,17,24,25]		
Medical Interventions	**Potential Concerns and Complications**	**Recommendations**
IV tPA without mechanical neurothrombectomy	Increased risk of hemorrhage and bleeding after tPA administration	Wait 24 hours to look for hemorrhage[24] New retrospective data may indicate minimal adverse events with initiation of mobilization within 24 hours; prospective trial is in progress[25]
IA tPA and/or mechanical neurothrombectomy	Femoral sheath may be limiting factor for mobility, depending on the type of sheath and patient presentation	Do not mobilize with femoral sheath, otherwise mobilization as tolerated
No tPA or mechanical neurothrombectomy	Standard risk of hemorrhage	Mobilize within 24 hours[16]

Abbreviations: IA, intra-arterial; IV, intravenous; tPA, tissue plasminogen activator.

monitoring for development of signs and/or symptoms associated with post-acute stroke complications. In this case, the physical therapist and speech/language pathologist mutually agreed to have the physical therapist examine the patient shortly after arrival to the Neurosciences floor because information about his mobility level, tolerance for upright positioning, and ability to follow basic commands could help determine the patient's ability to participate in the videofluoroscopy study ordered.

During the examination, the therapist should take into account any monitors, lines, and/or tubes the patient may have in place. While mobilization can occur with most monitors, lines, and tubes, specific precautions or contraindications for movement may be indicated.[23] Depending on the skills of the therapist, additional assistance from others on the medical team may be indicated to prevent adverse events such as pulling out a line. Common lines encountered in acute stroke patients may include a nasogastric (NG) tube for feeding, IV lines for fluids and medication delivery, Foley catheter for urinary drainage, and intracranial pressure monitors to track changes in intracranial pressure. At the time of initial examination, this patient had only an IV line and Foley catheter. Later during his acute hospitalization, he had an NG tube placed to deliver his nutritional needs.

There are several reliable and valid outcome measures used in persons post-stroke. The Orpington Prognostic Scale and Functional Reach can be used to document progress over time. The Postural Assessment Scale for stroke patients can be used to measure balance deficits. The Timed Up and Go (TUG) test and 10-Meter Walk Test can be used to measure common gait deficits post-CVA. The Neurology Section of the American Physical Therapy Association developed StrokEDGE, a website listing standardized outcome measures that are recommended or highly recommended measures. In addition, they identified specific measures that may be useful in acute care settings for persons post-stroke.[26] The choice of which particular standardized outcome measure may be determined by initial assessment of the individual patient's activity limitations, patient/family goals, and the availability of the measure. Appropriate use of standardized outcome measures within the initial examination may represent a change in practice for acute care physical therapists. A survey by Jette and colleagues[27] in 2009 found that only 16.9% of acute care therapists in their sample (acute care therapists were 15.4% of the total 456 therapists in the study) routinely used a standardized outcome measure in practice, representing the practice setting with the lowest implementation percentage. The top six reasons that physical therapists (regardless of practice setting) gave for not regularly using standardized outcome measures are listed in Table 1-5.

Changes in the technology available in most hospital settings, especially the advent of integrated electronic health records, may help decrease the barriers to using standardized outcome measures in acute care practice. With medical applications that incorporate standardized outcome measures available on smartphones and tablet computers, calculation and analysis time may be reduced because these functions are already integrated into the application. With electronic health records becoming more mainstream and available, especially for therapists working in a large health system where access to the patient's entire health record across settings is possible, it is recommended that one or more standardized tools such as those mentioned be used periodically to assess the patient's long-term change over the episode

Table 1-5   TOP SIX REASONS GIVEN BY PHYSICAL THERAPISTS FOR WHY THEY DID NOT USE STANDARDIZED OUTCOME MEASURES

Reason	n	Percentage
Takes too much time for patients/clients to complete	102	43.0
Takes too much of therapists' time to analyze/calculate/score	71	30.0
Are difficult for patients/clients to complete independently	69	29.1
Require support system that I do not have (e.g., technology, staffing)	64	27.0
Often are not completed at discharge, so are not useful in determining patients'/clients' response to treatment	58	24.5
Do not contain the types of items or questions that are relevant for the types of patients/clients who I see	57	24.1

Modified with permission from Jette DU, Halbert J, Iverson C, Miceli E, Shah P. Use of standardized outcome measures in physical therapist practice: perceptions and applications. Phys Ther. 2009;89:125-35. American Physical Therapy Association.

of care. This should begin in the acute care setting whenever possible to establish each patient's baseline activity and function. Even if the acute care therapist does not gain immediately useful information on the patient's response to treatment, these baseline data can help show progress over longer time periods in the episode of care, especially in patients who routinely need longer courses of rehabilitation (e.g., persons post-CVA). Comparisons throughout the episode of care can then be made to assist in prognostication, evaluation of patient response to therapy intervention, and determination of discharge disposition. At this patient's hospital, all the patients with stroke have the Orpington Prognostic Scale administered before discharge and the physical therapist can choose to include other appropriate standardized outcome measures. The patient scored a 5 on the Orpington Prognostic Scale on day 4 after admission (hospital day 4), indicative of a moderate to moderately severe stroke that generally responds to acute rehabilitation and correlates with high likelihood of discharge to acute rehabilitation after acute hospitalization.[28] Because of the patient's large CVA, severe hemiparesis, and decreased functional mobility, the therapist had to account for floor effects when selecting additional measures. For patients with more severe functional deficits after stroke, finding a reliable and valid functional measure to document status and track changes, especially in the short time period of the acute care stay, can be difficult. The Function in Sitting Test (FIST) has been found reliable and valid for measurement of sitting dysfunction in persons post-acute stroke.[29] The FIST has a total possible score of 56 and a minimal detectable change of greater than 5 points, allowing the therapist to assess changes in sitting balance.[30] The physical therapist used the FIST to document baseline function in sitting. The patient scored a 32/56 and the results on individual FIST test items helped in decision making to select appropriate interventions in sitting for the patient during the remainder of his hospital stay.

Abnormal muscle tone is an impairment commonly seen in persons post-stroke. Changes in muscle tone are seen during the acute post-stroke period, with many patients initially presenting with hypotonia or flaccidity that evolves into hypertonia and/or spasticity.[31] Because these changes can occur even during the 4-to-5 day average acute hospital stay, accurate assessment of abnormal muscle tone can be an important measure of early change in a person post-stroke. A valid and reliable scale such as the Modified Ashworth Scale (MAS) can document spasticity throughout the episode of care and is easily understood by both physical therapists and other rehabilitation team members. If medications, nerve blocks, or other medical procedures are trialed or required to manage emerging increases in muscle tone, a baseline tone assessment using the MAS can help determine the relative value of such medical interventions. This patient presented at initial examination with complete right upper extremity flaccidity and right lower extremity spasticity in the hip flexors, knee flexors, and plantarflexors rating a 2 (increase in muscle tone with minimal resistance to passive movement through the range) on the MAS.[32] Positioning and interventions may need to be adapted to help normalize the patient's muscle tone during therapy interventions.

Plan of Care and Interventions

Specific, individualized goals are set after the initial examination and must reflect considerations of common post-acute stroke complications and discharge recommendations. In addition to specific findings from the initial examination, physical therapy interventions should include: patient/family education and training regarding skin protection in areas with decreased sensation and/or attention, therapeutic exercises to prevent loss of ROM on the involved side, joint protection techniques and strategies, and a positioning program to enhance these areas. Goals related to joint and skin protection should be incorporated with other healthcare providers such as nursing and may involve the assistance of family, as appropriate. Interventions to increase activity, such as bed mobility training, transfer training, and pre-gait/gait training should be initiated as soon as feasible. Neuromuscular re-education incorporating task-specific activities and using motor learning principles can be used to work on impairments and activity limitations. Intensity and duration of these activities should be based on the physiologic response of the patient to increases in mobility and activity, laboratory values impacting physiologic tolerance of increased activity, and patient's subjective response.

In the acute phase after ischemic CVA, patients are often hypertensive. Without treatment, this hypertension declines over the next 24 hours and may continue to decline for up to 7 days after the stroke.[33] To ensure adequate cerebral perfusion to the ischemic penumbra region after stroke, American Heart Association/American Stroke Association guidelines recommend during initial treatment that arterial hypertension not be treated unless it *exceeds* 220 mm Hg systolic or 120 mm Hg diastolic.[34] Because of the risk of hemorrhage with tPA administration, the guidelines for management of initial hypertension in patients receiving thrombolytics is more conservative; hypertension is treated if systolic BP *exceeds* 180 mm Hg, diastolic is *above* 105 mm Hg, or mean arterial pressure *exceeds* 130 mm Hg.[34] Physical therapists should be familiar with the patient's presentation and medical management, because these values need to be considered during patient mobilization and exercise. This patient, who did not receive thrombolytic therapy, should be monitored before, during, and after therapy sessions to ensure his blood pressure remains under 220 mm Hg systolic and 120 mm Hg diastolic. This will ensure adequate cerebral perfusion pressures and decrease the risk for hemorrhage. In addition, he should be monitored for signs of hemorrhagic conversion and development of cerebral edema, as evidenced by increasing intracranial pressure. One small study ($n = 8$) by Hunter and colleagues[35] used transcranial Doppler imaging to map cerebral blood flow with position changes (0° head of bed angle vs. 30° head of bed angle) at 24 hours post-acute ischemic stroke. In persons with incompletely recanalized arteries (arteries not completely reopened), they found decreased cerebral blood flow velocity when the head of bed angle was at 30° versus 0°. In contrast, there was no difference in cerebral blood flow velocity with head of bed angle position in persons with completely recanalized arteries (arteries completely open). Emerging research may help determine optimal timing to initiate physical therapy and/or optimal patient positioning based on patient-specific factors such as recanalization of involved arteries or restoration of the individual's cerebral blood flow.

Another common complication in persons with stroke is the development of a hemiplegic painful shoulder syndrome. Pain can be detrimental to recovery after stroke as it may inhibit movement, delay initiation of therapy, lead to poor tolerance of movement during therapy, and is associated with decreased motor recovery.[36] Hemiplegic shoulder pain syndrome develops in 5% to 84% of all stroke patients.[36] Symptoms can occur as early as the first week after stroke, and in one study ($n = 46$) more than one third of participants had shoulder pain immediately after their stroke.[36] Risk factors include glenohumeral subluxation, hemineglect, spasticity, flaccidity, and prior shoulder pathology.[36] During the acute phase after stroke, patients commonly have hypotonicity or flaccidity present, putting them at risk for development of a subluxation due to abnormally low muscle tone in the biceps brachii and rotator cuff musculature.[36,37] This inability to stabilize the humeral head in the glenoid fossa, especially when coupled with body positions in which gravity pulls inferiorly on the arm or when the humerus is internal rotated, can lead to an inferior glenohumeral subluxation.[36,37] The plan of care must incorporate both early recognition of the risk for developing subluxation and of **hemiplegic shoulder pain syndrome** as well as early intervention to prevent pain. Proper alignment of the scapula can greatly enhance comfort and reduce the risk for shoulder subluxation. Scapular exercises (as tolerated) should begin early, with particular attention to strengthening supporting muscles such as the serratus anterior as soon as possible.[19,32,37] Range of motion exercises should occur through the pain-free range, ensuring adequate scapular mobility in conjunction with glenohumeral joint mobility, and emphasizing shoulder external rotation and optimal glenohumeral alignment.[32,37,38] When upright, the patient should be positioned to encourage active weightbearing through the hemiparetic limb to help keep the humeral head positioned in the glenoid fossa while avoiding the pull of gravity on the limb.[37,38] Facilitation or handling may need to be provided by the therapist or a supportive sling or brace may be needed to keep the humeral head positioned optimally. Additional interventions during the acute phase can include functional electrical stimulation to the vertical stabilizers of the glenohumeral joint (e.g., long head of the biceps, supraspinatus).[32]

Due to this patient's right upper extremity flaccidity, he is at risk for developing hemiplegic painful shoulder syndrome. His positioning program addressed maintenance of both scapular and glenohumeral joint range of motion (ROM), prevention of contractures, potential for edema development, and support for the glenohumeral joint to avoid pain and subluxation. Figs. 1-3 and 1-4 show positioning strategies for the patient in the supine and sitting positions, respectively. All healthcare providers as well as the patient's family/caregivers were instructed in the positioning program to increase effectiveness and adherence. To prevent subluxation and development of pain in the right shoulder during the acute phase of recovery, careful attention must be paid to maintaining glenohumeral joint approximation through supported weightbearing of the right upper extremity when in antigravity positions such as sitting or standing.[32,37] His acute care rehabilitation team implemented a rigorous program of positioning to support the right arm, instructed

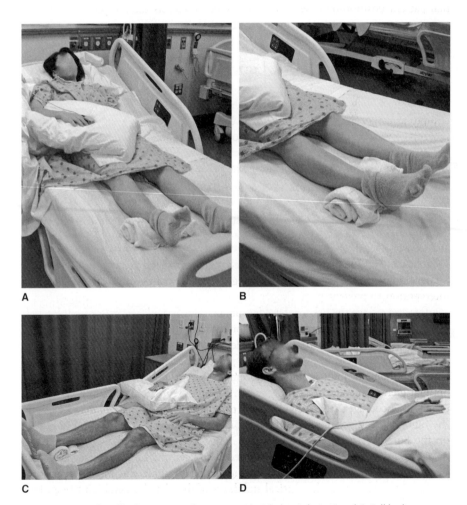

Figure 1-3. Examples of bed positioning for person with right hemiplegia. **A** and **C.** Full body positioning of hemiplegic right side. **B.** Close-up of heel floating using towel roll. **D.** Close-up of pillow placement for right upper extremity support and elevation.

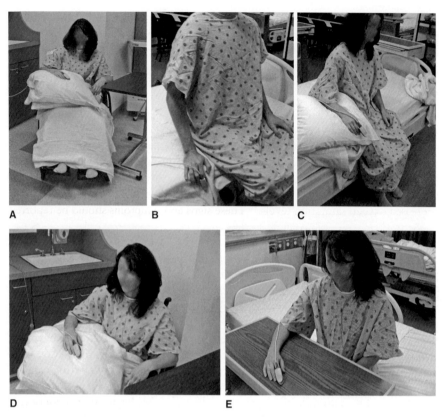

Figure 1-4. Examples of seated positioning for person with right hemiplegia with variations of right upper extremity support. **A.** Wheelchair positioning. **B.** Active support at edge of bed. **C.** Pillows for glenohumeral support at edge of bed. **D.** Close-up of upper extremity positioning with pillows in wheelchair. **E.** Bedside table for glenohumeral support at edge of bed.

his wife in proper positioning and ROM, and incorporated active weightbearing for the right upper extremity during all therapy sessions. They monitored the patient through self-report of right shoulder pain and periodic re-examination for development of pain and subluxation,[36] and the patient did not develop any problems with right shoulder pain or subluxation during his acute hospitalization.

In the first few months after CVA, nearly one quarter to one third of patients develop lower respiratory tract infections.[39] Development of pneumonia after stroke is associated with the need for endotracheal intubation and mechanical ventilation, increased morbidity and mortality, significantly longer hospital lengths of stay, and higher costs of care.[39,40] Interventions that increase the risk of pneumonia after stroke include tracheostomies, feeding tubes, proton pump inhibitors, or H2 blocker medication use for the treatment of gastroesophageal reflux disease, and dysphagia.[39] In persons poststroke with dysphagia, aspiration is a common cause of pneumonia, and "if not immediately recognized may be the pivotal factor that precipitates a significant decline in a patient's outcome."[40] Dysphagia after stroke has been associated with increased likelihood of a length of stay greater than 7 days and is considered a bad prognostic indicator.[40] Early diagnosis of dysphagia often includes videofluo-roscopy studies so that appropriate interventions and diet can be started to prevent unnecessary aspiration. The physical therapist should be attentive to any feeding recommendations from speech/language pathology after videofluoroscopy. During therapy interventions, emphasis on trunk posture and optimal upright posture can benefit patients with dysphagia, because optimal posture can produce more efficient swallowing mechanisms.[37] Liquid feeding via NG tubes is commonly used in the acute phase after stroke to ensure adequate nutrition and to decrease the risk of aspiration.[37] Therapists working with persons with dysphagia should monitor the patient for signs and symptoms of aspiration pneumonia, regardless of placement of an NG tube. Signs and symptoms include elevated respiratory rate, elevated heart rate, accessory muscle use, possible pleuritic chest pain, thick tenacious mucus, and decreased oxygen saturation levels.[41] These signs and symptoms should be reported to the medical team immediately so they can investigate potential development of aspiration pneumonia and institute treatment as soon as possible. The patient in this case had a videofluoroscopy demonstrating a high risk for aspiration with thin and thick liquids, so an NG tube was placed and the patient was started on bolus tube feedings throughout the day. Relevant considerations for physical therapy included waiting for radiographic confirmation of correct NG tube placement before resum-ing physical therapy, protection of the NG tube to keep it from dislodging or migrat-ing during intervention sessions, and keeping his head elevated ≥ 30° above the horizontal during bolus feedings and for approximately 30 minutes afterward.[23,41,42] The therapist also included interventions to maximize the patient's sitting balance abilities and worked with the speech/language pathologist to ensure good position-ing when working on swallowing to further address his dysphagia and risk for devel-opment of aspiration pneumonia.

Evidence-Based Clinical Recommendations

SORT: Strength of Recommendation Taxonomy

A: Consistent, good-quality patient-oriented evidence

B: Inconsistent or limited-quality patient-oriented evidence

C: Consensus, disease-oriented evidence, usual practice, expert opinion, or case series

1. Maintaining hypertension as prescribed by the medical team in the immediate post-stroke period improves patient outcomes. **Grade B**

2. Early mobility post-stroke in appropriately selected individuals is safe and benefi-cial to overall prognosis. **Grade A**

3. Physical therapy interventions including positioning, scapular exercises, progres-sive weightbearing to the involved upper extremity, and functional electrical stimulation decrease complaints of shoulder pain and protect the glenohumeral joint from subluxation in persons with stroke. **Grade B**

COMPREHENSION QUESTIONS

1.1 Which of the following signs or symptoms is *most* indicative of changes seen in the *later stages* of increasing intracranial pressure?

   A. Headache

   B. Vomiting

   C. Lethargy

   D. Sluggish pupil responses

1.2 In a patient with stable vital signs, which of the following describes the *most* suitable scenario to initiate early mobility after stroke?

   A. Patient who received tPA 8 hours ago

   B. Patient with positive bleed on head CT scan in ED

   C. High-intensity exercise focusing on uninvolved limbs in first 24 hours after stroke

   D. Patient with negative head CT scan who was not a PA candidate 20 hours after stroke

ANSWERS

1.1 **B.** Vomiting is only seen in the later stages of increasing intracranial pressure. Headache is seen in both early and late stages and cannot be used to differentiate between early and later stages without consideration of other signs and symptoms (option A). Lethargy and sluggish pupil responses to light are all seen during the early stages of increasing intracranial pressure (options C and D).

1.2 **D.** This patient does not have a hemorrhagic CVA, is not at risk for hemorrhage development because he did not receive tPA, and has had 20 hours pass since the onset of CVA symptoms. The patient is stable for initiation of physical therapy examination. While there is a paucity of evidence indicating when activity, and specifically physical therapy, should be initiated after delivery of tPA, many facilities and neurology teams hold initiation of physical therapy for up to 24 hours after tPA administration to monitor the patient for adverse events such as development of intracranial hemorrhage (option A). Patients need to be evaluated for intracranial hemorrhage. Until the patient has been stabilized and neurosurgery has made a determination as to whether surgical intervention is indicated, the physical therapist should not initiate an initial examination (option B). Cerebral recovery is impeded by high intensity, ipsilesional activity extremely early after stroke (option C).

REFERENCES

1. Dugdale D, Zieve D. Hypertension; June 10, 2011. Available at: http://www.nlm.nih.gov/medlineplus/ency/article/000468.htm. Accessed October 20, 2011.

2. Marino P. *The ICU Book*. 3rd ed. Philadelphia, PA: Lippincott Williams & Wilkins; 2007.

3. Stroke NINDS. What you need to know about stroke. Available at: http://www.ninds.nih.gov/disorders/stroke/. Accessed October 20, 2011.

4. Goodman C, Fuller K. *Pathology: Implications for the Physical Therapist*. 3rd ed. Philadelphia, PA: WB Saunders; 2008.

5. Stroke NINDS. Stroke risk factors and symptoms. Available at: http://www.ninds.nih.gov/disorders/stroke/stroke_bookmark.htm. Accessed October 20, 2011.

6. Sacco RL, Benjamin EJ, Broderick JP, et al. American Heart Association Prevention Conference on prevention and rehabilitation of stroke: risk factors. *Stroke*. 1997;28:1507-1517.

7. The NINDS t-PA Stroke Study Group. Generalized efficacy of t-PA for acute stroke. Subgroup analysis of the NINDS t-PA stroke study. *Stroke*. 1997;28:2119-2125.

8. Albers GW, Amarenco P, Easton JD, Sacco RL, Teal P. Antithrombotic and thrombolytic therapy for ischemic stroke: American College of Chest Physicians Evidence-Based Clinical Practice Guidelines. 8th ed. *Chest*. 2008;133:630S-669S.

9. Fonarow GC, Smith EE, Saver JL, et al. Improving door-to-needle times in acute ischemic stroke: the design and rationale for the American Heart Association/American Stroke Association's Target: stroke initiative. *Stroke*. 2011;42:2983-2989.

10. Baker W, Colby J, Tongbram V, et al. Neurothrombectomy devices for the treatment of acute ischemic stroke: state of the evidence. *Ann Internal Med*. 2011;154:243-252.

11. Internet Stroke Center. Hemorrhagic conversion. Available at: http://www.strokecenter.org/professionals/brain-anatomy/cerebral-embolism-formation/hemorrhagic-conversion/. Accessed October 27, 2011.

12. Fischer U, Rothwell PM. Blood pressure management in acute stroke: does the Scandinavian Candesartan Acute Stroke Trial (SCAST) resolve all of the unanswered questions? *Stroke*. 2011;42:2995-2998.

13. Hankey GJ. Lowering blood pressure in acute stroke: the SCAST trial. *Lancet*. 2011;377:696-698.

14. Jeffery S. SCAST: no benefit, possible harm, from lowering BP in acute stroke. *Medscape Medical News*. Available at: http://www.medscape.com. Accessed October 13, 2011.

15. Bernhardt J, Dewey H, Collier J, et al. A Very Early Rehabilitation Trial (AVERT). *Int J Stroke*. 2006;1:169-171.

16. Bernhardt J, Dewey H, Thrift A, Collier J, Donnan G. A Very Early Rehabilitation Trial for stroke (AVERT): phase II safety and feasibility. *Stroke*. 2008;39:390-396.

17. Cumming T, Thrift AG, Collier JM, et al. Very early mobilization after stroke fast-tracks return to walking: further results from the phase II AVERT randomized controlled trial. *Stroke*. 2011;42:153-158.

18. Alberts MJ, Latchaw RE, Jagoda A, et al. Revised and updated recommendations for the establishment of primary stroke centers: a summary statement from the brain attack coalition. *Stroke*. 2011;42:2651-2665.

19. Winstein C, Rose DK, Tan SM, Lewthwaite R, Chui HC, Azen SP. A randomized controlled comparison of upper-extremity rehabilitation strategies in acute stroke: a pilot study of immediate and long-term outcomes. *Arch Phys Med Rehabil*. 2004;85:620-628.

20. Jette DU, Grover L, Keck CP. A qualitative study of clinical decision making in recommending discharge placement from the acute care setting. *Phy Ther*. 2003;83:224-236.

21. Jette DU, Brown R, Collette N, Friant W, Graves L. Physical therapists' management of patients in the acute care setting: an observational study. *Phys Ther*. 2009;89:1158-1181.

22. Gorman SL, Wruble Hakim E, Johnson W, et al. Nationwide acute care physical therapist practice analysis identifies knowledge, skills, and behaviors that reflect acute care practice. *Phys Ther*. 2010;90:1453-1467.

23. Paz J, West M. *Acute Care Handbook for Physical Therapists*. 2nd ed. Boston, MA: Saunders; 2008.

24. Covil L, Ronnebaum J. Mobilization of patients status post-acute ischemic stroke treated with tissue plasminogen activator: using the evidence for clinical decision making. *Acute Care Perspectives*. 2008;17:7-9.

25. Arnold S, Chavez O, Freeman W, Meschia J, Mooney L. Early mobilization of ischemic stroke patients within 24 hours after intravenous-tissue plasminogen activator (IV-tPA) (EMISTPA); April 6, 2011. Available at: http://www.clinicaltrials.gov/ct2/show/NCT01331200. Accessed October 25, 2011.

26. Force ST. StrokEDGE outcome measures for acute care. Available at: http://ww.neuropt.org/files/StrokEDGE_acute_care_recs.pdf. Accessed October 13, 2011.

27. Jette DU, Halbert J, Iverson C, Miceli E, Shah P. Use of standardized outcome measures in physical therapist practice: perceptions and applications. *Phys Ther*. 2009;89:125-135.

28. Rehabilitation Measures Database. Rehab measures: Orpington Prognostic Scale. Available at: http://www.rehabmeasures.org/Lists/RehabMeasures/PrintView.aspx?ID=915. Accessed October 25, 2011.

29. Gorman S, Radtka S, Melnick ME, Abrams G, Byl NN. Development and validation of the Function In Sitting Test in adults with acute stroke. *J Neuro Phys Ther*. 2010;34:150-160.

30. Gorman S. Function In Sitting Test (FIST) web-based training. Available at: http://www.samuelmerritt.edu/fist. Accessed October 13, 2011.

31. Sanger TD, Delgado MR, Gaebler-Spira D, Hallet M, Mink JW. Task force on childhood motor disorders classification and definition of disorders causing hypertonia in childhood. *Pediatrics*. 2003;111:89-97.

32. Chancler C, Dillon H. Neurologic and neurosurgical diseases and disorders. In: Malone D, ed. *Physical Therapy in Acute Care: A Clinician's Guide*. Thorofare, NJ: Slack; 2006:317-384.

33. Owens WB. Blood pressure control in acute cerebrovascular disease. *J Clin Hypertens*. 2011;13: 205-211.

34. Adams HP, del Zoppo G, Alberts MJ, et al. Guidelines for the early management of adults with ischemic stroke: a guideline from the American Heart Association/American Stroke Association Stroke Council, Clinical Cardiology Council, Cardiovascular Radiology and Intervention Council, and the Atherosclerotic Peripheral Vascular Disease and Quality of Care Outcomes in Research Interdisciplinary Working Groups. *Stroke*. 2007;38:1655-1711.

35. Hunter AJ, Snodgrass SJ, Quain D, Parsons MW, Levi CR. HOBOE (Head-of-Bed Optimization of Elevation) Study: association of higher angle with reduced cerebral blood flow velocity in acute ischemic stroke. *Phys Ther*. 2011;91:1503-1512.

36. Dromerick AW, Edwards DF, Kumar A. Hemiplegic shoulder pain syndrome: frequency and characteristics during inpatient stroke rehabilitation. *Arch Phys Med Rehabil*. 2008;89:1589-1593.

37. Ryerson S. Hemiplegia. In: Umphred D, ed. *Neurological Rehabiliation*. 5th ed. St. Louis, MO: Mosby Elsevier; 2007:857-901.

38. Baum N. Proprioceptive neuromuscular facilitation shoulder progression for patients with spinal cord injury resulting in quadriplegia. *Phys Ther Case Reports*. 1998;1:296-300.

39. Marciniak C, Korutz AW, Lin E, Roth E, Welty L, Lovell L. Examination of selected clinical factors and medication use as risk factors for pneumonia during stroke rehabilitation: a case-control study. *Am J Phys Med Rehabil*. 2009;88:30-38.

40. Altman KW, Yu GP, Schaefer SD. Consequence of dysphagia in the hospitalized patient: impact on prognosis and hospital resources. *Arch Otolaryngol Head Neck Surg*. 2010;136:784-789.

41. Lindsay K, Malone D. Pulmonary diseases and disorders. In: Malone D, ed. *Physical Therapy in Acute Care: A Clinician's Guide*. Thorofare, NJ: Slack; 2006:212-273.

42. Harris K. Critical care competency program development and implementation. *Acute Care Perspectives*. 2006;15(1):16-19.

Respiratory Failure

Scott M. Arnold

CASE 2

One week ago, a 64-year-old female was admitted to the intensive care unit (ICU) through the hospital Emergency Department in respiratory distress with chief complaints of nonproductive cough and progressively worsening dyspnea on exertion (DOE). Two years ago, she underwent right single lung transplantation due to idiopathic pulmonary fibrosis (IPF). Her postoperative course since transplantation has been complicated by multiple hospitalizations for recurrent respiratory infections and acute graft rejection. For the past month, she has required increased home supplemental oxygen (O_2) to 3 L per minute (LPM) via nasal cannula from her typical 2 LPM. Upon ICU admission, her vital signs were: heart rate 90 beats per minute, blood pressure 120/81 mm Hg (mean arterial pressure 94 mm Hg), body temperature 38°C (101°F), oxygen saturation per pulse oximetry (SpO_2) 87% at rest on 3 LPM O_2 (which dropped to 82% with minimal exertion), and respiration rate 33 breaths per minute with notable distress. Chest radiograph revealed right upper lobe infiltrates; the patient was placed on non-rebreather mask at 10 LPM of O_2 and started on broad-spectrum antibiotics. Differential diagnosis upon admission was acute respiratory distress secondary to infection versus acute graft rejection. She has no underlying cardiac disease and her only significant comorbidities are a large hiatal hernia and gastroesophageal reflux disease (GERD) for which she takes omeprazole daily. Other relevant medications include tacrolimus, mycophenolate mofetil, prednisone, and alendronate. Her respiratory status since hospitalization has continued to deteriorate with cultures confirming bronchiolitis obliterans syndrome (BOS). Arterial blood gases show a trend of increasing hypercapnia with worsening hypoxia. The patient has been intubated for the past 2 days and now requires mechanical ventilatory support of pressure control mode, 0.4 fraction of inspired oxygen (FiO_2), and positive end-expiratory pressure (PEEP) of 5 cm/ H_2O. Her critical care team is discussing plans for possible tracheostomy if her status remains unchanged or worsens over the next few days. A physician referral for physical therapy consultation has been made today. The patient lives with her adult daughter.

- ▶ Based on the patient's health condition, what do you anticipate will be the contributors to activity limitations?
- ▶ What are the physical therapy examination priorities?
- ▶ What are the most appropriate physical therapy interventions?
- ▶ What precautions should be taken during physical therapy examination and interventions?
- ▶ What are possible complications interfering with physical therapy?
- ▶ How would this individual's contextual factors influence or change your patient/client management?

KEY DEFINITIONS

BRONCHIOLITIS OBLITERANS SYNDROME: Clinical diagnosis for chronic lung graft rejection

ENDOTRACHEAL TUBE: Artificial airway made of plastic tubing orally inserted into a patient's trachea to facilitate maintenance of respiratory activity via a mechanical ventilator

IDIOPATHIC PULMONARY FIBROSIS: Progressive, life-threatening lung disease characterized by alveolar scarring, reduced pulmonary compliance, and diminished capacity to breathe

IMMUNOSUPPRESSION: Deactivation or diminution of the body's ability to fight disease or infection; intentionally achieved pharmacologically in individuals with transplanted organs to reduce rejection of grafted organs

LUNG TRANSPLANTATION: Surgical replacement of one or both diseased lungs with those from a deceased donor

MECHANICAL VENTILATION: External support of adequate respiratory gas exchange by an automated apparatus via natural or artificial airway

Objectives

1. Describe the medical treatment plan for ventilator-dependent patients with respiratory failure.
2. Understand the indications for drugs prescribed post–lung transplantation.
3. Identify potential adverse drug reactions (ADRs) that may affect physical therapy examination or interventions and describe possible therapy solutions.
4. Recognize signs and symptoms of inadequate oxygenation.
5. List the anticipated deficits resulting from long-term mechanical ventilation.
6. List typical precautions when working with patients status/post organ transplant as well as those for mobilizing mechanically ventilated patients and discuss their rationale.
7. Design an appropriate plan of care for the patient on mechanical ventilation.

Physical Therapy Considerations

PT considerations during management of the mechanically ventilated lung transplant recipient experiencing chronic lung graft rejection:

- **General physical therapy plan of care/goals:** Prevent or minimize loss of range of motion, strength, and aerobic functional capacity; screen for readiness and facilitate early activity and mobility; maximize functional independence and safety while minimizing secondary impairments; facilitate ventilator weaning

- **Physical therapy interventions:** Early patient mobilization and resumption of any prior exercise regimen in preparation for the next phase of patient care

- **Precautions during physical therapy:** Airway protection precautions; close physical supervision to decrease risk of injury; consistent monitoring of vital signs, especially oxygen saturation (SpO_2); recognize potential signs and symptoms of decreased cardiac and respiratory reserves

- **Complications interfering with physical therapy:** Patient sedation, critical illness acquired weakness, intolerance to functional activity, complications and ADRs of long-term immunosuppressant therapy, lack of interprofessional understanding for the physical therapist's contributions to patient management

Understanding the Health Condition

Idiopathic pulmonary fibrosis (IPF) is a progressive and irreversible lung disease and the second leading indication for lung transplantation. The disease is characterized by scarring and thickening of alveolar tissue and surrounding interstitial space that leads to reduced lung compliance, hindered ability to breathe, and restricted physical function. Primary clinical presentation of IPF is progressive DOE and a dry, nonproductive cough. Average age of onset is 55 years or older. Although the exact etiology of IPF is unknown, links to both inflammatory and autoimmune disorders have been suggested. GERD, which is known to cause lung inflammation secondary to microaspiration of gastric acid, is an over-represented comorbidity in most individuals with IPF—present in 79% to 87% of patients.[1,2] Prognosis for IPF is poor, with an average life expectancy after diagnosis of 2 to 5 years.[3] Progression of the disease is nonlinear and patients often experience sudden acute episodes of respiratory deterioration requiring hospitalization; these exacerbations lead to over half of all IPF deaths.[4] Conventional medical management includes glucocorticoids for controlling inflammation and/or immunosuppressant therapy for controlling fibroblast proliferation.[5] Secondary consequences of long-term drug therapies can be severe and may result in diminished quality of life.

Lung transplantation remains the best option for increased survival and improved quality of life for patients diagnosed with IPF. Due to the unpredictable course of the disease process and poor prognosis, individuals with IPF are referred for transplantation evaluation soon after confirmed diagnosis. Mean waiting time for lung transplantation is 4.9 months in the United States,[6] with donor lungs coming from brain-dead patients. Patients with IPF may have either both lungs or only one lung replaced, depending on disease severity and patient age. Post–lung transplant complications are numerous and include graft rejection, frequent infections, and medication-related adverse effects. Of all solid organ transplant recipients, lung transplant recipients have the highest mortality, with rates approaching 49% and 75% at 5 and 10 years post-transplant, respectively. However, for reasons not well understood, post-transplant survival for patients with IPF is slightly lower, having mortality rates at 52% and 76% at 5 and 10 years, respectively.[5,7] Although single lung transplantation (SLT) is routinely performed in 63% of transplants for IPF,[8] the evidence appears to favor double lung transplantation (DLT) for optimal outcomes.[7] Three- and 5-year patient survival rates for DLT versus SLT are 76.3% versus 59.3% and 73.2% versus 43.8%, respectively.[9] Recipients of SLT are at greater risk for complications from infections and ventilation–perfusion mismatches occurring in the nontransplanted native lung. One study looking at outcomes of SLT versus DLT in IPF patients found median survival after SLT of 3.8 years compared to 5.2 years after DLT in recipients under age 60.[10]

Organ transplant recipients must adhere to a life-long regimen of immunosuppressive (antirejection) medication to improve graft survival and optimize lung function. Most transplant recipients (85%) will go through at least one episode of graft rejection during their first year after their transplants.[11] Infections and acute graft rejection remain the primary causes of death in the first post-transplant year. However, it is chronic rather than acute rejection that presents the greater risk of long-term morbidity and mortality.[12] Chronic rejection is clinically diagnosed as bronchiolitis obliterans syndrome (BOS) and leads to the inflammation and scarring of small airways in the transplanted lung. BOS occurs in up to 70% of lung transplant patients by the fifth post-transplant year.[13] By the time the condition is diagnosed, it is usually well advanced. As with IPF, BOS is also irreversible. Effective treatment for BOS has proven elusive. Median survival after onset is 2.4 to 4.8 years,[14] and BOS will usually first be detected by a progressive decline in the patient's forced expiratory volumes (e.g., FEV_1) of greater than 20% over several weeks of testing.[7] Cultures from bronchoalveolar lavage via bronchoscopy confirm the diagnosis of BOS. Causes of BOS are not well understood, but appear to be related to the frequency of past acute rejection episodes. GERD is also a common risk factor for both BOS and IPF. Treatment of GERD with proton pump inhibitors (PPIs) is a standard practice; however, fundiplication (esophageal wrap) surgery to reduce acid reflux has been shown to improve lung function post-transplant[15] and may be recommended by physicians. Adjustments in dosages and choices of immunosuppressants coupled with antibiotic therapies are the prevailing treatment regimens for BOS; some hospitalized patients may need mechanical ventilatory support. In a small number of cases (less than 5%), patients with advanced graft rejection may be listed for retransplantation. Survival in retransplanted patients is 59% at 1 year and 32% at 5 years. This compares with 79% and 45%, respectively, for 1 and 5 years for primary lung transplants.[16] Of note to the physical therapist, maintaining maximal physical function during any newly relisted waiting period is essential to improve future recovery and outcomes.

BOS - most common form of et Chronic LT rejection

Physical Therapy Patient/Client Management

Caring for critically ill patients in the ICU involves a multidisciplinary team approach. For the patient in respiratory failure requiring mechanical ventilation, the care team typically includes pulmonologists, critical care intensivists (MDs), registered nurses (RNs), respiratory therapists (RTs), pharmacists, case managers/social workers, and rehabilitation specialists such as physical and occupational therapists. If the patient is also an organ recipient, the team may also include transplant critical care specialists with knowledge and training specific to transplanted patients. Some hospitals have a separate respiratory ICU for ventilator-dependent patients where needed resources and specialists are centrally located.

The role of the physical therapist in the ICU is to assess the patient's current functional capabilities, readiness for activity and mobilization, and to prepare for the next phase of care after discharge from the unit. The specific roles of the physical therapist are to: prevent or minimize complications of immobility; assess range of motion, strength, neurologic function, functional endurance, dynamic balance and safety during transfers and gait within the indicated precautions; anticipate potential ADRs and modify interventions as appropriate to minimize their occurrence, and educate the patient and her daughter regarding postdischarge rehabilitation needs.

Frequent and prolonged hospitalizations resulting from infections and/or episodes of rejection may place a great deal of stress on both the patient and her family members. It is important for the physical therapist to be sensitive to the emotional or psychological impact the patient's medical condition may be having on her and her family members or caregivers. Family members may be a long way from home, work, family, and friends and may also face unforeseen financial burdens associated with their family member's health condition such as lost wages and unexpected expenses. Medication adverse effects, periods of immobilization, feelings of loss of independence, and uncertainty about the future are all issues that may affect the patient's motivation and compliance with therapeutic interventions. The incidence of affective mood disorders such as depression and anxiety is high in pre–lung transplant and post–lung transplant patients, and the physical therapist must be aware of signs or symptoms of any suspected mood changes and make appropriate professional referrals as needed.[17]

Finally, when considering clinical management of the critically ill patient, the physical therapist must be aware of the extent of practice patterns such as early ICU activity and mobilization currently in use in his or her own hospital. Although not a new concept, early patient mobility in the ICU population has been inconsistently utilized over the last few decades, partly due to real and perceived obstacles inherent in the care of critically ill patients. Studies have shown ICU patients often are not mobilized out of bed due to a multitude of factors, including staff fears of causing patient harm and the lack of time and needed personnel.[18] While current critical care medicine has made the most of breakthrough innovations in medical technologies, pharmaceuticals, clinical procedures, and treatment protocols that have resulted in higher survival rates, some more "common sense" practices (*e.g.*, getting patients up and moving sooner) have given way to over-reliance on patient sedation for patient management. This has contributed to a culture of patient immobility in many ICUs.[19] Because evidence-based protocols have only recently surfaced demonstrating the safety and feasibility of early mobilization of the medically complex ICU patient,[20] a cultural paradigm shift at the organizational level may be needed for the universal inclusion of early mobility as an established practice pattern in critical care physical therapy.[21] The acute care physical therapist can play an important role as an advocate for the immobilized patient in the ICU and for the advancement of physical therapy in this setting. An essential part of this role is to inform key ICU team members and hospital administrators about the growing body of evidence that inclusion of early mobility contributes to successful patient outcomes.

Examination, Evaluation, and Diagnosis

Prior to seeing the patient, the physical therapist should acquire information from her chart including: medications, lab values, ventilator settings, recent progress notes, and any activity or mobility restrictions. Critical lab values to check include: trends in hemoglobin, hematocrit, and blood gases. Exercise or mobilization should be discussed with the physician/s, if lab values and levels of ventilator support are not within safe limits.

The medication list should be reviewed to predict potential ADRs and to strategize possible therapy solutions to mitigate their effect on patient management. Antirejection drugs work by reducing the immune system's responsivity. Table 2-1 lists common ADRs of immunosuppressants as well as long-term complications that occur in individuals who must take these drugs for life. To minimize the incidence and severity of some of these ADRs, transplant physicians frequently employ a three-drug regimen consisting of a glucocorticoid (e.g., prednisone) in combination with a calcineurin inhibitor (e.g., tacrolimus or Prograf) or cyclosporine (Neoral, Sandimmune, Gengraf) plus a lymphocyte antiproliferation drug, (e.g., mycophenolate mofetil [CellCept] or azathioprine [Imuran]). Studies have shown that tacrolimus and mycophenolate mofetil perform better at preventing rejection when compared to cyclosporine or azathioprine[22,23]; however, specific immunosuppressive strategies vary by transplant center and individual patient effectiveness and tolerance.

Table 2-1   COMMON ADVERSE DRUGS REACTIONS OF IMMUNOSUPPRESSIVE DRUGS
Anemia
Coronary artery disease
Fetal malformation (teratogenesis)
Gastroesophageal reflux disease
Hypertension
Increased risk for infections
Liver and kidney damage
Malignancies
Myopathies
New-onset diabetes
Obesity
Osteoporosis

When reviewing ADRs, the physical therapist must consider those most relevant to the examination and subsequent treatment of the patient. Osteoporosis, for example, is a well-documented ADR that occurs in up to one half of the post-transplant population[24-27] and has been shown to increase risk for fractures of the vertebrae and long bones.[28] As a consequence of prolonged glucocorticoid use, osteoporosis is also prevalent in most patients waiting lung transplants, with estimates of abnormal bone mass density occurring in nearly 85% of lung transplant candidates.[29] Osteoporosis is of particular relevance to the physical therapist working with the lung transplant and pretransplant population due to its high prevalence and potential ADRs of the drugs prescribed to treat it.[25-27] Physicians often prescribe bisphosphonates such as alendronate (Fosamax) to prevent or reverse bone loss in pre- and post-transplant patients. The physical therapist should be alert to the potential ADRs of these drugs and modify therapy interventions as needed. Bisphosphonates, ironically, carry an ✓ increased risk for rare, spontaneous subtrochanteric and diaphyseal femoral fractures in some long-term users.[30] Moreover, severe joint, bone, and muscle pain has been reported in some new and long-term bisphosphonate users.[31] Long-term use of other drugs such as omeprazole (the PPI taken by this patient for control of her GERD symptoms) has been shown to heighten the risk for femoral neck fractures in osteoporotic patients.[32] The physical therapist treating patients on these drugs must monitor for signs and symptoms of potential fractures as well as be alert to the ADRs of any pain medication that might be prescribed for the patient.

The physical therapist should perform a comprehensive review of information in the patient medical record in advance of the examination. Assessment of the patient and her surrounding environment begins immediately upon arrival in the patient's room. Modifications to standard physical therapy examination may be needed due to the unique setting and circumstances in the care of the critically ill patient. For example, the patient on mechanical ventilation via endotracheal tube (ETT) or tracheostomy will be unable to speak, so other means of communication (gestures, communication boards, etc.) may need to be employed by the therapist to elicit reliable information during the examination. Provided that the patient has given permission for others to discuss her situation, family members or visitors may be valuable sources of patient information regarding the patient's prior level of function, home situation, assistive, and adaptive equipment. Pain levels in the nonverbal patient can be assessed using the 10-point Numeric Rating Scale (NRS) or the Wong–Baker Faces Pain Scale (Fig. 2-1). The nurse should be alerted to any pain

Wong-Baker FACES Pain Rating Scale

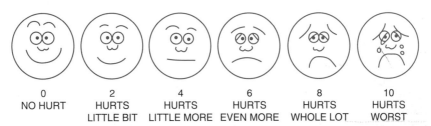

0	2	4	6	8	10
NO HURT	HURTS LITTLE BIT	HURTS LITTLE MORE	HURTS EVEN MORE	HURTS WHOLE LOT	HURTS WORST

Figure 2-1. Wong-Baker FACES Pain Rating Scale. (Reproduced with permission from Hockenberry MJ, Wilson D, Winkelstein ML. *Wong's Essentials of Pediatric Nursing.* 7th ed. St. Louis, MO: Mosby; 2005)

complaint that the physical therapist considers will interfere with the patient's participation in therapy. Some hospitals or rehabilitation departments may have *specific* policies regarding patients' pain complaints. For example, it is the policy of the Rehabilitative Services Department of Mayo Clinic Florida that the treating therapist notifies the nurse with any inpatient pain rating of 5 or greater using the NRS. However, policies may vary by facility and no universally agreed upon, evidence-based research exists that establishes a maximal level of pain as a contraindication to participation with therapy.

The physical therapist should explore the patient's level of function regarding general activity level, tolerance to activities of daily living, and participation and extent of any daily exercise routines prior to hospital admission. Because the lung transplant recipient is usually required to participate in a structured pulmonary rehabilitation program before or after transplantation, details of most recent sessions (e.g., treatment durations and intensities, familiarity with dyspneic and exertion-level rating scales) can provide useful baseline information for use in setting goals and predicting responses to future treatments. The physical therapist should also be familiar with common signs and symptoms of rejection that might occur during therapy sessions. These include DOE, fatigue, nonproductive cough, fever, flu-like symptoms, decreased oxygen saturations, and diminished lung function tests.

All invasive lines, monitoring equipment, and patient attachment points must be verified, and the logistics of safely moving the patient with lines and equipment must be considered in the therapist's overall decision-making process regarding planned interventions. Ancillary equipment such as ventilator, monitors, hemodialysis machine, various catheters, tubes, and drains represent potential limitations to patient assessment and intervention. Mobilizing the patient in the ICU requires communication and collaboration between the patient care team, and in some cases may require a doctor's written order before mobilization of the patient can occur. For example, patients receiving *intermittent* hemodialysis (usually 2-3 hours in duration) are attached to equipment that is sensitive to changes in vascular resistance; physical therapy is contraindicated during these sessions due to the potential of interference with the proper operation of the dialysis machine. However, patients receiving *continuous* dialysis, such as continuous renal replacement therapy or continuous veno-venous hemodialysis, can usually be mobilized out of bed to a chair (after permission from the physician) with the only contraindication to patient mobilization being the presence of a femoral intravenous access point. Specific equipment limitations and contraindications are reviewed in the next section.

Plan of Care and Interventions

Mobilizing the ventilator-dependent patient requires extreme caution, and represents an advanced practice pattern by the physical therapist[33] in which risks must be weighed against benefits. Presence of mechanical ventilation in itself is *not* a contraindication to patient mobilization, but it does signify an underlying state of reduced patient respiratory reserve. Patient mobilization demands the highest level of clinical knowledge, judgment, and decision-making skills to minimize risks to patient safety. Critically ill patients vary in their needs, and clinical management is a dynamic process requiring a thorough understanding of the underlying disease and physiological processes, significance of lab values, presence and effects of administered medications, and excellent communication skills. Although consensus among clinical experts on safe patient selection and monitoring parameters for early mobilization is evolving,[34] no evidence-based standard of care has been established. Currently, less than 10% of hospitals in the United States have existing guidelines for physical therapy interventions of any kind in their ICUs.[35] Suggested early mobilization guidelines found here and in the literature must not be taken in isolation but rather should be used as part of a well-reasoned process to support clinical decision-making based on the patient's overall condition and safety concerns in mind.

The key to effective and safe patient mobilization is developing and communicating a coordinated strategy of appropriate patient selection and monitoring, using a multidisciplinary, goal-oriented approach focused on the specific needs of each patient. Communication, collaboration, and close coordination between the appropriate team members are essential to preventing patient harm. The plan of care for mobilizing a patient in the ICU should be individualized and based on goals derived from specific deficits uncovered through the examination process, and developed through collaboration with the patient, family, and members of the multidisciplinary care team.

The hospital course for the patient requiring mechanical ventilatory support will vary depending on the underlying medical condition, and it may be complicated by a number of potential issues if an extended period of immobilization is involved.[36,37] Immobilization for even relatively short periods of time has been shown to have deleterious effects on lower extremity strength and lean body mass in healthy older adults representative of the age cohort of many hospitalized ICU patients. A study of 12 healthy, moderately active older individuals (mean age 67 years) subjected to 10 days of continuous bedrest showed decreases of 15.6% in mean knee extension strength and 6.3% in lower extremity lean body mass.[38] Immobilization, coupled with the physiological stress in some critically ill, bed-bound patients, can lead to longer-term complications. These include the onset of persistent neuromuscular weakness resulting from enhanced systemic inflammatory response mechanisms associated with critical illness[39-41] and neurocognitive and psychological problems that may be linked to protracted immobilization and sedation.[42,43] Such complications may contribute to patients' subsequent failure to regain their preadmission levels of function.[44,45] Early patient activity and mobility is fundamental to avoiding potential complications.[46,47] Evidence has demonstrated that **early mobilization of the mechanically ventilated patient** is safe,[20,48] may facilitate ventilator weaning,[49] and can lead to decreased hospital lengths of stay.[50]

Long-term physical therapy goals for this ventilator-dependent patient include improving musculoskeletal conditioning, optimizing aerobic capacity, and preparing her for eventual discharge to the next level of care. Short-term physical therapy goals should include early mobilization to prevent complications of immobility and resumption of any preadmission exercise regimen. Patient mobilization should be considered as soon as the patient is physiologically stable; exercise for the recipient of a lung transplant should include both progressive aerobic and strength training components. **Exercise benefits for the lung-transplanted patient** include increased

Table 2-2 COMMON CRITERIA FOR MOBILIZING THE CRITICALLY ILL PATIENT	
Indications (Safe to Mobilize)	Contraindications (Do Not Mobilize)
Stable blood pressure with mean arterial pressure (MAP) between 60 and 110 mm Hg	Standard contraindications and precautions
Resting heart rate < 110 beats per minute	New onset of cardiac arrhythmias or signs/symptoms of myocardial infarction
Acceptable respiratory patterns	New additions or adjustments to vasoactive medications
No contraindicated patient attachments	Femoral sheath
Fraction of inspired oxygen (FiO_2) < 0.6	Intra-aortic balloon pump
Positive expiratory end-pressure (PEEP) < 10 cm/H_2O	Intermittent hemodialysis
Oxygen saturation via pulse oximetry (SpO_2) > 90%	

muscle strength, partial reversal of glucocorticoid-related myopathy, restoration of bone mineral density toward pretransplant levels, and reduction of immuno-suppressant-related osteoporosis risks.[51] Progression of physical therapy interventions is based on patient safety, tolerance of previous interventions, and medical stability.

Three physiologic conditions necessary for safe, early patient mobilization are hemodynamic stability with adequate cardiovascular reserve, sufficient oxygenation with adequate respiratory reserve, and a cognitive ability allowing participation in therapy. Table 2-2 lists specific selection criteria for critically ill patients to be able to participate in physical therapy.[39,52]

Optimal patient safety is the guiding principle when mobilizing the ventilator-dependent patient. Prior to the intervention, all necessary team members and equipment should be assembled. Appropriate staff may include the patient's nurse (RN), RT, and any additional support personnel, such as rehabilitation or nursing aides, needed for patient safety. The physical therapist should receive an update on the patient's current condition from the nurse. Any activity restrictions that may limit patient mobilization (e.g., bedrest orders after a procedure) should be clarified prior to mobilizing the patient; the therapist may need to contact the ordering physician to have activity orders modified.

To the extent that breakdowns in communications occurring among healthcare providers has been identified as the primary cause of medical mistakes and unintended patient (and staff) injuries in hospitals,[53] the physical therapist must accept responsibility for effectively communicating the goals and objectives of each planned intervention, and for insuring that all team members understand their specific roles and duties prior to and during the intervention.

Upon entering the patient's room, the physical therapist should review the planned intervention with the patient and obtain permission to proceed. The patient's pain level should be assessed and the RN alerted to pain complaints that may hinder patient participation. Vital signs should be confirmed and retaken if necessary (*e.g.*, blood pressure). The treatment environment should be inspected and made ready: all patient lines and attachments should be located, inspected, and properly secured *prior* to patient mobilization; the nurse should disconnect any unneeded equipment. Many pieces of equipment used in the ICU (*e.g.*, intravenous infusion pumps) are designed with internal power supplies for portability. Patients on continuous monitoring (electrocardiogram, pulse oximetry, blood pressure) must continue to be monitored by portable monitoring equipment (*i.e.*, telemetry box or transport monitor) if taken outside the room. Portable monitors with screens are preferable to telemetry boxes from a patient safety standpoint because they provide the therapist with immediate information regarding the patient's physiological changes occurring during the treatment session, and may offer additional information (SpO_2, BP) without the need for extraneous equipment. The central monitor technician should be alerted when the patient is transferred to the portable equipment to allow for uninterrupted patient monitoring.

Any ETT or tracheostomy connections should be inspected by the physical therapist and secured; location of the ETT should be noted and confirmed by the RN or RT prior to and after the treatment session. An RT's assistance is needed for mobilizing the ventilator-dependent patient beyond the bedside chair.[19,54] The RT may either connect the existing ventilator to portable oxygen tanks or use a portable ventilator for transport from the room, depending on the ventilator's capabilities. Some investigators of early mobilization have suggested increasing FiO_2 by 0.2 during mobilization to ensure adequate patient oxygenation[54]; however, the physical therapist should discuss any changes to FiO_2 settings with the RT or physician prior to the proposed activity. Some ventilators in transport mode are unable to regulate FiO_2 and can only deliver 100% oxygen; this necessitates the need for spare oxygen tanks due to the relatively rapid exhaustion of oxygen from the tank. Patients with recent organ transplants may be required to wear a mask outside the room depending on the transplant program or institutional infection control policies. Some ICUs may have specialized air filtration that eliminates the need for a patient mask. All isolation precautions must be observed.

During the mobilization session, the physical therapist should closely observe for signs and symptoms of patient intolerance. Vital signs, including continuous pulse oximetry, should be monitored before, during, and after mobilization. Pulse oximetry fingertip probes are sensitive to changes in skin temperature or perfusion. A firm patient grip on an assistive device (*e.g.*, walker) can result in a lack of readout or erroneously low readings. Oximetry probes may need to be relocated if inaccuracies are suspected. Alternate locations include the patient's uninvolved hand (if using a cane), the forehead, or the earlobe. The patient should be frequently questioned during mobilization about exertion and dyspnea levels using the Borg Rating of Perceived Exertion scale or an alternate suitable dyspneic scale. For added safety during ambulation, the patient should be followed from the rear by a wheelchair in the event of excessive fatigue or an emergent need to sit. At the end of the mobilization session, the patient's response to treatment should be assessed. The nurse call bell should be placed within the reach of the patient. The physical therapist should reinspect all patient lines and attachments and reconnect and resume all lines and equipment to their original state. The monitor technician should be alerted and the RN updated if he/she was not part of the treatment. Details of the mobilization session should be documented including vital signs before, during, and after the session, the patient's response to treatment, any significant changes to monitored signs and symptoms, the position of any ETTs before and after mobilizing, and ventilator settings (e.g., mode, FiO_2, PEEP).

Evidence-Based Clinical Recommendations

SORT: Strength of Recommendation Taxonomy

A: Consistent, good-quality patient-oriented evidence

B: Inconsistent or limited-quality patient-oriented evidence

C: Consensus, disease-oriented evidence, usual practice, expert opinion, or case series

1. If precautions are followed, early mobilization by physical therapists of patients on ventilatory support is safe, well tolerated, and decreases overall hospital length of stay. **Grade A**

2. Early patient mobilization promotes earlier ventilator weaning. **Grade B**

3. Structured physical therapy interventions improve functional endurance and quality of life in patients with chronic lung graft rejection. **Grade B**

COMPREHENSION QUESTIONS

2.1 A physical therapist has created a physical therapy goal of early mobilization for a patient on mechanical ventilatory support in the ICU. Which of the following is an appropriate rationale for mobilizing a critically ill patient?

    A. Prevention of muscle weakness including critical illness myopathy/polyneuropathy

    B. Improvement of respiratory function

    C. Prevention of skin breakdown

    D. All of the above

2.2 Normal hemoglobin and hematocrit (H&H) levels for an adult range from 9.0 to 14.0 g/dL and 36% to 50%, respectively. Is the patient awaiting a lung transplant with a diagnosis of idiopathic pulmonary fibrosis (IPF) safe for activity and mobilization with a hemoglobin level of 7.2 and a hematocrit level of 23.6%?

    A. Yes, but the physical therapist must monitor for signs and symptoms of activity intolerance.

    B. No, hemoglobin levels < 8.0 g/dL and hematocrit levels < 25.0% are contraindications for physical therapy.

    C. Possibly, depending on other factors.

    D. Physical therapists are not qualified to treat patients with lung transplants.

2.3 Complications of post-transplantation immunosuppressant drugs include:

A. Osteoporosis

B. Increased risk for infections

C. New onset of type 2 diabetes mellitus

D. Malignancies

E. All of the above

2.4 Which of the following medical conditions is commonly found both in patients with IPF and in cases of bronchiolitis obliterans syndrome (BOS) post-transplant?

A. Osteoarthritis

B. Gastroesophageal reflux disease (GERD)

C. Peripheral vascular disease

D. Ischemic cardiomyopathy

ANSWERS

2.1 **D.** All of the choices are appropriate rationales for early mobilization in the ICU. Early patient mobilization may prevent critical illness-acquired weakness, improve lung function, prevent skin breakdown, and may also decrease the risk for Ventilator-Acquired Pneumonia due to earlier extubation from mechanical ventilation.

2.2 **C.** Decreased H&H levels signify a decreased ability to capture and transport oxygen at the cellular level. Activity and mobilization of the anemic patient is a precaution to initiating therapy; the decision should be based on recent and past trends in H&H levels and oxygen saturations. A *sudden* drop in hemoglobin, hematocrit, or both may indicate a potential bleeding problem and therapy may need to be withheld until the issue is resolved; in contrast, patients with chronic anemia may be asymptomatic and tolerate normal activity. In the case of the patient awaiting an organ transplant, physicians may avoid transfusing blood products due to the added complications of tissue-matching when searching for prospective donor grafts. Patients in these cases may receive erythropoietin to boost their own production of red blood cells. The physical therapist must monitor for signs and symptoms of exercise intolerance (e.g., shortness of breath, increased respiration rate, dizziness, lightheadedness, increased fatigue) in all patients with low oxygen-carrying capacity.

2.3 **E.** All of the above are complications of immunosuppressant drugs. Osteoporosis develops in half of transplant patients, and the incidence of vertebral fractures is 1 in 3.[26] Immunosuppression diminishes the body's ability to fight infections, and infections are one of the leading causes of death in the first year after transplantation. New onset of diabetes mellitus occurs in 13.4% of solid organ transplant patients.[55] Over one half of Caucasian transplant recipients will develop skin cancers as a result of long-term immunosuppressive medications.[56]

2.4 **B.** Gastroesophageal reflux disease has a higher prevalence in pretransplant patients with IPF and in post-transplant BOS. One study of 66 patients with established IPF revealed a prevalence of 87% for abnormal acid reflux levels with almost half (47%) of patients unaware of symptoms of GERD.[1] Osteoarthritis, peripheral vascular disease, and ischemic cardiomyopathy are not in themselves identified with patients with lung transplants. Gout, a form of arthritis, does occur in 7.6% of renal transplant patients by the third year.[57]

REFERENCES

1. Raghu G, Freudenberger TD, Yang S, et al. High prevalence of abnormal acid gastro-oesophageal reflux in idiopathic pulmonary fibrosis. *Eur Respir J.* 2006;27:136-142.

2. Morehead RS. Gastro-oesophageal reflux disease and non-asthma lung disease. *Eur Respir Rev.* 2009;18:233-243.

3. Frankel SK, Schwarz MI. Update in idiopathic pulmonary fibrosis. *Curr Opin Pulm Med.* 2009;15:463-469.

4. Agarwal R, Jindal SK. Acute exacerbation of idiopathic pulmonary fibrosis: a systematic review. *Eur J Intern Med.* 2008;19:227-235.

5. American Thoracic Society. Idiopathic pulmonary fibrosis: diagnosis and treatment. International consensus statement. American Thoracic Society (ATS), and the European Respiratory Society (ERS). *Am J Respir Crit Care Med.* 2000;161:646-664.

6. 2009 Scientific Registry of Transplant Recipients Annual Report. Available at: http://www.ustransplant.org/annual_reports/current/105_dh.pdf. Accessed May 16, 2012.

7. Mason DP, Brizzio ME, Alster JM, et al. Lung transplantation for idiopathic pulmonary fibrosis. *Ann Thorac Surg.* 2007;84:1121-1128.

8. Christie JD, Edwards LB, Aurora P, et al. Registry of the International Society for Heart and Lung Transplantation: twenty-fifth official adult lung and heart/lung transplantation report 2008. *J Heart Lung Transplant.* 2008;27:957-969.

9. Neurohr C, Huppmann P, Thum D, et al. Potential functional and survival benefit of double over single lung transplantation for selected patients with idiopathic pulmonary fibrosis. *Transpl Int.* 2010;23:887-896.

10. Thabut G, Christie JD, Ravaud P, et al. Survival after bilateral versus single-lung transplantation for idiopathic pulmonary fibrosis. *Ann Intern Med.* 2009;151:767-774.

11. DeVito Dabbs AD, Hoffman LA, Iacono AT, et al. Pattern and predictors of early rejection after lung transplantation. *Am J Crit Care.* 2003;12:497-507.

12. Christie JD, Edwards LB, Aurora P, et al. The registry of the International Society for Heart and Lung Transplantation: twenty-sixth official adult lung and heart-lung transplantation report-2009. *J Heart Lung Transplant.* 2009;28:1031-1049.

13. Zhang Y, Wroblewski M, Hertz MI, et al. Analysis of chronic lung transplant rejection by MALDI-TOF profiles of bronchoalveolar lavage fluid. *Proteomics.* 2006;6:1001-1010.

14. Finlen Copeland CA, Snyder LD, Zaas DW, et al. Survival after bronchiolitis obliterans syndrome among bilateral lung transplant recipients. *Am J Respir Crit Care Med.* 2010;182:784-789.

15. Murthy SC, Nowicki ER, Mason DP, et al. Pretransplant gastroesophageal reflux compromises early outcomes after lung transplantation. *J Thorac Cardiovasc Surg.* 2011;142:47-52.

16. Keshavjee S. Retransplantation of the lung comes of age. *J Thorac Cardiovasc Surg.* 2006;132:226-228.

17. Fusar-Poli P, Lazzaretti M, Ceruti M, et al. Depression after lung transplantation: causes and treatment. *Lung.* 2007;185:55-65.

18. Morris PE. Moving our critically ill patients: mobility barriers and benefits. *Crit Care Clin.* 2007;23:1-20.

19. Hopkins RO, Spuhler VJ. Strategies for promoting early activity in critically ill mechanically venti-lated patients. *AACN Adv Crit Care*. 2009;20:277-289.

20. Bailey P, Thomsen GE, Spuhler VJ, et al. Early activity is feasible and safe in respiratory failure patients. *Crit Care Med*. 2007;35:139-145.

21. Hopkins RO, Spuhler VJ, Thomsen GE. Transforming ICU culture to facilitate early mobility. *Crit Care Clin*. 2007;23:81-96.

22. Hachem RR, Yusen RD, Chakinala MM, et al. A randomized controlled trial of tacrolimus versus cyclosporine after lung transplantation. *J Heart Lung Transplant*. 2007;26:1012-1018.

23. Palmer SM, Baz MA, Sanders L, et al. Results of a randomized, prospective, multicenter trial of mycophenolate mofetil versus azathioprine in the prevention of acute lung allograft rejection. *Transplantation*. 2001;71:1772-1176.

24. Maalouf NM, Shane E. Osteoporosis after solid organ transplantation. *J Clin Endocrinol Metab*. 2005;90:2456-2465.

25. Aris RM, Neuringer IP, Weiner MA, et al. Severe osteoporosis before and after lung transplantation. *Chest*. 1996;109;1176-1183.

26. Cohen A, Shane E. Osteoporosis after solid organ and bone marrow transplantation. *Osteoporos Int*. 2003;14:617-630.

27. Rodino MA, Shane E. Osteoporosis after organ transplantation. *Am J Med*. 1998;104:459-469.

28. Van Staa TP, Leufkens HG, Abenhaim L, et al. Use of oral corticosteroids and risk of fractures. *J Bone Miner Res*. 2000;15:993-1000.

29. Lu BS, Bhorade SM. Lung transplantation for interstitial lung disease. *Clin Chest Med*. 2004;25: 773-782.

30. Shane E, Burr D, Ebeling PR, et al. Atypical subtrochanteric and diaphyseal femoral fractures: report of a task force of the American Society for Bone and Mineral Research. *J Bone Miner Res*. 2010;25:2267-2294.

31. FDA Patient Safety News. *Severe pain with osteoporosis drugs*. Show #73, March 2008. Available at: http://www.accessdata.fda.gov/scripts/cdrh/cfdocs/psn/transcript.cfm?show=73. Accessed May 16, 2012.

32. Targownik LE, Lix LM, Metge CJ, et al. Use of proton pump inhibitors and risk of osteoporosis-related fractures. *CMAJ*. 2008;179:319-326.

33. Perme C, Chandrashekar R. Early mobility and walking program for patients in intensive care units: creating a standard of care. *Am J Crit Care*. 2009;18:212-221.

34. Hanekom S, Gosselink R, Dean E, et al. The development of a clinical management algorithm for early physical activity and mobilization of critically ill patients: synthesis of evidence and expert opinion and its translation into practice. *Clin Rehab*. 2011;25:771-787.

35. Hodgin KE, Nordon-Craft A, McFann KK, et al. Physical therapy utilization in intensive care units: results from a national survey. *Crit Care Med*. 2009;37:561-568.

36. MacIntyre NR. Mechanical ventilator dependency: etiologies, management, and outcome. Program of the 12th European Respiratory Society Annual Congress; September 14-18, 2002; Stockholm, Sweden. Retrieved March 2, 2009 from Medline database.

37. Dock W. The evil sequelae of complete bed rest. *JAMA*. 1944;125:1083-1085.

38. Kortebein P, Ferrando A, Lombeida J, et al. Effect of 10 days of bed rest on skeletal muscle in healthy adults. *JAMA*. 2007;297:1772-1774.

39. De Jonghe B, Lacherade JC, Durand MC, et al. Critical illness neuromuscular syndromes. *Crit Care Clin*. 2007;23:55-69.

40. Bercker S, Weber-Carstens S, Deja M, et al. Critical illness polyneuropathy and myopathy in patients with acute respiratory distress syndrome. *Crit Care Med*. 2005;33:711-715.

41. Johnson KL. Neuromuscular complications in the intensive care unit: critical illness polyneuromyopathy. *AACN Clinical Issues*. 2007;18:167-180. Available at: http://www.nursingcenter.com/library/JournalArticle.asp?Article_ID=714674. Accessed May 16, 2012.

42. Desai SV, Law TJ, Needham DM. Long-term complications of critical care. *Crit Care Med.* 2011;39:371-379.

43. Davydow DS, Desai SV, Needham D, et al. Psychiatric morbidity in survivors of the acute respiratory distress syndrome: a systematic review. *Psychosomatic Med.* 2008;70:512-519.

44. Dowdy DW, Eid MP, Dennison CR, et al. Quality of life after acute respiratory distress syndrome: a meta-analysis. *Intensive Care Med.* 2006;32:1115-1124.

45. Combes A, Costa MA, Trouillet JL, et al. Morbidity, mortality, and quality-of-life outcomes in patients requiring > or =14 days of mechanical ventilation. *Crit Care Med.* 2003;31:1373-1381.

46. Needham DM, Chandolu S, Zanni J. Interruption of sedation for early rehabilitation improves outcomes in ventilated, critically ill adults. *Aust J Physiother.* 2009;55:210.

47. Griffiths RD, Hall JB. Intensive care unit-acquired weakness. *Crit Care Med.* 2010;38:779-787.

48. Needham DM. Mobilizing patients in the intensive care unit: improving neuromuscular weakness and physical function. *JAMA.* 2008;300;1685-1690.

49. Burns RJ, Jones FL. Letter: early ambulation of patients requiring ventilatory assistance. *Chest.* 1975;68:608.

50. Morris PE, Goad A, Thompson C, et al. Early intensive care unit mobility therapy in the treatment of acute respiratory failure. *Crit Care Med.* 2008;36:2238-2243.

51. Mitchell MJ, Baz MA, Fulton MN, et al. Resistance training prevents vertebral osteoporosis in lung transplant recipients. *Transplantation.* 2003;76:557-562.

52. Stiller K, Phillips A. Safety aspects of mobilising acutely ill inpatients. *Physiotherapy Theory and Practice.* 2003;19:239-257.

53. Rose L. Interprofessional collaboration in the ICU: how to define? *Nurs Crit Care.* 2011;16:5-10.

54. Korupolu R, Gifford JM, Needham DM. Early mobilization of critically ill patients: reducing neuromuscular complications after intensive care. *Contemp Crit Care.* 2009;6:1-11.

55. Heisel O, Heisel R, Balshaw R, et al. New onset diabetes mellitus in patients receiving calcineurin inhibitors: a systematic review and meta-analysis. *Am J Transpl.* 2004;4:583-595.

56. Euvrard S, Kanitakis J, Claudy A. Skin cancers after organ transplantation. *N Engl J Med.* 2003;348:1681-1691.

57. Abbott KC, Kimmel PL, Dharnidharka V, et al. New-onset gout after kidney transplantation: incidence, risk factors and implications. *Transplantation.* 2005;80:1383-1391.

Delirium

Laura White
Jeremy Fletcher

A 78-year-old male was admitted to the hospital 2 days ago with complaints of right hip pain after falling in his home. Notable previous medical history includes coronary artery disease, glaucoma, and moderate hearing loss. He was diagnosed with a right intertrochanteric femur fracture and underwent an open reduction internal fixation (ORIF) of the fracture without surgical complications. Relevant new inpatient medications include Percocet, Lovenox, Colace, and Benadryl. You are asked to evaluate and treat the patient on postoperative day (POD) 1. Based on a review of his medical chart, you note that the patient has several risk factors for delirium. The patient is expected to be discharged to a skilled nursing facility for continued physical rehabilitation in the next few days. The patient is a retired accountant who lives alone in a single-story home. He ambulates independently within his community and has no history of previous falls.

▶ What examination signs may be associated with the diagnosis of delirium?
▶ What are the most appropriate examination tests?
▶ What are possible complications interfering with physical therapy?
▶ What is his rehabilitation prognosis?
▶ What are the most appropriate physical therapy interventions?
▶ What precautions should be taken during physical therapy examination and interventions?

KEY DEFINITIONS

PRECIPITATING FACTOR: Temporal event that increases the risk for developing a particular disease or disorder

PREDISPOSING FACTOR: Intrinsic characteristic of an individual that increases his/her vulnerability of developing a particular disease or disorder

PSYCHOMOTOR AGITATION: Excessive and purposeless mental and motor activity

PSYCHOMOTOR RETARDATION: Generalized slowing of mental and motor activity

Objectives

1. List predisposing and precipitating factors for delirium in the acute care setting.
2. Recognize signs and symptoms of hyperactive, hypoactive, and mixed subtypes of delirium.
3. Identify a reliable and valid clinical tool that can be used to screen for delirium in the acute care setting.
4. Describe preventative clinical interventions for acute care patients at risk for developing delirium.
5. Discuss interventions that should be included in the physical therapy plan of care for patients with delirium in the acute care setting.
6. Recognize the potential effects of adverse drug reactions (ADRs) that may affect physical therapy management of patients with delirium.

Physical Therapy Considerations

PT considerations during management of the individual with delirium:

▶ **General physical therapy plan of care/goals:** Prevent or minimize loss of range of motion, strength, and aerobic functional capacity; maximize functional independence; reduce risk of falls and movement-related injuries

▶ **Physical therapy interventions:** Patient and caregiver training regarding reorientation techniques and cognitive stimulation; caregiver training for safe guarding during mobility; seating and positioning interventions to reduce the use of physical and chemical restraints; communication and coordination of care with multidisciplinary team to decrease severity and duration of delirium

▶ **Precautions during physical therapy:** Monitor for physical and emotional distress; close physical supervision to reduce risk of falls; recognize potential ADRs; monitor for pain; closely monitor vital signs and oxygen saturation levels

▶ **Complications interfering with physical therapy:** Impaired memory, inattention, altered level of consciousness, impaired sensory perception, psychomotor retardation, psychomotor agitation, falls, violent behavior to self and others

Understanding the Health Condition

Delirium is a complex neuropsychiatric syndrome that is prevalent, yet underdiagnosed, in the acute care setting. The prevalence of delirium in hospitalized patients varies based on patient population and clinical setting, with the highest prevalence in elderly patients who have undergone a surgical procedure or who are in the intensive care unit (ICU).[1] The incidence of delirium ranges from 14% to 42% of older patients admitted to general internal medicine or acute geriatric units and from 28% to 61% of older patients treated for hip fractures.[2] Delirium is also more prevalent in the post-anesthesia period after surgery and in the ICU for younger adult and pediatric patients, although the clinical presentation of delirium may be somewhat different in younger patient populations.[3,4] Delirium has also been reported in hospitalized patients with advanced cancer, stroke, and post-cardiac surgery.[5,6]

The key clinical features of delirium are *acute* changes in level of consciousness and cognitive function that fluctuate throughout the day.[7] Inattention, perceptual disturbances, psychomotor agitation or retardation, and disturbed sleep–wake cycles are other common features.[8] The clinical presentation can be quite varied, so delirium is categorized into three clinical subtypes based on motoric signs: hyperactive, hypoactive, and mixed.[9,10] The hyperactive subtype is characterized by psychomotor agitation, manifested by behaviors such as restlessness, frequently changing positions, constantly tapping fingers, and combativeness. The hypoactive subtype is characterized by psychomotor retardation, which may present as a slowed or absent response to verbal stimuli, generalized slow movement, and staring into space. Individuals with the mixed subtype fluctuate in their motor behavior, demonstrating features of hyperactive and hypoactive subtypes.

Delirium is caused by an underlying medical condition, substance intoxication or withdrawal, adverse effect of medication use, toxin exposure, or combination of these factors.[7] A diagnosis of delirium is based on findings of the history, physical examination, and laboratory tests. Findings should confirm that delirium is a direct physiological result of one or more of the aforementioned etiologic factors. The exact physiological mechanisms by which delirium develops are not well understood, although it appears that all etiologic factors cause an abnormality in central nervous system (CNS) neurotransmitter synthesis and function.[11,12] The presence of one or more factors does not guarantee that an individual will develop delirium. Rather, a complex interaction between predisposing (vulnerability) factors and precipitating (clinical) factors increases the risk of developing delirium. Predisposing factors for delirium in the acute care setting include age 65 years and older, pre-existing cognitive impairment, presence of severe illness, and current hip fracture.[13] Vision impairment and abnormal blood urea nitrogen (BUN) and creatinine levels at admission are additional predisposing factors in elderly patients.[14]

Precipitating factors include disorientation, constipation, dehydration, hypoxia, immobility, infection, multiple medications (*i.e.*, three or more added during hospitalization), pain, poor nutrition, sensory impairment, and sleep deprivation.[13] Because the predisposing factors are unmodifiable, interventions to reduce the incidence of delirium in the acute care setting focus on minimizing the occurrence of precipitating factors.

Addressing delirium through prevention and treatment in the acute care setting can improve patient outcomes. Delirium is associated with several adverse clinical outcomes including increased mortality rates, increased rates of institutionalization, and increased risk for developing dementia.[15] Hospital costs are higher for patients with delirium, as delirium is associated with increased nursing care time and increased length of stay.[12] It appears that the most effective means of reducing the incidence and the adverse effects of delirium is prevention. **Multicomponent intervention programs** aimed at identifying patients at high risk and reducing the number of precipitating factors in the acute care setting may be more effective than single interventions.[13,16,17] Prevention programs include interventions such as daily medical assessment by a geriatric specialist, early mobilization after surgery, monitoring fluid intake (to avoid dehydration), and reorientation and specialized communication by healthcare providers. A multidisciplinary team approach is required to address the multiple components of these preventative interventions. In patients who have been diagnosed with delirium, initial treatment usually focuses on identifying and treating the underlying etiologies.[2,13] Nonpharmacological interventions, such as reorientation and mobilization, should be initiated in an effort to reduce the duration and severity of the episode of delirium. In cases of extreme physical or emotional distress in which the patient may harm himself or others, the short-term use (1 week or less) of an antipsychotic agent, such as haloperidol or olanzapine, may be indicated.[13,18]

Physical Therapy Patient/Client Management

The physical therapist in the acute care setting plays an important role within the multidisciplinary team in screening, preventing, and treating delirium. During the course of the physical therapy examination and subsequent patient visits, the physical therapist assesses the patient for changes in cognition, motor function, and mobility. In some cases, the acute and fluctuating changes in consciousness, cognition, and psychomotor function that characterize delirium may be more readily and easily identified by the physical therapist than other members of the team. Because mobilization appears to be a key factor in preventing and treating delirium, the expertise and clinical skills of the physical therapist are often needed to educate family members and other multidisciplinary team members on safe mobilization of patients with serious medical conditions and/or multiple comorbidities. The primary roles of the physical therapist for a patient with an episode of delirium are to: (1) prevent or minimize loss of range of motion, strength, and aerobic functional capacity; (2) promote safe and frequent mobility; and (3) prevent, assess for, and treat pain using nonpharmacological interventions.

Examination, Evaluation, and Diagnosis

Prior to initiating any tests or measures, the physical therapist should review the medical chart and interview the patient and caregivers, if possible, to determine the patient's risk for developing delirium.[19] The physical therapist must be familiar with the common causes and predisposing and precipitating factors for delirium (Table 3-1). In the patient who has not been diagnosed with delirium but who presents with signs and symptoms, the underlying etiology may not have been identified yet by the medical specialists on the multidisciplinary team.

During the examination, the physical therapist should screen for delirium in those patients who are at high risk based on the information provided in the medical chart and patient/caregiver interviews. Patients who do not have a significant number of predisposing and precipitating factors but who demonstrate any signs consistent with delirium should also be screened. For example, examination findings such as lethargy and slow physical response to verbal commands should be "red flags" to the physical therapist that further screening for delirium is indicated. The physical therapist should be especially attentive to the signs of hypoactive delirium, as this subtype is particularly underdiagnosed.[9] Healthcare providers often mistakenly assume that a decreased level of consciousness and psychomotor retardation are normal signs of an aging or disease process. Based only on information gathered from the chart review, the patient in this case study presents with at least seven predisposing and precipitating factors for delirium: coronary artery disease (underlying medical condition), more than three drugs added during hospitalization, medication ADRs (Percocet and Benadryl),[11] older age, hip fracture, glaucoma (vision impairment), and moderate hearing loss (sensory impairment). It can also be reasonably assumed that on POD 1 for hip fracture repair, the patient would present with at least a few precipitating factors for delirium: pain, decreased mobility, and constipation.

Several standardized delirium screening tools have been validated for use in the acute care setting.[20,21] One of the most commonly used tools is the **Confusion**

Table 3-1   COMMON ETIOLOGIES AND PREDISPOSING AND PRECIPITATING FACTORS FOR DELIRIUM

Etiologies[1,7,23]	Predisposing Factors[13,14]	Precipitating Factors[13,14]
Underlying medical condition (infectious, metabolic, endocrine, cardiovascular, and/or cerebrovascular)	Age ≥ 65 years	Disorientation
	Pre-existing cognitive impairment	Constipation
	Presence of severe illness	Dehydration
	Current hip fracture	Hypoxia
Substance abuse	Vision impairment	Immobility
Substance withdrawal	BUN/creatinine ratio > 18	Infection
Medication ADRs		Multiple medications (≥ 3 new added during hospitalization)
Toxin exposure		Pain
Combination of any of the above		Poor nutrition
		Sensory impairment
		Sleep deprivation

Assessment Method (CAM), which was developed for use by trained nonpsychiatric clinicians.[8] The CAM can be used for both screening and diagnosis of delirium but should not be used as a measure of symptom severity either before or after diagnosis. The CAM is a brief screening tool that can be completed in 5 minutes based on observation of the patient during a structured interview. The tool includes two parts: an assessment instrument that contains items related to nine clinical features of delirium and a diagnostic algorithm that focuses on the four features that have the greatest ability to differentiate delirium from other psychiatric diagnoses (e.g., depression and dementia). These four differentiating features are: (1) acute onset and fluctuating course, (2) inattention, (3) disorganized thinking, and (4) altered level of consciousness. The diagnosis of delirium based on results of the CAM requires the presence of *both* features 1 and 2, and *either* feature 3 or 4. Although multidisciplinary teams may choose to screen and diagnose for delirium using a variety of methods or protocols, the physical therapist can screen for delirium by administering the assessment instrument section of the CAM and report the findings to the medical specialist, who would then use the criteria of the diagnostic algorithm to determine the diagnosis. The CAM–ICU is an adaptation of the CAM that can be used with nonspeaking mechanically ventilated patients.[22] Patients must be responsive to verbal commands because an auditory or visual test is used to assess attention.

A patient may develop delirium at any time during a hospitalization, so the physical therapist should informally assess cognitive status and level of consciousness during each encounter with the patient. The physical therapist should be especially vigilant when working with patients on hospital units that have no protocol for delirium screening by nursing on each shift.

Plan of Care and Interventions

When developing the physical therapy prognosis, goals, and discharge recommendations for patients with delirium, the physical therapist should consider the negative effects of delirium on both cognitive and functional outcomes. Patients with delirium tend to rehabilitate at a slower rate than those without delirium, and the adverse outcomes may persist 12 months post-hospitalization or longer.[24,25] Patients with a hip fracture who develop delirium postoperatively are less likely to return to prefracture (baseline) ambulatory and activities of daily living (ADLs) status than those without postoperative delirium.[26-28] The timeframes for physical therapy goals should reflect anticipated slower progress toward baseline function and longer hospital lengths of stay. Recommendations for discharge setting should reflect whether the patient's delirium has resolved at the time of discharge. If the patient is discharged to a familiar setting, such as the patient's home, this may be more beneficial than transfer to an unfamiliar rehabilitation setting.[29]

The physical therapist should use specialized communication skills and modify the physical environment when treating patients who have been diagnosed with, or who are at risk of developing, delirium. The goals of communication throughout the physical therapy visit are reorienting the patient and maintaining his perception of a calm, safe environment. Specific communication strategies are listed in Table 3-2.

Table 3-2   STRATEGIES FOR COMMUNICATING WITH THE PATIENT WITH OR AT RISK OF DEVELOPING DELIRIUM[13,30,31]
• Ensure the patient is wearing any needed visual or hearing aids • Reorient the patient to name, place, date, situation • Introduce self by name and role • Communicate clearly and concisely • Avoid medical jargon • Offer verbal and nonverbal reassurance • Maintain eye contact • Promote conversation between the patient and family/friends • Initiate reminiscence activities

The physical therapist should instruct the patient's family and friends to frequently reorient the patient and participate in cognitive activities with the patient, such as reminiscence activities and discussing current events.[13,30]

The physical therapist should also modify the patient's environment in an effort to reorient and calm the patient, provide an unambiguous environment, and promote safe and frequent mobilization. Transporting the patient with or at risk for delirium to a noisy treatment gym should be minimized, if possible. Clinical guidelines include several suggestions for **nonpharmacological interventions for treating delirium**[13,30,31] (Table 3-3).

The physical therapist may need to educate caregivers of patients with or at risk of developing delirium to assist with frequent mobilization of the patient. Ambulatory patients should walk at least three times per day, and nonambulatory patients should perform range of motion for at least 15 minutes, 3 times per day.[13,30] Because hypoxia is a precipitating factor for developing delirium and may contribute to prolonged delirium, the physical therapist should closely monitor and optimize oxygen saturation during physical therapy interventions.[13] Addressing patients' needs for both frequent mobility and optimal oxygen saturation may require communication and coordination with other team members.

Assessment and nonpharmacological management of pain in the patient with or at risk for developing delirium is a major role of the physical therapist. Pain is a precipitating factor and may contribute to a prolonged episode of delirium. Identifying pain in the patient who is unable to speak or is confused can be quite challenging.

Table 3-3   SUGGESTED ENVIRONMENTAL/TREATMENT MODIFICATIONS FOR THE PATIENT WITH OR AT RISK OF DEVELOPING DELIRIUM
• Place clock, calendar within view of patient • Provide lighting consistent with the time of day • Place familiar objects, photographs within view of patient • Place walking aids within the patient's reach (only if indicated) • Remove unneeded objects, clutter from patient's room • Minimize transport of patient outside of room or unit • Minimize noise, especially during sleeping hours • Schedule treatments to allow for longer periods of uninterrupted sleep • Provide positioning devices to improve patient comfort/quality of sleep

The physical therapist should be vigilant to identify and recognize nonverbal signs of pain, such as grimacing, agitation, and frequent position changes. Nonpharmacological interventions for pain should be maximized because opioids, nonsteroidal anti-inflammatory drugs, and polypharmacy in general may contribute to the onset or prolonged duration of delirium.[11,23]

Evidence-Based Clinical Recommendations

SORT: Strength of Recommendation Taxonomy

A: Consistent, good-quality patient-oriented evidence

B: Inconsistent, limited-quality patient-oriented evidence

C: Consistent, disease-oriented evidence, usual practice, expert opinion, or case series

1. Preventative multicomponent interventions delivered by a multidisciplinary team reduce the incidence of delirium in acute care patients at risk. **Grade B**

2. The CAM and CAM–ICU are valid screening tools for delirium when administered by trained healthcare professionals. **Grade A**

3. Nonpharmacological interventions (*e.g.*, optimizing oxygen saturation and walking at least 3 times per day) reduce the mortality and morbidity associated with delirium. **Grade C**

COMPREHENSION QUESTIONS

3.1 A physical therapist examines an older patient in the acute care setting who is inattentive during the examination. Which of the following additional findings would lead the therapist to suspect delirium rather than dementia or depression?

  A. Chronic memory loss

  B. Feeling of hopelessness

  C. Fluctuating disorientation

  D. Agitation

3.2 A patient in the acute care setting who has been diagnosed with delirium reports a new onset of low back pain that interferes with mobility. What is the physical therapist's *most* appropriate recommendation to the multidisciplinary team, given the patient's diagnosis of delirium?

  A. Recommend that the patient be prescribed a pain medication.

  B. Recommend multidisciplinary evaluation for nonpharmacological pain management.

  C. Recommend that the patient remain immobilized until the pain resolves.

  D. Recommend that the patient's current report of pain be ignored by the team, given the patient's fluctuating mental status.

ANSWERS

3.1 **C.** A key feature of delirium that differentiates it from dementia and depression is an acute and fluctuating change in mental status. Other key differentiating features, as indicated in the CAM tool, are: inattention, disorganized thinking, and altered level of consciousness. Although individuals with chronic memory loss due to dementia or depression may develop delirium, an *acute and fluctuating change in memory from baseline* would be expected in a patient with delirium (option A). Altered mood, such as a feeling of hopelessness (option B), may be present in a patient with delirium, but this is often a symptom of depression and therefore does not differentiate delirium from depression. Patients with hyperactive delirium may demonstrate agitation; however, agitation is also common in individuals with depression and dementia as well. Therefore, agitation is not a key differentiating feature of delirium (option D).

3.2 **B.** Pain, immobility, and additional medications are precipitating factors for delirium and may contribute to more severe and prolonged episodes of delirium. Therefore, nonpharmacological intervention is the optimal first approach to pain management in individuals with or at risk for delirium.

REFERENCES

1. Saxena S, Lawley D. Delirium in the elderly: a clinical review. *Postgrad Med J.* 2009;85:405-413.

2. Lundström M, Karlsson S, Brännström B, et al. A multifactorial intervention program reduces the duration of delirium, length of hospitalization, and mortality in delirious patients. *J Am Geriatr Soc.* 2005;53:622-628.

3. Smith HA, Fuchs DC, Pandharipande PP, et al. Delirium: an emerging frontier in the management of critically ill children. *Crit Care Clin.* 2009;25:593-614.

4. Turkel SB, Trzepacz PT, Tavare CJ. Comparing symptoms of delirium in adults and children. *Psychosomatics.* 2006;47:320-324.

5. Bush SH, Bruera E. The assessment and management of delirium in cancer patients. *Oncologist.* 2009;14:1039-1049.

6. Koster S, Hensens AG, Schuurmans MJ, et al. Risk factors of delirium after cardiac surgery: a systematic review. *Eur J Cardiovasc Nurs.* 2011;10:197-204.

7. Michael B, First, MD, ed. In: *Diagnostic and Statistical Manual of Mental Disorders. 4th Ed. (DSM-IV-TR™, 2000).* American Psychiatric Association; 2000.

8. Inouye SK, van Dyck CH, Alessi CA, et al. Clarifying confusion: the confusion assessment method: a new method for detection of delirium. *Ann Intern Med.* 1990;113:941-948.

9. Peterson JF, Pun BT, Dittus RS, et al. Delirium and its motoric subtypes: a study of 614 critically ill patients. *J Am Geriatr Soc.* 2006;54:479-484.

10. Robinson TN, Raeburn CD, Tran ZV, et al. Motor subtypes of postoperative delirium in older adults. *Arch Surg.* 2011;146:295-300.

11. Maldonado JR. Pathoetiological model of delirium: a comprehensive understanding of the neurobiology of delirium and an evidence-based approach to prevention and treatment. *Crit Care Clin.* 2008;24:789-856, ix.

12. Mittal V, Muralee S, Williamson D, et al. Review: delirium in the elderly: a comprehensive review. *Am J Alzheimers Dis Other Demen.* 2011;26:97-109.

13. National Collaborating Centre for Acute and Chronic Conditions. Delirium: diagnosis, prevention and management. London (UK): National Institute for Health and Clinical Excellence (NICE); 2010 Jul 29 (Clinical guideline; no. 103).

14. Inouye SK. Predisposing and precipitating factors for delirium in hospitalized older patients. *Dement Geriatr Cogn Disord*. 1999;10:393-400.

15. Witlox J, Eurelings LS, de Jonghe JF, et al. Delirium in elderly patients and the risk of postdischarge mortality, institutionalization, and dementia: a meta-analysis. *JAMA*. 2010;304:443-451.

16. Inouye SK, Bogardus ST Jr, Baker DI, et al. The Hospital Elder Life Program: a model of care to prevent cognitive and functional decline in older hospitalized patients. Hospital Elder Life Program. *J Am Geriatr Soc*. 2000;48:1697-1706.

17. Vidan MT, Sanchez E, Alonso M, et al. An intervention integrated into daily clinical practice reduces the incidence of delirium during hospitalization in elderly patients. *J Am Geriatr Soc*. 2009;57: 2029-2036.

18. Seitz DP, Gill SS, van Zyl LT. Antipsychotics in the treatment of delirium: a systematic review. *J Clin Psychiatry*. 2007;68:11-21.

19. Flaherty JH. The evaluation and management of delirium among older persons. *Med Clin North Am*. 2011;95:555-577.

20. Adamis D, Sharma N, Whelan PJ, et al. Delirium scales: a review of current evidence. *Aging Ment Health*. 2010;14:543-555.

21. Kean J, Ryan K. Delirium detection in clinical practice and research: critique of current tools and suggestions for future development. *J Psychosom Res*. 2008;65:255-259.

22. Ely EW, Margolin R, Francis J, et al. Evaluation of delirium in critically ill patients: validation of the Confusion Assessment Method for the Intensive Care Unit (CAM-ICU). *Crit Care Med*. 2001;29:1370-1379.

23. Fong TG, Tulebaev SR, Inouye SK. Delirium in elderly adults: diagnosis, prevention and treatment. *Nat Rev Neurol*. 2009;5:210-220.

24. McCusker J, Cole M, Dendukuri N, et al. Delirium in older medical inpatients and subsequent cognitive and functional status: a prospective study. *CMAJ*. 2001;165:575-583.

25. Murray AM, Levkoff SE, Wetle TT, et al. Acute delirium and functional decline in the hospitalized elderly patient. *J Gerontol*. 1993;48:M181-M186.

26. Marcantonio ER, Flacker JM, Michaels M, et al. Delirium is independently associated with poor functional recovery after hip fracture. *J Am Geriatr Soc*. 2000;48:618-624.

27. Edelstein DM, Aharonoff GB, Karp A, et al. Effect of postoperative delirium on outcome after hip fracture. *Clin Orthop Relat Res*. 2004;422:195-200.

28. Givens JL, Sanft TB, Marcantonio ER. Functional recovery after hip fracture: the combined effects of depressive symptoms, cognitive impairment, and delirium. *J Am Geriatr Soc*. 2008;56:1075-1079.

29. Caplan GA, Coconis J, Board N, et al. Does home treatment affect delirium? A randomised controlled trial of rehabilitation of elderly and care at home or usual treatment (The REACH-OUT trial). *Age Ageing*. 2006;35:53-60.

30. Kyziridis TC. Post-operative delirium after hip fracture treatment—a review of the current literature. *Psychosoc Med*. 2006;3:1-12.

31. American Psychiatric Association. Practice guideline for the treatment of patients with delirium. *Am J Psychiatry*. 1999;156:1-20.

Total Hip Arthroplasty

Sharon L. Gorman

CASE 4

A 71-year-old female was admitted to the hospital yesterday after an unwitnessed fall in her driveway that resulted in a left hip fracture. Her husband attempted to help her up but called emergency medical services due to the excessive pain in her left hip. She was transported to the Emergency Department (ED) via ambulance. Presentation in the ED included 9/10 left hip pain (on numeric rating scale, with 10 being the worst pain possible) and a shortened and externally rotated left lower extremity. Radiographs confirmed left displaced intertrochanteric femur fracture. The patient stated that she did not trip and she did not report any loss of consciousness. Prior medical history includes hypertension for 9 years treated with Lopressor (metoprolol/hydrochlorothiazide), osteopenia diagnosed last year and treated with Boniva (ibandronate), and remote history of appendectomy as a teenager. This morning, the patient was scheduled for a minimally invasive anterolateral approach total hip arthroplasty (THA) with regional anesthesia via psoas compartment block and local anesthetic infiltration postoperatively. She lives with her older husband who is debilitated and on portable oxygen due to emphysema. They live in a house with two steps to enter with a rail on the right when ascending the stairs. The patient had surgery this morning and would be transferred from the postanesthesia care unit to the orthopaedic floor this afternoon. Physical therapy is ordered starting on the day of surgery, with weightbearing as tolerated on the left lower extremity.

- ▶ Based on her surgical procedure and health condition, what do you anticipate will be the contributors to activity limitations and impairments?
- ▶ What are the examination priorities?
- ▶ What are the most appropriate physical therapy interventions?
- ▶ What precautions should be taken during physical therapy interventions?
- ▶ What are possible complications interfering with physical therapy?
- ▶ How would this individual's contextual factors influence or change your discharge recommendations?

KEY DEFINITIONS

ANTEROLATERAL APPROACH, MINIMALLY INVASIVE TECHNIQUE: Surgical approach using a substantially smaller incision intended to limit local surgical trauma to muscle and tissue

INTERTROCHANTERIC HIP FRACTURE: Fracture of the femur in intertrochanteric region

NERVE BLOCK: Local anesthetic drugs injected onto or near peripheral nerves for temporary pain control; commonly performed during orthopaedic surgical procedures, which results in decreased pain and motor function during surgery and in the postoperative period

OSTEOPENIA: Loss of bone density resulting in potentially weakened bone strength; defined as 1.0 to 2.5 standard deviations below normal bone density[1]

TOTAL HIP ARTHROPLASTY (THA): Replacement of both the acetabulum and the head and neck of the femur with titanium and/or plastic components

Objectives

1. Describe total hip precautions, including relating the precautions to the type of surgical procedure used.

2. Identify screening tools used in physical therapy practice to detect deep vein thrombosis (DVT).

3. Perform a fall risk screening and assessment in an acutely ill patient.

4. Describe your discharge recommendations taking personal and contextual issues into account.

Physical Therapy Considerations

PT considerations during management of the individual immediately after THA with an anterolateral minimally invasive surgical technique and a psoas nerve block:

▶ **General physical therapy plan of care/goals:** Decrease pain; increase activity and participation; increase hip strength; prevent or minimize loss of range of motion, strength, and aerobic functional capacity; improve quality of life

▶ **Physical therapy interventions:** Functional training; gait training including stairs; patient/family education and training on postoperative issues; assistive device prescription and fitting; progressive exercise program; coordination of care with interdisciplinary team; provision of discharge recommendations, taking into account patient safety, ability of spouse and/or family to assist, environmental and contextual issues at home, and availability of follow-up physical therapy care

▶ **Precautions during physical therapy:** Monitor vital signs, pain management in coordination with medical team, review of lab values, progressive weightbearing

▶ **Complications interfering with physical therapy:** Pathological fractures, hip prosthesis dislocation, postoperative complications (*e.g.*, DVT, pneumonia, urinary tract infection)

Understanding the Health Condition

Falls are one of the most pervasive and serious health concerns facing older adults.[2-4] Fall rates are as high as 30% to 40% in community-dwelling adults over 65 years of age, with rates for institutionalized adults even higher.[3] In the United States, more than 2.2 million older adults have a fall resulting in an injury needing medical treatment,[4] and between 20% and 30% of older adults who fall suffer serious injuries such as head trauma or hip fracture.[3] Falls in elders result in increased morbidity, mortality, and utilization of healthcare services, including premature skilled nursing facility (SNF) admissions.[2,5] One study of Medicare beneficiaries found that persons who fell had higher Medicare cost utilization than nonfallers.[4] In addition, only 48% of fallers reported talking to a healthcare provider after a fall, and only 60% of those who reported a fall received any fall prevention information or intervention.[4] Healthcare providers need to assess and intervene to prevent falls and their recurrence in older adults.[3,4,6]

In the United States, more than 300,000 hip fractures occur each year[5,7,8]; 90% of these fractures occurred in persons over 65 years of age.[9] Hip fracture rates rise 12% to 13% per year of age over 65 years.[8] As the population of older adults rises, the number of hip fractures could triple in the next 40 years.[8] Women have nearly twice the incidence of hip fracture as men, 612.7 per 100,000 to 333.4 per 100,000, respectively.[8] Hip fractures in the elderly population are more likely to be caused by pathological conditions such as osteoporosis or osteopenia of the head and neck of the femur or due to mechanical falls.[9] This differs from the younger population in which femur fractures are due to high-energy trauma. The disability burden and economic cost of hip fracture is estimated to cost more than US$8.7 billion annually.[8] In the year after hip fracture, individuals have a two-fold increased risk of mortality compared to controls without hip fracture. This was significant for two specific age groups: all women aged 65 to 79 years and exceptionally healthy women over 80 years of age.[5]

Surgery is indicated for hip fractures in the elderly unless the individual has other medical comorbidities that place her at high risk for anesthesia or surgery-related complications.[9] Nonambulatory patients or patients with severe dementia may also be treated nonoperatively.[9] Extracapsular femur fractures are commonly treated with open reduction internal fixation (ORIF) that uses surgical hardware to secure the fracture. Intracapsular fractures can be nondisplaced or displaced. Displaced intracapsular fractures, such as the one that occurred when this patient fell, are treated with a THA or hemiarthroplasty due to the disruption of circulation to the femoral head and risk of osteonecrosis that can occur with other fixation methods.[9]

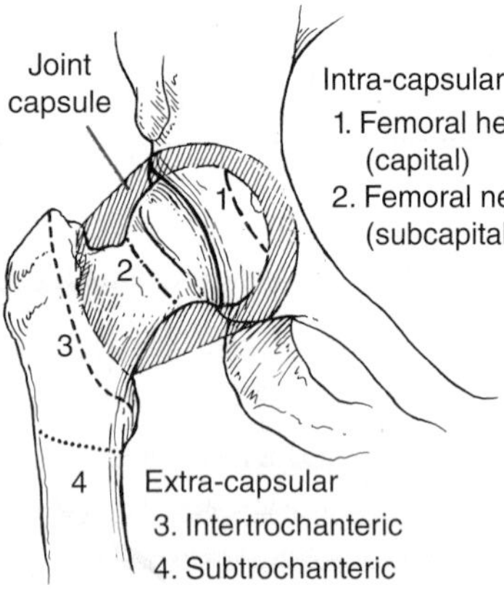

Figure 4-1. Proximal femoral fracture sites and their relationship to the joint capsule. (Reproduced with permission from Knoop KJ, Stack LB, Storrow AB, et al. *The Atlas of Emergency Medicine*, 3rd ed. http://www.accessmedicine.com. Copyright © The McGraw Hill Companies, Inc. All rights reserved.)

Nondisplaced intracapsular hip fractures can be treated with ORIF or THA. Figure 4-1 shows common femoral fracture sites and their anatomical relationship to the hip capsule. Recent research shows older adults with hip fracture treated with THA have better functional outcomes and quality of life with fewer complications compared to those receiving ORIF.[9]

THA is a surgical technique that involves replacing the head and neck of the femur and the acetabulum with artificial components (Fig. 4-2). Hip hemiarthroplasty, in which only the femoral head and neck are replaced and the patient retains the acetabulum, is a related surgical technique. Recent advances in surgical approach have allowed for smaller surgical incisions.[10] Compared to traditional surgical approaches, minimally invasive techniques are associated with less disruption of muscle and tissue, less postoperative pain, less use of assistive devices, faster return to daily activities and function, and earlier hospital discharge.[10] However, minimally invasive approaches do not seem to make a difference in recovery 3 months after surgery.[10] Anesthesia and postoperative pain control are also important surgical factors to be considered by the physical therapist. Anesthesia protocols using regional or local peripheral nerve blocks, psoas compartment blocks, lumbar plexus blocks, and local infiltration techniques have resulted in reduced nausea, vomiting, and hospital length of stay.[10]

Hip precautions may be implemented after a THA. Surgical approach, incision site, and surgeon preference listed in the postoperative orders, determine whether hip precautions are implemented after THA. After a posterolateral surgical approach, hip precautions include avoiding: hip adduction past neutral, internal rotation past neutral, and hip flexion greater than 90°. Posterolateral hip replacements nearly always require hip precautions for at least 4 to 6 weeks after THA due to the location of the capsular incision site.[11] The rationale for these movement restrictions is that they can cause significant stress to the sutured capsule, causing it to open and the hip joint to dislocate. These functional movements do not stress the hip joint capsule incision with recent surgical techniques involving minimally invasive approaches using anterolateral surgical incisions. In fact, recent evidence indicates

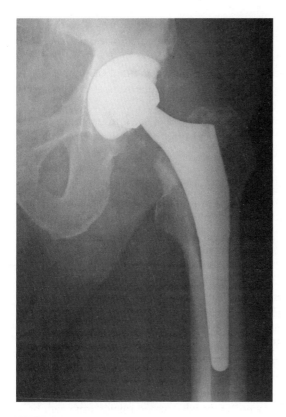

Figure 4-2. Radiograph of total hip arthroplasty that was implanted using press-fit technique for both acetabular and femoral components. Cement and screws were not utilized. (Reproduced with permission from Tintinalli JE, Stapczynski JS, et al. *Emergency Medicine: A Comprehensive Study Guide.* 7th ed. New York, NY: McGraw-Hill; 2004:105.)

the actual risk of dislocation is extremely low in patients with anterolateral surgical approaches (4 known dislocations in 2386 patients with 2612 hips, or 0.15%)[11] and conclude **no hip replacement precautions are required after primary THA with an anterolateral approach.**[11]

The overall complication rate after THA is approximately 7%.[12] Common THA postoperative complications seen in the hospital include fractures (0.6%), DVT (0.6%), and bleeding complications (0.5%).[12] Postdischarge complications include reoperation due to bleeding, wound necrosis, wound infection, and DVT.[12] General postoperative complications common in hospitalized patients also include pneumonia, urinary tract infection, and skin breakdown.[13]

Physical Therapy Patient/Client Management

Functional mobility and activity limitations are of primary concern for the physical therapist working with hospitalized patients.[14] Working on resolution of activity limitations will allow the patient the best chance of a safe discharge back to her home setting, while any necessary follow-up physical therapy care can be conducted via home health or outpatient services. Because this patient had an unplanned THA due to a fall, her hospital course and discharge disposition may be different from an individual who had an elective THA. Compared to individuals with elective THAs, individuals with THAs due to falls may have more medical comorbidities, pre-existing functional mobility limitations, and an increased fear of falling. Preoperative classes for individuals scheduled for total joint replacements are common. A recent nationwide pilot survey of physical therapists working with patients after total joint replacement found that 84% of respondents had preoperative classes for these patients.[15] Preoperative physical therapy or THA classes often include education about the surgical procedure and expected outcomes, exercise prescription, and other specific training. A systematic review found that a course of preoperative physical therapy had a modest effect on patient gait, stamina, strength, and health status in the preoperative and immediate postoperative period.[10] The key finding was that participation in preoperative physical therapy increased the potential for discharge to home and reduced the risk of discharge to a rehabilitation facility.[10] If the patient is not able to return home from the hospital, the physical therapist is uniquely suited to recommend more appropriate levels of care such as skilled nursing (either for short-term rehabilitation or residential care), board and care facility placement, or an acute rehabilitation stay. Medical stability is usually the primary concern for the medical team and is used to determine the first opportunity for discharge. Once the patient is adequately stabilized, discharge should proceed quickly. The physical therapist's examination and evaluation of movement dysfunction related to the patient's ability to either tolerate requirements for therapy (*i.e.*, acute rehabilitation settings, skilled nursing settings) and/or safety of the patient in her home environment (*i.e.*, home health, board, and care) form the foundation for safe and expedient discharge recommendations.[16]

Examination, Evaluation, and Diagnosis

Prior to seeing this patient, a full chart review should be completed. The therapist should pay particular attention to all pertinent physician orders, postoperative pain medication, movement or mobility precautions, and/or weightbearing restrictions. Nursing documentation should be reviewed to establish the patient's last pain medication, pain medication plan, and any options for breakthrough pain medication. Laboratory test results should be reviewed with specific attention to values commonly affected by surgery and associated blood loss such as hemoglobin, hematocrit, and platelets; white blood cell count should be reviewed to assess development of postsurgical infection complications. Mobilization, and possibly even bed-level exercise, should be adjusted appropriately, including holding intervention if indicated, if values fall into the critical range. Determining whether to hold physical therapy intervention should be based on risk versus benefit of the proposed interventions both for that session and for the overall episode of care. The emergency medical services transfer and/or ED notes should be reviewed briefly to determine if the cause of the fall could be ascertained. This information could help determine if a fall risk assessment is indicated, and whether any environmental reasons contributed to the fall. Social work or case management notes (if available this early in the patient's hospitalization) could provide valuable insight into the home environment and situation as well as any third-party payer issues that may affect discharge planning, such as insurance coverage for SNF rehabilitation.

During the examination, the therapist should take into account any monitors, lines, and/or tubes the patient may have in place postoperatively. While mobilization can occur with most monitors, lines, and tubes, specific precautions or contraindications for movement may be indicated.[17] Depending on the skills of the individual physical therapist, additional assistance from medical team members may be indicated to prevent adverse events such as pulling out a line. Consideration of anesthesia and postoperative pain control must be incorporated into the examination. During the surgical procedure, this patient had a nerve block to the psoas region for regional anesthesia. It is likely that she will have decreased sensation and motor function in the affected peripheral nerve distribution in the immediate postoperative period. The therapist should consistently monitor the return of sensation and motor function, incorporating this information into the plan of care. For example, the therapist may need to advise the patient to refrain from weightbearing on the involved limb until sensation and motor function have recovered substantially to ensure patient safety. Even though the patient may be *allowed* to bear weight on the involved lower extremity, weightbearing on a numb and weak limb could lead to unsafe buckling of the limb or a fall.

The physical therapist should choose a standardized tool for functional mobility and gait assessment. The Acute Care Index of Function (ACIF) is a reliable and valid tool for use in acute orthopaedic populations and collects data related to a patient's mentation, mobility, transfers, and locomotion (including stairs).[18] Most of the items on the ACIF are routinely examined in acute care, but completion of the ACIF results in a score that can allow comparisons and give a standardized result easily understood by therapists. The results from the ACIF may also help discharge prognosis formulation.[19,20] A descriptive gait examination may include: device used, weightbearing status, surface, and distance ambulated. If the therapist also calculates gait speed (which requires only a stopwatch and no additional time), this can provide valuable normative data that can be routinely assessed throughout the patient's episode of care and through a variety of care settings (hospital, skilled nursing, home health, outpatient) for continuous data on patient improvement and ability to approach age- and gender-based normative values.[21] Other standardized outcome measures may be used by other team members within the hospital to gather data on patient outcomes. Common measures used in postoperative hip surgery populations include: SF-12, SF-36, Harris Hip Score, Oxford Hip Score, and Western Ontario and McMaster Universities Osteoarthritis Index.[22]

Vital signs (heart rate, respiratory rate, blood pressure, and oxygen saturation) and pain should be carefully monitored postoperatively. Many inpatient facilities use the same pain measurement tool across disciplines, such as the Numeric Pain Rating Scale.[23] For best interdisciplinary care, the therapist should use this tool. Vital signs, especially in conjunction with lab values, are critical to ensure that the physical therapist is prescribing an appropriate dose of exercise, whether in the form of mobilization or therapeutic exercises.[24] Vital signs used in combination with the patient's report of fatigue and/or pain can help the therapist adjust the intensity of activity or exercises, ensuring the patient is maximizing her activity levels safely.[25]

Given the unclear nature of this patient's fall and history of osteopenia, the therapist should consider a fall risk assessment.[6] At initial examination, other priorities and the patient's limited postoperative endurance may not make this feasible. However, prior to hospital discharge, this should be completed so the therapist can make appropriate discharge recommendations through identification of any modifiable risk factors for falls. If the acute care stay is very short, this may be deferred to other physical therapists caring for the patient later in the episode of care. For example, should the patient require short-term rehabilitation in a SNF, the therapist in that setting should complete a fall risk assessment prior to the patient's discharge to home.

The therapist needs to obtain details about the home environment and ability of the patient's spouse to assist with care-giving and/or management of the household. Without comprehensive knowledge of these factors, the therapist cannot determine appropriate discharge recommendations.[16] For less experienced therapists, discussion or collaboration with other team members or colleagues may be required if complex contextual issues are present.[16] Communication of the initial discharge recommendations needs to occur in a coordinated and timely fashion with the interdisciplinary team, as well as any adjustments based on intervention, patient response, or patient progress.[16]

Plan of Care and Interventions

Individualized physical therapy anticipated goals, expected outcomes, and discharge recommendations are determined after the examination and evaluation. Goals related to improvement of functional mobility and gait, including stairs for this patient, need to be incorporated. Additional goals may include performance of an independent exercise program ("home" exercise program for hospitalized patient), caregiver training, and strengthening of specific muscles affected by the THA procedure. During the immediate postoperative period, assessment of sensory and motor function impaired by the psoas nerve block will guide decisions about the safety of weightbearing on the affected limb during transfer and gait training.

In addition to addressing specific deficits noted on initial examination, physical therapy intervention should include daily review of patient's lab results, monitoring the patient's physiologic status during intervention, and monitoring for postoperative complications common after THA such as DVT, pneumonia, urinary tract infection due to Foley catheterization, infection at the suture site, and skin breakdown.

Development of a DVT is a common postoperative complication that is exacerbated by prolonged immobility and decreased activity. The incidence of DVT without prophylaxis after joint replacement and hip fracture ranges from 41% to 85%.[26] After THA, DVT incidence varies between 20% and 27.3%.[27] Even with postsurgical prophylactic anticoagulation (usually with low molecular weight heparins such

Table 4-1 RISK FACTORS FOR DEVELOPMENT OF DVT	
Risk Categories	**Specific Risks**
Damage to veins	Previous DVT Surgery* Trauma Lower extremity fracture(s)* Varicose veins Postoperative sepsis Childbirth
Stasis	Prolonged bedrest Congestive heart failure (CHF) Myocardial infarction (MI) Neurologic disorders leading to lack of skeletal muscle activity (stroke, spinal cord injury, etc.) Chronic venous insufficiency Postoperative immobilization (limb or whole body)* Prolonged air travel
Hypercoaguability states	Cancer Autoimmune disorder Oral contraceptives Late pregnancy
Others	Age > 60 years* Obesity

as Lovenox), DVT may still occur in persons after THA.[28] Patients who are reluctant to mobilize need to be educated on the benefits of increased activity and mobilization against the development of DVT.[29] Other risk factors for DVT are presented in Table 4-1. The risk factors present in this patient's case are noted by asterisks (*).

Physical therapists should be skilled at assessment for a possible DVT.[30] Historically, a positive Homan's sign (pain in posterior calf with passive dorsiflexion) was considered adequate for screening DVT. However, because Homan's sign has poor sensitivity and specificity, it has been recommended that it be removed from the clinical examination for DVT.[31] A newer assessment, based on data pooled from 14 studies involving more than 8000 patients, is the **Modified Wells Clinical Prediction Rule (CPR) for DVT**. The Modified Wells CPR for DVT has good to excellent sensitivity and specificity for DVT, is simple to administer, and provides likelihood data about the presence of DVT that can assist the patient's physician in determining appropriate subsequent medical testing and interventions.[32] Because this is a clinical prediction rule, it should be used on a patient that the therapist suspects may have a DVT. Thus, initial screening must include the presence of any signs or symptoms of DVT (Table 4-2). If any signs and symptoms are present, then the Modified Wells CPR should be used.

If a patient exhibits *any* of the signs or symptoms of DVT, the therapist should use the Modified Wells CPR for DVT to ascertain the likelihood of DVT.[32] This patient presented for her afternoon therapy session on postoperative day (POD) 1 with

Table 4-2 SIGNS AND SYMPTOMS OF DVT	
Symptoms	Signs
Pain*	Erythema
Dull ache	Edema*
Tightness	Positive Homan's sign* (not recommended, high rate of false positives)

complaints of pitting edema on the involved lower limb and pain in her left proximal posterior calf that increased with passive dorsiflexion (positive Homan's sign). Given her risk factors for DVT (recent surgical procedure, lower extremity fracture, immobilization of the left leg postoperatively, and patient's age) and current signs and symptoms of DVT (edema, pain, and positive Homan's sign), the therapist used the Modified Wells CPR to assess her likelihood of a DVT. Table 4-3 outlines the Modified Wells CPR for DVT. The predictors in this patient are indicated by asterisks (*). To calculate a score using the Modified Wells CPR: 0 is given if the predictor is not present and 1 is given for each predictor that is present during the examination. For the last item titled "alternative diagnosis as least as likely," a score of

TABLE 4-3 MODIFIED WELLS CLINICAL PREDICTION RULE FOR DVT		
Predictor	Points If Present	Score for This Patient
Active cancer (treatment in last 6 months or palliative)	1	0
Calf swelling (> 3 cm vs. other calf; measured 10 cm below tibial tuberosity)*	1	1
Pitting edema (confined to symptomatic leg)*	1	1
Collateral superficial veins (non-varicose)	1	0
Swelling of entire leg	1	0
Localized pain (along distribution of deep vein system)*	1	1
Paralysis, paresis, or recent cast immobilization (LEs)	1	0
Recently bedridden > 3 days (or major surgery requiring general anesthesia or regional anesthesia in past 4 weeks)*	1	1
Alternative diagnosis at least as likely*	−2	−2
Score interpretation: High if score is ≥ 3; 75% probability of DVT (95% CI = 63%-84%) Moderate if score is 1-2; 17% probability of DVT (95% CI = 12%-23%) Low if score is ≤ 0; 3% probability of DVT (95% CI = 1.7%-5.9%) In patients with symptoms in both legs, the more symptomatic leg is used.		

Abbreviations: cm, centimeters; LEs, lower extremities.

Reproduced with permission from Wells PS, Owen C, Doucette S, Fergusson D, Tran H. Does this patient have deep vein thrombosis? JAMA. 2006;295:199-207.

−2 is given if the patient has a diagnosis that could account for lower extremity signs and symptoms. In this case, the patient's THA is a possible alternative diagnosis to the potential DVT, therefore 2 points are subtracted from the other 4 points for positive predictors present (calf swelling, pitting edema, localized pain, and recently bedridden) for a total score of 2. Based on the CPR, this patient's results (summated score of 2) predict that she has a moderate likelihood of a DVT. This should be communicated immediately to the medical team and/or physician, as well as clearly documented in the therapist's daily documentation. In this case, the physician selected a D-dimer blood test, which tests for the presence of a small fragment of fibrin from a blood clot. Negative D-dimer results can rule out a DVT, while a positive D-dimer requires additional testing.[33] This patient had a positive D-dimer test that prompted a Doppler ultrasound of the lower extremities that confirmed a DVT in the left popliteal region.

Should the patient have a distal lower extremity DVT confirmed via lab tests (positive D-dimer) or Doppler ultrasound scan, anticoagulation will be started. Depending on the type of anticoagulation medication administered to the patient, physical therapy intervention may have to be delayed or held to ensure adequate anticoagulation and stabilization of the clot.[34] Table 4-4 describes how the method of anticoagulation influences the activity level of the patient, and how lab values can provide information regarding the success of anticoagulation.

This patient was treated with Lovenox, and physical therapy was resumed 4 hours after medication administration by nursing. This timeframe was based on the onset time for Lovenox of 3 to 5 hours and no need to wait for confirmatory lab testing to verify therapeutic level.

Physical therapists, as experts in movement dysfunction, are uniquely suited to recommend safe discharge disposition. A recent study in the acute care environment showed that **physical therapists' discharge recommendations** were implemented 83% of the time; when the therapists' recommendations were *not* implemented, there was an increased likelihood of patient readmission.[40] A complex clinical decision-making process occurs in the acute care setting, as described by Jette et al.[16] This model describes the process where the patient's function and disability, wants

Table 4-4 ANTICOAGULATION FACTORS AND CHARACTERISTICS[26,35-39]			
	Heparin	Coumadin	Lovenox
Delivery route	IV or SQ	PO or IV	SQ
Onset	20-60 min	12-14 h	3-5 h
Duration	8-12 h	3-5 d	
Therapeutic time	2-3 d	1.5-4 d	3-5 h
Test for therapeutic level	aPTT or PTT	INR	No test commonly used
Purpose	Treatment	Treatment, especially long term	Prophylaxis and treatment

Abbreviatons: IV, intravenous; SQ, subcutaneous; PO, oral; aPTT, activated partial thromboplastin time; PTT, partial thromboplastin time; INR, international normalized ratio.

and needs, ability to participate, and context are considered in light of the physical therapist's experience to form an initial impression of discharge recommendations. Next, considerations of healthcare regulation, including insurance information, and opinion sharing with other healthcare providers results in a discharge recommendation. Often, due to the short hospital stays common in the United States, this process is started after the initial examination and further honed during subsequent interventions with the patient.

An important part of the initial physical therapy examination includes a preliminary discharge recommendation that includes the recommended discharge location, any equipment that may be needed, and specific physical therapy follow-up, if any, that may be needed. These recommendations may be adapted through the acute care stay based on additional information the therapist gathers, the patient's performance of required or necessary skills, and third-party payor information. Because this patient functions as a caregiver for her husband and it does not appear as if the husband could provide physical assistance for her, the therapist made an initial determination that she may need short-term rehabilitation after acute hospitalization to ensure that she can perform activities of daily living (ADLs) independently prior to discharge home. Her insurance may play a role in the determination of which SNFs she may select for a short-term rehabilitation stay. Equipment she will need on discharge may be deferred to the therapists at the SNF, since the patient will not yet be returning home. However, it is likely that she will need a raised toilet seat and mobility aid such as a walker; these needs may be mentioned in the documentation during the acute care stay. Because it is anticipated that this patient will need continued rehabilitation prior to going home, recommendations for continued physical therapy and occupational therapy should be stated clearly. The acute care therapist may also provide a recommendation that the patient will need more

Table 4-5   AGS/BGS FALL RISK SCREENING CRITERIA[6,41]
All older individuals should be asked whether they have fallen (in the past year).
An older person who reports a fall should be asked about the frequency and circumstances of the fall(s).
Older individuals should be asked if they experience difficulties with walking or balance.
Older persons who present for medical attention because of a fall, report recurrent falls in the past year, or report difficulties in walking or balance (with or without activity curtailment) should have a multifactorial fall risk assessment.
Older persons presenting with a single fall should be evaluated for gait and balance.
Older persons who have fallen should have an assessment of gait and balance using one of the available evaluations. Older persons who cannot perform or perform poorly on a standardized gait and balance test should be given a multifactorial fall risk assessment.
Older persons who have difficulty or demonstrate unsteadiness during the evaluation of gait and balance require a multifactorial fall risk assessment.
Older persons who report only a single fall and reporting or demonstrating no difficulty or unsteadiness during the evaluation of gait and balance do not require a fall risk assessment.
The multifactorial fall risk assessment should be performed by a healthcare provider (including therapists) with appropriate skills and training.

Abbreviations: AGS, American Geriatric Society; BGS, British Geriatric Society.

physical therapy after her SNF stay, potentially including home health and/or outpatient physical therapy.

The physical therapist should perform a **fall risk assessment** for this patient due to the circumstances of her fall in conjunction with her age and past medical history of osteopenia. The American Geriatric Society (AGS) and British Geriatric Society (BGS) have recommended all older adults be screened for fall risk. Table 4-5 (see page 62) describes the levels of screening and recommended follow-up actions. These screening criteria are based on best current evidence and expert consensus, and help to ascertain basic history about falls and to recommend appropriate follow-up assessment. For those at highest risk after screening, a multifactorial fall risk assessment is recommended to identify problems with body structures/functions and activities to help the healthcare provider tailor appropriate interventions to prevent falls.

Based on AGS/BGS screening recommendations, a multifactorial fall risk assessment is indicated for this patient because of her presentation with hip fracture due to a fall.[6] This assessment should occur before discharge or immediately upon discharge

Table 4-6   AGS/BGS RECOMMENDATIONS FOR MULTIFACTORIAL FALL RISK ASSESSMENT[6]

Focused history	History of falls: detailed description of the circumstances of the fall(s), frequency, symptoms at the time of fall, injuries, other consequences Medication review: all prescribed and over-the-counter medications with dosages History of relevant risk factors: acute or chronic medical problems (*e.g.*, osteoporosis, urinary incontinence, cardiovascular disease)
Physical examination	Detailed assessment of gait, balance, and mobility levels and lower extremity joint function Neurologic function: cognitive evaluation, lower extremity peripheral nerves, proprioception, reflexes, tests of cortical, extrapyramidal, and cerebellar function Muscle strength (lower extremities) Cardiovascular status: heart rate and rhythm, postural pulse, blood pressure, and if appropriate, heart rate and blood pressure responses to carotid sinus stimulation Assessment of visual acuity Examination of the feet and footwear
Functional assessment	Assessment of ADLs including use of adaptive equipment and mobility aids, as appropriate Assessment of the individual's perceived functional ability and fear related to falling (assessment of current activity levels with attention to the extent which concerns about falling are protective [*i.e.*, appropriate given abilities] or contributing to deconditioning and/or compromised quality of life [*i.e.*, individual is curtailing involvement in activities he or she is safely able to perform due to fear of falling.])
Environmental assessment	Environmental assessment including home safety

Reproduced with permission from the American Geriatrics Society for "AGS/BGS Clinical Practice Guideline: Prevention of Falls in Older Persons. Available at: http://www.americangeriatrics.org/health_care_professionals/clinical_practice/clinical_guidelines_recommendations/prevention_of_falls_summary_of_recommendations/) from the Journal of the American Geriatrics Society.

to the home. For this patient, this process could be initiated during her acute hospitalization but may be deferred to her SNF rehabilitation stay. Further delay of a fall risk assessment until the patient is at home and being seen by home health physical therapy would be acceptable in this case. However, it would be ideal to perform the fall assessment during the acute hospitalization or SNF rehabilitation period to allow the patient and family the opportunity to plan and schedule any recommended environmental adjustments to the home. Physical therapists are uniquely suited to conduct a multifactorial fall risk assessment in patients due to their ability to examine gait, balance, function, and physical examination skills pertinent to balance and fall reduction. Table 4-6 (see page 63) outlines recommendations for comprehensive multifactorial fall risk assessment from the American and British Geriatric Societies.[6]

Evidence-Based Clinical Recommendations

SORT: Strength of Recommendation Taxonomy

A: Consistent, good-quality patient-oriented evidence

B: Inconsistent or limited-quality patient-oriented evidence

C: Consensus, disease-oriented evidence, usual practice, expert opinion, or case series

1. Total hip precautions are not required for patients who have total hip arthroplasties with an anterolateral approach and minimally invasive surgical technique. **Grade B**

2. The Modified Wells CPR can be used to screen for likelihood of DVT. **Grade A**

3. Physical therapist discharge recommendations play an important role in discharge planning in acutely ill persons. **Grade B**

4. Prevention of falls in older adults includes appropriate screening and, as indicated, multifactorial fall risk assessment. **Grade A**

COMPREHENSION QUESTIONS

4.1 Which of the following lab tests results can be used to verify a therapeutic level of anticoagulation in a patient on Coumadin?

    A. aPTT (activated partial thromboplastin time)

    B. INR (international normalized ratio)

    C. D-dimer

    D. Lovenox

4.2 A 67-year-old patient presents in an outpatient physical therapy clinic. His health history form states he has fallen once in the past year when walking on wet leaves, and he reports no problems currently with gait or balance. What is the *most* appropriate fall risk assessment the physical therapist should perform?

A. Conduct a multifactorial fall risk assessment.

B. Conduct an environmental assessment of the patient's home.

C. Determine if the patient is curtailing his ADLs or activities because of fear of falling.

D. Perform a standardized test of gait and balance to see if the patient can perform without unsteadiness.

ANSWERS

4.1 **B.** INR results can indicate therapeutic levels of Coumadin. aPTT is a blood test used to determine if therapeutic levels of heparin have been achieved (option A). D-dimer is a diagnostic blood test wherein a positive result indicates a high likelihood of DVT (option C). Lovenox is a form of low molecular weight heparin commonly used for DVT prophylaxis and treatment postoperatively (option D). Lovenox does not require the use of aPTT to determine therapeutic levels. Instead, a 3- to 5-hour period of time after administration is used to allow Lovenox to become therapeutic.

4.2 **D.** Based on the AGS/BGS recommendations, a person who has had one fall but no reports of gait or balance problems should be screened with a standardized gait and balance test to see if he can complete the test and/or if he is unsteady when completing the test. It is not yet clear if the patient needs a multifactorial fall risk assessment. Only if the patient is unable to complete the standardized gait and balance test or is unsteady should a multifactorial fall risk assessment be conducted (option A). The environment assessment is part of the multifactorial fall risk assessment (option B). Determining if the patient is curtailing his ADLs or activities because of fear of falling is part of the functional assessment of the multifactorial fall risk assessment (option C). Physical therapists have the appropriate skills and training to conduct screenings and multifactorial fall risk assessments. They should involve the primary care physician in the patient's care, but they can conduct these screenings and assessments. Education materials may be useful, but do not negate the need to complete a screening on this patient.

REFERENCES

1. Goodman C, Snyder T. Screening for endocrine and metabolic disease. In: Goodman C, Snyder T, eds. *Differential Diagnosis for Physical Therapists: Screening for Referral.* 4th ed. St. Louis, MO: Saunders; 2007.

2. Rubenstein LZ. Falls in older people: epidemiology, risk factors and strategies for prevention. *Age Ageing.* 2006;35:ii37-ii41.

3. Rao SS. Prevention of falls in older patients. *Am Fam Physician.* 2005;72:81-88.

4. Shumway-Cook A, Ciol MA, Hoffman J, et al. Falls in the Medicare population: incidence, associated factors, and impact on health care. *Phys Ther.* 2009;89:324-332.

5. LeBlanc ES, Hillier TA, Pedula KL, et al. Hip fracture and increased short-term but not long-term mortality in healthy older women. *Arch Intern Med.* 2011;171:1831-1837.

6. American Geriatric Society, British Geriatric Society. AGS/BGS Clinical Practice Guideline: Prevention of Falls in Older Persons. Available at: http://www.americangeriatrics.org/health_care_professionals/clinical_practice/clinical_guidelines_recommendations/prevention_of_falls_summary_of_recommendations/. Accessed May 16, 2012.

7. Melton LJ, Kearns AE, Atkinson EJ, et al. Secular trends in hip fracture incidence and recurrence. *Osteoporosis Int.* 2009;20:687-694.

8. Melton LJ, Therneau TM, Larson DR. Long-term trends in hip fracture prevalence: the influence of hip fracture incidence and survival. *Osteoporosis Int.* 1998;8:68-74.

9. Antapur P, Mahomed N, Gandhi R. Fractures in the elderly: when is hip replacement a necessity? *Clin Interv Aging.* 2011;6:1-7.

10. Sharma V, Morgan PM, Cheng EY. Factors influencing early rehabilitation after THA: a systematic review. *Clin Orthop Relat Res.* 2009;467:1400-1411.

11. Restrepo C, Mortazavi SM, Brothers J, et al. Hip dislocation: are hip precautions necessary in anterior approaches? *Clin Orthop Relat Res.* 2011;469:417-422.

12. Cushner F, Agnelli G, FitzGerald G, et al. Complications and functional outcomes after total hip arthroplasty and total knee arthoplasty: results from the Global Orthopaedic Registry (GLORY). *Am J Orthop.* 2010;39:22-28.

13. Tidy C. Common post-operative complications. August 18, 2009. Available at: http://www.patient.co.uk/doctor/Common-Post-Op-Complications-to-Look-Out-For.htm. Accessed October 7, 2011.

14. Jette DU, Brown R, Collette N, et al. Physical therapists' management of patients in the acute care setting: an observational study. *Phys Ther.* 2009;89:1158-1181.

15. Gorman SL, Curry A. A pilot study exploring the variability of physical therapy practices of members of the total joint replacement listserv. *J Acute Care Phys Ther.* 2010;1:46-53.

16. Jette DU, Grover L, Keck CP. A qualitative study of clinical decision making in recommending discharge placement from the acute care setting. *Phys Ther.* 2003;83:224-236.

17. Biggs Harris K. Critical care competency program development and implementation. *Acute Care Perspectives.* 2006;15:16-19.

18. Roach KE, Dillen LV. Development of an Acute Care Index of Function status for patients with neurologic impairment. *Phys Ther.* 1988;68:1102-1108.

19. Roach KE, Ally D, Finnerty B, et al. The relationship between duration of physical therapy services in the acute care setting and change in functional status in patients with lower-extremity orthopedic problems. *Phys Ther.* 1998;78:19-24.

20. Scherer SA, Hammerich AS. Outcomes in cardiopulmonary physical therapy: acute care index of function. *Cardiopulm Phys Ther J.* 2008;19:94-97.

21. Hayes KW, Johnson ME. Measures of adult general performance tests: Berg Balance Scale, Dynamic Gait Index, gait velocity, Physical Performance Test, Timed Chair Stand Test, Time Up and Go, and Tinetti Performance-Oriented Mobility Assessment. *Arthritis Rheumatism.* 2003;49:S28-S42.

22. Ostendorf M, van Stel HF, Buskens E, et al. Patient-reported outcome in total hip replacement. A comparison of five instruments of health status. *J Bone Joint Surg Br.* 2004;86:801-808.

23. Salaffi F, Stancati A, Silvestri CA, et al. Minimal clinically important changes in chronic musculoskeletal pain intensity measured on a numeric rating scale. *Eur J Pain.* 2004;8:283-291.

24. Goodman C, Fuller K. *Pathology: Implications for the Physical Therapist.* 3rd ed. Philadelphia, PA: WB Saunders; 2008.

25. Stiller K. Safety issues that should be considered when mobilizing critically ill patients. *Crit Care Clin.* 2007;23:35-53.

26. Hardwick ME, Colwell CW Jr. Advances in DVT prophylaxsis and management in major orthopaedic surgery. *Surg Technol Int.* 2004;12:265-268.

27. Kim YH, Oh SH, Kim JS. Incidence and natural history of deep-vein thrombosis after total hip arthroplasty. A prospective and randomised clinical study. *J Bone Joint Surg Br.* 2003;85:661-665.

28. Buller HR, Agnelli G, Hull RD, et al. Antithrombotic therapy for venous thromboembolic disease: the Seventh ACCP Conference on Antithrombotic and Thrombolytic Therapy. *Chest.* 2004;126:401S-428S.

29. Aissaoui N, Martins E, Mouly S, et al. A meta-analysis of bed rest versus early ambulation in the management of pulmonary embolism, deep vein thrombosis, or both. *Int J Cardiol.* 2009;137:37-41.

30. Aldrich D, Hunt DP. When can the patient with deep vein thrombosis begin to ambulate? *Phys Ther.* 2004;84:268-273.

31. Ebell MH. Evaluation of the patient with suspected deep vein thrombosis. *J Fam Pract.* 2001;50:167-171.

32. Wells PS, Owen C, Doucette S, et al. Does this patient have deep vein thrombosis? *JAMA.* 2006;295:199-207.

33. Kruip MJ, Slob MJ, Schijen JH, et al. Use of a clinical decision rule in combination with D-dimer concentration in diagnostic workup of patients with suspected pulmonary embolism: a prospective management study. *Arch Intern Med.* 2002;162:1631-1635.

34. Anderson CM, Overend TJ, Godwin J, et al. Ambulation after deep vein thrombosis: a systematic review. *Physiother Can.* 2009;61:133-140.

35. Costello E, Elrod C, Tepper S. Clinical decision making in the acute care environment: a survey of practicing clinicians. *JACPT.* 2011;2:46-54.

36. Bauer K. Therapeutic Use of Fondaparinux. May 2011. Available at: http://www.uptodate.com/contents/therapeutic-use-of-fondaparinux. Accessed May 17, 2012.

37. Kim E, Bartholomew J. Venous thromboembolism. Available at: http://www.clevelandclinicmeded.com/medicalpubs/diseasemanagement/cardiology/venous-thromboembolism/#bib42#bib42. Accessed October 30, 2011.

38. A Patient's Guide to Antithrombotic and Thrombolytic Therapy: Comprehensive Guide. Available at: http://accptstorage.org/newOrganization/patients/AT8/AT8ComprehensiveGuidePatient.pdf. Accessed October 30, 2011.

39. Panus PC, Katzung B, Jobst EE, et al. *Pharmacology for the Physical Therapist.* New York: McGraw-Hill; 2009.

40. Smith BA, Fields CJ, Fernandez N. Physical therapists make accurate and appropriate discharge recommendations for patients who are acutely ill. *Phys Ther.* 2010;90:693-703.

41. National Committee for Quality Assurance (NQMC). Fall risk management: the percentage of Medicare members 75 years of age and older or who are 65 to 74 years of age with balance or walking problems or a fall in the past 12 months who were seen by an MAO practitioner in the past 12 months and who discussed falls or problems with balance or walking with their current practitioner. Available at: http://www.qualitymeasures.ahrq.gov. Accessed 10/27/2011.

Dizziness

Anne K. Galgon
Heather Dillon Anderson

CASE 5

A 73-year-old female was admitted to the hospital 2 days ago for an elective right total hip replacement due to severe osteoarthritis and pain in her right hip. The surgery involved a posterior surgical approach with replacement of both the acetabulum and the femoral head. Notable past medical history includes osteoporosis, complaints of positional dizziness, hypercholesterolemia, and type 2 diabetes mellitus. The surgical team stated that she must follow hip precautions (no hip flexion past 90°, no internal rotation/crossing of legs) and she could bear weight as tolerated. The physical therapist is asked to evaluate and treat the patient before she is discharged to her two-story home in 2 to 3 days with her husband, who is retired but limited in his physical ability to assist her due to a recent history of back surgery. She will have a few home physical therapy and nursing visits following discharge and then she plans to attend outpatient physical therapy to continue postsurgical treatment of her hip. Her current complaints are pain in her right hip and short duration complaints of dizziness associated with positional changes.

▶ Based on her health condition, what do you anticipate will contribute to her symptoms of dizziness?
▶ What are the examination priorities?
▶ What are the most appropriate examination tests?
▶ What are the most appropriate physical therapy interventions?
▶ What precautions should be taken during physical therapy interventions?
▶ What are possible complications interfering with physical therapy?
▶ How would this individual's contextual factors influence or change your patient/client management?

KEY DEFINITIONS

DIZZINESS: Symptoms that can have several meanings to different individuals; may include sensations of lightheadedness, disorientation, imbalance, or vertigo; may be related to increased heart rate (HR), a vasovagal event, syncope, nystagmus, and/or feelings of anxiety

NYSTAGMUS: Repeated rapid alternating eye movements that include slow (one direction) and fast phases (opposite direction); direction of nystagmus is named for the fast phase movements

TRIAD OF HEAD ORIENTATIONS SIGNS: Three cardinal signs associated with acute unilateral vestibular hypofunction. Signs include: (1) ocular skew deviation (or tilt) where one eye is deviated up and one eye is deviated down, (2) ocular torsion where eyes roll away from head orientation, and (3) head tilt toward the side of unilateral vestibular imbalance.

UNIDIRECTIONAL NYSTAGMUS FOLLOWING ALEXANDER'S LAW: Spontaneous and gaze-holding nystagmus usually seen in acute stage of unilateral vestibular hypofunction; nystagmus is horizontal, with the fast phase beating away from the ear with decreased sensory function. Alexander's law indicates that the nystagmus will decrease in intensity when the eyes gaze toward the involved side and increase in intensity when they gaze away.

VERTIGO: Sensation of rotation or spinning; person either feels like she is spinning or as if her surroundings are rotating around her

VESTIBULAR OCULAR REFLEX (VOR): Three-neuron reflex connecting sensory information (angular head acceleration) from the semicircular canals of the vestibular apparatus to the oculomotor system to control eye movements when the head is moving; VOR allows for gaze stabilization when the head is moving during functional tasks; disruptions of these neurons can cause osillopsia (world appears unsteady or jumpy) and dizziness with head movements

Objectives

1. Outline the procedures and clinical decision-making process for differentiating between causes of dizziness in an acute care setting.
2. Identify reliable and valid tests and measures to differentiate the causes of dizziness.
3. Identify critical lab values, medication(s), and vital sign responses that should be checked prior to treating the patient.
4. Interpret examination findings to diagnose the cause of dizziness.
5. Determine appropriate physical therapy interventions based on diagnostic outcome.

Physical Therapy Considerations

PT considerations during management of dizziness in the individual post-surgery:

▶ **General physical therapy plan of care/goals:** Minimize loss of range of motion, strength, and aerobic functional capacity; decrease symptoms of dizziness and pain; maximize functional independence while minimizing secondary impairments to improve quality of life

▶ **Physical therapy interventions:** Patient and caregiver education regarding postoperative precautions and weightbearing restrictions, complications related to the surgical procedure, and recommendations for follow-up care for dizziness and continued care of total hip replacement; positioning during modified mobility training and treatment of positional dizziness while maintaining hip precautions; lower extremity exercises; functional mobility training; caregiver training

▶ **Precautions during physical therapy:** Adherence to hip precautions during all functional mobility; close supervision to decrease risk of falls; monitor blood pressure, blood glucose, medications, and lab values

▶ **Complications interfering with physical therapy:** Dizziness, increased pain, hip precautions, deep vein thrombosis

Understanding the Health Condition

Total hip arthroplasty (THA), also referred to as total hip replacement (THR), is a common surgical procedure often chosen when conservative treatment does not successfully relieve chronic hip pain and dysfunction. Although there are many variations of hip surgeries, THA involves replacement of the femoral head as well as the hip socket (acetabulum) with prosthetic components. Approximately 285,000 THA surgeries took place in the United States in 2005.[1] As the elderly population continues to grow, the annual incidence of THA is expected to rise. One of the most common reasons for performing a THA is severe osteoarthritis causing chronic pain.[2] Additional causes include rheumatoid arthritis, avascular necrosis of the hip, childhood hip disease, and prior trauma.[3]

There are different approaches and techniques for hip replacement surgery with varying postoperative instructions and precautions. Prior to mobilizing a person following hip replacement surgery, it is important to know which surgical approach was used and the corresponding postoperative precautions. Traditionally, the posterior or posterolateral approach has been credited with preserving hip abductor function and providing good exposure to the proximal femur and acetabulum.[4] In the past, the main disadvantage associated with this technique was a higher dislocation rate.[5] However, a 2009 study conducted by Palan et al.,[4] compared the anterolateral approach to the posterior approach and found no differences in dislocation rates. The usual precautions following the posterior approach include avoidance of hip flexion beyond 90° and restriction from hip adduction and internal rotation beyond 45° for at least 6 weeks postoperatively.[6]

Weightbearing restrictions are also common following hip surgery and are typically dependent on the specific type of surgical procedure. When cement is used to fixate the femoral prosthesis into the acetabulum, the patient is typically permitted to bear weight as tolerated.[3] However, in more complex surgical procedures, or a prosthesis fixed without cement, the patient may be limited in how much weight can be loaded through the affected extremity.[3] The therapist must always confirm the postoperative protocol and any associated precautions with the surgical team prior to mobilization because precautions vary by surgical case.

Physical therapy is an essential component of the postoperative care for persons who receive a THA. A study in 2000 conducted by Freburger[7] demonstrated that increased utilization of physical therapy in the acute care setting for persons who received a THA was associated with decreased total cost of care and increased probability of discharge to home. The main objectives of physical therapy interventions following THA are to mobilize the patient, provide patient and caregiver education on the postsurgical precautions, recommend appropriate exercises, and assist in discharge planning.

While providing physical therapy interventions for persons in the acute care setting following surgery, common patient symptoms include pain, dizziness, and fatigue. Coordination of pain management with the interdisciplinary team following surgery is essential in order to effectively implement physical therapy interventions. Similarly, evaluating patient complaints of dizziness is critical. According to Post and Dickerson,[8] dizziness is the primary symptom in approximately 3% of primary care visits for persons over 25 years of age and is present in close to 3% of emergency department visits. Dizziness is also a common complaint in the acute care setting. Determining the cause of dizziness as well as the actual symptoms associated with the term can be challenging. Perceptions and definitions of dizziness often vary from person to person. Classifying dizziness into one of four identified main types (vertigo, disequilibrium, presyncope, or lightheadedness) is helpful in determining its cause.[8]

Vertigo is described as the false sense of spinning or motion.[9] Vertigo is most often associated with an otologic or vestibular cause of dizziness.[8] Disequilibrium is typically described as a sense of imbalance. Presyncope is associated with the feeling(s) a person experiences prior to fainting and may be associated with a significant drop in blood pressure (orthostatic hypotension).[8] Orthostatic, or postural hypotension, occurs when the body is not able to adequately compensate for the reduction of blood coming to the heart when a person moves from a supine to sitting or standing position. Common factors that may lead to orthostatic hypotension include: age-associated physiological changes, elevated blood pressure (BP), blood volume depletion, vasodilating medications, immobility, and autonomic insufficiency.[10] The diagnostic criteria for orthostatic hypotension varies depending on the reference or resource. Criteria often include a decrease in systolic blood pressure (SBP) of 20 mm Hg, or a decrease of 10 mm Hg in diastolic blood pressure (DBP), or an increase in heart rate of 30 beats per minute at least 1 minute after the person changes from a supine to upright position.[8] Lightheadedness is often described as feeling faint or disoriented. Research indicates that psychiatric causes of lightheadedness are common.[8] If a patient describes symptoms of dizziness as being lightheaded in nature, inquiry about anxiety and depression is warranted.

Positional dizziness or vertigo could be caused by positional nystagmus. Understanding the various disorders that cause positional nystagmus will assist in diagnosis and interventions that may be part of the plan of care. The most common cause of positional vertigo is benign paroxysmal positional vertigo (BPPV).[11] BPPV causes nystagmus and complaints of vertigo that is usually provoked when an individual moves from supine to sitting or from sitting to supine, rolls in bed, or bends forward or reaches overhead. The complaints of vertigo are often reported as episodic; an individual may have many bouts of short-duration vertigo over a period of weeks or months. The symptoms may resolve and then reoccur. Patients may be fearful and avoid positions that might provoke vertigo.

BPPV may account for 20% to 30% of vestibular-related dizziness seen in individuals undergoing treatment in balance clinics and is more prevalent in older individuals.[12] Oghalai et al.[13] found that 61% of 100 older adults (mean age 74 ± 1 years) had dizziness and 71% had complaints of imbalance. The majority did not seek intervention for dizziness or imbalance. Nine percent of these individuals had unrecognized BPPV. Older individuals with BPPV have decreased independence in activities of daily living (ADLs) and have an increased prevalence of falls in the 3 months prior to being diagnosed with BPPV.[13] Because of these negative consequences, BPPV should always be screened for in this susceptible older population. The complaint of a spinning sensation in the *absence* of lightheadedness has been shown to be predictive of BPPV (sensitivity 59% and specificity 98%).[13] Positional testing, however, is required to make the appropriate diagnosis.

BPPV is considered a mechanical disorder involving the peripheral vestibular apparatus. Figure 5-1 shows the normal anatomy of the vestibulocochlear apparatus within the inner ear. In BPPV, calcium carbonate crystals (otoconia) are dislodged from the utricle macula, and become displaced into the endolymph of a semicircular canal (canalithiasis). Because otoconia are microscopic, this condition is not visible with imaging. In some cases, the otoconia adhere to the cupula of a semicircular canal (cupulolithiasis). The semicircular canal becomes sensitive to gravitational force as the head is positioned in relation to the gravitational field. The hydrodynamic drag of the otoconia (canalithiasis) or the weight of the otoconia (cupulolithiasis) during positional changes causes the cupula to bend (Fig. 5-2). This stimulates the VOR associated with the involved semicircular canal and manifests as stereotypical abnormal nystagmus and complaints of vertigo. Posterior canal involvement is the mostly likely presentation occurring in about 76%[11] to 94%[14] of individuals with BPPV. Systematic testing for BPPV and identification of canal involvement and type (canalithiasis vs. cupulolithiasis) are presented in Table 5-4 and will be reviewed in the differential diagnosis section of this case. Correct diagnosis of which semicircular canal(s) are involved (anterior, posterior, horizontal) and type of BPPV (canalithiasis or cupulolithiasis) is critical because interventions to reduce nystagmus and symptoms of vertigo have been shown to be highly effective when applied appropriately.[15,16]

Other vestibular conditions that result in positional vertigo can be categorized as peripheral or central in nature. These conditions are less common than BPPV

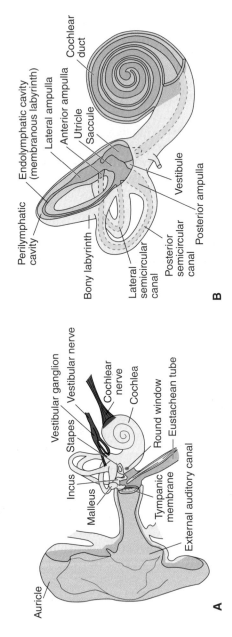

Figure 5-1. Normal anatomy of the vestibulocochlear apparatus within the inner ear. **A.** The right ear showing the external ear, auditory canal, middle ear, and the inner ear with its semicircular canals. **B.** The main parts of the inner ear. (Reproduced with permission from Ropper AH, Samuels MA, eds. *Adams and Victor's Principles of Neurology.* 9th ed. New York, NY: McGraw-Hill; 2009. Figure 15-1.)

(a) Canalithiasis

(b) Cupulolithiasis

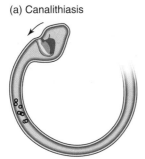
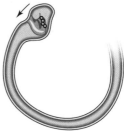

Figure 5-2. Mechanisms of benign paroxysmal positional vertigo (BPPV). When the semicircular canal (SCC) is placed in the gravitational field: **A.** displacement of the otoconia (black dots) creates a drag on the endolymph that deflects the cupula and results in nystagmus of less than 1 minute; or **B.** otoconia lodged on the cupula cause deflection and result in nystagmus lasting longer than 1 minute or until the SSC is moved out of the gravitational field.

and present with a different history of onset and with additional signs and symptoms, which assist in the differential diagnosis. Peripheral disorders that might cause positional vertigo include perilymphatic fistula,[17] superior (anterior) semicircular canal dehiscences,[18] and acute vestibular hypofunction due to neuritis. Positional nystagmus and vertigo also commonly occur during acute vestibular migraines.[19] Central nervous system (CNS) lesions in the medial cerebellum, nodulus, and vermis, or the connecting pathways with vestibular and ocular brainstem structures can also cause positional nystagmus and vertigo. These CNS lesions may be caused by stroke, tumor, multiple sclerosis, or degenerative disorders of the brainstem or cerebellum. The most common presentation of nystagmus for vertigo with a CNS (central) cause is pure up-beating or down-beating nystagmus that may be present in multiple head positions.[20] Table 5-1 reviews the common presentations of peripheral versus central positional vertigo based on latency, duration, fatigability, direction, and intensity of nystagmus and vertigo. An individual presenting with positional nystagmus with either a history of a CNS disorder or new CNS signs and symptoms must be immediately referred to a neurologist. In some elderly individuals, central positional nystagmus may be present *without* symptoms of vertigo. In these benign cases, the etiology is unknown, there are no findings on MRI, and intervention is not provided because they are asymptomatic.[20]

The first occurrence of BPPV may be sudden and severe and provoke a great deal of anxiety. The vertigo associated with BPPV can mimic an acute vestibular neuritis of the eighth cranial nerve. Although these conditions may be present at the same time, they are distinct in nature. One common cause of acute vestibular neuritis is a reactivation of a latent herpes simplex virus.[21] A unilateral peripheral vestibular hypofunction (UVH) resulting from neuritis presents with sudden and severe vertigo and imbalance that last for days (> 72 hours). Head movement provoked oscillopsia, dizziness, and imbalance continue for weeks to months.[22] Vestibular neuritis is the third most common cause of peripheral vestibular pathology and its annual incidence is about 3.5 per 100,000.[21] Acutely, the UVH creates an imbalance in tonic vestibular sensory inputs to the vestibular nuclei. This aberrant sensory

Table 5-1 COMMON PRESENTATIONS OF PERIPHERALLY PROVOKED (BPPV) VERSUS CENTRALLY PROVOKED POSITIONAL VERTIGO THAT CAN BE USED IN DIFFERENTIAL DIAGNOSIS

Symptom or Sign	Peripheral Cause	Central Cause
Latency		
Time to onset of vertigo or nystagmus	0-40 s (mean 7.8 s)	No latency—begins immediately
Duration of vertigo or nystagmus		
Single episode	< 1 min (canalithiasis) > 1 min (cupulolithiasis)	More likely persistent (*i.e.*, continues as long as position is maintained)
Fatigability		
Lessening of vertigo or nystagmus with repeated maneuvers	Yes	No
Direction of nystagmus	Direction fixed torsional to testing side plus up- or down-beating	Variable: may change directions, or be pure up-beating or down-beating
Intensity	Severe vertigo Marked nystagmus Nausea more likely Symptoms worse in the morning & variable throughout the day	Usually mild vertigo Less intense nystagmus Nausea rare Symptoms more constant throughout the day
Reproducibility	Inconsistent	More consistent

information affects the oculomotor and postural control systems resulting in a horizontal (unidirectional) spontaneous nystagmus, loss of perception of upright, and a triad of head orientations signs including: ocular skew deviation, ocular torsion, and head tilt response. In the first days to weeks following onset, the CNS will compensate to the new sensory information and reduction of these signs and symptoms are expected. Because the UVH affects the ability to detect head movement, the VOR and balance become disrupted when the head is moving. Central compensation is expected to improve VOR and balance as the individual begins to move and returns to normal activity. Management of acute vestibular neuritis includes methylprednisone to improve peripheral vestibular function, an antivertiginous drug to reduce symptoms of nausea and vertigo, and physical therapy for central compensation to improve VOR function and balance.[21,22] Some individuals with UVH present with positional nystagmus.[20] Of note, BPPV is more likely in individuals with a history of UVH.[23] Understanding the physiology of the vestibular system and CNS changes associated with UVH helps in the differential diagnosis between UVH and BPPV. Schubert and Minor[22] provide a thorough review of this topic.

Physical Therapy Patient/Client Management

Postoperative hip management in the acute care setting involves early mobilization, pain management, patient education, and assessment of functional mobility to initiate discharge planning. The physical therapist works with the surgical team to implement the required postoperative surgical precautions and weightbearing instructions. The physical therapist initially coordinates with the nurses to optimize pain control and plan for early mobilization out of bed. The physical therapist also coordinates with discharge planners to determine the most appropriate discharge setting and what type of equipment and/or services the patient will require.

For patients in the acute care setting that report dizziness in addition to their primary diagnosis, the physical therapist must also investigate the cause of the dizziness. The patient's history and presentation are essential in determining which tests and measures are incorporated into the physical therapy examination. Depending on the results of the examination and evaluation, a diagnosis of dizziness may be established and appropriate physical therapy interventions will be incorporated into the patient's plan of care. If the cause is more medical in nature, the physical therapist coordinates with the medical team and follows the appropriate guidelines for dizziness when incorporating other physical therapy interventions.

Examination, Evaluation, and Diagnosis

Before initiating the patient examination, the physical therapist must acquire information from the chart to understand the patient's past medical history, recent surgical procedure(s), and any complications during the hospitalization. Additional information that must be reviewed in the chart prior to mobilizing the patient includes: medication list, recent lab values, weightbearing restrictions, postoperative precautions, and any exercise or mobility restrictions.

When reviewing the medication list, specifically examine: new medication(s) that may decrease BP or have the known adverse drug reaction (ADR) of causing dizziness, potential interactions of multiple medications, withdrawal of medications that the patient had taken previously, and recent changes in dosage of medications. Medications known to cause damage to the vestibular system, referred to as ototoxicity, must be recognized. Aminoglycosides, a class of antibiotics including tobramycin, kanamycin, and gentamicin, are well known to cause oxotoxic ADRs.[24] However, these antibiotics are still used to treat some bacterial infections due to their effectiveness and low cost. Gentamicin, the most frequently used of these medications, is sometimes used to purposely disrupt vestibular function to treat dizziness in severe cases of Meniere's disease.[24]

When reviewing the patient's most recent lab values, it is important to consider the hemoglobin, hematocrit, white blood cell, and platelet counts. If the patient is receiving anticoagulation therapy following surgery to prevent thromboembolism (e.g., Coumadin), the international normalized ratio (INR) level should be reviewed. If any of the lab values are not within normal limits, the physical therapist should check with the surgical team prior to mobilizing the patient.[25] Table 5-2 outlines a process to examine a patient complaining of dizziness in the acute care setting.

During the initial part of the physical examination, the physical therapist should evaluate the patient's level of pain and knowledge of surgical precautions and weightbearing restrictions. If the patient's pain is not adequately controlled,

Table 5-2   EVALUATION OF THE "DIZZY" PATIENT IN THE ACUTE CARE SETTING

Procedure	Considerations
Review the patient's chart	Past medical history Recent events Complication(s) during hospitalization
Review the medication list	New medications that decrease the BP or have known ADR of causing dizziness Interaction of multiple medications Withdrawal of medication the patient has taken previously Change(s) in dosage
Review the patient's most recent lab values	Hemoglobin and hematocrit
Gather the patient's history, especially in assessing dizzy symptoms	Determine: **What** "dizzy" means to the patient (light-headedness vs. actual vertigo) **When** exactly the patient feels dizzy: specific movement(s) vs. when the patient is still (spontaneous) **How** often the patient's symptoms occur (*e.g.*, every hour vs. once per week) and how long symptoms last (*e.g.*, seconds, minutes, hours) **Whether** the patient has a history of similar symptoms and what exactly occurred at that time **Which** positions provoke the dizzy symptoms and which positions eliminate them
Rule out orthostatic hypotension by taking patient's BP and heart rate (HR) in the following sequence: supine, sitting on the edge of the bed, and standing. Wait at least 1 minute once the new position is obtained prior to assessing the vital sign response.	Orthostatic hypotension: SBP drops 20 mm Hg or, DBP drops 10 mm Hg or, HR increases 30 beats per min
Examine functional mobility, balance, and gait	Assess bed mobility, gait on level surfaces and on steps; static and dynamic balance
Oculomotor and vestibulo-ocular interaction testing	Refer to Table 5-3
Positional testing	Refer to Table 5-4 and Figs. 5-2 to 5-4

coordination of pain medicine with the nurse is helpful for successful mobilization. If the patient is unaware of her precautions and weightbearing restrictions, it may be helpful to post signs in the room as a reminder. It is also helpful to educate a family member to ensure guidelines are followed all the time.

Next, the patient's lower extremities should be examined for edema, pulses, and positioning. Following a THA, most patients will be positioned supine with their lower extremities (in thromboembolic disease, or TED hose) abducted with a triangular hip abductor pillow between them. If the patient's wound is visible, it should be inspected; however, the physical therapist should not remove the original surgical dressing unless instructed to do so by the surgical team.

A basic strength assessment for the uninvolved lower extremity and both upper extremities should be completed as well as sensory and proprioception testing for both lower extremities. Next, the patient should be carefully mobilized to assess bed mobility, transfers, ambulation, and balance. All functional mobility and balance testing must be completed within the boundaries of the postoperative precautions and weightbearing restrictions. If the patient is suspected to have a vestibular cause of dizziness (*i.e.*, no episodes of orthostatic hypotension noted in chart, no suspicion of medication-induced dizziness, the patient reports positional vertigo with specific changes in her head position during subjective assessment), it is important to complete the mobility assessment *before* assessing for positional dizziness. This is because it is common for individuals with positional dizziness to experience an increase in symptoms following a vestibular examination, which will likely affect their ability to participate in the examination of functional mobility and balance. Prior to and during initial mobilization, the patient's vital sign response and pain level must be carefully monitored. If the patient complains of feeling dizzy during mobilization, testing for orthostatic hypotension is warranted (procedure described in Table 5-2).

If testing for orthostatic hypotension is negative and the patient's history suggests vestibular involvement, the physical therapist should conduct systematic screening for peripheral vestibular hypofunction or central-related disorders. Oculomotor testing and vestibular-ocular interaction tests are the best screening tools and can be performed at the bedside within 5 minutes. Key examination findings for normal, peripheral vestibular, or central disorders for these tests are presented in Table 5-3. The patient should be sitting upright with eyes open in a well-lit environment. Glasses should be worn, if required for normal distant vision. First, observe eye position in the orbits and inspect for presence of spontaneous nystagmus. Spontaneous nystagmus in sitting is always considered pathological and warrants further medical investigation. Next, test convergence by having the patient focus on a small target (*e.g.*, tip of a finger or pen) a few feet from her face and slowly bring the target forward to the bridge of her nose. The eyes should adduct and pupils should constrict as the target moves closer to the face. The therapist should instruct the patient to report when the object appears blurred or double. To test ocular range of motion, ask the patient to track the target right, left, up, and down as far as possible. The therapist should observe the eyes for symmetry and range of motion. The tests of gaze holding nystagmus and smooth pursuit can be combined by having the patient track a slowly moving target starting from midline to approximately 30° in each direction (right, left, up, and down). At approximately 30° from midline, the therapist holds each position and asks the patient to continue to fixate on the target. The therapist should note whether the eyes smoothly follow the target and remain still when the target is held in place. To measure saccadic ocular control, the therapist presents two targets in front of the patient at approximately 30° right and left or up and down from the midpoint of the visual field. The patient is asked to quickly look back and forth between the targets. The therapist should observe a quick movement of the eyes and fixation on the targets without deviation.

If vestibular hypofunction is suspected, the physical therapist can perform the two bedside tests for vestibular-ocular interaction: the head thrust test (Halmagyi) and the dynamic visual acuity test. To perform the head thrust test, the therapist rapidly rotates the patient's head right and then left about 1 in from midline as the

Table 5-3   KEY EXAMINATION FINDINGS OF BEDSIDE OCULOMOTOR AND VESTIBULAR–OCULAR INTERACTION TESTS

Test and Measures	Normal Findings	Positive Findings	
		Peripheral Disorder	Central Disorder
Oculomotor examination In room light, assess eye position (visual fixation)	Eyes neutral position	Triad of head orientations signs (skew deviation, ocular torsion, and head tilt toward the side of lesion)	Single or bilateral eye deviation: CN III, IV, or VI disorder Central insults may show the triad of head orientations signs
Spontaneous nystagmus	No nystagmus	Unidirectional nystagmus	Vertical or nystagmus that changes direction
Ocular ROM and convergence	Full ROM convergence to 6 in of nose	Normal ROM and convergence Unidirectional nystagmus may be noted	Eyes are not able to move fully throughout the range or do not move together and/or symmetrically
Gaze holding nystagmus	Hold gaze 30° from midline without deviation	Unidirectional nystagmus (follows Alexander's law)	Directional changing nystagmus or vertical nystagmus
Smooth pursuit	Eyes smoothly track moving target	Eyes smoothly track Unidirectional nystagmus may be noted	Eyes are not able to smoothly follow target Increased saccades
Saccadic eye movements	Eyes move precisely from one target to another	Eyes move precisely Unidirectional nystagmus may be noted	Overshooting or undershooting targets
Vestibular–ocular interaction (VOR function)			
Head thrust (Halmagyi) or fast VOR	Eyes maintain fixation on target when head rapidly moved	Saccadic correction after quick movement Unilateral or bilateral	False positives: VOR can be disrupted with oculomotor deficits
Dynamic visual acuity (DVA)	1-2 line loss	>2 lines lost	Central VOR loss will show lost DVA

Abbreviation: CN, cranial nerve.

patient focuses on a central target (the bridge of the therapist's nose). The therapist should observe the patient's eyes, which should stay fixed on the target during movement of the patient's head (the "head thrust"). A positive test occurs when the patient's head is turned *toward* a dysfunctional semicircular canal, and the patient's eyes are not able to stay focused on the target and then make a "catch-up" saccade to return to the target. When performed correctly, the head thrust test can identify peripheral vestibular hypofunction (sensitivity 71% and specificity 82%).[26] Dynamic visual acuity is a functional test of the VOR and can be screened at bedside using a handheld Snellen (or E-directional) eye chart. The therapist places the chart at a distance determined by the chart scale. The patient is first tested with the head fixed for static visual acuity and then with the head moving back and forth horizontally at about 2 Hz for dynamic visual acuity. The difference in lines that the patient can read correctly between the static versus dynamic test is recorded (Table 5-3).

When testing oculomotor and vestibular-ocular function in older individuals, it is important to consider that smooth pursuits, saccadic control, and VOR function may decline with age. Healthy and active individuals over the age of 75 years are more likely to show declines in VOR function, but maintain normal oculomotor function. Kerber et al.[27] found that older individuals who demonstrate declines in oculomotor and VOR function also frequently have impairments on balance and gait measures. Occasional saccadic correction during smooth pursuit and additional saccades to reach targets during the test of saccadic control may be considered normal for age, if no other CNS signs are found. However, individuals showing these signs should be examined for balance and gait deficits.

Testing for positional nystagmus is the next step in the examination to determine cause of positional dizziness. Posterior and anterior semicircular canal (SCC) BPPV is tested with the **Dix-Hallpike test.** This test has been shown to have high sensitivity (82%) and specificity (71%) for identifying posterior SCC BPPV.[16] Figure 5-3 shows the Dix-Hallpike test for otoconia in the left anterior or posterior SCCs (left Dix-Hallpike). This test is performed by first placing the patient in a long sitting position. The physical therapist rotates the patient's head 45° to right (to test the right side) or left (to test left; Fig. 5-3A) and then quickly moves the patient to the supine position with her head hanging over the edge of bed in about 20° of neck extension (Fig. 5-3B). The therapist observes the patient's eyes for nystagmus; if observed, the therapist notes onset latency, direction, and duration of the nystagmus to identify the canal of involvement (anterior or posterior) and type of BPPV (canalithiasis or cupulolithiasis) as indicated in Table 5-4. The end position is held for at least 30 seconds; if nystagmus is not observed, the patient must be returned to upright sitting before testing the other side. Both sides should be tested; the test can be repeated to confirm the nystagmus. However, frequent repetitions with little rest in between tests will cause the intensity of the response to diminish or fatigue. Resting between tests also decreases anxiety for individuals with severe symptoms. Contraindications for performing the Dix-Hallpike test include recent neck surgery, recent neck trauma, severe rheumatoid arthritis, atlantoaxial or occipitoatlantal instability, cervical myelopathy or radiculopathy, carotid sinus syncope, Chiari malformations, and vascular dissection syndrome.[11,28] In the absence of medical screening to rule out these contraindications, if the patient can perform the combined position of 45° active neck rotation with 20° of cervical extension in sitting without neck pain or neurologic symptoms, then the test is considered safe.[11]

Although sensitivity and specificity have not been reported, the **supine roll test** is the preferred method to test for horizontal SCC BPPV (Fig. 5-4).[11,16] Other types of positional nystagmus may be observed in this test as well. If present, nystagmus should be evaluated for additional causes. To perform the supine roll test, the patient is placed in supine with neck flexed approximately 30°. The therapist rapidly moves the patient's head 90° to one side and observes the eyes for horizontal nystagmus. After 30 seconds, the therapist returns the patient's head to the starting position and the test is repeated on the other side. A positive supine roll test includes horizontal nystagmus when the head is rolled both toward the right and the left. Direction of the nystagmus in relation to the ground (geotropic, toward the ground; or, ageotropic, away from the ground) determines the type of BPPV (canalithiasis vs. cupulolithiasis) and intensity of the nystagmus and symptoms determine the side of involvement (Table 5-4).

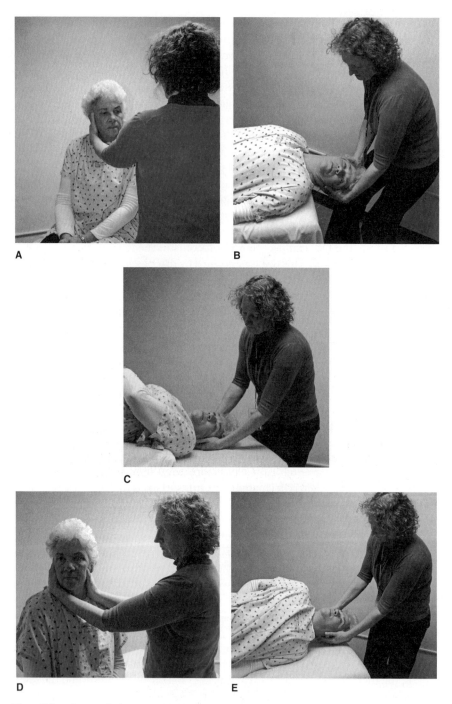

Figure 5-3. Left Dix-Hallpike Test. **A.** Start position: long sitting with head rotated 45° to the left. **B.** End position: supine with head extended 20° off end of surface. **C.** *End position modification*: to support head and avoid neck extension. **D.** Modified Dix-Hallpike Start position: sitting with head rotated 45° to the right. **E.** Modified Dix-Hallpike end position: sidelying to left; maintain head rotation.

	Direction of Nystagmus *Duration*	SCC Involvement *Type of BPPV*	*Side of Involvement*
Positional test			
Dix-Hallpike test	Up-beating torsional to side of head rotation <1 minute >1 minute	Posterior SCC *Canalithiasis* *Cupulolithiasis*	Side of head rotation during positional test (typically the side with nystagmus and symptoms)
	Down-beating torsional to side of head rotation <1 minute >1 minute	Anterior SCC *Canalithiasis* *Cupulolithiasis*	
Roll test	Horizontal (or lateral) Geotropic (toward the ground) Ageotropic (away from the ground) *Duration not significant for diagnosis*	Horizontal SCC *Canalithiasis* *Cupulolithiasis*	*Canalithiasis:* Side with strongest nystag-mus and symptoms *Cupulolithiasis:* Side with less nystagmus and symptoms

Table 5-4   DIFFERENTIAL DIAGNOSIS OF SEMICIRCULAR CANAL (SCC) INVOLVEMENT, TYPE OF BPPV, AND SIDE OF INVOLVEMENT BASED ON DIRECTION AND DURATION OF NYSTAGMUS AND INTENSITY OF SYMPTOMS

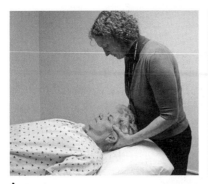
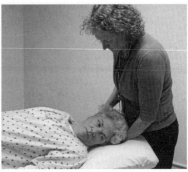

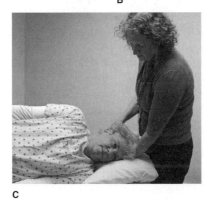

Figure 5-4. Left supine roll test. **A.** Start position: supine, neck flexed 30°. **B.** End position: head rotated 90° to the left. **C.** End position modification: add trunk rotation for limited cervical rotation ROM.

In the current patient who is 2 days status/post THA, these tests can be performed. However, modifications must be made to prevent breaking hip precautions and causing excessive hip discomfort. In addition, in an older individual there are likely postural alignment changes (*e.g.*, thoracic kyphosis, loss of cervical ROM) that limit the ability to attain precise test positions. The essential considerations in performing these tests are that the head is moved into the correct position(s) to place the SCC into the gravitational field and that there is adequate movement of the otoconia to provoke the nystagmus. If range of motion (ROM) is limited or if increased neck extension should be avoided, modifications to the test can be made. Common modifications to avoid the head-hanging position in the Dix-Hallpike test include placing a towel roll under the patient's shoulders to achieve cervical extension or using a tilt table or hospital bed with the head reclined below the body to support the head in the down position. Figure 5-3C shows an example of an end position modification. A sidelying test is an option for patients with low back discomfort or poor trunk mobility. In this modified Dix-Hallpike test, the patient is moved from short sitting to sidelying at the edge of bed with the head rotated 45° away from the side she is moved onto (Fig. 5-3D-E). For the supine roll test, rolling with the trunk toward sidelying can be added, if 90° of neck rotation is unavailable (Fig. 5-4C).

In this case, the patient's history was significant for prior experiences of brief positional vertigo 1 year ago, which seemed to resolve without intervention. Her lab values were within normal limits and her medication list did not contain any drugs known to cause dizziness or vertigo. Following her THA surgery, the patient reported experiencing vertigo (spinning sensation without lightheadedness) lasting less than a minute when she changed the position of her head, especially turning her head toward the left. Her symptoms were more severe when initiating lying down than when coming up to sitting.

Considering the blood loss associated with THA and the limited mobility of this patient following surgery, the therapist assessed her for orthostatic hypotension early during the examination and found her vital signs to be stable and within normal limits. Next, because persons with positional vertigo often do not tolerate extensive mobilization following positional vertigo testing, a standard postoperative THA physical therapy examination (as previously described) was conducted including assessment of functional mobility, gait, and balance. Oculomotor and head thrust tests were conducted next and revealed normal results. Finally, the Dix-Hallpike maneuver was performed to test for positional nystagmus and vertigo. The therapist modified the test position by declining the head of the hospital bed and maintained her hip precautions throughout the test. Because the patient seemed to have more symptoms when turning her head toward the left, a test was completed on the *right* first to rule it out. The right Dix-Hallpike positional test was negative (*i.e.*, no nystagmus and no vertigo). In the end position of the left Dix-Hallpike test, the therapist observed left, torsional, up-beating nystagmus lasting less than 30 seconds accompanied by the patient's complaints of vertigo. After allowing a few minutes for the patient to recover, the therapist performed a supine roll test in both directions to rule out the right and left horizontal canals. No symptoms or nystagmus were provoked. The physical therapist made the diagnosis of left, posterior canalithiasis BPPV.

Plan of Care and Interventions

When treating a person post-THA in the acute care setting, the physical therapist typically completes the examination on postoperative day 1 (POD 1) and treats the patient 1 to 3 times per day during the acute hospital stay, which averaged just over 4 days in 2009.[29] Physical therapy interventions for individuals following THA include: extensive patient education, gentle hip exercises, out of bed mobilization, and functional mobility tasks.

Because patients are often groggy and distracted by pain following surgery, many need constant reminders to adhere to postoperative precautions and weightbearing restrictions. Educating family members and supplementing patient education with visual information is important. In this case, the patient's husband is home and able to remind her about the hip precautions, but his ability to physically assist her is limited due to his own health condition. Therefore, the patient needs to be functioning at a supervision level prior to discharge to home.

The typical exercises initiated immediately following THA include ankle pumps, quadriceps sets, and gluteal sets at a level of submaximal exertion with a frequency of 10 times per hour.[3] As the patient's tolerance for out of bed activity improves, supported standing exercises for the involved lower extremity such as hip flexion, abduction, and extension may be initiated within the surgical precautions. Upper extremity exercises may be initiated as well as functional activities such as walking and standing to complete ADLs.

To treat the patient's left posterior canalithiasis, the physical therapist should use a left canalith repositioning maneuver (CRM, Fig. 5-5). The purpose of the CRM is to progressively move the otoconia through the posterior SCC canal, relocating the otoconia back into the utricle, thereby eliminating symptoms of vertigo and nystagmus associated with gravitational influences on the SCC. The patient starts in a long sitting position with head rotated 45° to the left (Fig. 5-5A). Next, the therapist moves the patient to the head-hanging position similar to the Dix-Hallpike test (Fig. 5-5B). The therapist should wait until the symptoms and nystagmus resolve plus an additional 30 seconds before moving to each subsequent position. The therapist turns the patient's head 90°, so the neck is positioned in 45° of right rotation (Fig. 5-5C). The therapist should ensure that the head stays down (or neck does not flex) during the movement. Next, the therapist rotates the patient's head 90° again, so the head is facing 45° down toward the floor. This position requires that the patient rolls into sidelying to the right as the therapist moves the patient's head (Fig. 5-5D). The patient is then moved to upright sitting on the side of the bed to end the maneuver. The head should remain rotated 45° to right as the patient comes up to sitting (Fig. 5-5E). Careful handling and guarding of the patient should be performed when coming to sitting, since patients may feel dizzy and lose balance at the end of the maneuver. Throughout the maneuver, the therapist should observe the patient's eyes; if nystagmus occurs, it should continue to be up-beating and left torsional in relationship to the orbit of the eyes whenever the patient has symptoms. A reversal of the direction of the nystagmus (*e.g.*, down-beating and right torsional) would indicate the otoconia moved the wrong direction within the SCC rather than moving through the SCC and out into the utricle. This would indicate a failed

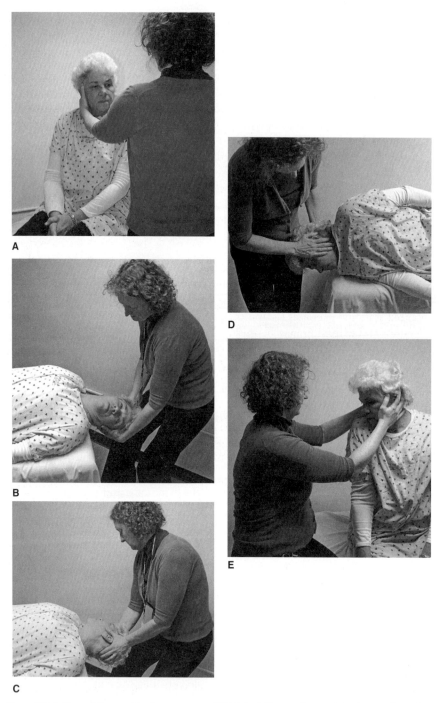

Figure 5-5. Left canalith repositioning maneuver (CRM) for left posterior semicircular canal canalithiasis. **A.** Start position: long sit with head rotated 45° to left. **B.** Supine with head extended 10° off end of surface. **C.** Supine with head 45° to right. **D.** Sidelying with head 45° toward ground. **E.** End position: sitting, maintain head position until full upright.

treatment and the maneuver should be stopped and repeated, starting from the initial position. If performed correctly, the maneuver can be completed within about 5 minutes, but the patient should be given several minutes to recover at the end of the maneuver before beginning any other mobility task.

Although BPPV may resolve spontaneously without intervention, symptoms may take months to resolve. In 72% of BPPV cases, a single CRM resolved symptoms within a day to a week.[15] Several systematic reviews have determined that the **CRM (also referred to as the modified Epley maneuver) is the treatment of choice for posterior canalithiasis.**[15,16,30,31] One meta-analysis calculated the odds ratio for resolution of symptoms and nystagmus using the CRM versus no treatment or sham to be 4.42 and 6.40, respectively.[30] Across several studies, the number needed to treat (NNT) to resolve BPPV with the CRM was calculated to be between 1.3 and 3.4.[16]

In the current patient case, the CRM for left posterior canalithiasis was performed following the initial examination that included the Dix-Hallpike test. The maneuver required two persons to complete to ensure the patient's lower extremities were positioned to maintain her hip precautions throughout the maneuver. This was accomplished by maintaining the hip abductor pillow between her lower extremities as she was rolled onto her right side. Resolution of her symptoms was a priority because her vertigo would likely have interfered with the exercise and mobility progression required for a timely discharge to home. Optimal improvement of her balance and ADL function would likely be limited by the coexistence of BPPV. Performing the CRM during her initial treatment session is important to provide the opportunity to reassess for resolution of the nystagmus in her continued physical therapy sessions before discharge. This will also help to determine if follow-up testing should be incorporated into her future plan of care. The incidence of BPPV is more likely in individuals who have had a previous episode of BPPV; however, the rate of having additional episodes or reoccurrences of BPPV may be decreased when treated less than 24 hours as compared to greater than 24 hours after onset.[32]

Following the CRM, the patient was provided with standard post-maneuver instructions which include: avoid sleeping or lying flat for the first 24 hours (which can be accomplished by elevating the head of the bed or using an extra pillow); avoid bending the head down to the floor when picking up objects; and, avoid extreme neck extension (no looking up to the ceiling). Twenty-four hours after the CRM, patients should not restrict head movements or positions, if symptoms have resolved. Following **post-maneuver restrictions** for 3 days after a CRM was once thought to improve success of the maneuver and prevent reoccurrence of BPPV. However, current evidence does not support the need for any restricting movements for any length of time after CRM.[16] In this patient's case, 24-hour restrictions were provided based on therapist preference, to decrease the patient's anxiety, and to promote engagement in functional mobility.

Ideally, following the CRM, the BPPV will be resolved so that she no longer experiences positional vertigo and nystagmus. Even if this patient has complete resolution of symptoms during this episode of care, it is important to educate her on how to recognize future occurrences because BPPV is known to reoccur.[32] As part of her plan of care, additional education about her positional vertigo should be provided to her and her husband. This education should include the nature and cause of BPPV, purpose of the CRM, likelihood of reoccurrences, and relationship of BPPV to balance and mobility deficits. She should also be provided with resources to seek services so any reoccurrences can be treated promptly and appropriately. Her history of BPPV should also be described to her providers at the next level of care.

Evidence-Based Clinical Recommendations

SORT: Strength of Recommendation Taxonomy

A: Consistent, good-quality patient-oriented evidence

B: Inconsistent or limited-quality patient-oriented evidence

C: Consensus, disease-oriented evidence, usual practice, expert opinion, or case series

1. The Dix-Hallpike test can be used to identify posterior canal BPPV. **Grade A**

2. The supine roll test is the preferred method to identify horizontal canal BPPV. **Grade B**

3. The canalith repositioning maneuver is the treatment of choice to reduce symptoms and nystagmus associated with posterior canalithiasis BPPV. **Grade A**

4. There is no difference in BPPV recurrence rates in individuals who follow post-CRM restrictions compared to those who do not follow post-CRM restrictions. **Grade B**

COMPREHENSION QUESTIONS

5.1 A patient in the hospital complains of positional dizziness following surgery. Prior to mobilizing the patient, the physical therapist completes testing for orthostatic hypotension. Which of the following represents a vital sign response consistent with orthostatic hypotension?

    A. Vital sign change from BP 130/70 and HR 100 to 120/80 and HR 120

    B. Vital sign change from BP 130/70 and HR 100 to 110/60 and HR 100

    C. Vital sign change from BP 130/70 and HR 100 to 130/80 and HR 120

    D. Vital sign change from BP 130/70 and HR 100 to 115/70 and HR 70

5.2 After ruling out other causes of dizziness, the therapist tests a patient for BPPV by completing the Dix-Hallpike test. In the end position of the right Dix-Hallpike test, the patient has right up-beating, torsional nystagmus that lasts less than 30 seconds. What is this patient's diagnosis?

    A. Right anterior canalithiasis

    B. Right posterior cupulolithiasis

    C. Right posterior canalithiasis

    D. Left posterior canalithiasis

ANSWERS

5.1 **B.** The diagnostic criteria for orthostatic hypotension is a decrease in systolic blood pressure of 20 mm Hg, or diastolic blood pressure decrease of 10 mm Hg, or an increase in heart rate of 30 beats per minute after a person changes from a supine to upright position. The other options (A, C, and D) do not present vital sign changes that meet the parameters defined for orthostatic hypotension.

5.2 **C.** The nystagmus described represents that for right posterior canalithiasis. Right anterior canalithiasis would be represented by right torsional, down-beating nystagmus with a duration of less than 1 minute (option A). Right posterior cupulolithiasis would be represented by right torsional, up-beating nystagmus lasting more than 1 minute (option B). Left posterior canalithiasis would be represented by left torsional, up-beating nystagmus lasting less than 1 minute (option D).

REFERENCES

1. Swanson EA, Schmalzried TP, Dorey FJ. Recommendations after total hip and knee arthroplasty: a survey of the American Association for Hip and Knee Surgeons. *J Arthroplasty*. 2009;24:120-126.

2. Vissers MM, Bussmann JB, Verhaar JAN, et al. Recovery of physical functioning after total hip arthroplasty: systematic review and meta-analysis of the literature. *Phys Ther*. 2011;91:615-629.

3. Maxey L, Magnusson J. *Rehabilitation for the Postsurgical Orthopedic Patient*. St. Louis, MO: Mosby, Inc.; 2001;172-187.

4. Palan J, Beard DJ, Murray DW, et al. Which approach for total hip arthroplasy: anterior or posterior? *Clin Orthop Relat Res*. 2009;467:473-477.

5. Pellicci PM, Potter HG, Foo LF, et al. MRI shows biologic restoration of posterior soft tissue repairs after THA. *Clin Orthop Relat Res*. 2009;467:940-945.

6. Crow JB, Gelfand B, Su EP. Use of joint mobilization in a patient with severely restricted hip motion following bilateral hip resurfacing arthroplasty. *Phys Ther*. 2008;88:1591-1600.

7. Freburger JK. An analysis of the relationship between the utilization of physical therapy services and outcomes of care for patients after total hip arthroplasty. *Phys Ther*. 2000;80:448-458.

8. Post RE, Dickerson LM. Dizziness: a diagnostic approach. *Am Fam Physician*. 2010;82:361-368.

9. Tarnutzer AA, Berkowitz AL, Robinson KA, et al. Does my dizzy patient have a stroke? A systematic review of bedside diagnosis in acute vestibular syndrome. *CMAJ*. 2011;183:1025-1032.

10. Luukinen H, Koski K, Laippala P, et al. Prognosis of diastolic and systolic orthostatic hypotension in older persons. *Arch Intern Med*. 1999;159:273-280.

11. Herdman SJ, Tusa RJ. Physical therapy management of benign positional vertigo. In: Herdman SJ, ed. *Vestibular Rehabilitation*. 3rd ed. Philadelphia, PA: F.A. Davis; 2007: 235.

12. von Brevern M, Radtke A, Lezius F, et al. Epidemiology of benign paroxysmal positional vertigo: a population based study. *J Neurol Neurosurg Psychiatry*. 2007;78:710-715.

13. Oghalai JS, Manolidis S, Barth JL, et al. Unrecognized benign paroxysmal in elderly patients. *Otolaryngol Head Neck Surg*. 2000;122:630-634.

14. Honrubia V, Baloh RW, Harris MR, et al. Paroxysmal positional vertigo syndrome. *Am J Otol* 1999;20:465-470.

15. White J, Savvides P, Cherian, N, et al. Canalith repositioning for benign paroxysmal positional vertigo. *Oto Neurotol*. 2005;26:704-710.

16. Bhattacharyya N, Baugh RF, Orvidas L, et al. Clinical practice guideline: benign paroxysmal positional vertigo. *Otolaryng Head Neck Surg.* 2008;139:S47-S81.

17. Al Felasi M, Pierre G, Mondain M, et al. Perilymphatic fistula of the round window. *Euro Annals Otorhinolaryngol Head Neck Dis.* 2011;128:139-141.

18. Minor LB, Solomon D, Zinreich JS, et al. Sound and/or pressure-induced vertigo due to dehiscence of the superior semicircular canal. *Arch Otolaryngol Head Neck Surg.* 1998;124:249-258.

19. Polensek SH, Tusa RJ. Nystagmus during attacks of vestibular migraine: an aid in diagnosis. *Audio Neurootol.* 2010;15:241-246.

20. Tusa JT. Differential diagnosis mimicking BPPV (Appendix 17A). In: Herdman SJ, ed. *Vestibular Rehabilitation.* 3rd ed. Philadelphia, PA: F.A. Davis; 2007.

21. Strupp M, Brandt T. Vestibular neuritis. *Semin Neurol.* 2009;29:509-519.

22. Schubert MC, Minor LB. Vestibulo-ocular physiology underlying vestibular hypofunction. *Phys Ther.* 2004;84:373-385.

23. Mandalà M, Santoro GP, Awrey J, et al. Vestibular neuritis: recurrence and incidence of secondary benign paroxysmal positional vertigo. *Acta Otolaryngol.* 2010;130:565-567.

24. Reiter RJ, Tan DX, Korkmaz A, et al. Drug-mediated ototoxicity and tinnitus: alleviation with melatonin. *J Physiol Pharmacol.* 2011;62:151-157.

25. Goodman CC, Fuller KS. *Pathology: Implications for the Physical Therapist.* 3rd ed. Philadelphia, PA: Saunders; 2009:1650.

26. Schubert MC. Tusa RJ, Grine LE, et al. Optimizing the sensitivity of the head thrust test for identifying vestibular hypofunction. *Phys Ther.* 2004;84:151-158.

27. Kerber KA, Ishiyama GA, Baloh RW. A longitudinal study of oculomotor function in normal older people. *Neurobio Aging.* 2006;27:1346-1353.

28. Humphriss RL, Baguley DM, Sparkes V, et al. Contraindications to the Dix-Hallpike manoeuvre: a multidisciplinary review. *Int J Audiol.* 2003;42:166-173.

29. U.S. Department of Health and Human Services, Agency for Healthcare Research and Quality. Available at: http://hcupnet.ahrq.gov/HCUPnet.jsp. Accessed January 27, 2012.

30. Hilton MP, Pinder D. The Epley (canalith repositioning) maneuver for benign paroxysmal positional vertigo. *Cochrane Database Syst Rev.* 2002; CD003162.

31. Helminski JO, Zee DS, Janssen I, et al. Effectiveness of particle repositioning maneuvers in the treatment of benign paroxysmal positional vertigo: a systematic review. *Phys Ther.* 2010;90:663-678.

32. Do YK, Kim J, Park DY, et al. The effect of early canalith repositioning on benign paroxysmal positional vertigo on recurrence. *Clin Exp Otorhinolaryngol.* 2011;4:113-117.

Total Knee Arthroplasty

Alisa L. Curry

CASE 6

A 69-year-old female presents to her orthopaedic surgeon's office with pain and swelling in her left knee. She has been experiencing pain on the medial side for the past 2 years; however, she has been independent in all activities of daily living (ADLs) and has been able to exercise regularly until the last 3 months. Her primary complaint was pain with descending stairs. Visual examination showed overall effusion and palpable warmth with greater valgus deformity of the left knee than the right. Passive range of motion of the left knee was 5° to 125° with pain in the last 10° of flexion. X-rays showed tricompartmental arthritis with approximation of the medial femoral condyle and tibial plateau on the anteroposterior view. Merchant view showed a loss of joint space with lateral shift of the patella out of the patellar groove. Her relevant medical history includes: hypertension, hiatal hernia, and non-insulin–dependent diabetes mellitus. Surgical history includes two previous left knee arthroscopies (5 and 20 years ago) and hysterectomy 12 years ago. Daily preoperative medications are pantoprazole (Protonix), valsartan/hydrochlorothiazide (Diovan HCT), and ibuprofen (two to four 200 mg tablets, as needed). The patient has been retired for 4 years and maintained an active lifestyle. Prior to this recent 3-month onset of increased knee pain, she played golf, exercised regularly at a gym, and participated in a variety of volunteer activities 5 days per week. After discussion of the x-ray findings with the orthopaedic surgeon, she was scheduled for a total knee arthroplasty (TKA). The patient received educational materials regarding the surgery and the predicted hospital course. She also attended a preoperative education class prior to surgery. The patient is a widow and lives alone; however, she has two adult children living nearby who will be able to assist her after hospital discharge. She was admitted to the hospital and had a left TKA with no complications. According to the ordered TKA protocol, physical therapy is ordered to begin postoperative day 1 (POD 1).

► What are the most appropriate physical therapy outcome measures for gait and balance?
► What are the most appropriate physical therapy interventions?

▶ What are the possible complications that may limit the effectiveness of physical therapy?

▶ Identify referrals to other medical team members.

KEY DEFINITIONS

RAPID RECOVERY PROTOCOLS: Protocols or clinical pathways designed to decrease length of stay and accelerate patient recovery postoperatively; typically include a combination of preoperative education materials, surgical technique, multimodal pain management, and focused rehabilitation interventions

TOTAL KNEE ARTHROPLASTY (TKA): Resurfacing of the articulating surfaces of the knee joint; comprised of four components including a distal femoral component, tibial plateau tray, patellar button, and polyethylene liner

VENOUS THROMBOSIS: Development of a blood clot in a vein

Objectives

1. Define osteoarthritis (OA) and its pharmacologic management.
2. Understand the indications for TKA.
3. List the complications of immobility.
4. Describe rapid recovery protocols for TKA.
5. Describe the Modified Bromage scale to measure motor function of the lower extremities in a patient with epidural or continuous femoral nerve blockade.
6. Describe the normal phases of the healing process and how they influence rehabilitation of the individual post-TKA.

Physical Therapy Considerations

PT considerations during management of the individual status/post TKA:

▶ **General physical therapy plan of care/goals:** Increase range of motion (ROM), control edema, visually inspect and monitor wound; maximize functional independence and safety; improve quality of life, establish home exercise program

▶ **Physical therapy interventions:** Patient and caregiver education regarding expected progression of healing, decreasing risk of deep vein thromboses, and risk of falls; gait training; caregiver training for safe guarding during ambulation; prescription of a home exercise program; referral to home health or outpatient physical therapy

▶ **Precautions during physical therapy:** Wound precautions; close physical supervision to decrease risk of falls; consistent monitoring of vital signs, especially blood pressure (BP); recognize adverse drug reactions (ADRs) of pain medications and make appropriate changes to interventions, as needed

▶ **Complications interfering with physical therapy:** Uncontrolled pain, deep vein thromboses, pulmonary embolism, falls, wound healing

Understanding the Health Condition

Osteoarthritis, the primary type of arthritis causing the "wear and tear" of joint surfaces, develops in many adults over the age of 45 years and its progression is affected by age, obesity, injury, overuse, genetics, and/or muscle weakness.[1] Conservative treatment (*i.e.*, nonsurgical) is often attempted before making the decision to proceed with surgical intervention. Pharmacologic management includes oral non-opioid and opioid medications for pain and nonsteroidal anti-inflammatory medications for pain and inflammation. Some medications are injected intra-articularly, which decreases the likelihood of systemic ADRs. These include glucocorticoids to reduce swelling, hyaluronan (a glycosaminoglycan) to lubricate the joint, and opioids to reduce joint pain. Additional conservative treatment of OA includes physical therapy, activity modification, and weight management.[2] Surgeons may initially perform less invasive surgical options, such as arthroscopy, to address knee OA and to remove degenerative or loose cartilage that interferes with joint kinematics. These interventions can relieve pain and improve joint motion and alignment. A TKA is designed to replace the lost articular cartilage on the weightbearing and approximating surfaces with nonorganic materials. Femoral and tibial components are often made of cobalt chrome metal and the patella is resurfaced with a button of polyethylene plastic. The primary indication for a TKA is loss of knee articular cartilage, decreased ROM, decreased joint function, and pain that is no longer tolerable and is associated with a decrease in functional abilities. The incidence of TKA procedures is expected to continue rising in years to come. Kurtz et al.[3] have predicted that by 2030 in the United States "the demand for primary total hip arthroplasties is estimated to grow by 174% to 572,000. The demand for primary total knee arthroplasties is projected to grow by 673% to 3.48 million procedures."

Osteoarthritis can change the alignment of joint surfaces. In some cases, there can be a greater degree of wear on the medial or lateral compartments of the joint, causing valgus or varus deformities, respectively. Prolonging surgery can contribute to overstretching of the medial or lateral collateral ligaments that stabilize the knee, as well as the posterior capsule of the knee joint. While knee joint deformity can occur without painful arthritis, patients may wait to seek surgical intervention until pain is intolerable. Surgeons may elect to use other knee joint realignment or resurfacing techniques, such as tibial osteotomy or unicompartmental knee arthroplasty. These surgical techniques have specific indications.[4,5] By directly addressing the cartilage wear on a specific weightbearing surface of the joint, these surgical techniques can provide temporary or long-term pain relief. However, patients may still continue to have progressive degeneration of the remaining articular cartilage, which can lead to the need for a TKA. When radiological evidence demonstrates articular cartilage degradation, bone approximation and joint deformity, joint realignment or resurfacing techniques will inevitably cease to provide long-term relief.

Prior to the surgical procedure, the surgeon selects the appropriate component sizes using preoperative radiographic templates. Templating can be performed manually or with computer assistance. The surgical procedure consists of a variety of cutting jigs and alignment rods to determine proper alignment and placement of the components. Surgical approaches involve dissection of the medial aspect of the knee via medial parapatellar, subvastus, midvastus, or quadriceps-sparing techniques.[6] Each technique has advantages and disadvantages and the surgeon chooses a technique based on preference for exposure.[4,7,8] The particular surgical approach impacts the rate of recovery of knee function. The extent of the dissection around the patella and the vastus medialis oblique during surgery can lead to inhibition of the quadriceps and impact knee control during gait training activities in rehabilitation.[9] A minimally invasive TKA is defined as a procedure with a smaller incision, averaging 4 to 6 in, compared to the traditional incision of 8 to 10 in. The quadriceps-sparing technique involves less extensive surgical dissection, use of smaller instrumentation, and lack of patellar eversion.[10] Weinrauch et al.[7] noted that both the subvastus and midvastus surgical approaches in minimally invasive TKAs were associated with excellent short-term clinical results. The average lifespan of the TKA in the United States has been determined to be greater than 20 years.[11] Factors that can decrease the lifespan of the TKA include[12]: the patient, surgical technique, knee kinematics, perioperative or postoperative complications, and the quality or lack of postoperative physical therapy.

While there are numerous studies assessing management of patients with a TKA in inpatient rehabilitation settings, skilled nursing facilities, and outpatient rehabilitation settings, few articles exist on physical therapy rehabilitation in the acute care hospital. In a 2003 review of rehabilitation after joint surgery, Roos[13] concluded that early mobilization was the gold standard for achieving functional mobility after arthroplasty. Physical therapy for any patient in the acute care setting helps to prevent complications associated with immobility (e.g., deep vein thrombosis, pulmonary embolism, loss of joint mobility, skin breakdown). These potential complications are compounded in the patient with a TKA due to pain management and immobility induced by postsurgical lower extremity surgery. After orthopaedic surgery, a multidisciplinary approach focused on multimodal pain control and mobilization is beneficial. Without a coordinated plan of action, disjointed treatment of this patient may result in a prolonged length of stay (LOS) in the acute care setting. According to the Agency for Healthcare Research and Quality's 2009 results, the average hospital length of stay for individuals with TKA was 3.0 days.[14] For those patients moving to a secondary level of care (e.g., skilled nursing facility) from the hospital, this timeframe correlates with Medicare requirements for a 3-day hospital qualifying stay. A patient who demonstrates near independent or independent ability to transfer, safe ambulation with proper assistive device, and the ability to move the operative knee in flexion and extension can be deemed safe enough to return home within this timeframe.

Physical Therapy Patient/Client Management

The physical therapist can participate as part of the multidisciplinary team to educate the patient before the patient is admitted to the hospital. This surgery is elective; therefore, it is possible to anticipate predictable outcomes. The **provision**

of preoperative patient education has been questioned regarding its benefits. A 2003 Cochrane Review of nine randomized controlled trials found little evidence that preoperative education decreases pain, improves function, or decreases length of acute hospital stay. However, presurgery education may decrease anxiety and improve recovery in patients with limited social support or who have significantly limited mobility prior to surgery.[15] More recent evidence has shown that education provided prior to TKA surgery was associated with decreased number of falls in the hospital.[16] Once the TKA is completed, the therapist's training and professional judgment determine how the patient functionally progresses. The rehabilitation focus is on increasing knee ROM, ambulation, and functional mobility and helping to provide and maintain adequate pain control.

In the last 10 years, there has been increased attention focused on determining the best practice in caring for the postsurgical TKA population. Studies have examined daily versus twice-daily physical therapy treatments, use of the continuous passive motion (CPM) machine, group exercise classes, and discharge disposition. Many inpatient acute care programs have shifted toward the development of clinical pathways and "rapid recovery protocols" to give patients a designated course of treatment. This has helped to streamline all aspects of treatment from the operating room to the unit-based care. While the term "rapid recovery protocol" has not been specifically defined in the literature, many clinicians describe the combination of preoperative education, multimodal pain management, surgical technique, and aggressive, focused rehabilitation as essential components to a successful program.[17] A 2008 review evaluating five studies indicated that rapid recovery protocols are correlated with decreased length of stay, better active and passive knee ROM at discharge, decreased need to send patients to secondary levels of care (e.g., skilled nursing facilities), and higher patient satisfaction scores.[18-20] Currently, there is inconsistent evidence to determine what should be the recommended frequency of physical therapy treatments during the hospital stay. The National Institutes of Health Consensus statement supports the need for further research into the most effective frequency.[21] In the physical therapy community, researchers have compared a once per day (QD) versus twice daily (BID) physical therapy intervention model. Lawson[22] (2009) found that BID physical therapy sessions resulted in decreased LOS and better functional outcomes, whereas QD physical therapy sessions resulted in less pain and increased knee ROM. An interesting point regarding the comparison between QD and BID physical therapy sessions is that the *average* time of treatment and *total* number of treatments was comparable between the two groups (i.e., the amount of time required to achieve the goals). Thus, the controversy regarding the ideal treatment schedule for this population remains unanswered. Therapists need to consider what is in the best interests of their patients. It is important to recognize that patients want outcomes that will enable them to resume their previously active lifestyles because individuals are now having total knee arthroplasties before qualifying for Medicare (i.e., less than 65 years old). The number of "baby boomers" (people born between 1943 and 1960) reaching the age to qualify for Medicare benefits is increasing and this population is living longer and becoming and staying increasingly active. The challenge is to help this population regain function and return to an active lifestyle in the fastest manner possible. The American Association of

Orthopaedic Surgeons has published guidelines for the activities recommended and not recommended following total joint replacement surgery.[23] Therapists should familiarize themselves and their patients with these recommendations to allow optimal return to an active, healthy lifestyle after a TKA.

Examination, Evaluation, and Diagnosis

The initial chart review of the patient's medical history, lab values, medications, postoperative precautions, and activity restrictions gives the therapist guidelines to follow when initiating the examination. In the acute care environment, the physical therapist must be familiar with these values in order to physically challenge patients safely. Pertinent lab values to review for any patient after surgery include hematocrit and hemoglobin (H&H), prothrombin time/international normalized ratio (PT/INR), and platelets. Patients with a hemoglobin value below 8 g/dL may experience dizziness and decreased endurance, which can increase the fall risk. Patients with an INR value above 3.0 may be at an increased risk for bleeding. In this case, aggressive physical therapy could cause increased bleeding into the replaced knee; in addition, a fall could prompt uncontrolled bleeding, including intracranial, if the fall was serious enough. The INR and potential for increased risk of bleeding can be affected by anticoagulation medications, which are commonly used to prevent development of blood clots postoperatively. Management of swelling and pain are important in the immediate recovery process, as these can be roadblocks to achieving therapy goals. The therapist must monitor the patient's edema, incision healing, and be aware of the possibility of a deep vein thrombosis (DVT). Symptoms of a DVT can mimic typical postoperative complaints after a total joint arthroplasty—pain, swelling, and joint stiffness. The gold standard for diagnosis of DVT is venography or Doppler ultrasound.[24] However, the physical therapist can use Wells Clinical Prediction Rule for DVT.[25] The likelihood of a patient having a DVT can be predicted by the total score based on the clinical criteria that were outlined in Case 4 (Table 4-3). A patient scoring ≥3 points is at high risk (75%); 1 to 2 points at moderate risk (17%), and <1 point at low risk (3%). All patients having lower extremity joint arthroplasty are at least at a moderate risk for DVT.[26,27]

A multimodal approach to pain control is recommended for this patient population. Beginning with intraoperative anesthesia, the options for pain management include spinal anesthesia, analgesics, and/or anesthetics administered via epidural catheter, and single injection or continuous peripheral nerve blocks. Peripheral nerve blocks have been shown to more effectively control pain for the patient status/post total joint replacement; however, these nerve blocks can impact leg function during rehabilitation.[28] Peripheral nerve blocks involve using an anesthetic such as ropivacaine to interrupt action potentials in the sensory nerve pathway. Blockade of the femoral nerve provides sensory and motor anesthesia to the anterior thigh, knee, and medial aspect of the calf, ankle, and foot. As the epidural analgesia or continuous femoral nerve block medications are decreased during the first postsurgical days, oral medications are integrated into the pain management. The use of short- and long-acting oral opioids and selective COX-2 inhibitors (*e.g.*, Celebrex) are used to replace the need for intravenous opiates.[29,30] Although there remains some concern regarding the possibility of opiate addiction when patients are using multiple opioid medications, a 2009 Cochrane Review concluded that the use of opiates in patients with no history of substance addiction or abuse is effective for long-term pain relief for some patients with a very small (though not zero) risk of developing addiction, abuse, or other serious adverse effects.[31] Many patients express a desire to discontinue oral opiates too quickly (particularly after hospital discharge), which may slow the rehabilitation process due to intolerance to postoperative exercise. Medications should be utilized as a tool to tolerate initial physical therapy and are tapered by the multidisciplinary team (and/or by the patient) as knee ROM and functional goals are reached.

The physical therapist must take care to monitor muscle control in the legs when beginning to mobilize the patient. Epidural or femoral nerve blockades decrease sensation and motor control to the quadriceps muscle, thereby decreasing the patient's ability to use that limb functionally. The patient may not appreciate the lack of control she has over her operative leg. If she attempts to stand and the quadriceps are not completely contracting, she is at high risk for a fall. A fall could result in a partial or complete dehiscence of the incision and/or disruption of the capsular repair or the quadriceps tendon, either of which could lead to another surgical intervention. For patients with an epidural or continuous femoral blockade, the physical therapist can use the **Modified Bromage Scale** (developed by Breen from the original Bromage scale) to determine the degree of motor function of the lower extremities.[32] The original Bromage scale is the most frequently used measure of motor blockade and has been used for labor anesthesia for years. The physical therapist can use the Modified Bromage Scale to predict the degree of anesthetic motor blockade based on the patient's ability to move her lower extremities in designated ways.[33] The Modified Bromage Scale is a scale from 1 to 6. A score of "1" indicates complete block with the patient unable to move feet or knees. A score of "2" indicates almost complete motor block in which the patient can only move the feet. A score of "3" indicates that the patient is just able to move the knees. A score of "4" indicates that the patient is able to fully flex the knees, but has detectable hip flexion weakness. A score of "5" indicates no hip flexion weakness when tested in the supine position. Finally, a score of "6" indicates that the patient is able to perform a partial knee bend. By using this scale, the multidisciplinary team can comparably rate the quality of lower extremity motion. The physical therapist can use the scoring to assist in determining the patient's fall risk and when the patient would be safe to begin assisted sit to stand transfers and begin taking steps.

Once the epidural or peripheral nerve anesthetic is discontinued, manual muscle testing and other standardized tools can be integrated into assessments of function. With each treatment session, therapy goals should be re-assessed and revised, if necessary, to maximize the patient's functional ability, ambulation distance, and pain management through various modalities. The more commonly used standardized measures and tests for patients with TKA include, but are not limited to: Timed Up and Go,[34] Tinetti Performance-Oriented Scale (POMA),[35] Berg Balance Scale, goniometry,[36] Western Ontario and McMaster Universities Osteoarthritis Index

(WOMAC),[37] pain Visual Analog Scale,[38] Short Form (SF)-12,[39] or SF-36,[40] and the Functional Independence Measure (FIM).[40] All of the above tests can provide subjective and objective data regarding patient outcomes and support the clinical decision-making process for safe discharge to home. Kennedy et al.[41] reported a higher slope of recovery in self-reported outcomes and physical functioning in the initial recovery phase for patients with total knee replacements compared to those with total hip replacements.

Plan of Care and Interventions

The therapist prepares the patient for her home environment and obstacles and introduces the home exercise program. Interviewing the patient and anyone who will be helping the patient after discharge helps the therapist establish a goal-specific plan of care based on concerns regarding the home environment. Common exercises utilized after a TKA include knee flexion and extension, hip abduction and adduction, ankle plantarflexion and dorsiflexion, and reinforcement of the normal gait sequence. The exercises can also be integrated into a group exercise class. This method provides patients with the opportunity to begin practicing their home exercise program, perform exercises in the hospital environment with feedback from the physical therapist, and observe other patients' techniques to improve knee ROM. Group classes can also provide motivation and encouragement. A 2007 study with adults with chronic low back pain found higher adherence to active group exercise than to individual manual techniques; this study may provide insight into continued compliance with a home exercise program.[42] Patients can review the home exercise program with each session, perform the exercises under the therapist's guidance and see how other patients perform, which may improve their own techniques. There is no consensus on precise knee ROM goals prior to discharge from acute care. However, the physical therapist must be aware of the knee ROM required to participate in various functional activities (Table 6-1).[43] Goals should be set to help the patient achieve the ROM necessary to perform the activities she needs to do.

	Standing Erect	Descending Stairs (flexed leg)	Descending Stairs (lead leg)	Tying Shoe	Squatting with Back Straight	Bathtub Use	Normal Gait as Leg Advances Forward
ROM	0° extension	86°-107° flexion	0° extension	106° flexion	117° flexion	135° flexion	0° extension

Table 6-1 FUNCTIONAL KNEE RANGE OF MOTION REQUIREMENTS FOR ACTIVITIES OF DAILY LIVING

Reproduced with permission from Kolber MJ, Brueilly KE. Arthofibrosis following total knee arthroplasty: Considerations for the acute care physical therapist. Acute Care Perspectives. 2006;15:11-16.

Whether or not to use **continuous passive motion (CPM) machines in postoperative rehabilitation after TKA** is another long-standing debate in the physical therapy community. Surgeons may prescribe the use of a CPM machine as an adjunct or substitution for physical therapy intervention within the hospital and/or after hospitalization. There is strong evidence from a Cochrane Review[44] and a randomized controlled trial by Denis et al.[45] that while CPM machines increased passive and active knee flexion when used in conjunction with a standardized TKA rehabilitation protocol, these effects were too small to be clinically worthwhile and had no effect on length of stay in the hospital.

With progression in ambulation distance, activity tolerance, and pain management, the team makes decisions regarding the patient's readiness to discharge from the hospital. Patients may be discharged to an inpatient acute rehabilitation center or skilled nursing facility to ensure that they continue to receive physical therapy services. Recent research suggests that discharge directly to home from the hospital after total joint arthroplasty correlates with decreased readmission rates to the hospital.[46] The primary benefits of discharge to home include decreased infection risk and discharge to a familiar environment, which allows the patient to return to normal eating and resting habits. The three phases of healing—inflammatory, regeneration, and remodeling—take place after a TKA and can be used by the physical therapist to guide activity progression.[47] During the inflammatory phase (up to 72 hours postsurgery), modalities, medications, and mobilization are important. In the regenerative phase (3 to 6 weeks postsurgery), patients have loose scar tissue (Type I collagen fibers that are not entirely cross-linked) and increased knee ROM is still attainable. Over weeks to months postsurgery, highly vascularized granulation tissue develops. Collagen fibers remain mobile enough to manipulate until 6 to 8 weeks after surgery. After this time, the collagen fibers mature to the point that attempts to manipulate any scar adhesions could potentially damage healthy soft tissues, such as muscle, tendon, or ligament. Based on this expected healing timeline, the therapist should encourage the patient to attain maximum ROM and flexibility in the first 6 to 8 weeks after surgery. After 6 weeks, it is nearly impossible for patients to independently alter scar tissue. At this point, if the existing ROM is not functional, the patient may need manipulation under anesthesia. Active use of the surgical leg should be encouraged with all activities. Research supports closed chain activities, such as occurs during functional transfers, to facilitate knee flexion and extension. Management of this patient's non-insulin dependent diabetes mellitus is also a concern postoperatively because sustained increases in glucose levels can impact wound healing. The stressors associated with pain and rehabilitation after a TKA promote hyperglycemia and insulin suppression.[48] This secondary problem can have a deleterious effect during the rehabilitation process, especially on wound healing. Possible complications of poor glycemic control include increased risk of infection,[49] morbidity and mortality, and length of stay.[50] Close monitoring of blood glucose, good dietary control, and possible short-term use of anti-diabetic medications can ensure that the patient weathers the storm of surgical stress to the body. Early discharge to home can help the patient to re-establish normalcy in diet and sleep patterns, which also helps the healing process.

Evidence-Based Clinical Recommendations

SORT: Strength of Recommendation Taxonomy

A: Consistent, good-quality patient-oriented evidence

B: Inconsistent or limited-quality patient-oriented evidence

C: Consensus, disease-oriented evidence, usual practice, expert opinion, or case series

1. Education provided prior to total knee arthroplasty is beneficial for patients with anxiety, those with limited social support, and/or those who have significantly limited mobility. **Grade B**

2. In patients with peripheral nerve blockades, physical therapists can use the Modified Bromage Scale to predict the degree of lower extremity anesthetic motor blockade and the level of assistance that may be needed to perform functional activities and gait. **Grade B**

3. The addition of CPM machines to standard rehabilitation protocols after a TKA does not affect hospital length of stay and any increased knee ROM that is attained is not clinically significant. **Grade A**

COMPREHENSION QUESTIONS

6.1 A patient asks if she can return to the swimming pool 5 weeks after her TKA. Which is the *most* appropriate answer?

　　A. The wound closure is not complete and immersion in a swimming pool will increase the chance of infection.

　　B. Swimming is a viable option to increase flexibility due to thermal effects of the water; it can begin after the wound closure is complete, which is usually three to four weeks postoperatively.

　　C. Swimming does not promote full flexion of the knee joint.

　　D. The patient will very likely still be in the hospital 5 weeks after a TKA.

6.2 Which of the following is *not* a component of a rapid recovery protocol for TKA?

　　A. Surgical techniques of the orthopaedic surgeon

　　B. Age and sex of the patient

　　C. Preoperative education and multimodal pain management

　　D. Physical therapy beginning on POD 1

6.3 A patient with a continuous femoral nerve blockade has a score of 2 on the Modified Bromage Scale. What does this score *most* accurately indicate?

A. Possibility of compromised motor control of the femoral nerve; moderate fall risk

B. Complete femoral nerve return; minimal fall risk

C. Complete femoral nerve block; severe fall risk

D. The Modified Bromage Scale cannot be used for patients with continuous femoral nerve blockades.

ANSWERS

6.1 **B.** The wound should be closed by 5 weeks status/post TKA (option A). The buoyancy and thermal effects of water can promote increased knee ROM with decreased pain. The average length of stay after TKA in the United States is only 3 to 4 days. (option D).

6.2 **B.** Age and sex of the patient are not considered components of TKA rapid recovery protocols.

6.3 **A.** The Modified Bromage Scale has a grading system of 1 to 6 and it is used to predict the degree of anesthetic motor blockade based on the patient's ability to move the lower extremities in designated ways. A score of 2 indicates that the patient is only able to move her foot on the affected side, thus she would present a moderate fall risk. Complete femoral nerve return would reflect the highest score of 6 (option B). Complete femoral nerve block would indicate that the patient could not move her foot or knee, and would therefore be a severe fall risk (option C).

REFERENCES

1. Arthritis Foundation. Who Gets Osteoarthritis? 2012. Available at: http://www.arthritis.org/who-gets-osteoarthritis.php. Accessed May 17, 2012.
2. Walker-Bone K, Javaid K, Arden N, et al. Medical management of osteoarthritis. BMJ. 2000;321: 936-940.
3. Kurtz S, Ong K, Lau E, et al. Projections of primary and revision hip and knee arthroplasty in the United States from 2005 to 2030. J Bone Joint Surg Am. 2007;89:780-785.
4. Bonutti PM, Zywiel MG, Ulrich SD, et al. A comparison of subvastus and midvastus approaches in minimally invasive total knee arthroplasty. J Bone Joint Surg Am. 2010; 92:575-582.
5. Dalury DF, Mulliken BD, Adams MJ, et al. Early recovery after total knee arthroplasty performed with and without patellar eversion and tibial translation: a prospective randomized study. J Bone Joint Surg Am. 2009;91:1339-1343.
6. Brander V, Stulberg SD. Rehabilitation after hip- and knee-joint replacement: an experience- and evidence-based approach to care. Am J Phys Med Rehabil. 2006;85:S98-S118.
7. Weinrauch P, Myers N, Wilkinson M, et al. Comparison of early postoperative rehabilitation outcome following total knee arthroplasty using different surgical approaches and instrumentation. J Orthop Surg. 2006;14:47-52.

8. Jung YB, Lee YS, Lee EY, et al. Comparison of the modified subvastus and medial parapatellar approaches in total knee arthroplasty. *Int Orthop.* 2009;33:419-423.

9. Scuderi GR, Tenholder M, Capeci C. Surgical approaches in mini-incision total knee arthroplasty. *Clin Orthop Relat Res.* 2004;428:61-67.

10. American Academy of Orthopedics Surgeons Website. Minimally Invasive Total Knee Arthroplasty. 2007. Available at: http://orthoinfo.aaos.org/topic.cfm?topic=a00405. Accessed May 17, 2012.

11. Rodriguez JA, Bhende H, Ranawat CS. Total condylar knee replacement: a 20-year follow up study. *Clin Orthop Relat Res.* 2001; 388:10-17.

12. Dennis DA, Komistek RD, Scuderi GR, et al. Factors affecting flexion after total knee arthroplasty. *Clin Orthop Relat Res.* 2007;464:53-60.

13. Roos EM. Effectiveness and practice variation of rehabilitation after joint replacement. *Cur Opin Rheumatol.* 2003;15:160-162.

14. Agency for Healthcare Research and Quality. National and regional estimates on hospital use for all patients from the HCUP Nationwide Inpatient Sample (NIS)—2009 Data. Available at: http://hcupnet.ahrq.gov/HCUPnet.jsp. Accessed May 17, 2012.

15. McDonald S, Hetrick SE, Green S. Pre-operative education for hip or knee replacement. *Cochrane Database of Syst Rev.* 2004;1:CD003526.

16. Clarke HD, Timm VL, Goldberg BR, et al. Preoperative patient education reduces in-hospital falls after total knee arthroplasty *Clin Orthop Relat Res.* 2012;470:244-249.

17. Breusch SJ, Malchau H, eds. *The well-cemented total hip arthroplasty: theory and practice.* Heidelberg, Germany: Springer; 2005.

18. Khan F, Ng L, Gonzalez S, et al. Multidisciplinary rehabilitation programmes following joint replacement at the hip and knee in chronic arthropathy. *Cochrane Database Syst Rev.* 2008;2:CD004957.

19. Husni ME, Losina E, Fossel AH, et al. Decreasing medical complications for total knee arthroplasty: effect of critical pathways on outcomes. *BMC Musculoskeletal Disorders.* 2010;11:160.

20. Cook JR, Warren M, Ganley KJ, et al. A comprehensive joint replacement program for total knee arthroplasty: a descriptive study. *BMC Musculoskeletal Disord.* 2008;9:154.

21. NIH Consensus Statement on total knee replacement. *NIH Consens State Sci Statements.* 2003; 20:1-34.

22. Lawson D. Comparing outcomes of patients following total knee replacement: does frequency of physical therapy treatment affect outcomes in the acute care setting? A case study. *Acute Care Perspectives.* 2009. Available at: http://www.thefreelibrary.com/. Accessed May 17, 2012.

23. Healy WL, Sharma S, Schwartz B, et al. Athletic activity after total joint arthroplasty. *J Bone Joint Surg Am.* 2008;90:2245-2252.

24. Ramzi DW, Leeper KV. DVT and pulmonary embolism: Part I. Diagnosis. *Am Fam Physician.* 2004;69: 2829-2836.

25. Wells PS, Anderson DR, Rodger M, et al. Derivation of a simple clinical model to categorize patients probability of pulmonary embolism: increasing the models utility with the SimpliRED D-dimer. *Thromb Haemost.* 2000;83:416-420.

26. Geerts WH, Heit JA, Clagett GP, et al. Prevention of venous thromboembolism. *Chest.* 2001;119:132S-175S.

27. Agnelli G. Prevention of venous thromboembolism in surgical patients. *Circulation.* 2004;110:IV4-IV12.

28. Gandhi K, Viscusi ER. Multimodal pain management techniques in hip and knee arthroplasty. *J New York School of Regional Anesthesia.* 2009;13:1-10.

29. Duellman TJ, Gaffigan C, Milbrandt JC, et al. Multi-modal, pre-emptive analgesia decreases the length of hospital stay following total joint arthroplasty. *Orthopedics.* 2009; 32:167.

30. Maheshwari AV, Blum YC, Shekhar L, et al. Multimodal pain management after total hip and knee arthroplasty at the Ranawat Orthopaedic Center. *Clin Orthop Relat Res.* 2009;467:1418-1423.

31. Noble M, Treadwell JR, Tregear SJ, et al. Long-term opioid management for chronic noncancer pain. *Cochrane Database Syst Rev.* 2010;1:CD006605.

32. Bromage PR. *Epidural Analgesia.* Philadelphia, PA: WB Saunders; 1978: 144.

33. Breen TW, Shapiro T, Glass B, et al. Epidural anesthesia for labor in an ambulatory patient. *Anesth Analg.* 1993;77:919-924.

34. Podsiadlo D, Richardson S. The timed "Up & Go": a test of basic functional mobility for frail elderly persons. *J Am Geriatr Soc.* 1991;39:142-148.

35. Raiche M, Herbert R, Prince F, et al. Screening older adults at risk of falling with the Tinetti balance scale. *Lancet.* 2000;356:1001-1002.

36. Watkins MA, Riddle DL, Lamb RL, et al. Reliability of goniometric measurements and visual estimates of knee range of motion obtained in a clinical setting. *Phys Ther.* 1991;71:90-97.

37. Bombardier C, Melfi CA, Paul J, et al. Comparison of a generic and a disease-specific measure of pain and physical function after knee replacement surgery. *Med Care.* 1995;33:AS131-AS144.

38. Bergh I, Sjostrom B, Oden A, et al. An application of pain rating scales in geriatric patients. *Aging.* 2000;12:380-387.

39. Ware JJR, Kosinski M, Keller SD. A 12-item short-form health survey: construction of scales and preliminary tests of reliability and validity. *Med Care.* 1996;34:220-233.

40. Stineman MG, Shea JA, Jette A, et al. The functional independence measure: tests of scaling assumptions, structure, and reliability across 20 diverse impairment categories. *Arch Phys Med Rehabil.* 1996;77:1101-1108.

41. Kennedy DM, Stratford PW, Hanna SE, et al. Modeling early recovery of physical function following hip and knee arthroplasty. *BMC Musculoskelet Disord.* 2006;7:100.

42. Hough E, Stephenson R, Swift L. A comparison of manual therapy and active rehabilitation in the treatment of non specific low back pain with particular reference to a patient's Linton & Hallden psychological screening score: a pilot study. *BMC Musculoskelet Disord.* 2007;8:106.

43. Kolber MJ, Brueilly KE. Arthrofibrosis following total knee arthroplasty: considerations for the acute care physical therapist. *Acute Care Perspectives.* 2006;15:11-16.

44. Harvey LA, Brosseau L, Herbert RD. Continuous passive motion following total knee arthroplasty in people with arthritis. *Cochrane Database Syst Rev.* 2010;3:CD004260.

45. Denis M, Moffet H, Caron F, et al. Effectiveness of continuous passive motion and conventional physical therapy after total knee arthroplasty: a randomized clinical trial. *Phys Ther.* 2006;86: 174-185.

46. Bini SA, Fithian DC, Paxton LW, et al. Does discharge disposition after primary total joint arthroplasty affect readmission rates? *J Arthroplasty.* 2010;25:114-117.

47. International Associations of Athletics Federations. (1996-2009). Soft Tissue and Healing: Theory and Techniques. Available at: http://www.iaaf.org/mm/Document/imported/42032.pdf. Accessed May 17, 2012.

48. Rizvi AA, Chillag SA, Chillag KJ. Perioperative management of diabetes and hyperglycemia in patients undergoing orthopaedic surgery. *J Am Acad Orthop Surg.* 2010;18:426-435.

49. Lamloum SM, Mobasher LA, Karar AH, et al. Relationship between postoperative infectious complications and glycemic control for diabetic patients in an orthopedic hospital in Kuwait. *Med Princ Pract.* 2009;18:447-452.

50. Kittelson K. Glycemic control: a literature review with implications for perioperativen. Nursing practice. *AORN J.* 2009;90:714-730.

Lumbar Spinal Fusion

Christina N. Brown
Nicholas S. Testa

CASE 7

A 78-year-old male was admitted to the hospital for a scheduled L2-S1 posterior decompression, posterolateral fusion with autograft, and posterior instrumented fusion. The patient has a history of chronic low back pain and lumbar radiculopathy into bilateral lower extremities with failed conservative management that included medications and physical therapy. Diagnostic imaging revealed L2-S1 spinal stenosis. During surgery, the patient sustained significant blood loss of 2000 mL. Past medical history is significant for hypertension, gastroesophageal reflux disease, and anemia. Past surgical history is significant for appendectomy. The patient's inpatient hospital medication list includes Vicodin (for moderate pain), Demerol and morphine (for breakthrough pain), Flexeril, Tramadol, acetaminophen, Protonix, and Enalapril. Due to adverse drug reactions, Vicodin, Demerol, and morphine were recently discontinued and the patient was placed on Ultram. Chart review revealed the following significant values: hemoglobin 9.3, hematocrit 26.7, and heart rate around 120 beats per minute. Due to these values and the patient being symptomatic of anemia, a blood transfusion was ordered. The patient was on bedrest for the first 8 hours postsurgery, and he stood at the edge of the bed the previous evening with help from the nursing staff. The orthopaedic surgeon indicated that the patient should ambulate with a thoracolumbosacral orthosis (TLSO) and follow postoperative spine precautions. The patient lives with his wife in a two-story home, with both the bedroom and bathroom located on the second floor. There are four steps to enter the home with bilateral railings and 12 stairs to the second floor with one railing. The patient owns the following durable medical equipment (DME): standard walker, rolling walker, commode, crutches, and TLSO. The patient's wife expressed concerns about her ability to care for her husband at home. A physical therapy consultation was ordered by the orthopaedic surgeon on postoperative day 1 (POD 1).

▶ Based on the patient's diagnosis and surgery, what do you anticipate will be the contributors to activity limitations?
▶ What are the examination priorities?

▶ What are the most appropriate physical therapy interventions during the acute phase of healing?

▶ What precautions should be taken during physical therapy examination and interventions?

▶ What are the possible complicating factors presented that could impact the patient management process?

KEY DEFINITIONS

AUTOGRAFT: Graft that is harvested from the patient

DECOMPRESSION: Surgical procedure involving removal of the lamina or surrounding structures to relieve pressure on the spinal cord or nerve roots

DURAL TEAR: Complication of spine surgery in which the dura mater is torn

FUSION: Surgical procedure in which two or more adjacent vertebrae are fused together with or without instrumentation

THORACOLUMBOSACRAL ORTHOSIS (TLSO): Rigid back brace that may be used postoperatively to protect the spine by limiting excessive motion

Objectives

1. Describe conservative and surgical management for chronic low back pain (LBP) and lumbar spinal stenosis (LSS).

2. Understand the signs, symptoms, and implications of a dural tear.

3. Identify possible adverse drug reactions (ADRs) that may affect physical therapy examination or interventions and describe possible therapy solutions.

4. Identify critical lab values that should be checked prior to seeing the patient and physical therapy implications of abnormal values.

5. Design an appropriate plan of care for a patient status/post lumbar fusion.

6. Describe the factors influencing the discharge planning process and the role of the physical therapist.

Physical Therapy Considerations

PT considerations during management of the individual status/post lumbar spinal fusion:

▶ **General physical therapy plan of care/goals:** Prevent or minimize loss of range of motion (ROM), strength, and aerobic functional capacity; maximize functional independence and safety while minimizing secondary impairments; improve quality of life

▶ **Physical therapy interventions:** Patient and caregiver education regarding spine precautions, TLSO use, decreasing risk of deep vein thrombosis (DVT), and decreasing risk of falls; bed mobility, transfer, gait, and stair training; ROM activities for bilateral upper and lower extremities; coordination with social worker regarding discharge planning

▶ **Precautions during physical therapy:** Postoperative spinal precautions; close physical supervision to decrease risk of falls; close monitoring of vital signs (blood pressure, heart rate, oxygen saturation, respiratory rate) and laboratory values (hemoglobin and hematocrit); recognize potential ADRs

▶ **Complications interfering with physical therapy:** Spinal headache, anemia, DVT, falls

Understanding the Health Condition

Injury or damage to any of the structures associated with the lumbar spine (vertebrae, discs, ligaments, meninges, spinal cord) can result in LBP. It is estimated that 70% of adults will experience acute LBP at some point in their lifetime.[1] In 10% to 30% of these cases, the pain becomes chronic as demonstrated by relapse or symptom persistence greater than 1 year.[2] Chronic pain is defined as pain persisting greater than 3 months. The economic impact of LBP is significant; it is estimated that LBP costs 12.2 to 90.6 billion dollars annually in the United States.[3]

Over 85% of individuals presenting to primary care for LBP do not have a definitive causal factor for their symptoms.[4,5] Of the 15% where the cause is identifiable, common diagnoses of mechanical LBP are disc herniation, spinal stenosis, osteoporotic fractures,[2,5] lumbar strain/sprain, and trauma-related fractures.[5] Common causes of nonmechanical LBP are neoplasms, infection, and inflammatory diseases.[2,5] Mechanical disorders account for 97% of LBP, nonmechanical disorders account for 1%, and visceral disease (pelvic organ or renal disorders, aortic aneurysm, and gastrointestinal disorders) accounts for the remaining 2%.[5] Risk factors for mechanical LBP include obesity, pregnancy, and activities that require heavy lifting or prolonged sitting. Fibromyalgia is another cause of chronic LBP.[6]

Diagnosis of LBP is often complex. It is based upon a thorough and accurate patient history, physical examination, psychosocial assessment, diagnostic imaging, and ruling out other nonmusculoskeletal (systemic) causes of pain.[3,4] For individuals presenting with nonspecific LBP, diagnostic imaging is not routinely recommended.[4] Treatment aimed at symptomatic management is indicated for individuals younger than 50 years of age in the absence of red flags or systemic disease. If systemic disease is suspected or the individual is older than 50 years of age, plain film radiography and laboratory tests are recommended.[5] The use of radiographs in the presence of nonspecific pain should be reserved for those with symptoms persisting 1 to 2 months.[3] Diagnostic imaging, typically magnetic resonance imaging (MRI) or in certain cases computed tomography (CT) scan, is recommended in when individuals present with red flags, severe and rapid symptom progression, persistent pain, and radicular symptoms for > 6 weeks,[3,4] or those who are considering injections[4] or surgery.[4,5] Imaging can also be used postoperatively to assess success of surgical procedure, disease progression, new bone formation, hardware failure or fracture, and complications including hematoma, infection, and instability.[7]

Conservative treatment of LBP is multifaceted and must take into consideration the individual's unique needs. Pharmacological management includes acetaminophen, nonsteroidal anti-inflammatory drugs (NSAIDs), opioid analgesics, tramadol, tricyclic antidepressants,[2-4] skeletal muscle relaxants,[3,4] and selective serotonin reuptake inhibitors (SSRIs).[2] Other potential interventions are therapeutic exercise, yoga, massage, acupuncture, cognitive behavioral therapy, progressive relaxation, spinal manipulation,[2,3,4,8] and epidural glucocorticoid injections.[3] Physical therapy is often indicated for individuals with LBP and may consist of patient education, therapeutic exercise, manipulation, and mobilization. In a systematic literature review, Morris and Louw[1] tried to determine whether conservative treatment of LBP by a general practitioner or a physical therapist was more effective and concluded that the evidence is insufficient and further research is needed.

Surgical management is considered in individuals who have pain that is consistent with diagnostic findings, severe functional limitations and disability, and persistent pain despite conservative measures. There are a variety of surgical options including spinal fusion, decompression, and disc arthroplasty.[3] Multiple approaches can be used for spinal fusion including anterior interbody fusion (AIF), posterior interbody fusion (PIF), transforaminal interbody fusion (TIF), and extreme lateral interbody fusion (XLIF).[7] In 2005, Bhandari et al.[9] reviewed the results of the Spine Stabilisation Trial Group in which 349 individuals with chronic LBP of ≥ 12 months who were potential surgical candidates were randomized to receive lumbar spinal fusion or rehabilitation led by physical therapists. The participants were followed for 2 years after treatment. At the conclusion of the study, there were no significant benefits of fusion over conservative methods noted on the Oswestry Disability Index, walking test, or secondary outcome measures.

Lumbar spinal stenosis is a common cause of LBP. LSS is the narrowing of the vertebral canal, lateral recess, or intervertebral foramina.[10-13] It may be hereditary[14] or due to congenital narrowing of the spinal canal.[12,13] Other causes include age-related degenerative changes, facet hypertrophy, disc herniation,[5,10,11,13] spondylolisthesis,[11,12] and thickening of the ligamentum flavum.[5,10,12,13] In the United States, over 1 million individuals suffer from LBP and neurogenic claudication associated with spinal stenosis.[11] It is more common in older adults[5] affecting 5 of 1000 adults older than 50 years of age.[15] It affects men more than women at a 2:1 ratio.[12] LSS is the leading cause of spine surgery in the geriatric population.[13,15]

LSS usually develops insidiously in middle age.[12] The hallmark symptom is neurogenic claudication, which presents as leg pain (and sometimes paresthesias) in the posterolateral thigh/s that radiates distally in a dermatomal distribution. Pain is often worse in positions that promote spinal extension (prolonged standing and ambulation) and is usually relieved by positions favoring spinal flexion (sitting).[5,10,11,12,15] Other distinguishing factors of LSS include lower extremity fatigue, weakness, and heaviness,[11,12,15] limited ambulation and exercise tolerance,[11,15] urinary incontinence,[11] diminished or absent patellar or Achilles reflexes,[10] and stooped standing posture.[10,15] When diagnosing spinal stenosis, it is imperative to distinguish between neurogenic and vascular claudication. Vascular claudication is associated with peripheral vascular disease and the pain is aggravated by activity and relieved with rest *regardless* of spine position. It is also important to rule out osteoarthritis of the hip.[12]

Radiographs are often the initial diagnostic imaging choice to delineate bony changes such as spondylolisthesis, scoliosis, fracture, and facet pathology, as well as decreased disc space, neoplasm, or infection.[12] CT or MRI is recommended if symptoms of spinal stenosis persist longer than 6 weeks.[5] MRI is ideal for assessing neural compression and extent of spinal stenosis of the central canal and lateral recesses. MRI should be reserved for use until symptoms are so severe that they are interfering with daily life and spinal stenosis is strongly suspected. For diagnosing spinal stenosis, MRI has a sensitivity of 90% and specificity of 72% to 100%, while CT scan has a sensitivity of 90% and specificity of 80% to 96%.[5] It is important to note that 20% of individuals older than 60 years of age have spinal stenosis as evidenced by diagnostic imaging, but are asymptomatic.[5]

For individuals with LSS and mild symptoms, treatment is often aimed at **conservative measures focusing on pain management.** Conservative management includes modalities (heat, ice, transcutaneous electrical nerve stimulation, ultrasound, massage, traction, acupuncture), patient education and activity modification, pharmacological management (NSAIDs, tricyclic antidepressants, oral glucocorticoids, muscle relaxants), chiropractic care, epidural glucocorticoid injections, selective nerve root blocks, and physical therapy (modalities, flexion-based exercises, cardiovascular training, strengthening core muscles and stretching tight muscles, and patient education).[12] When moderate to severe symptoms of LSS persist despite various attempts at conservative treatment, surgery may be indicated.[2,11] Indications for surgery include severe symptoms (*e.g.*, unrelenting pain, cauda equina syndrome), significant functional limitations affecting ambulation and activities of daily living, and neurogenic claudication not responsive to conservative measures.[12]

Common **surgical interventions for LSS include decompression and decompression with fusion with or without instrumentation**.[12] Decompression via laminectomy is the most common surgical intervention for individuals with LSS.[16] This procedure is performed to reduce pressure on the spinal cord nerve roots and promote stability.[10] Decompression may consist of a laminotomy, laminectomy, and/or discectomy. A laminotomy is a partial removal of the laminae to free the nerve root. A laminectomy is the removal of partial or whole laminae and possibly a portion of the ligamentum flavum, facet joints, and any osteophytes to allow room for nerve roots. A discectomy is the removal of the nucleus pulposus portion of the disc that has herniated through the annulus and may be causing pressure on a spinal nerve root.[17] Techniques involving laminectomy with foraminotomy can potentially cause trauma and instability, which would require a spinal fusion. Decompression with elevation and retraction of the multifidi muscles can lead to paraspinal muscle weakness and atrophy. Decompression can also involve removal of the interspinous or supraspinous ligaments, leading to spinal instability. Bilateral lumbar decompression can be completed through a unilateral approach consisting of a laminectomy or laminotomy and focuses on soft tissue dissection with minimal bone removal to allow for greater stability. Cavusoglu et al.[18] conducted a prospective study of 100 patients who underwent bilateral decompression with unilateral approach. At follow-up (mean of 5.4 years postsurgery), significant improvements were noted in Oswestry Disability Index scores compared to preoperative scores and no spinal instability was evident. A lumbar spinal fusion with or without instrumentation (pedicle screws and metal implants such as threaded cages, plates, and rods)[17] may also be indicated for individuals with complex LSS.[12] A fusion often utilizes a bone graft—either an autograft (typically obtained from the individual's iliac crest or surgically detached laminae) or allograft (from a cadaver). The bone graft is positioned over the portion of the spine to be fused, and is further stabilized with the use of metal implants.[17] In a posterolateral approach, a bone graft is used to achieve fusion or a bone graft can be used in conjunction with instrumentation such as pedicle screws. A posterior approach may be used with bone grafts and cages.[19] Anderson et al.[20] followed 125 patients who underwent a posterolateral lumbar fusion with or without instrumentation using pedicle screws to assess long-term results. After 10 years, the majority had improved functional outcomes and there were no significant differences with or without instrumentation. After lumbar spine fusion, bracing may be used to provide stabilization and minimize movement at the surgical site to promote healing. It may take 6 to 12 months for complete healing to occur following a fusion.[17]

Newer minimally invasive surgical techniques are being investigated. The use of interspinous spacers (X-STOP) to prevent spinal extension is an option for individuals with LSS.[12] At 2-year follow-up, X-STOP was found to be successful in patients with LSS and neurogenic claudication.[21] However, this technique has also been found to have a high failure rate, requiring further surgical intervention when spinal stenosis results from degenerative spondylolisthesis.[22]

There are many complications of spinal surgeries. In 211 patients who underwent a lumbar fusion (noninstrumented posterolateral fusion, instrumented posterolateral fusion, or interbody fusion with bone grafts), Fritzell et al.[23] found that the 2-year complication rates were 12%, 22%, and 40%, respectively. Major complications included deep infection (2.4%), new nerve root pain (7.1%), pulmonary disorder or respiratory distress syndrome (0.9%), and thrombosis or pulmonary embolism (0.9%). Minor complications included donor site pain (4.3%), dural tear (5.6%), gastrointestinal disorder (1.4%), and superficial infection (0.9%).[23] After bilateral decompression surgeries, Cavusoglu et al.[18] noted complications including dural tear, wrong site procedure, and infection. The incidence of dural tears with associated subsequent leakage of cerebrospinal fluid (CSF) with surgical interventions for LSS is estimated to be 8.5%.[24] Adverse effects associated with dural tears include increased length of hospitalization, worse neurologic outcome, and the development of CSF fistulae.[25] To treat the dural tear, fibrin glue may be used in conjunction with sutures to reduce CSF leakage.[25] Khan et al.[26] examined 2024 cases of lumbar spine surgery consisting of lumbar decompression with and without fusion, and estimated the incidence of dural tears to be 7.6%, increasing to 15.9% when subsequent revisions were performed. Failed back syndrome, where symptoms and functional limitations persist despite surgical interventions, occurs in 10% to 40% of patients following spinal surgery.[27]

Up to 80% of individuals with LSS who undergo decompression surgery experience good to excellent outcomes.[12] However, roughly 25% of those who undergo surgery have no symptom relief or have reoccurrence of symptoms. A poor prognosis is associated with delayed surgery in individuals with severe symptoms or leg symptoms present for at least 1 year.[12] Weinstein et al.[28] studied over 600 individuals with LSS having ≥ 12-week history of leg symptoms with no radiographic evidence of spondylolisthesis. The authors concluded that patients who underwent surgery had significantly better outcomes than those who received conservative treatment.

Physical Therapy Patient/Client Management

Postoperative management of a patient following lumbar decompression and fusion includes a team approach typically consisting of the orthopaedic surgeon, nurses, social worker, physical therapist, and occupational therapist. A respiratory therapist and dietician may also be involved. The physical therapist works with the patient and members of the team to promote optimal functional outcomes while the patient is in the inpatient setting. During this immediate postoperative phase, the role of the physical therapist includes: conducting an initial assessment of the patient's functional status; developing, implementing, and modifying an appropriate plan of care based on the patient's response and potential complicating factors; educating the patient and family; communicating and collaborating with members of the interdisciplinary team; providing concise and accurate documentation; and preparing the patient and family for discharge.

Examination, Evaluation, and Diagnosis

Examination is the first component of the patient management process. Before seeing the patient in an acute care setting, the physical therapist should conduct a thorough chart review to gather all necessary information. Laboratory testing is often performed preoperatively to ensure the patient is stable for surgery; however, lab values can be altered as a result of surgery. The physical therapist must interpret lab values with respect to the patient's ability to safely participate in activity. Lab values of particular note to review in the patient who has recently had surgery include the international normalized ratio (INR), hematocrit, hemoglobin, blood glucose, white blood cell count, and oxygen saturation level.

Garritan et al.[29] stated that individuals with levels *out* of the normal ranges may present with fatigue, cardiac arrhythmias, weakness, dyspnea on exertion, confusion, hyper/hypotension and states of diaphoresis. If the patient presents with any of these signs or symptoms, the therapist should modify or discontinue treatment and notify appropriate nursing and medical staff. Other pertinent information that can be gathered from the chart review includes past medical and surgical history, social history, history of present condition, surgical procedure and any complications, previous vital signs, and any mobility restrictions or precautions.

The physical therapist should review the inpatient medication list. Table 7-1 provides an overview of the current patient's medications including drug class, indications, and common ADRs.[30,31] Of the eight medications he has been taking since surgery, six are given to provide postoperative analgesia. The sedation, dizziness, nausea, and constipation these drugs cause are common barriers to a patient's

Table 7-1	OVERVIEW OF THE PATIENT'S MEDICATIONS		
Drug Name	**Drug Class**	**Indications**	**Common ADRs**
Meperidine (Demerol) Morphine (MS Contin)	Opioid analgesic	Moderate to severe pain	Sedation, euphoria, respiratory depression, nausea/vomiting, constipation, tolerance, dizziness, headache
Tramadol (Ultram)	Opioid analgesic and weak norepinephrine/ serotonin reuptake inhibitor	Moderate to severe pain	Nausea, headache, dizziness
Cyclobenzaprine (Flexeril)	Skeletal muscle relaxant polysynaptic inhibitor	Muscle spasms	Sedation and drowsiness, dizziness, lightheadedness, nausea, headache, confusion, weakness, dyspepsia
Acetaminophen (Tylenol)	Non-NSAID analgesic and antipyretic	Mild to moderate pain, fever	Nausea, rash, headache
Hydrocodone/ acetaminophen (Vicodin)	Non-NSAID analgesic and opioid combination	Moderate to moderately severe pain	Sedation, dizziness, nausea/vomiting, constipation
Pantoprazole (Protonix)	Proton pump inhibitor (PPI)	Gastroesophageal reflux disease (GERD), gastric and duodenal ulcers	Diarrhea, abdominal discomfort, headache
Enalapril (Vasotec)	ACE inhibitor	Hypertension, congestive heart failure	Persistent dry cough, hypotension, dizziness, fatigue, hyperkalemia

ability to fully participate in physical therapy sessions. Because of significant sedation, Vicodin, Demerol, and morphine were discontinued on POD 1 and the patient was placed on Ultram. The therapist may need to schedule treatment sessions when pain medications have reached peak effect to allow the patient to mobilize with tolerable pain levels, but the therapist must also closely monitor for ADRs that can inhibit the patient's ability to safely mobilize after surgery. The therapist must communicate with other members of the interdisciplinary team regarding ADRs that are inhibiting the patient's progress and be flexible enough to change therapy session times to find the best time for the patient. The physical therapist should be aware that medication changes are common in the acute care setting and be cognizant of such changes.

Next, the physical therapist conducts the patient interview. During this process, the physical therapist begins to develop a trusting relationship while obtaining information that may not have been evident in the chart review. Family or caregivers may be present and included in the process of history taking. Information that needs to be gathered includes: family/caregiver support, home set-up (including stairs, ramps, railings, number of stories, location of bedroom and bathroom), if the patient has any assistive devices or other DME, whether the patient needs DME prior to discharge, and the patient's goals for physical therapy. The physical therapist should also ask the patient about his *optimal* discharge plan. Based on the patient's functional progress and hospital course, the discharge plan may change. Once this component of the examination is completed, the physical therapist conducts a systems review consisting of a brief examination of the cardiovascular/pulmonary, integumentary, musculoskeletal, and neuromuscular systems, and the patient's communication abilities.[32]

Depending on the orthopaedic surgeon, the patient may be on bedrest for up to 8 hours following surgery or longer, if a dural tear was sustained. Typically, the patient stands at the bedside the evening of surgery with nursing staff. Physical therapy is initiated on POD 1. When the therapist sees the patient, he is typically supine. The patient may be repositioned in sidelying for pressure relief. This position also assists in pulmonary hygiene and allows for visualization of the surgical dressing. Clear drainage, possibly surrounded by a ring of yellow, can indicate a CSF leak. If this is noted, the physical therapist should immediately notify the patient's nurse and/or appropriate medical staff. The patient will also have a drain from the surgical incision site for 48 to 72 hours postsurgery.[17] Patients can be mobilized with drains in place; typically, it is easiest to attach the drain to the patient's gown with a safety pin to prevent tension on the tubing during mobilization. The therapist needs to be aware of patient monitoring devices, intravenous lines, and catheters. The patient is connected to monitors that assess heart rate, blood pressure, and oxygen saturation for the first 24 hours or until the medical team decides they are no longer needed. The physical therapist should monitor blood pressure, heart rate, and oxygen saturation throughout the treatment session since these values can change quickly.

During the examination, the therapist is assessing the individual's cognitive state. To do so, the physical therapist can ask questions such as the time of day/date, location, and reason for admission. The reason for asking these basic questions is that general anesthesia affects individuals differently. Common post-anesthesia adverse effects include hypotension, lightheadedness, sedation, ataxia, delirium, confusion, and muscle weakness. These symptoms may persist in patients who are debilitated or have impaired drug elimination.[30,31]

Preoperatively, patients may have impaired sensation as a result of spinal stenosis. To determine if sensation has improved as a result of the surgery, the therapist must thoroughly assess sensation of the lower extremities. Range of motion (ROM) and strength of upper and lower extremities should be tested in the supine and sitting positions. It is critical to assess strength and ROM of the upper extremities because the individual must be able to don and doff his TLSO, use an assistive device, and transfer in and out of the bed properly and safely. Prior to mobilizing the patient, the physical therapist educates the patient on spinal precautions, TLSO use, and assistive device use.

The physical therapist slowly assists the individual in transitioning from supine to sitting at the edge of the bed to assess strength and ROM of the lower extremities. To move from the supine to the sitting position, a log roll technique is used in which the patient adopts a hooklying position (hips and knee bent to 90°) and then rolls to the sidelying position by moving the knees and shoulders at the same time. This technique allows the individual to use stabilizing muscles of the spine and abdomen without twisting the spine. This movement decreases the stress placed on the surgical site. Once on his side, the patient then pushes up with the arm that is closest to the bed to get into the sitting position. Initially, the therapist needs to assist the person in transitioning from sidelying to sitting. Once in sitting, the TLSO is donned (though some surgeons may indicate that the TLSO should be donned in the supine position). Not all spinal surgeons request that their patients wear a TLSO after surgery. Use of a TLSO has been shown to decrease pain, protect the spine against further injury, correct deformity,[33] correct posture, and reduce the mobility of the thoracolumbar spine.[34]

An important precaution that is reiterated to individuals following lumbar fusion is that they are not allowed to sit for longer than 20 to 30 minutes until advised by the surgeon. This restriction results from the concept that there is a higher load on the lumbar spine in the sitting position that will put unwanted stress on the surgical site, which could potentially disrupt the healing process. For the 70-kg (154 lb) individual, the load on the lumbar spine (L3) is 25 kg in supine, 150 kg in standing, 175 kg in sitting, 200 kg in sitting while bending forward, and 225 kg in standing while bending at the waist.[19] Thus, after spine surgery, patients are taught spinal precautions that include avoiding activities that place increased stress or load on the surgical site. Spinal precautions include avoidance of: spinal flexion and rotation, lifting, pushing, and pulling (usually restricted to no more than 10 lb). Ambulation is assessed using an assistive device as needed for patient safety and stability. Because the current patient has been on bedrest and is taking several opioid and non-opioid medications, it is important to slowly transition him to an upright position and monitor for symptomatic orthostatic hypotension.

When mobilizing this patient, the physical therapist needs to monitor for signs and symptoms associated with a dural tear or anemia. An individual who has sustained a dural tear would most likely present with a severe headache that does not subside when the head is elevated.[26] If this is the case, the best approach would be to return the patient back to bed and immediately notify the nurse and/or surgeon. After any surgery, there is some amount of blood loss but the physical therapist should be aware of signs and symptoms of anemia: dyspnea, headache, lightheadedness, fatigue, insomnia, and pallor.[35] If these are noticed by the physical therapist and/or other support personnel, the individual should be returned to bed and the patient's symptoms brought to the physician's attention immediately. The physical therapist should defer treatment until signs and symptoms are stabilized. The patient may require a blood transfusion. Post-transfusion, laboratory testing is performed to reassess hemoglobin and hematocrit levels. The physical therapist should frequently review the chart to determine if physical therapy treatment is safe and appropriate. Throughout the examination, the physical therapist evaluates the patient's response and identifies any factors that may indicate referral to another member of the healthcare team. The therapist should also encourage the patient to use the incentive spirometer between physical therapy sessions to reduce the risk of postoperative atelectasis.[17]

Plan of Care and Interventions

In the acute care setting, the main goals of physical therapy are to promote the healing process and prepare patients for return home. Short-term goals are based on the patient's functional status at the time of the initial examination and optimal discharge plans. Physical therapy goals often focus on achieving independence in transfers, ambulation, and stairs. To assist the patient in attaining these goals, the plan of care should include patient and caregiver education regarding spinal precautions, TLSO use, decreasing risk of deep vein thrombosis (DVT), and decreasing risk of falls; bed mobility, transfer, and gait training; ROM activities for bilateral upper and lower extremities and coordination with the social worker regarding discharge planning. If there are no postsurgical complications, most individuals who have lumbar fusions return home within 2 to 4 days postsurgery, though this can vary based on facility. The first few days are vital to ensure that patients have the knowledge and equipment they will need to be safe and successful when they return home. It is for this reason that the physical therapist continues to assess the patient for any equipment needs as well as the appropriateness of discharge plans. The physical therapist communicates with the social worker if the patient needs an assistive device or assistance with discharge planning (*e.g.*, home vs. short-term rehabilitation in a skilled nursing facility). Physical therapists play an essential role in the discharge planning process that is initiated during the initial examination. Smith et al.[36] retrospectively studied the role of physical therapists in discharge planning of 72 patients in the acute care setting of a large academic medical center. They found that physical therapists' discharge recommendations were followed 83% of the time. In those cases in which the recommendations were *not* followed, the readmission was 2.9 times more likely.

One of the major postoperative precautions taken in the acute care setting is DVT prevention. Risk factors for acquiring a DVT are advanced age, fractures to the lower extremities, paralysis or prolonged immobility, prior DVTs, operations, obesity, congestive heart failure, myocardial infarction, and stroke.[37] In a review by Kehl-Pruett,[38] the incidence of DVT was 40% to 60% in patients hospitalized after orthopaedic surgery. Up to 18% of individuals undergoing elective spine surgery experience a DVT.[39] In addition to the postoperative spinal precautions, patients are educated on the importance of performing ankle pumps while in bed. This consists of the patient actively plantarflexing and dorsiflexing their ankles bilaterally for about 1 in minute every hour that they are awake. This action promotes venous return and circulation, which helps prevent a DVT. Each patient uses bilateral **intermittent pneumatic compression devices** that have been shown to reduce the incidence of DVT by 7% to 15%.[38] For patients who have undergone elective spine surgery, **early and progressive ambulation is recommended.** For individuals with DVT risk factors such as advanced age and the presence of neurologic deficits, additional prophylactic methods are recommended including heparin, intermittent pneumatic compression, and/or graded compression stockings.[40] Physician orders for DVT prophylaxis for the patient presented in this case included intermittent pneumatic compression devices and antiembolism compression stockings (*e.g.*, TED hose).

The physical therapist helps the patient practice the activities performed in the examination and evaluation with an emphasis on demonstrating spinal precautions. These activities include log-rolling into and out of bed and transferring from supine to sitting, sitting to standing, and sitting to supine. The patient must practice donning and doffing his TLSO (with assistance from his wife, if possible) and he must wear the TLSO any time he is out of bed, including during ambulation. With any walking speed, wearing the TLSO helps reduce pelvic obliquity and rotation as well as axial force on the spine.[33] The patient must be educated on inspecting his skin to monitor for any areas of persistent redness or skin breakdown due to the TLSO or due to infection at the incision site. When patients begin ambulating after spinal surgery, it is recommended that a rollator walker (front-wheeled walker or four-wheeled walker) be used to provide greater stability if the patient presents with significant postoperative pain or decreased standing balance. The patient presented in this case is at an increased risk for falls due to pain, decreased standing balance, and generalized weakness. Therefore, it is critical that the therapist trains the patient in using both the TLSO and the walker multiple times before hospital discharge. Vogt et al.[41] compared three groups of geriatric inpatients at a rehabilitation clinic: those issued a four-wheeled walker for the first time, those who used a four-wheeled walker in the community prior to admission, and those who ambulated without an assistive device. The authors observed similar improvements in mobility, strength, and balance among the groups during rehabilitation. The authors concluded by recommending walker use during inpatient stays to improve patient confidence and mobility. Once the patient is able to ambulate safely, stair training should be initiated. During gait and stair training, it is important to provide appropriate levels of supervision and assistance for patient safety and fall prevention.

A group in Denmark has recently demonstrated the value of including physical therapy interventions in the spinal surgery population. Nielson et al.[42] studied 60 patients who underwent spine surgery and assigned them to one of two groups: (1) exercise and optimization of pain management 2 months before surgery with early postoperative pain management and physical therapy for exercises and ambulation twice per day, or (2) postoperative pain management and ambulation once per day. The authors found that individuals in the group that included the more intense exercise program had a shorter length of hospital stay, higher satisfaction, and achieved goals for mobility and activities of daily living more quickly than those in the other group.

When the patient's pain is under control and physical therapy goals have been met, the patient is ready for discharge (from a physical therapy standpoint). Factors that may suggest placement into a rehabilitation facility instead of discharge to home include a lack of mobility independence, decreased assistance at home, delay in postoperative progress, and postoperative complications. In this case, the patient continued to require moderate assistance for bed mobility and transfers, minimal assistance for ambulation due to unsteadiness, and total assistance to don and doff the TLSO. The patient's wife felt she would be unable to manage the patient at home. Due to all these factors, the physical therapist recommended discharge to a short-term rehabilitation facility prior to discharge to home.

Evidence-Based Clinical Recommendations

SORT: Strength of Recommendation Taxonomy

A: Consistent, good-quality patient-oriented evidence

B: Inconsistent or limited-quality patient-oriented evidence

C: Consensus, disease-oriented evidence, usual practice, expert opinion, or case series

1. Conservative nonsurgical management is effective for individuals with mild symptomatic lumbar spinal stenosis. **Grade B**

2. Surgical interventions for patients with LSS are associated with improvement in function. **Grade B**

3. Intermittent pneumatic compression devices reduce the incidence of deep vein thromboses following elective spine surgery. **Grade B**

4. Early and progressive ambulation is an effective measure to decrease the risk of deep vein thrombosis following elective spine surgery. **Grade C**

COMPREHENSION QUESTIONS

7.1 One of the possible complications of undergoing a spinal surgery is sustaining a dural tear. An individual who has sustained a dural tear would *most* likely present with:

  A. Severe headache that does not subside

  B. Night sweats

  C. Dyspnea on exertion (DOE)

  D. Sputum production

7.2 The log roll technique allows an individual to transfer in and out of bed by:

  A. Using the stabilizing muscles of the spine as well as the abdominal muscles to roll from supine to sidelying with the knees bent to avoid twisting the spine

  B. Using the strength of the upper and lower extremities

  C. Using the help of a family member or caregiver

  D. Both B and C

7.3 Which of the following has *not* been described as an indication for a thoracolumbosacral orthosis (TLSO)?

  A. To control pain

  B. To protect the spine against further injury

  C. To reduce the mobility of the thoracolumbar spine

  D. To promote lumbar spine rotation

ANSWERS

7.1 **A.** When an individual sustains a dural tear, there are two signs and/or symptoms that are most common. One is that clear fluid is seen in the postoperative drain that the individual is usually required to wear for the first 24 hours. This clear fluid is CSF that has leaked secondary to the dural tear. The second most common sign and/or symptom seen is a persistent headache that does not subside when the head is elevated.[26]

7.2 **A.** The spine itself has many smaller deep muscles that play multiple roles. These various muscles can help extend, rotate, and stabilize the spine. When lying supine, these smaller muscles in conjunction with the abdominal muscles allow an individual to rotate in the sagittal plane without the use of his/her upper or lower extremities. This technique also minimizes the amount of stress that is put on the surgical site.

7.3 **D.** The TLSO has been indicated to control pain (option A), protect the spine against further injury (option B), correct deformity,[33] correct posture, and reduce the mobility of the thoracolumbar spine (option C).[34] Because it is indicated to *decrease* thoracolumbar mobility, it would not be used to promote lumbar spine rotation.

REFERENCES

1. Morris LD, Louw QA. Physiotherapists and general practitioners as first-line of management for acute low back pain: which is better? A systematic review. *JBI Library of Systematic Reviews*. 2010; 8:382-404.

2. Balague F, Dudler J. An overview of conservative treatment for low back pain. *Int J Clin Rheumatol*. 2011;6:281-290.

3. Last AR, Hulbert K. Chronic low back pain: evaluation and management. *Am Fam Physician*. 2009;79:1067-1074.

4. Horsely L. ACP Guidelines for the diagnosis and treatment of low back pain. *Am Fam Physician*. 2008;77:1607-1610.

5. Jarvik JG, Deyo RA. Diagnostic evaluation of low back pain with emphasis on imaging. *Ann Intern Med*. 2002;137:586-597.

6. Ehrlich GE. Low back pain. *Bull World Health Organ*. 2003;81:671-676.

7. Hayeri MR, Tehranzadeh J. Diagnostic imaging of spinal fusion and complications. *Applied Radiology*. 2009;38:14-28.

8. Atlas SJ. Nonpharmacological treatment for low back pain. *J Muscoloskel Med*. 2010; 27:20-27.

9. Bhandari M, Petrisor B, Busse JW, et al. Does lumbar surgery for chronic low back pain make a difference? *CMAJ*. 2005;173:365-366.

10. Strayer A. Lumbar spine: common pathology and interventions. *J Neurosci Nurs*. 2005;37:181-193.

11. Snyder DL, Doggett D, Turkelson C. Treatment of degenerative lumbar spinal stenosis. *Am Fam Physician*. 2004;70:517-520.

12. Yuan PS, Albert TJ. Managing degenerative lumbar spinal stenosis. *J Musculoskel Med*. 2009;26: 222-231.

13. Tran de QH, Duong S, Finlayson RJ. Lumbar spinal stenosis: a brief overview of nonsurgical management. *Can J Anesth*. 2010;57:694-703.

14. Moore KL, Dalley AF. *Clinically Oriented Anatomy*. 4th ed. Philadelphia, PA: Lippincott Williams & Wilkins; 1999.

15. Iverson MD, Choudhary VR, Patel SC. Therapeutic exercise and manual therapy for persons with lumbar spinal stenosis. *Int J Clin Rheumatol*. 2010;5:425-437.

16. Jakola AS, Sorlie A, Gulati S, et al. Clinical outcomes and safety assessment in elderly patients undergoing decompressive laminectomy for lumbar spinal stenosis: a prospective study. *BMC Surg*. 2010;10:34.

17. Harvey CV. Spinal surgery patient care. *Orthop Nurs*. 2005;24:426-440.

18. Cavusoglu H, Kaya RA, Turkmenoglu ON, et al. Midterm outcome after unilateral approach for bilateral decompression of lumbar spinal stenosis: 5 year prospective study. *Eur Spine J*. 2007;16: 2133-142.

19. Dutton M. *Orthopaedic Examination, Evaluation, and Intervention*. 2nd ed; 2008. Available at: http://www.accessphysiotherapy.com/content/55589198. Accessed January 13, 2012.

20. Anderson T, Videbaek TS, Hansen ES, et al. The positive effect of posterolateral lumbar spinal fusion is preserved at long-term follow-up: a RCT with 11-13 year follow-up. *Eur Spine J*. 2008;17:272-280.

21. Kuchta J, Sobottke R, Eysel P, et al. Two-year results of interspinous spacer (X-Stop) in 175 patients with neurologic intermittent claudication due to lumbar spinal stenosis. *Eur Spine J*. 2009;18: 823-829.

22. Verhoof OJ, Bron JL, Wapstra FH, et al. High failure rate of the interspinous distraction device (X-stop) for the treatment of lumbar spinal stenosis caused by degenerative spondylolisthesis. *Eur Spine J*. 2008;17:188-192.

23. Fritzell P, Haag O, Nordwall A. Complications in lumbar fusion surgery for chronic low back pain: comparison of three surgical techniques used in a prospective randomized study. A report from the Swedish lumbar spine study group. *Eur Spine J*. 2003;12:178-189.

24. Tafazal SI, Sell PJ. Incidental durotomy in lumbar spine surgery: incidence and management. *Eur Spine J*. 2005;14:287-290.

25. Jankowitz BT, Atteberry DS, Gerszten PC, et al. Effect of fibrin glue on the prevention of persistent cerebral spinal fluid leakage after incidental durotomy during lumbar spine surgery. *Eur Spine J*. 2009;18:1169-1174.

26. Khan MH, Rihn J, Steele G, et al. Postoperative management protocol for incidental dural tears during degenerative lumbar spine surgery. A review of 3,183 consecutive degenerative lumbar cases. *Spine*. 2006;31:2609-2613.

27. Bokov A, Istrelov A, Skorodumov A, et al. An analysis of reasons for failed back surgery syndrome and partial results after different types of surgical lumbar nerve root decompression. *Pain Physician*. 2011;14:545-557.

28. Weinstein JN, Tosteson TD, Lurie JD, et al. Surgical versus nonsurgical therapy for lumbar spinal stenosis. *N Engl J Med*. 2008;358:794-810.

29. Garritan S, Jones P, Kornberg T, et al. Laboratory values in the intensive care unit. *Acute Care Perspectives*. 1995;3:7-11.

30. Ciccone CD. *Pharmacology in Rehabilitation*. 4th ed. Philadelphia, PA: FA Davis; 2007.

31. Panus PC, Jobst EE, Masters SB, et al. *Pharmacology for the Physical Therapist*. New York, NY: McGraw-Hill; 2009.

32. American Physical Therapy Association. *Guide to Physical Therapist Practice*. 2nd ed. Alexandria, VA; 2003.

33. Konz R, Fatone S, Gard S. Effect of restricted spinal motion on gait. *J Rehabil Res Dev*. 2006;43:161-170.

34. van Leeuwen PJ, Bos RP, Derksen JC, et al. Assessment of spinal movement reduction by thoracolumbar-sacral orthoses. *J Rehabil Res Dev*. 2000;37:395-403.

35. Lasch KF, Evan CJ, Schatell D. A qualitative analysis of patient-reported symptoms of anemia. *Nephrol Nurs J*. 2009;36:621-633.

36. Smith BA, Fields CJ, Fernandez N. Physical therapists make accurate and appropriate discharge recommendations for patients who are acutely ill. *Phys Ther.* 2010; 90:693-703.

37. Lieberman JR, Hsu WK. Prevention of venous thromboembolic disease after total hip and knee arthroplasty. *J Bone Joint Surg Am.* 2005;87:2097-2112.

38. Kehl-Pruett, W. Deep vein thrombosis in hospitalized patients: a review of evidence-based guidelines for prevention. *Dimens Crit Care Nurs.* 2006;25:53-59.

39. Nicolaides AN, Fareed J, Kakkar AK, et al. Prevention and treatment of venous thromboembolism International Consensus Statement (Guidelines according to scientific evidence). *Int Angiol.* 2006;25:101-161.

40. Becker RC. Focus on thrombosis applying management guidelines in clinical practice. *J Thromb Thrombolysis.* 2007;24:183-222.

41. Vogt L, Lucki K, Bach M, et al. Rollator use and functional outcome of geriatric rehabilitation. *J Rehabil Res Dev.* 2010;47:151-156.

42. Nielson PR, Jorgensen LD, Dahl B, et al. Prehabilitation and early rehabilitation after spinal surgery: randomized clinical trial. *Clin Rehabil.* 2010;24:137-148.

Brain Tumor Status/Post Craniotomy

Erin E. Jobst

A 62-year-old right-hand dominant male went to the hospital with complaints of persistent headaches that were getting progressively worse, increasing left-sided weakness, and gait instability. Magnetic resonance imaging revealed a large enhancing mass within the right parietal lobe with extensive surrounding vasogenic edema. Differential diagnoses include a solitary metastasis or a primary central nervous system (CNS) neoplasm. The patient was admitted to the hospital and the tumor was grossly resected the next day. Relevant inpatient medications include dexamethasone, insulin, ondansetron, oxycodone, acetaminophen, bisacodyl, and senna-docusate. Physical therapy evaluation was ordered on the third postoperative day (POD 3). The patient is expected to be discharged home tomorrow. He is a retired schoolteacher and lives in a single-story house with his wife, who will be available as a full-time caregiver.

▶ Based on his health condition, what do you anticipate will be the contributors to activity limitations?
▶ What are the examination priorities?
▶ What are the most appropriate physical therapy interventions?
▶ What precautions should be taken during physical therapy examination and interventions?
▶ What are possible complications interfering with physical therapy?
▶ How would this individual's contextual factors influence or change your patient/client management?

KEY DEFINITIONS

CRANIOTOMY: Most common surgical procedure to resect (remove) a brain tumor; part of the skull is removed to gain access to the brain; after brain tumor is biopsied and/or removed, bone flap is secured back in position

METASTASIS: Spread of cancer cells to one or more areas elsewhere in the body, usually by the lymph or vascular system

NEOPLASM (TUMOR): Abnormal mass of tissue resulting from neoplasia; tumors can be cancerous (malignant) or noncancerous (benign)

Objectives

1. Describe the medical treatment plan for benign and malignant brain tumors.
2. Understand the indications for the drugs prescribed to a patient post-craniotomy.
3. Identify potential adverse drug reactions (ADRs) that may affect physical therapy examination or interventions and describe possible therapy solutions.
4. Recognize signs and symptoms of rising intracranial pressure (ICP).
5. List the anticipated deficits resulting from parietal lobe damage or dysfunction.
6. List typical craniotomy precautions and discuss their rationale.
7. Design an appropriate plan of care for the patient status/post brain tumor resection, in the absence of knowing the prognosis.

Physical Therapy Considerations

PT considerations during management of the individual status/post craniotomy due to brain tumor:

▶ **General physical therapy plan of care/goals:** Prevent or minimize loss of range of motion, strength, and aerobic functional capacity; maximize functional independence and safety while minimizing secondary impairments; improve quality of life

▶ **Physical therapy interventions:** Patient and caregiver education regarding craniotomy precautions, decreasing risk of deep vein thromboses, and decreasing the risk of falls; gait training; caregiver training for safe guarding during ambulation; prescription of a home exercise program; and, if indicated, referral to home health or outpatient physical therapy

▶ **Precautions during physical therapy:** Craniotomy precautions; close physical supervision to decrease risk of falls; consistent monitoring of vital signs, especially blood pressure (BP); recognize potential ADRs

▶ **Complications interfering with physical therapy:** Brain edema, headaches, deep vein thromboses, seizures, falls, unknown prognosis (if histopathology from biopsy sample not completed prior to patient's participation in physical therapy)

Understanding the Health Condition

Brain tumors are uncontrollably growing solid growths that originate either from tissue within the brain itself (primary brain tumor) or result from a metastasis from cancer elsewhere in the body (secondary, or metastatic brain tumor). Primary brain tumors can originate from neural tissue, meninges, glandular tissue, choroid plexi, cranial nerves, or blood vessels. Primary brain tumors are named for the primary cell type involved (*e.g.*, astrocytomas arise from astrocytes; oligodendrogliomas arise from oligodendrocytes) and they can be benign or malignant. However, the distinction between benign and malignant brain tumors is not as clear-cut as it is for tumors in other parts of the body. For example, even though a primary brain tumor may be histologically benign, the treatment, prognosis, and impact on the patient's function may be very similar to that of a malignant tumor if the benign tumor is not completely resectable. This is because brain tumors can grow and spread within the brain, compressing and damaging nearby normal brain tissue, with resulting disruption of essential brain function. In general, benign brain tumors grow slowly, have distinct borders, and rarely spread. In contrast, malignant brain tumors grow rapidly, can be invasive, and are life-threatening.

In adults, metastatic brain tumors are much more common than primary brain tumors. Brain metastases occur in 10% to 30% of adults with systemic cancers;[1] each year, approximately 250,000 Americans develop metastatic brain tumors during the course of their illness.[2] The origin of brain metastases is usually primary cancers of the lung, breast, skin (melanoma), kidney, and colon. In contrast, fewer than 65,000 cases of primary brain (and CNS) tumors were expected to be diagnosed in the United States in 2011.[3] Of these primary CNS tumors, approximately 22,000 will be malignant. In adults, the median age at diagnosis for a primary brain tumor is 57 years[3] and more than 60% of these tumors are located in the cerebral hemispheres.[4] The most common primary brain tumor is the typically benign meningioma (34.4% of all primary brain and CNS tumors).[3] Glioblastoma multiforme is the most common malignant primary brain tumor (16.7% of all primary brain and CNS tumors).[3]

Signs and symptoms of brain tumors can be the result of direct infiltration or compression of specific brain structures as well as increased ICP from edema surrounding the tumor. One of the most common symptoms is a deep, dull headache that recurs often and persists without relief. The headache may increase with activities that raise ICP such as exercising, placing the head below the heart, and coughing or sneezing.[5] While the location of the tumor determines the specific deficits, other general signs and symptoms include: seizures, vomiting, vision changes (hemianopsias, double vision), weakness or paralysis, difficulties with walking and balance, speaking difficulties, changes in mental acuity or personality, and altered states of consciousness (lethargy, somnolence). The severity of many signs and symptoms depends on tumor size and location.

If a brain tumor is suspected after clinical and laboratory investigations have ruled out other causes for presenting signs and symptoms (*e.g.*, infections, medications), imaging is the essential tool for diagnosis. Magnetic resonance imaging is the gold standard because it provides excellent anatomical detail and can detect tumors near bones, slow-growing tumors, and tumors that are only a few millimeters in size.[6] Definitive diagnosis of the type and grade of brain tumor must be confirmed by histological examination of the tissue obtained by biopsy. Brain tumors are then classified based on predominant cell type and graded based on the presence of any pathological features (e.g., degree of cell differentiation, presence of necrotic cells in tumor). There are many classification systems for brain tumors, but the universal method for CNS tumors is the World Health Organization (WHO) grading system.[7,8] The WHO grading system is a four-tiered tumor guideline that assigns grades from I to IV; the grade indicates the degree of malignancy. In general, higher-grade malignancies (e.g., glioblastoma multiforme) are expected to grow faster and have poorer prognoses than lower-grade malignancies (e.g., oligodendroglioma). Depending on the classification system used, brain tumors may have more than one name or a different grade. This can be confusing for patients, family members, and clinical staff. Although it would be impossible to be knowledgeable about the over 100 types of brain tumors, it is important to understand the most prevalent types and be as consistent as possible in classification names and grades.

Treatment options are usually multifaceted. The standard approach is to reduce the tumor size as much as possible using surgery, radiation therapy, or chemotherapy. These treatments are used alone, or more commonly, in combination. Medical treatment (and prognosis) depends on tumor resectability, tumor location, age of patient, and tumor histology. For most brain tumors, surgery is usually the first and most desirable option to remove all of the tumor (complete resection) or as much as possible (debulking) without affecting normal brain function. To gain access to the brain, a neurosurgeon performs a craniotomy in which the skin, subcutaneous tissue, galea, and muscle (depending on incision site) are cut and several burr holes are drilled into the skull. Bone between the burr holes is cut and then bone, muscle, and dural flaps are turned back to expose the brain.[9] After the tumor is removed, the bone flap is replaced and fixed in place and the scalp is closed with stitches or staples. Some low-grade tumors may be successfully treated by surgical removal alone (e.g., meningiomas, pituitary adenomas). If surgical removal is impossible due to the location of the tumor, radiation may be used as the main treatment. Radiation therapy may also be given after surgery if a benign tumor is not entirely resectable. To focus radiation on the tumor site and minimize radiation dose to the entire brain, radiosurgery may be used. Gamma knife, external beam radiation therapy, and stereotactic radiotherapy are examples of unique radiosurgery techniques. For metastatic brain tumors, radiation therapy is the most common intervention. Often, the brain metastasis will usually be treated first due to its life-threatening nature and because the treatment may be incompatible with treatment of tumors in the rest of the body. In adults, chemotherapy is generally reserved for higher-grade tumors and is usually administered following surgery or radiation therapy. Most chemotherapy agents given via traditional routes cannot cross the blood-brain barrier. Therefore, chemotherapy drugs may be administered directly into the brain, intrathecally, intra-arterially, or into the cerebrospinal fluid via a ventricular access catheter.

The most important prognostic factors for patients with brain tumors are primary cell type, aggressiveness of the tumor cells (i.e., how quickly they are growing), and the patient's age. For example, the 5-year relative survival rate for a 50-year-old adult with a low-grade astrocytoma is 40%. This rate drops to 6% for a 50-year-old adult with a high-grade glioblastoma.[3] For all brain tumors, survival rates drop with increasing age.[3]

Physical Therapy Patient/Client Management

For the postoperative patient diagnosed with a brain tumor, the treatment team generally includes: neurologists, neurosurgeons, endocrinologists, nurses, psychologists, social workers, and rehabilitation specialists. If the tumor is malignant, radiation and medical oncologists are also included. It is important to be aware that a patient may be admitted to the hospital with the diagnosis of a brain tumor, undergo brain surgery, but not yet know the type of tumor he has when the therapist performs an evaluation. When this is the case, all members of the team must remember that future medical intervention and long-term prognosis is *unknown*. Sometimes, the physical therapist may read a recent neuropathology chart note describing the histology of the brain tumor; however, unless it is clear that the patient and family members have been made aware of the definitive diagnosis, discussions regarding diagnosis (with respective prognosis and medical treatment plan) should generally be deferred to the neurosurgeon or primary physician. If the tumor is malignant and the patient and his family are aware of this diagnosis, the physical therapist must recognize and gently inform patient and family members that the patient's current presentation may not accurately reflect his future function. Sensitive therapists strive to prepare the patient and the family for the potential of progressive neurologic and functional decline, while avoiding being unrealistically optimistic or pessimistic regarding the patient's ability to have an independent lifestyle. Regardless of the patient's prognosis, the role of the physical therapist in the acute postoperative phase after craniotomy is to assess the patient's current functional capabilities and to prepare for discharge. The specific roles of the physical therapist are to: prevent or minimize postoperative complications; assess range of motion, strength, neurologic function, dynamic balance and safety during transfers and gait within the indicated postoperative precautions; anticipate potential ADRs and modify interventions as appropriate to minimize their occurrence; and, educate the patient and his wife regarding postoperative precautions, mobility training, and the effects of the diagnosis on current and future mobility.

Examination, Evaluation, and Diagnosis

Prior to seeing the patient, the physical therapist needs to acquire information from his chart, including: medications, lab values, postoperative precautions, and any exercise or mobility restrictions. Critical lab values to check include: hemoglobin, hematocrit, platelet count, and trends in blood pressure. Exercise or mobilization should be withheld if hemoglobin, hematocrit, and cell counts are not within safe limits.

The medication list should be reviewed to predict potential ADRs and to strategize possible therapy solutions to mitigate their effect on patient management. Dexamethasone is a systemic glucocorticoid given to limit cerebral edema. It may also help decrease nausea and headaches after surgery. Dosage is usually progressively tapered to nothing over a few weeks, if the patient is not having radiation therapy after surgery.[8,10] Common ADRs of systemic glucocorticoids that may affect inpatient rehabilitation include changed effect (depression, mood swings) and increased BP. Even though this patient is not diabetic, patients often need insulin to maintain normoglycemia because dexamethasone tends to increase blood glucose concentration. Therapy sessions should not be closely timed with insulin administration because insulin and physical activity both decrease blood glucose concentration, increasing the risk of hypoglycemia. Ondansetron is given to prevent nausea and vomiting in the postoperative phase. It may be helpful for the patient to receive a dose prior to the initial physical therapy examination, since early mobilization frequently increases nausea. Oxycodone and acetaminophen are analgesics taken for mild-to-severe headaches that occur due to stretching and irritation of scalp nerves post-craniotomy.[11] Orthostatic hypotension and sedation are common ADRs. Slow transfers to upright positions decrease the likelihood of symptomatic orthostatic hypotension and subsequent falls. Bisacodyl and senna-docusate are laxatives to keep stool soft, allowing patients to avoid straining during bowel movements, which increases ICP. A helpful incentive to encourage patients to participate in physical therapy is to inform them that increasing mobility as much as possible after surgery also promotes laxation, decreasing the need to strain during bowel movements.

Maintenance of normal ICP and prompt recognition of elevated ICP are of paramount importance in the postoperative phase. Increased ICP can cause neurologic damage by reducing blood flow (and thus, oxygen) to the brain; increased ICP can also cause brain herniation. ICP is the pressure that the cerebrospinal fluid exerts within the ventricles. The determinants of ICP are brain volume, cerebrospinal fluid, and intracranial blood. Normally, ICP ranges from 4 to 15 mm Hg.[12] Physiological elevations of ICP have been documented with coughing, head-down tilt, Valsalva maneuver, compression of neck veins, increased body temperature, increased cerebral metabolism, increases in arterial, venous, and intrathoracic pressures,[13,14] and even with increased anxiety and anger.[15,16] Although elevations in ICP associated with these stimuli can be large, they do not normally cause brain damage because the pressure is distributed equally throughout the craniospinal axis.[14,17] After brain surgery, cerebral edema is controlled with fluid restriction and glucocorticoids to avoid dangerous increases in ICP (sustained pressure elevations > 15-20 mm Hg).[14] In addition, an upper limit for systolic blood pressure (SBP) is usually set by the neurosurgeon (e.g., SBP < 160 mm Hg) to minimize increases in ICP. The physical therapist should know the patient's recent BP trends in order to be able to make reasonable judgments as to whether changes in BP (and ICP) are related to medical interventions (e.g., intravenous fluid changes or medications), physical therapy interventions (e.g., position changes and physical exertion), or if trends are signaling neurologic decline (e.g., intracranial hemorrhage).

Not all patients who have undergone brain surgery have invasive ICP monitoring devices (e.g., epidural sensor, subarachnoid bolt, intraventricular catheter). In addition, when patients are moved from the intensive care unit to the main hospital floor, ICP monitoring is often discontinued. Thus, changes in neurologic status due to evolving cerebral edema should be anticipated in the first days after surgery and **signs and symptoms of rising ICP** must be assessed vigilantly. One of the first signs of rising ICP is a change in mentation, ranging from confusion to lethargy to restlessness.[18] Other signs include changes in vision, headache, progressive impairment of motor function contralateral to side of the lesion, and abnormal respiratory rate and depth.[4,12,19] The therapist should continually monitor vital signs and neurologic status, especially during changes in the patient's position and with increases in physical exertion.

Although the precise location of the tumor and the extent of the tumor removed may not be known, general tumor location determines the cognitive and physical deficits the therapist should anticipate. The parietal lobes process and integrate somatosensory input with visual information, forming a type of map which guides interactions with the environment.[20] Parietal lobe dysfunction that can easily be assessed in the acute care examination includes: impaired proprioception, sensory extinction, impaired hand-eye coordination, inability to multitask, reading problems (alexia), apraxia, denial of deficits (anosognosia), and contralateral neglect.[21,22] Damage to the right parietal lobe in particular often results in neglect of the left side of the body or the left side of the extrapersonal space.

During introductions, the physical therapist assesses the patient's level of alertness, mental status, and orientation. Specific questions should be asked regarding the patient's prior level of function and current activity level since surgery. To assess reading problems (alexia), the therapist can ask the patient to read out loud the written craniotomy precautions. Active range of motion, strength, and sensation testing are most easily tested with the patient seated at the edge of the bed. The patient should be instructed to breathe (i.e., not hold his breath) during manual muscle testing to avoid performing a Valsalva maneuver. Special attention should be paid to symmetry during strength and sensation testing. If the patient has intact sensation to light touch on each extremity, the therapist should also test extremities on either side simultaneously (double simultaneous stimulation). The patient should be able to attend and identify a tactile stimulus that is applied to both sides of the body simultaneously. If the patient consistently fails to report *contralesional* touch (on the left side, in this case) with bilateral stimulation, despite reporting the same stimulation when given in isolation, this is sensory extinction (or, extinction to simultaneous stimulation).[23] Sensory extinction, most common after right hemisphere stroke, may indicate dysfunction of the posterior parietal lobe.[24] In stroke survivors, tactile extinction on the left side of the body is an important predictor of functional outcome.[25] Proprioception (joint movement and position sense) of the lower extremity joints should be tested. If the patient cannot accurately detect distal movement (of a toe), the therapist should progressively test more proximal joints until he can identify the movement correctly. Apraxia is the inability to perform voluntary learned movements despite a lack of deficits in sensation, strength, coordination, attention, or comprehension. In other words, a person knows how to do to a task, but cannot perform the necessary sequence of activities to allow him to perform the task correctly. Two basic tests for apraxia can be done while the patient is still in his room. To test for dressing apraxia, the therapist can turn the patient's gown or robe inside out and ask the patient to put it back on correctly. For ideomotor apraxia, the therapist asks the patient to perform a common task such as waving or kicking something (e.g., an imaginary ball). The inability to make the proper movement in response to a command to pantomime demonstrates ideomotor apraxia.

While the patient dons his robe, pants, or shoes, the physical therapist should carefully observe for other indications of parietal lobe dysfunction: hand-eye coordination and spatial neglect. Accurate hand-eye coordination requires the patients to reach, grasp, and manipulate the clothing object. Spatial neglect can be observed in watching the patient get dressed. The patient may forget to put his sleeve or pant leg on the neglected (left) side.

To determine the impact of compromised lower extremity proprioception on static standing balance, the Romberg test can be performed.[26,27] The patient is asked to stand with feet together and eyes open, and then with eyes closed for 20 to 30 seconds. Patients with significant impairments in lower extremity proprioception have more difficulty maintaining their balance with their eyes *closed*—as noted by increased sway, stepping, opening the eyes, or even a fall (positive Romberg sign).[26] The sharpened Romberg (tandem Romberg) requires the patient to stand with one foot in front of the other in tandem stance for 60 seconds with eyes closed.[28] Because the base of support is narrower in the sharpened Romberg, it may be more sensitive than the Romberg.[29] **One-legged stance tests (OLSTs)** are also commonly used to test static standing balance.[24,28] In this case of a patient with a unilateral brain tumor, OLST may provide more discriminative information because it enables direct comparison between lower extremities. Both legs should be tested alternately and differences between sides noted. The patient stands on both legs, crosses his hands over his chest, then picks up one leg and holds it with the hip in neutral and knee flexed to 90°.[30] Criteria to stop the test include: legs touching each other, foot touches the ground, or arms move from start position. To determine the extent to which vision contributes to the patient's stability, the OLST can be repeated with eyes closed. Shorter stance times on the contralesional lower extremity with eyes closed may indicate impaired peripheral sensation and proprioception. The patient's timed performance on the sharpened Romberg and OLST can be compared to published norms for older non-institutionalized adults (Table 8-1). In the study by Briggs et al.[31] (sharpened Romberg and OLST in women), subjects had to be able to walk independently without an assistive device; Jedrychowski et al.[32] (OLST in men) did not state whether independent ambulation was an inclusion criterion.

Table 8-1 PERFORMANCE NORMS FOR QUIET STANDING BALANCE TESTS IN OLDER ADULTS			
Age (years)	Sharpened Romberg in Women[31] (sec) Eyes Open; Eyes Closed	OLST on Dominant leg in Women[31] (sec) Eyes Open; Eyes Closed	OLST in Men[32] (sec) Eyes Open
60-64	56; 24	38; 6	
65-69	56; 32	24; 4	58
70-74	49; 24	18; 4	32
75-79	40; 14	11; 2	22
80-86	45; 22	11; 3	17 (age 80-89)

In normal adults, leg dominance and shoe wear did not affect OLST results.[31] Thus, data from patients who often wear only hospital-issued socks can be confidently compared to published norms. Although results from the sharpened Romberg and OLSTs alone cannot accurately predict a patient's likelihood of future falls, the data can help the therapist determine the appropriateness of an assistive device and guide the prescription of a home exercise program.

Gait pattern in patients with parietal lobe dysfunction may present as a hemiplegic pattern (if one-sided weakness is predominant) or as a sensory ataxic pattern (if patient demonstrates significant deficits in proprioception).[26,29] In this case, the patient had normal and bilaterally equal extremity strength, moderate impairments in proprioception (left toes and ankle), and sensory extinction of the left lower extremity. His gait pattern was notable for a wide base of support with irregular step length, though he had no loss of balance when asked to walk in a straight line. The patient should be asked to make turns in either direction to assess the presence of any unilateral (left) neglect and to assess if the ataxic gait pattern increases to the degree that the patient loses his balance. During gait, the therapist can also determine whether the patient can multitask effectively and safely. A common example of an inability to multitask is the patient who needs to stop walking to engage in a conversation. Persons who stop walking while talking are at an increased risk of falling.[33]

Finally, the physical therapist should assess the patient's jaw range of motion. Most cranial surgery involves transection of the temporalis muscle; this can impair jaw mobility and cause myofascial pain that could last for up to 6 months.[34]

Throughout the examination, the physical therapist should ascertain whether the patient has insight into any of his deficits. Anosognosia is more common in patients with right brain dysfunction.[35] The presence of anosognosia may particularly impair the patient's participation in rehabilitation since he is unaware of or denies the presence of any deficits he demonstrated in the examination. Balance impairments and the inability to recognize these deficits place the patient at a high risk for falls. Anosognosia has also been shown to be a negative predictor for functional outcome in individuals post-stroke.[36]

Plan of Care and Interventions

Because this patient's brain tumor classification and grade are unknown, the physical therapist must be careful when interacting with the patient and his wife to avoid making statements about prognosis. Since treatment and prognosis vary dramatically depending on type of brain tumor, the patient may be returning to the hospital for radiation and chemotherapy. The short-term goal, however, remains the same: to determine whether the patient is safely able to return home tomorrow with his wife. While it is impossible to address all the patient's impairments in the acute care setting, the plan of care and interventions should always prioritize the patient's ability to safely perform functional tasks within medically prescribed precautions and to ensure the most optimal future functional outcome. Interventions for patients after craniotomy for brain tumor resection frequently include: patient and caregiver education regarding craniotomy precautions, decreasing risk

Table 8-2   COMMON CRANIOTOMY PRECAUTIONS

Restriction	Functional Considerations
Keep SBP < 160 mm Hg	Therapist should measure the patient's SBP response to most strenuous anticipated activity after discharge from hospital (e.g., ascending/descending flight of stairs) Educate the patient to keep physical exertion level below the exercise intensity that correlated with SBP near or at 160 mm Hg
No breath holding	Count or read out loud while having a bowel movement or performing a strenuous task (avoid Valsalva maneuver)
No stifling coughs or sneezes No blowing nose	Avoid vigorous coughs
Keep head above the level of the heart (In hospital bed, keep head of bed 30°-45° above the horizontal)[14]	Use pillow to elevate head in bed No bending over to don shoes or tie shoelaces; instead, bring legs up to knees to don shoes Use an assistive device (e.g., reacher) to pick objects off floor
No lifting, pushing, pulling > 10 lb	A gallon of milk weighs ~8 lb Consider weight of small children and pets
No end-range hip flexion	Avoid postures with *sustained* hip flexion, which can increase intrathoracic pressure and ICP
Minimize irritating environmental stimuli	Modify environment to minimize external stimulation (e.g., minimize strong emotions and loud noise; choose dim lights)

of deep vein thromboses, and decreasing the risk of falls; gait training; caregiver training for safe guarding during ambulation; prescription of a home exercise program; and, if indicated, referral to home health or outpatient physical therapy. Patients who have undergone brain surgery are taught **craniotomy precautions** (Table 8-2). The goal of these precautions is to avoid potentially dangerous increases in ICP after surgery. Restricted activities have been shown to produce elevations in ICP.[4,9,14,16,17,18] Typically, patients are advised to follow these precautions for 6 weeks following surgery. Table 8-2 lists craniotomy precautions with functional considerations for the physical therapist to highlight for the patient and caregiver. Written educational materials are highly recommended. One of the most difficult craniotomy precautions to follow is keeping SBP < 160 mm Hg. For the patient to understand what level of physical activity corresponds to a SBP of 160 mm Hg, two tasks are required: monitoring of vital signs during the therapy session and informing the patient about his SBP at various activity levels. Patients can be taught to use a rating of perceived exertion (RPE) scale to correlate exertion level with SBP. Another craniotomy precaution that often requires further education is the restriction against breath holding. While the patient may state that he never holds his breath, the therapist should directly inquire whether he typically holds his breath during bowel movements. This habit results in a Valsalva maneuver that increases BP and ICP.[37,38] Surgery, anesthesia, and decreased mobility increase the likelihood of constipation. To minimize the need for straining during bowel movements, patients should be encouraged to breathe during bowel movements, take prescribed stool softeners, increase physical activity as much as possible, decrease frequency of oral opiate medication as soon as possible, and stay hydrated within any prescribed fluid restrictions. The therapist should educate patient and caregiver to be aware of signs and symptoms of increased ICP. Because changes in neurologic status can be subtle and patients may not communicate or be insightful about their deficits or symptoms, special attention should be given to ensuring that caregivers observe and question patients closely.

Deep vein thrombosis (DVT) and pulmonary embolism are the most frequent complications following craniotomy for brain tumors. Because these patients are at risk for intracranial bleeding, anticoagulants are generally not given.[39] Three strategies to decrease the risk of DVT are employed in the inpatient setting: early mobilization, elastic lower extremity stockings and/or pneumatic pressure devices that simulate the muscle action that occurs during active ankle movement, and active ankle dorsiflexion ("ankle pumps"). While patients and caregivers should be taught to recognize the signs and symptoms of a DVT (i.e., calf pain or tightness, leg swelling, increased temperature in affected leg), DVTs are often asymptomatic.[4] This reinforces the importance of consistent use of each of the DVT prevention strategies.

To promote safety during ambulation, patients who demonstrate a sensory ataxic gait pattern can be taught to compensate for impaired processing of somatosensory information by relying more on vision. Techniques such as watching their feet while walking (especially during turns), making sure that environments are well-lit, and minimizing distractions (e.g., small pets running between feet) can improve balance during gait. Assistive devices should be prescribed, if the use of one increased stability or endurance during the gait examination. If indicated, caregivers can be provided with gait belts and taught how to safely guard the patient during ambulation. Because patients with anosognosia are at a higher risk of falls due to decreased insight into their functional deficits, following safety precautions for falls should be reinforced with care providers.

Patients should be told to expect increased fatigue, or an increased headache or short-temper with fatigue during the first 6 weeks after craniotomy.[10] Energy conservation techniques—especially incorporation of a rest in the middle of the day—may help. For patients with cancer, a walking program performed at moderate intensity (50%-70% of age-predicted heart rate maximum, or at an RPE of 12-13) improves quality of life, decreases cancer-related fatigue, and improves aerobic functional capacity in adults receiving chemotherapy and/or radiation.[40,41] Prescription of a walking program may also be beneficial for the post-craniotomy patient, as long as the exertion level does not exceed the prescribed SBP limit.

If the patient has impaired jaw opening and closing, home exercises should be prescribed to attain full jaw range of motion. **Jaw exercises**[42] include: (1) open mouth as wide as possible and hold for several seconds; (2) open mouth a small amount and move jaw side to side; (3) open mouth widely and move jaw side to side; (4) make exaggerated chewing movements for 30 seconds. Ten repetitions of each of these exercises should be performed 3 times per day. Chewing several sticks of gum at one time can also exercise the temporalis muscle. In a descriptive study of 71 patients 4 to 6 months post-craniotomy, many had limited jaw protrusion and 28% reported pain during normal jaw movements. Patients with post-craniotomy headaches also had more masticatory muscle tenderness on palpation than those without post-craniotomy headaches.[43] Whether prescription of a home exercise program to patients post-craniotomy decreases the incidence of jaw dysfunction and temporalis-related headache pain is unknown.

Evidence-Based Clinical Recommendations

SORT: Strength of Recommendation Taxonomy

A: Consistent, good-quality patient-oriented evidence

B: Inconsistent or limited-quality patient-oriented evidence

C: Consensus, disease-oriented evidence, usual practice, expert opinion, or case series

1. Some signs and symptoms of rising intracranial pressure can be detected without invasive ICP monitoring. **Grade A**

2. In patients with unilateral brain lesions, physical therapists can use the One-legged Stance Test to help determine differences between lower extremities in static standing balance. **Grade B**

3. Craniotomy precautions minimize increases in ICP. **Grade B**

4. Jaw exercises after craniotomy increase jaw mobility and decrease temporalis-related headache pain. **Grade C**

COMPREHENSION QUESTIONS

8.1 A therapist has prescribed a home exercise program for a patient going home 3 days after a craniotomy for brain tumor resection. Which is *not* an appropriate intervention to include as part of a home exercise program?

   A. Single limb squats with hand-held or countertop support for balance and safety

   B. Daily walking program at RPE of 12-13

   C. Resistance training with heavy weights on distal extremities

   D. Multiple repetitions of full jaw opening and closing 3 times per day

8.2 Signs of a localized lesion in the parietal lobe include:

   A. The patient cannot perform a specific task when asked to, but can perform the task when left on his own.

   B. The patient ignores the contralesional side of his body and environmental stimuli on that side.

   C. The patient denies or lacks awareness of deficits resulting from his condition.

   D. All of the above

8.3 Three days post-craniotomy, a patient becomes weak, dizzy, and diaphoretic when ambulating with the physical therapist. Which drug is *most* likely responsible for this adverse drug reaction?

  A. Insulin

  B. Dexamethasone

  C. Oxycodone

  D. Ondansetron

ANSWERS

8.1 **C.** Resistance training should be avoided because it can cause sharp increases in SBP. Increased SBP increases ICP, which is contraindicated in the early post-craniotomy phase. In addition, many individuals perform a Valsalva maneuver when performing resistance exercises, further increasing SBP and ICP. The other exercises listed appropriately address common deficits noted after craniotomy: single limb balance (option A), fatigue and decreased aerobic capacity (option B), and impaired jaw range of motion (option D).

8.2 **D.** All of the listed deficits are typically associated with parietal lobe dysfunction: ideomotor apraxia (option A), unilateral neglect (option B), and anosognosia (option C).

8.3 **A.** It is likely that the patient is experiencing hypoglycemia due to insulin administration and physical activity, both of which reduce blood glucose concentration. The opiate analgesic oxycodone may cause orthostatic hypotension, which can cause dizziness. However, the diaphoresis the patient experienced is more typical of hypoglycemia than orthostatic hypotension. The therapist should have the patient sit down, take his blood pressure and oxygen saturation (to rule out hemodynamic contributions), and ask the nurse to test his blood glucose. If the patient is hypoglycemic, he should be given a fast-acting oral glucose source (*e.g.*, fruit juice). To minimize recurrence of hypoglycemia, insulin administration and therapy interventions should not be timed closely together.

REFERENCES

1. Wen PY, Loeffler JS. Overview of the clinical manifestations, diagnosis, and management of patients with brain metastases. Available at: http://www.uptodate.com/contents/clinical-presentation-and-diagnosis-of-brain-tumors. Accessed June 25, 2011.

2. American Cancer Society. Available at: http://www.cancer.org/. Accessed June 07, 2011.

3. Central Brain Tumor Registry of the United States. Available at: http://www.cbtrus.org/factsheet/factsheet.html. Accessed June 07, 2011.

4. Goodman CC, Fuller KS. *Pathology—Implications for the Physical Therapist*. 3rd ed. St. Louis, MI: Saunders Elsevier; 2009.

5. Forsyth PA, Posner JB. Headaches in patients with brain tumors: a study of 111 patients. *Neurology*. 1993; 43:1678-1683.

6. University of Maryland Medical Center. Available at: http://www.umm.edu/patiented/articles/how_brain_tumors_diagnosed_000089_6.htm. Accessed June 08, 2011.

7. Louis DN, Ohgaki H, Wiestler OD, et al. The 2007 WHO classification of tumours of the central nervous system. *Acta Neuropathol.* 2007;114:97-109.

8. Christiansen CJ, Lopez RO, Phillips K, M. Ch 23: Brain tumors. In: Umphred DA, ed. *Neurological Rehabilitation.* 4th ed. St. Louis, MO: Mosby; 2001:696-716.

9. Moak E. Perioperative care of the craniotomy patient: a review. *Todays OR Nurse.* 1992;14:9-14.

10. Melbourne Neurosurgery Post Operative Information Leaflet Craniotomy. Available at: www.neurosurgery.com.au/pdfs/postop/postopcranipdf.pdf. Accessed June 7, 2011.

11. Quiney N, Cooper R, Stoneham M, et al. Pain after craniotomy. A time for reappraisal? *Br J Neurosurg.* 1996;10:295-299.

12. Paz JC, West MP. *Acute Care Handbook for Physical Therapists.* 3rd ed. St. Louis, MI: Saunders Elsevier; 2009.

13. Muwaswes M. Increased intracranial pressure and its systemic effects. *J Neurosurg Nurs.* 1985;17:238-243.

14. Lee EL, Armstrong TS. Increased intracranial pressure. *Clin J Oncol Nurs.* 2008;12:37-41.

15. Dandy WE. Intracranial pressure without brain tumor: diagnosis and treatment. *Ann Surg.* 1937;106:492-513.

16. Venes J. Intracranial pressure monitoring in perspective. *Childs Brain.* 1980;7:236-251.

17. Miller DJ, Piper IR. Raised intracranial pressure and its effect on brain function. In: Crockard A, Hayward R, Hoff JT, eds. *Neurosurgery: The Scientific Basis of Clinical Practice.* 2nd ed. Malden, MA: Blackwell Science; 1985:373-389.

18. Hammerschmidt M, Mulholland J. *Notes on ICU Nursing: FAQ Files from the MICU.* 2nd ed. PA: Infinity Publishing; 2003.

19. Flotte E. Neurosurgery Student Syllabus. Available at: neurosurgery.umc.edu/docs/StudentHandout.pdf. Accessed June 7, 2011.

20. Kandel E, Schwartz J, Jessell T. *Principles of Neural Science.* 4th ed. New York, NY: McGraw-Hill Professional; 2000.

21. Neurosurgical Case Discussions. Available at: http://www.neurosurvival.ca/ClinicalAssistant/Examinations/parietal%20lobe/parietal_lobe_testing.htm. Accessed June 08, 2011.

22. Culham JC, Valyear KF. Human parietal cortex in action. *Curr Opin Neurobiol.* 2006;16:205-212.

23. Kluger BM, Meador KJ, Garvan CW, et al. A test of the mechanisms of sensory extinction to simultaneous stimulation. *Neurology.* 2008;70:1644-1645.

24. NeuroLogic Examination Videos and Descriptions—an Anatomical Approach. Available at: http://library.med.utah.edu/neurologicexam/html/sensory_normal.html. Accessed June 26, 2011.

25. Rose L, Bakal DA, Fung TS, et al. Tactile extinction and functional status after stroke. A preliminary investigation. *Stroke.* 1994;25:1973-1976.

26. Lundy-Ekman L. *Neuroscience: Fundamentals for Rehabilitation.* 3rd ed. Philadelphia, PA: Elsevier Mosby/Saunders; 2007.

27. Lanska DJ, Goetz CG. Romberg's sign: development, adoption, and adaptation in the 19th century. *Neurology.* 2000;55:1201-1206.

28. Newton R. Review of tests of standing balance abilities. *Brain Inj.* 1989;3:335-343.

29. Fattal D, Lanska DJ. Balance and gait disorders. *Neurology MedLink* [serial online]. 2009:6/26/11. Available at: http://www.medlink.com/medlinkcontent.asp. Accessed September 5, 2011.

30. Stayner CJ, Lopez RM, Tuzzolino KM. Ch 25: Brain tumors. In: Umphred DA, ed. *Neurological Rehabilitation.* 5th ed. Philadelphia, PA: Elsevier/Mosby/Saunders; 2007:812-833.

31. Briggs RC, Gossman MR, Birch R, et al. Balance performance among noninstitutionalized elderly women. *Phys Ther.* 1989;69:748-756.

32. Jedrychowski W, Mroz E, Tobiasz-Adamczyk B, et al. Functional status of the lower extremities in elderly males. A community study. *Arch Gerontol Geriatr.* 1990;10:117-122.

33. Snijders AH, Verstappen CC, Munneke M, Bloem BR. Assessing the interplay between cognition and gait in the clinical setting. *J Neural Transm.* 2007;114:1315-1321.

34. de Andrade Junior FC, de Andrade FC, de Araujo Filho CM, et al. Dysfunction of the temporalis muscle after pterional craniotomy for intracranial aneurysms. comparative, prospective and randomized study of one flap versus two flaps dieresis. *Arq Neuropsiquiatr.* 1998;56:200-205.

35. Appelros P, Karlsson GM, Hennerdal S. Anosognosia versus unilateral neglect. coexistence and their relations to age, stroke severity, lesion site and cognition. *Eur J Neurol.* 2007;14:54-59.

36. Hartman-Maeir A, Soroker N, Oman SD, et al. Awareness of disabilities in stroke rehabilitation—a clinical trial. *Disabil Rehabil.* 2003;25:35-44.

37. Prabhakar H, Bithal PK, Suri A, et al. Intracranial pressure changes during valsalva manoeuvre in patients undergoing a neuroendoscopic procedure. *Minim Invasive Neurosurg.* 2007;50:98-101.

38. Matsuda M, Watanabe K, Saito A, et al. Circumstances, activities, and events precipitating aneurysmal subarachnoid hemorrhage. *J Stroke Cerebrovasc Dis.* 2007;16:25-29.

39. Freeman G. Brain tumors. In: Umphred DA, ed. *Neurological Rehabilitation.* 3rd ed. St. Louis, MI: Mosby; 1994.

40. Monga U, Garber SL, Thornby J, et al. Exercise prevents fatigue and improves quality of life in prostate cancer patients undergoing radiotherapy. *Arch Phys Med Rehabil.* 2007;88:1416-1422.

41. Windsor PM, Nicol KF, Potter J. A randomized, controlled trial of aerobic exercise for treatment-related fatigue in men receiving radical external beam radiotherapy for localized prostate carcinoma. *Cancer.* 2004;101:550-557.

42. Popovic E. Craniotomy: postoperative problems with chewing and talking. Available at: http://www.popovic.com.au/surgery_cranial.html#3. Accessed June 27, 2011.

43. Rocha-Filho PA, Fujarra FJ, Gherpelli JL, et al. The long-term effect of craniotomy on temporalis muscle function. *Oral Surg Oral Med Oral Pathol Oral Radiol Endod.* 2007;104:e17-e21.

Breast Cancer— Metastasis to Lumbar Spine

Erin E. Jobst

CASE 9

A 54-year-old female was admitted to the hospital 12 days ago with complaints of severe back pain with no identified mechanism of injury. Notable previous medical history includes breast cancer 4 years ago, treated with a partial mastectomy plus radiation. Imaging (x-rays and radionuclide bone scan) shows bone metastases (with lytic and blastic features) in the third and fourth lumbar vertebral bodies. The patient started radiation therapy and a bisphosphonate 5 days ago. The patient expects to be discharged to her single-level home with her husband in several days. She will be continuing cancer treatment as an outpatient. The oncologist stated that she has "spinal precautions," but no weightbearing restrictions and she can ambulate within pain tolerance. Her current complaints are back pain and fatigue.

▶ Based on her health condition, what do you anticipate may be the contributors to activity limitations?
▶ What are the examination priorities?
▶ What are the most appropriate physical therapy interventions?
▶ What are possible complications interfering with physical therapy?

KEY DEFINITIONS

BONE SCAN: Radionuclide imaging to detect presence and amount of metastatic lesions in bones

METASTASIS: Spread of cancer cells to one or more areas elsewhere in the body, usually by the lymph or vascular system

PARTIAL MASTECTOMY: Removal of the breast tumor and surrounding area

RADIATION THERAPY: Local cancer treatment involving use of high energy x-rays, electron beam, or radioactive isotopes to destroy cancer cells

Objectives

1. Describe cancer-related fatigue.
2. Identify a reliable and valid outcome tool to measure cancer-related fatigue.
3. Identify critical lab values that should be checked prior to physical therapy examination.
4. Prescribe an appropriate intensity aerobic exercise program to minimize cancer-related fatigue.
5. Describe benefits of aerobic exercise for patients receiving cancer therapies.

Physical Therapy Considerations

PT considerations during management of the breast cancer survivor with development of bone metastases in lumbar spine:

▶ **General physical therapy plan of care/goals:** Prevent or minimize loss of range of motion, strength, and aerobic functional capacity; decrease cancer-related fatigue; decrease risk of pathological fractures; improve quality of life

▶ **Physical therapy interventions:** Patient education regarding pathological fractures and complications; modified mobility training to decrease risk of pathological vertebral fractures; energy conservation techniques; light to moderate intensity aerobic walking program

▶ **Precautions during physical therapy:** Spinal precautions, close physical supervision to decrease risk of falls, monitor vital signs

▶ **Complications interfering with physical therapy:** Spinal cord compression, pathological fractures

Understanding the Health Condition

Breast cancer is one of the most common cancers in women in the United States, affecting approximately one in eight women during their lives.[1] Treatment of breast cancer can include surgery, radiation, chemotherapy, or hormonal therapy. Cancer recurrence—the detection of cancer after treatment and some period of time when the patient is considered "cancer-free"—can be local or distant. Metastases occur most often within 3 years of the initial cancer diagnosis.[1] The most common sites of cancer metastases (distant recurrences) are liver, lung, bone, and brain.

Bones are particularly common metastatic sites for breast and prostate cancers. Although metastases ("mets") can occur in any bone, the spine is the most common. Other common sites are the pelvis, femur, humerus, ribs, and skull. Skeletal complications of bone metastases include bone pain, pathological fractures, spinal cord compression, and hypercalcemia of malignancy. Usually, the first symptom of bone metastasis is deep, sharp, and severe bone pain. The pain pattern generally progresses from intermittent pain worsened by activity and weightbearing, increasing pain at night, to constant pain. Bone metastases may be lytic, blastic, or a mixture of both. When cancer cells begin to destroy the bone (lytic process), the bone may attempt to grow new bone (blastic process) to surround the cancer. Cancer cells that have invaded a bone can progressively weaken its structure to the point of fracture. These pathological fractures can result from an injury or fall, but can also occur during simple activities of daily living. As cancer cells damage bones, calcium is released into the blood; patients are monitored for hypercalcemia. The most serious complications of vertebral metastases are compression of the spinal cord (within cervical and thoracic regions) and stenosis or cauda equina syndrome (within lumbar region). Spinal cord compression can be due to the tumor encroaching into the spinal canal or due to bone lesions that weaken the vertebral body. The latter process creates a fragile vertebral body at high risk for an impending vertebral fracture, which can impinge into the spinal canal, compressing neural structures. Depending on the vertebral level involved, impingement of neural structures can cause pain, numbness, weakness, paralysis, and/or bowel and bladder signs.

Treatment options for bone metastases include radiotherapy to decrease bone pain and/or prevent impending fractures, surgery to stabilize weakened bones or repair pathological fractures, analgesics, and bisphosphonates.[2,3] One of the side effects of radiotherapy is decreased blood cell counts (primarily white blood cells and platelets), increasing the risk of infections and bleeding. Bisphosphonates are drugs given intravenously that significantly reduce the risk of fractures or delay the onset of pathological fractures. These agents inhibit both osteoclast-mediated bone resorption and tumor-associated osteolysis. In addition to being effective for fracture prevention, bisphosphonates have been shown to decrease narcotic requirements in those with metastatic breast cancer.[2] Prognosis of metastatic bone disease depends on the primary site, with breast and prostate cancers associated with a survival measured in years.[1]

Cancer-related fatigue—an extreme tiredness that does not abate with rest—is a common side effect of cancer or cancer treatment.[4] Cancer-related fatigue can be overwhelming, making it difficult for patients to maintain their normal activities, including being able to follow their treatment plan. Fatigue may also fluctuate in intensity and duration, so patients might find it difficult to plan activities. There are likely multiple causes of cancer-related fatigue, including cytokines released from malignant cells or immune cells, anemia, radiation treatment, chemotherapy, and deconditioning. If a particular cause can be identified (e.g., anemia), then it is usually treated (e.g., by a blood transfusion or drugs to increase red blood cell formation). However, in most cases, cancer-related fatigue is not easily treatable.

Physical Therapy Patient/Client Management

There are multiple cancer treatment options ranging from local to systemic interventions. Treatment regimens change frequently based on disease progression and the patient's tolerance of cancer treatments. The physical therapist works with the oncology team to create functional goals and improve quality of life for patients. The primary physical therapy goal is to enable patients to return to their functional level prior to cancer diagnosis. Regardless of prognosis, the aim of the entire rehabilitation team is to maintain the patient's quality of life as long as possible.

Examination, Evaluation, and Diagnosis

Prior to seeing this patient, the physical therapist needs to acquire information from her chart, including lab values, weightbearing restrictions, and any exercise or mobility restrictions. Critical lab values to check before seeing this patient include: hemoglobin, hematocrit, white blood cell count, and platelet count. Exercise or mobilization should be withheld if these values are not within safe limits.

During the examination, the physical therapist evaluates the patient's level of fatigue and pain as well as her knowledge of spinal precautions and fall risk precautions. The Brief Fatigue Inventory (BFI) is a quick, reliable tool to identify and measure severe fatigue in people with cancer.[5] The BFI is a 10-item self-report scale: 0 represents no fatigue or no fatigue interference with daily life; 10 represents the worst fatigue or worst fatigue interference with daily life imaginable. Pain can be rated on a numerical rating scale (NRS) that involves asking patients to rate their pain from 0 to 10, in which 0 represents no pain and 10 is the worst pain imaginable. The validity of the NRS has been well documented.[6] The NRS is sensitive to treatments that are expected to influence pain intensity.[7,8] A 30% change in NRS score (corresponding to a change of approximately 2 points) has been shown to represent a minimal clinically important difference (MCID) in pain.[9] Thus, the physical therapist can assess pain before and after an intervention to determine whether the patient had a *clinically significant* difference in pain (by noting whether her reported pain changed by at least 2 points). Pain can also be measured using a visual analog scale (VAS) that consists of a line (usually 10-cm long) with the left end labeled as "no pain" and the right end labeled as "unbearable pain." An advantage of the VAS is that it is independent of language and is usually easily understood by most patients. Pain and fatigue levels should be reassessed throughout the examination and physical therapy interventions.

Plan of Care and Interventions

Specific physical therapy goals are set after the evaluation and must take into consideration the patient's discharge plans. Goals related to cancer-related fatigue and decreased risk of pathological fracture must be incorporated.

In addition to specific findings from the examination, physical therapy interventions should include: patient education regarding pathological fractures and complications, modified mobility training to decrease risk of pathological vertebral fracture, energy conservation techniques, and prescription of an aerobic walking program.

To decrease the likelihood of vertebral pathological fractures, the patient should be taught to follow **spinal precautions.** During transitions from lying to sitting, she should be taught to "log roll"—that is, the entire spine should move at the same time like a stiff rolling log. The objective is to avoid spinal rotation, or twisting of the upper body with respect to the lower body. The patient should also be taught to avoid spinal flexion and rotation when lifting up objects from the floor or turning around. Instead, she should be taught to bend at the hips and knees and to pivot her feet to change direction. Lifting restrictions are generally set at no more than 10 lb (a gallon of milk weighs roughly 8 lb). Pain should not increase dramatically during movement. Increased pain could be indicative of a pathological fracture or a new bone metastasis[1]; this should be reported to the physician immediately.

Physical therapy interventions for cancer-related fatigue can include energy conservation techniques and prescription of an aerobic exercise program. Typical energy conservation principles include prioritization of activities and participation when the patient has the most energy. Placing frequently used items within reach (or in one location), pacing, and asking for assistance from caregivers should be emphasized. Consultation and coordination with an occupational therapist to reinforce these principles is recommended. Unless there are mobility restrictions, an aerobic exercise program should be included into the cancer treatment plan. To objectively estimate the patient's current functional activity level and aerobic capacity, the physical therapist can have her perform a **Six-Minute Walk Test** (6MWT).[10,11] This test is ideal for the inpatient setting, requiring only a 100-ft hallway and a period of 6 minutes. The patient is instructed to cover as much distance as possible during the 6 minutes; she should choose her own pace and she is allowed to stop and rest during the test, if needed. If fall risk is a concern, assistive devices can be used during the 6MWT. The physical therapist monitors blood pressure, heart rate, rating of perceived exertion (RPE) and any signs or symptoms before, during, and after the 6MWT. Oxygen saturation can also be measured by pulse oximetry (SpO_2). The patient's walking pace achieved without signs/symptoms of exercise intolerance can serve as a baseline exercise intensity prescription. Several recent studies with moderate to good methodological quality have supported the effectiveness of incorporating a formal aerobic exercise program during the inpatient treatment of individuals with cancer. Adults receiving chemotherapy and/or radiation who participated in an inpatient walking program (total of 3 to $\geq$ 24 hours) *clinically* improved their quality of life and decreased their cancer-related fatigue, and statistically improved their aerobic functional capacity (or mitigated significant decreases in aerobic functional capacity) compared to individuals who received usual cancer care.[12-17] In studies in which the exercise intensity was measured, the walking program was performed at moderate intensity (50%-70% of age-predicted heart rate maximum, or at an RPE of 12-13).[13,14,17] A study in women 1 to 3 years after breast cancer treatment demonstrated that 2 months of a moderate intensity aerobic exercise program (65%-85% of age-predicted heart rate maximum) may have been too vigorous, resulting in exercise-related fatigue that may have been misinterpreted as cancer-related fatigue.[17] Walking should be encouraged daily with a goal of at least 60 minutes of walking per week *during* cancer treatment. Since all studies to date have used walking interventions, results cannot be generalized to nonambulatory populations or to those who have other comorbidities that prevent walking at requisite heart rates.

Evidence-Based Clinical Recommendations

SORT: Strength of Recommendation Taxonomy

A: Consistent, good-quality patient-oriented evidence

B: Inconsistent or limited-quality patient-oriented evidence

C: Consensus, disease-oriented evidence, usual practice, expert opinion, or case series

1. Following "spinal precautions" decreases the risk of pathological fractures. **Grade C**

2. Physical therapists can use the Six-Minute Walk Test to prescribe a safe, appropriate intensity aerobic exercise program. **Grade B**

3. Light to moderate intensity walking programs (50%-70% of age-predicted heart rate maximum) for $\geq$ 60 minutes per week increase quality of life, decrease cancer-related fatigue, and improve aerobic functional capacity in individuals receiving chemotherapy or radiotherapy for cancer. **Grade A**

COMPREHENSION QUESTIONS

9.1 A physical therapist evaluates a patient in the hospital who is receiving chemotherapy for prostate cancer. Which of the following is *not* an adverse effect typically associated with chemotherapy?

   A. Numbness and tingling in hands and feet

   B. Hair loss

   C. Euphoria

   D. Nausea

9.2 A physical therapist has been working in the hospital with a patient with breast cancer. During the past several treatment sessions, the patient has complained of progressively increasing back pain. Today, the patient complains that her pain is worsened by walking and is spreading to both of her thighs. The *most* appropriate therapist action is to:

   A. Notify the physician immediately about the patient's symptoms and discontinue therapy until the physician has cleared the patient to resume physical therapy

   B. Provide the patient with a walker to decrease weightbearing on the lower extremities

   C. Advise the patient to slightly flex her spine and decrease gait speed when pain increases

   D. Notify the physician after therapy session and note the patient's symptoms in the chart

ANSWERS

9.1 **C.** Antineoplastic drugs are used in multiple combinations to treat cancer. Generally, chemotherapy acts by killing rapidly dividing cells. Normal cells that divide quickly are also affected. When cells in the bone marrow, hair follicles, and epithelial lining of the digestive tract are killed, the most common adverse effects of chemotherapy become evident: hair loss (alopecia), nausea, vomiting, diarrhea, anemia, and immunosuppression (options B and D). Chemotherapy can also have adverse effects on the nervous system as well. Peripheral neuropathies include numbness or paresthesias in the extremities (option A). Physical therapists should anticipate decreased balance and gait deviations if the patient experiences altered sensation in the extremities. Though neuropathies may improve or disappear after discontinuation of chemotherapy, the physical therapist should provide appropriate assistive devices to increase safety and normalize gait pattern. The most common mental and cognitive changes are fatigue and difficulties concentrating and remembering. The latter manifestation is sometimes referred to by patients as "chemo brain."

9.2 **A.** Increasing pain that is worsened by activity—especially weightbearing—should be a major concern in patients with cancer. Bone metastases to the vertebra can lead to pathological fractures. Increasing bilateral thigh pain could be indicative of a current or impending vertebral fracture impinging the spinal cord. The patient's pain complaints should be relayed to the physician immediately and physical therapy should be withheld until medical clearance is received.

REFERENCES

1. American Cancer Society. Available at: www.cancer.org. Accessed May 12, 2010.
2. Lipton A. Management of bone metastases in breast cancer. *Curr Treat Options Oncol.* 2005;6: 161-171.
3. McQuay HJ, Collins SL, Carroll D, et al. Radiotherapy for the palliation of painful bone metastases. *Cochrane Database Syst Rev.* 2000;2:CD001793.
4. Polich S, Paz JC. Oncology. In: Paz JC, West MP, eds. *Acute Care Handbook for Physical Therapists.* 3rd ed. St Louis, MO: Saunders Elsevier; 2009:199-217.
5. Mendoza TR, Wang XS, Cleeland CS, et al. The rapid assessment of fatigue severity in cancer patients: use of the brief fatigue inventory. *Cancer.* 1999;85:1186-1196.
6. Ong KS, Seymour RA. Pain measurement in humans. *Surgeon.* 2004;2:15-27.
7. Seymour RA. The use of pain scales in assessing the efficacy of analgesics in post-operative dental pain. *Eur J Clin Pharmacol.* 1982;23:441-444.
8. Keefe FJ, Schapira B, Williams RB. EMG-assisted relaxation training in the management of chronic low back pain. *Am J Clin Biofeedback.* 1981;4:93-103.
9. Farrar JT, Young JP, LaMoreaux L. Clinical importance of changes in chronic pain intensity measured on an 11-point numerical pain rating scale. *Pain.* 2001;94;149-158.
10. ATS statement: guidelines for the six-minute walk test. *Am J Respir Crit Care Med.* 2002;166: 111-117.
11. Swisher AK, Goldfarb AH. Use of the six-minute walk/run test to predict peak oxygen consumption in older adults. *Cardiopulm Phys Ther.* 1998;9:3-5.

12. Mock V, Frangakis C, Davidson NE, et al. Exercise manages fatigue during breast cancer treatment: a randomized controlled trial. *Psychooncology*. 2005;14:464-477.

13. Monga U, Garber SL, Thornby J, et al. Exercise prevents fatigue and improves quality of life in prostate cancer patients undergoing radiotherapy. *Arch Phys Med Rehabil*. 2007;88:1416-1422.

14. Windsor PM, Nicol KF, Potter J. A randomized, controlled trial of aerobic exercise for treatment-related fatigue in men receiving radical external beam radiotherapy for localized prostate carcinoma. *Cancer*. 2004;101:550-557.

15. Chang PH, Lai YH, Shun SC, et al. Effects of a walking intervention on fatigue-related experiences of hospitalized acute myelogenous leukemia patients undergoing chemotherapy: a randomized controlled trial. *J Pain Symptom Manage*. 2008;35:524-534.

16. Watson T, Mock V. Exercise as an intervention for cancer-related fatigue. *Phys Ther*. 2004;84: 736-743.

17. Daley A, Crank H, Saxton J, et al. Randomized trial of exercise therapy in women treated for breast cancer. *J Clin Oncol*. 2007;25:1713-1721.

Breast Cancer— Status/Post Mastectomy

Barbara E. Nicholson

CASE 10

A 38-year-old female was admitted to the hospital for bilateral modified radical mastectomies with right axillary lymph node dissection secondary to breast cancer. She had 10 right axillary lymph nodes removed. She opted for a prophylactic mastectomy on the left because she is positive for the BRCA1 gene mutation. She is going to have reconstructive breast surgery at a later date. She is a stay-at-home mom with two children who are 2 and 5 years old. She has a supportive husband and her parents live close by and they enjoy watching the children during the day. She has always experienced good health—running 5 times per week and taking yoga classes. Her cancer diagnosis came as quite a shock to her and she is anxious about her appearance, regaining her strength, lymphedema, and her prognosis.

- ▶ How would this individual's contextual factors influence or change your patient management?
- ▶ What precautions should be taken during physical therapy examination and interventions?
- ▶ Identify the psychological factors apparent in this case.
- ▶ Identify referrals to other medical team members.

KEY DEFINITIONS

AXILLARY LYMPH NODE DISSECTION: Surgical removal of lymph nodes from the axilla to remove cancerous cells and for diagnostic purposes

BRCA1 AND BRCA2 GENE MUTATIONS: Normal BRCA1 and BRCA2 genes repair breast cell damage and keep cells growing normally; when these genes mutate, they function abnormally and increase breast cancer risk; BRCA1 and BRCA2 gene mutations cause 5% to 10% of breast cancers[1]

CLASS I COMPRESSION GARMENT: Compression sleeve used in the treatment of upper extremity lymphedema that provides 20 to 30 mm Hg of pressure

LYMPHEDEMA: Abnormal increase of protein-rich fluid in the interstitium that can lead to inflammation, infection, and indurated tissue

MODIFIED RADICAL MASTECTOMY: Removal of breast, surrounding tissue, and lymph nodes that are affected by cancer

PROPHYLACTIC MASTECTOMY: Removal of breast that is not thought to contain cancerous cells in order to reduce the risk for cancer occurring in this region

SENTINEL LYMPH NODE DISSECTION: Biopsy of the first lymph nodes that receive lymphatic drainage from a tumor; if these lymph nodes contain cancerous cells, a more extensive axillary dissection may occur. If sentinel nodes do not contain cancerous cells, then additional nodes do not need to be removed.

SEROMA: Collection of clear serous fluid that may occur after surgery

Objectives

1. Describe lymphedema.
2. Explain appropriate guidelines to reduce the risk of lymphedema.
3. Prescribe an appropriate exercise program for the patient status/post bilateral mastectomy.
4. Identify appropriate medical referrals for the patient status/post mastectomy.

Physical Therapy Considerations

PT considerations during management of the breast cancer survivor status/post bilateral mastectomy with right axillary lymph node dissection:

▶ **General physical therapy plan of care/goals:** Prevent or minimize loss of shoulder range of motion (ROM), and strength; decrease cervical and thoracic pain; decrease scar tissue and fascial restrictions

▶ **Physical therapy interventions:** Patient education on lymphedema risk reduction and appropriate exercise program status/post bilateral mastectomy

▶ **Precautions during physical therapy:** Postsurgical lifting and shoulder ROM precautions

▶ **Complications interfering with physical therapy:** Poor wound healing of mastectomy scar, infection, drainage complications, seroma formation

Understanding the Health Condition

There are 2.6 million breast cancer survivors in the United States.[2] Five to ten percent of breast cancers are positive for the BRCA1 or BRCA2 gene mutations.[1] On average, a woman has a 12% to 13% chance of developing breast cancer. However, women with the BRCA1 or BRCA2 gene mutation have a 60% risk of developing breast cancer.[1] They are also at higher risk for other cancers such as ovarian, melanoma, colon, pancreatic, and thyroid.[1] This particular group of breast cancer survivors may have a prophylactic oophorectomy (to decrease the risk of ovarian cancer) after their breast cancer surgery. These survivors are seeking the best care possible to help them heal from the adverse effects of the disease as well as its treatment. The adverse effects of breast cancer treatment can create functional and physical impairments that can keep these women from doing simple activities such as reaching to turning off an alarm clock to more skilled activities such as tennis, golf, and yoga. Six to twelve months after breast cancer surgery, 50% of women report active shoulder ROM restrictions, pain, and lymphedema.[3] Breast cancer–related lymphedema is a protein-rich swelling that may occur after the removal of axillary lymph nodes. The incidence and severity of this type of lymphedema varies depending on the number of lymph nodes dissected and subsequent treatments. There are two types of axillary dissections a breast surgeon may choose to perform. The first is a sentinel lymph node dissection, which minimizes the number of lymph nodes removed and thus decreases the risk for lymphedema. If these lymph nodes contain cancerous cells, a surgeon will perform an axillary dissection to ensure removal of all cancerous lymph nodes. Risk factors for lymphedema include the number of axillary lymph nodes removed, radiation treatment, infection, lack of mobility, and obesity.[4] The risk for lymphedema with radiation and sentinel lymph node biopsy is 4% to 17%. This risk increases with axillary node dissection and radiation to 33% to 47%.[5] Lymphedema may affect the upper extremity (UE) on the side of the removed lymph nodes and the upper trunk, causing disfigurement, physical discomfort, functional impairments, and emotional distress. Recent research has shown that early treatment of lymphedema can decrease the progression of this chronic condition and allow the patient improved function and mobility.[4]

Physical Therapy Patient/Client Management

Preoperative assessment allows early education and intervention to address shoulder function in patients with breast cancer. A 2010 study with 94 women who underwent surgery for stages I to III breast cancer were preoperatively evaluated by a physical therapist for pain, fatigue, upper limb volume, UE ROM and strength.[6] Subjects were educated on lymphedema risk reduction and given a preoperative postsurgical exercise program to begin when cleared by their surgeon. The women were seen for a total of four visits: preoperatively, 1, 3 to 6, and 12 months after surgery. If a deficit was noted during any visit, then the subject received further physical therapy intervention. At 12 months, 92% of the subjects had full shoulder ROM.[6] Unfortunately, this study did not have a control group that did not receive the intervention. However, a recent Canadian study with 347 women with breast cancer who did *not* receive physical therapy intervention found that 50% of women had shoulder ROM restrictions 6 to 12 months after surgery.[3] Thus, it appears that early physical therapy intervention can be helpful in decreasing UE morbidity in women with breast cancer. Since physical therapists are not always included in the *preoperative* management of this patient population, it is imperative that physical therapists in the acute care setting educate patients on appropriate postsurgical exercise programs and lymphedema risk reduction aimed at reducing future functional limitations. The physical therapist should work closely with the surgeon to determine appropriate timeframes for exercise post-mastectomy and any additional specific precautions for each patient. The surgical removal of both breasts can be a shocking experience for breast cancer survivors. It is important for the physical therapist to work closely with the oncological social worker to refer patients as needed to counseling services and support groups. Patients may also need referrals to outpatient physical therapy for strengthening, ROM lymphedema, scar tissue adhesions, and pain. While there are many barriers to rehabilitation after surgery for breast cancer (*e.g.*, financial, logistical, travel), almost all manual therapies are beneficial to this patient population.[7] The inpatient physical therapist is perfectly poised to provide education about resources available after hospital discharge.

Examination, Evaluation, and Diagnosis

Prior to seeing this patient, the physical therapist should acquire information from her chart regarding mobility, exercise precautions, and lifting restrictions after surgery. If specific information is not in the chart, the therapist must speak with the surgeon for clarification. During the examination, the physical therapist assesses the patient's pain level and active cervical ROM. There is some controversy about *specific* recommendations for early post-mastectomy shoulder ROM as well as the intensity and timing of shoulder mobility exercises.[8] Early shoulder active ROM (usually limited to approximately 90° of flexion and abduction) is described in the literature as beginning the first few days after surgery.[7] The concerns regarding early aggressive ranging of the shoulder relate to potential increased risk of seroma formation, delayed wound healing, and interference with the early regeneration of damaged lymphatic vessels.[8] UE strength testing is contraindicated due to recent surgery and ROM restrictions. The physical therapist should evaluate the patient's understanding of her ROM and lifting precautions. Since the patient has lifting and bilateral UE ROM restrictions, taking care of her young children will be difficult. The physical therapist should ask direct questions regarding the tasks she needs to perform when she is discharged from the hospital. The physical therapist can help her strategize how to successfully perform these tasks, even if this entails advising the patient to have caregivers or family members take over the tasks that would cause her to break her postsurgical precautions. If family members are present during the examination or subsequent therapy sessions, therapists should take this opportunity to reinforce the need for the patient to follow her precautions and the need for assistance to be provided at home (*e.g.*, a family member to temporarily care for the children and cook meals). A patient with bilateral mastectomies will also likely be going home with drains in place. This patient is generally advised to limit her activity until the drains are removed. In the hospital, the physical therapist provides an appropriate exercise program that she can start after drain removal and with her surgeon's clearance. For optimal outcomes, a thorough review of lymphedema risk reduction must occur during the initial evaluation or subsequent treatment.

Plan of Care and Interventions

Specific physical therapy goals are set after the evaluation. Goals related to shoulder ROM and lymphedema risk reduction must be incorporated. Table 10-1 describes typical physical therapy guidelines for UE ROM and strength progression for individuals post-mastectomy.

The acute care physical therapist may be the first person to explain post-mastectomy exercise guidelines to the patient. **In the first few days after surgery, general activity**

Table 10-1   POST-MASTECTOMY UPPER EXTREMITY EXERCISE GUIDELINES[8,12]

Timeframe (Weeks Since Surgery)	Exercises	Precautions/Limitations
0-2	Active movements: shoulder circles, scapular retraction, neck rotation Active assisted shoulder flexion to 90° in supine Hand, wrist, and elbow ROM and strengthening exercises Deep breathing Postural education to limit protective posturing	Limit shoulder flexion to 90° of active assisted ROM for the first few days postsurgery and until the drains are removed, then gradually increase from postoperative day (POD) 3-14 No lifting > 8-11 lb
2-4	Slow progression to full shoulder active ROM Scapular stabilization exercises	No lifting > 11 lb for 2-8 wk postsurgery
4-8	Slow, sustained stretches to enhance full shoulder and trunk ROM Start gentle scar massage Progressive resistance exercise with light weights to increase UE and postural muscle strength	No lifting > 11 lb for2-8 wk postsurgery If full shoulder active ROM is not achieved, patient should consult outpatient physical therapist.

and ROM of the shoulder should be limited.[8] A typical exercise program from POD 3 to POD 14 may include: shoulder circles, active scapular retraction, active neck rotation, active assisted shoulder flexion to 90° in supine and deep breathing. Drains are usually removed when < 25 cc fluid is present over a 24-hour period. This time line varies from patient to patient, but surgeons generally do not leave drains in for longer than 1 month. The goals of these exercises are to maintain ROM of the UE and neck, prevent postural changes, and minimize muscle tension in the neck. The experience of breast cancer is very stressful. During stress, people often breathe shallowly. Encouraging the patient to breathe deeply and slowly can decrease stress and it also encourages rib mobility. Postural education is also important. After removal of a breast, a patient can develop *protective posturing* due to the aesthetic changes of her body. Protective posturing is a slouched position characterized by bilateral shoulder internal rotation, increased upper thoracic kyphosis, and a forward head position. Educating the patient on good posture is helpful to decrease the risk of shoulder impingement and cervical pain. From 2 to 8 weeks postsurgery, the patient can start to gradually progress her shoulder ROM.[8] Appropriate exercises include: active assisted ROM to achieve full shoulder ROM. Progression should emphasize active shoulder flexion, abduction, and external rotation. At 1 to 2 months after mastectomy, slow sustained stretches to enhance shoulder and trunk ROM are appropriate.[8] This is also an appropriate time to teach patients how to perform self-scar massage over the incision site.[8] Low-load resistive exercise can begin, but no lifting greater than 11 lb should occur until after 8 weeks.[8] The physical therapist should educate the patient that if she has not attained full shoulder ROM 8 weeks after surgery and/or if she still has pain and scar tissue tightness, she can get treatment from an outpatient physical therapist to improve these signs and symptoms. If shoulder ROM limitations are left untreated, they can progress to impingement syndrome, adhesive capsulitits, and/or shoulder tendonitis or bursitis. Decreased strength and ROM of the shoulder can also lead to lymphedema.[4]

The physical therapist should thoroughly educate the patient on the signs and symptoms of lymphedema, lymphedema risk reduction, and use of compression garments. Table 10-2 presents specific signs and symptoms that occur with each stage of lymphedema.

Table 10-2 LYMPHEDEMA STAGES[9,10]	
Stage	**Clinical Features**
Stage 0: Latency	Lymphatic vessels and/or nodes have been damaged. Lymphedema is not present.
Stage I: Spontaneously reversible	Limb is swollen and feels heavy. Pitting may occur. Swelling reduces with rest and/or elevation of limb.
Stage II: Spontaneously irreversible	Limb is swollen and spongy. Tissue fibrosis may develop and cause the limb to feel hard. Swelling does not go away with rest and elevation.
Stage III: Lymphostatic elephantiasis	Elephantiasis (extreme, gross enlargement of the limb due to lymphatic system impairment) is present. This rarely occurs in the breast cancer population.

The incidence of breast cancer-related lymphedema ranges from 7% to 47%.[5] It can occur at *any* time after lymph node removal; however, it usually appears 1 to 3 years postoperatively.[4,5] Lymphedema may present as a sensation of soreness, fullness, or heaviness of the UE; a change in size, shape, and/or tissue texture may occur in the affected arm.[5,9] Patients may notice that rings, clothes, or watchbands feel tighter than usual. The physical therapist should educate the patient that if she is noticing these sensations, she should follow-up with her healthcare provider immediately and ask about early treatment for lymphedema. Table 10-3 outlines risk reduction strategies designed by the National Lymphedema Network.

If lymphedema does occur, it is treated with manual lymph drainage, bandaging, compression garments, and exercise. The extent of treatment depends on the stage of lymphedema. If lymphedema is diagnosed early, there is mild

Table 10-3 NATIONAL LYMPHEDEMA NETWORK RISK REDUCTION STRATEGIES[11]	
Skin care Goal: avoid trauma/injury to reduce infection risk	Keep extremity clean and dry. Apply moisturizer daily to prevent chapping. Attention to nail care: do not cut cuticles. Protect skin with sunscreen and insect repellent. Use care with razors to avoid nicks. If possible, avoid punctures, injections and blood draws on affected limb. Wear gloves when doing activities that may cause injury. If scratches/punctures occur, wash with soap, water, apply antibiotic, and observe for signs of infection. With a rash, itching, redness, pain, increased skin temperature, fever or flu-like symptoms, contact physician immediately.
Activity/lifestyle	Gradually progress exercise. Take frequent rest periods during a new activity. Monitor the extremity for changes in size, shape, soreness, heaviness, firmness, and tissue texture. Maintain an optimal weight.
Avoid limb constriction	As possible, avoid having blood pressure taken on the affected side. Wear loose-fitting jewelry and clothing.
Compression garments	Should be well-fitting Support at-risk limb with a compression garment for strenuous activity (*e.g.*, weight-lifting, prolonged standing, running) except in patients with open wounds or with poor circulation in the at-risk limb. Consider wearing well-fitting compression garment for air travel. Avoid exposure to extreme cold, which can be associated with rebound swelling or chapping of skin. Avoid prolonged (> 15 min) exposure to heat, particularly hot tubs and saunas. Avoid placing limb in water temperatures above 102°F (38.9°C).

evidence that treatment can prevent progression to a more advanced stage.[4,5] The **efficacy of compression garments in reducing early stage I UE lymphedema** was recently tested. In 2007, Stout et al.[5] followed 196 female breast cancer survivors to determine the incidence of UE lymphedema and the effectiveness of class I UE compression garments in treating lymphedema. They assessed bilateral UE strength, ROM, and volume preoperatively and 1, 3, 6, 9, 12, and 18 months after breast cancer surgery. Forty-three subjects at some time point in the study were found to have subclinical lymphedema—defined as > 3% upper limb volume increase compared to preoperative measurements. The authors used a sensitive limb volume measuring tool called a Perometer to measure limb volume.[13] When lymphedema was diagnosed, a subject was prescribed a class I compression garment and hand gauntlet to use during the day for 1 month. Measurements were then repeated at 1 month; if edema was reduced, subjects could stop wearing the garment except with strenuous activity and when symptoms of heaviness or visible swelling were present. If symptoms worsened, subjects were advised to follow-up with their physical therapist. Otherwise, they were instructed to wait 3 months for their next limb volume assessment. Subjects who wore the garment daily for 1 month and subsequently later only with strenuous activity had a reduction in follow-up limb volume measurements of 4.1%. This study demonstrated that a short trial of compression garments was effective in treating early stage I lymphedema.[5]

Torres et al.[4] designed a randomized controlled trial to determine the effectiveness of **early physiotherapy in reducing the risk of breast cancer-related lymphedema.** They included 120 women who had breast surgery with axillary node dissection. Each participant was assessed preoperatively and between days 3 and 5 after hospital discharge. Four follow-up visits were scheduled at 1, 3, 6, and 12 months postsurgery. The control group received education on the lymphatic system and lymphedema risk reduction. The intervention group received education on the lymphatic system and lymphedema risk reduction, manual lymph drainage, scar tissue massage, and progressive active shoulder exercise. After 12 months of follow-up, 25% of the control group developed lymphedema, compared with only 7% in the intervention group. Thus, preoperative and postoperative physical therapy could be effective in the prevention of secondary lymphedema. Acute care physical therapists can be the bridge to providing education and key referrals to reduce the risk of breast cancer-related lymphedema.

Evidence-Based Clinical Recommendations

SORT: Strength of Recommendation Taxonomy

A: Consistent, good-quality patient-oriented evidence

B: Inconsistent or limited-quality patient-oriented evidence

C: Consensus, disease-oriented evidence, usual practice, expert opinion, or case series

1. Early shoulder range of motion exercises in the breast cancer population reduces functional impairments in UE ROM and strength. **Grade B**

2. Use of compression garments in early stage lymphedema decreases the risk of progression to more advanced lymphedema. **Grade B**

3. Physical therapy interventions such as shoulder ROM and strengthening exercises, manual lymph drainage, scar massage, and education on lymphedema risk reduction provided before or early after breast cancer surgery reduce the risk of breast cancer-related lymphedema. **Grade A**

COMPREHENSION QUESTIONS

10.1 A patient status/post right axillary lymph node dissection secondary to breast cancer and prophylactic mastectomy on the left is very worried about regaining her shoulder ROM. Her friend has had a frozen shoulder and she does not want this complication along with everything else she is dealing with right now. She has requested that she should begin exercise for her shoulder while she is in the hospital. The *most* appropriate course of action for the physical therapist is to:

A. Start her with full passive shoulder ROM in the hospital.

B. Explain to her that she has to leave her arm by her side for 2 weeks and then follow-up with outpatient physical therapy.

C. Explain to her that she needs to perform very little activity except for gentle hand, wrist, elbow shoulder ROM exercises for 2 to 3 days or until the drains are removed. Give her an appropriate exercise guideline handout.

D. Give her a compression garment.

10.2 The patient in 10.1 mentions that she is terrified about getting lymphedema. Before she had her surgery, she looked on the Internet and she said that the pictures were "horrible." What is the *best* education the physical therapist can provide to the patient to decrease her risk of lymphedema?

A. Stop using the affected arm during all activities.

B. Lymphedema risk reduction guidelines such as proper skin care, avoiding limb restriction, maintaining an active lifestyle and normal weight, and wearing compression garments.

C. Individuals who have mastectomies are not at risk for lymphedema.

D. Place ice on her arm if and when it looks swollen.

ANSWERS

10.1 **C.** There is a typical exercise progression for a patient status/post mastectomy. Passive shoulder ROM should not be performed beyond 90° of flexion in the first 2 to 3 days of surgery because it may interfere with proper healing of lymph vessels and surgical incisions (option A). For the first few days after surgery, the patient can begin gentle exercises, keeping the shoulder below 90° of flexion. An appropriate postoperative mastectomy program is outlined in Table 10-1. Telling a patient to leave her arm by her side for 2 weeks may lead to frozen shoulder and increased tightness throughout the upper trunk region (option B). Compression garments for the UE do not affect shoulder ROM (option D).

10.2 **B.** Explaining to the patient the anatomy and physiology of the lymphatic system, as well as a thorough review of lymphedema risk reduction guidelines may decrease this patient's fear of lymphedema. Education about the lymphatic system, the early signs of lymphedema, and how to get assistance with lymphedema in the early stages is the most beneficial advice. If the patient were to stop using the arm, she would become weak and be at greater risk for lymphedema (option A). Lymphedema risk is *not* dependent on type of breast surgery (option C). It does vary based on the number of lymph nodes removed. Lymphedema is not a swelling due to inflammation (option D). It can occur due to damage to the lymphatic system. Furthermore, cold can cause a rebound swelling that can increase lymphedema.

REFERENCES

1. National Cancer Institute Available at: http://www.cancer.gov/cancertopics/factsheet/Risk/BRCA. Accessed October 19, 2011.

2. National Cancer Institute. Available at: http://seer.cancer.gov/statfacts/html/breast.html. Accessed October 19, 2011.

3. Thomas-MacLean RL, Hack T, Kwan W, et al. Arm morbidity and disability after breast cancer: new directions for care. *Oncol Nurs Forum.* 2008;35:65-71.

4. Torres Lacomba M, Yuste Sanchez MJ, Zapico Goni A, et al. Effectiveness of early physiotherapy to prevent lymphoedema after surgery for breast cancer: randomised, single blinded, clinical trial. *BMJ.* 2010;340:1-8.

5. Stout Gergich N, Pfalzer L, McGarvey C, et al. Preoperative assessment enables the early diagnosis and successful treatment of lymphedema. *Cancer.* 2008;112:2809-2819.

6. Springer BA, Levy E, McGarvey C, et al. Preoperative assessment enables early diagnosis and recovery of shoulder function in patients with breast cancer. *Breast Cancer Res Treat.* 2010;120: 135-147.

7. Cheville AL, Tchou J. Barrier to rehabilitation following surgery for primary breast cancer. *J Surg Oncol.* 2007;95;409-418.

8. Harris S, Campbell K, McNeeley M. Upper extremity rehabilitation for women who have been treated for breast cancer. *Physiother Can.* 2004;56;202-214.

9. National Lymphedema Network. Available at: http://www.lymphnet.org/lymphedemaFAQs/overview.htm. Accessed October 19, 2011.

10. National Cancer Institute. Available at: http://www.cancer.gov/cancertopics/pdq/supportivecare/lymphedema/Patient/page1. Accessed October 19, 2011.

11. National Lymphedema Network. Available at: http://www.lymphnet.org/pdfDocs/nlnriskreduction.pdf. Accessed October 19, 2011

12. Providence Health Systems. Post Breast Surgery Exercise Program: Patient Handouts. Portland, Oregon. Accessed November 2011.

13. Lee MJ, Boland RA, Czerniec S, et al. Reliability and concurrent validity of the perometer for measuring hand volume in women with and without lymphedema. *Lymphat Res Biol*. 2011;9:13-18.

Head and Neck Cancer Status/Post Neck Dissection

Margaret L. McNeely

A 46-year-old male was diagnosed with squamous cell carcinoma of the head and neck. He was admitted to the hospital for surgical excision of the cancerous tumor in the right tonsil region and a right-sided anterolateral selective neck dissection (SND) including Levels I to IV. He works as a manager for a large company, is married, and has a grown son and a teenage daughter. Prior to his diagnosis, he was otherwise healthy, a nonsmoker, and only drank alcohol on an occasional basis. He enjoys running and plays on a men's soccer team. He is right-hand dominant. Testing confirmed that the cancer was positive for human papilloma virus (HPV) P16. The patient is expected to be discharged within the next 5 to 10 days. It is anticipated that the patient will be referred for adjuvant radiation therapy as an outpatient. The physical therapist is asked to evaluate and treat the patient on postoperative day 3 (POD 3).

▶ What are the examination priorities?
▶ What examination signs must be assessed prior to discharge that may indicate spinal accessory nerve damage?
▶ What is his rehabilitation prognosis in terms of neck and shoulder recovery?
▶ Describe a physical therapy plan of care for the shoulder based on the patient's current stage of recovery.

KEY DEFINITIONS

HEAD AND NECK CANCER: Cancers that occur in the head or neck region, including the nasal cavity, sinuses, lips, mouth, salivary glands, throat, or larynx (voice box)[1]

NECK DISSECTION: Surgery to remove lymph nodes and other tissues in the neck[2]

RADIATION THERAPY: Local cancer treatment involving use of high energy x-rays, γ-rays, neutrons, protons, or other sources to destroy cancer cells[2]

SQUAMOUS CELL CARCINOMA: Cancer that begins in the thin, flat squamous cells that are found in tissue that forms the surface of the skin, lining of the hollow organs of the body, and the passages of the respiratory and digestive tracts[2]

Objectives

1. Describe the key sequelae associated with a neck dissection procedure.

2. Identify a valid and reliable outcome tool that can be used to evaluate impairments related to neck dissection.

3. Prescribe appropriate exercises that help minimize impairments in the neck and shoulder in the early rehabilitation period.

4. Describe the goals and objectives of patient education for an individual recovering from neck dissection that involved spinal accessory nerve damage.

Physical Therapy Considerations

PT considerations during management of the individual status/post neck dissection:

▶ **General physical therapy plan of care/goals:** Prevent postsurgical complications (*e.g.*, pneumonia, deep vein thrombosis); prevent or minimize loss of range of motion (ROM) in the neck and shoulder; prevent or minimize pain/discomfort in the region

▶ **Physical therapy interventions:** Patient education regarding sequelae associated with surgery and neck dissection; early mobilization to prevent postsurgical complications; appropriately prescribed exercises for the region based on stage of healing

▶ **Precautions during physical therapy:** Monitor vitals, healing of incision and surgical site; increased swelling; worsening of pain or fatigue; close supervision of exercises

▶ **Complications interfering with physical therapy:** Infection, seroma formation, poor wound healing, pain

Understanding the Health Condition

Head and neck cancer (HNC) is a cancer that develops in the mucosal lining of the oral cavity, oropharynx, hypopharynx, larynx, sinuses, or nasopharynx. The most common histological type is squamous cell carcinoma.[3] In North America, HNCs account for approximately 3% of all malignant tumors.[4] The mean age at diagnosis is 62 years, with more than 90% of cases occurring in individuals over the age of 40 years,[5,6] and a current male-to-female ratio of 3:1.[4] The etiology of most HNC is related to lifestyle factors such as smoking and heavy alcohol consumption.[7] The use of alcohol in conjunction with smoking is estimated to increase the risk of HNC by 2.5 times that of nonsmokers/nondrinkers.[8] Additional risk factors for HNC include viruses, exposure to dust and chemicals, chronic candidal infection, and nutritional and vitamin deficiencies.[7]

The overall incidence of HNC has decreased in the United States over the last number of years, in parallel with the decrease in smoking rates across the country.[3] Over the same time period, however, there has been an increase in the incidence of squamous cell carcinomas of the tonsil and tongue base associated with HPV 16 infection.[3] This trend in increased incidence of HPV-associated HNC has been seen predominantly in white men younger than 50 years of age who have no history of excessive alcohol or tobacco use.[3] Thus, there has been a growing population of patients with HNC who have a less typical demographic and behavioral profile.

The prognosis for HNC depends on the stage at diagnosis and the site of the tumor.[9,10] The 5-year survival rates for early stage (I and II) range from 60% to 95%[9] and late stage (III and IV) range from 0% to 50%.[10] The overall survival rates for HNC have not changed significantly in the last few decades; however, in individuals with HPV-positive HNC, survival and progression-free survival rates are considerably more favorable when compared to HNCs resulting from other etiologies.[3]

Signs and symptoms of HNC normally occur in the region of the primary cancer and are consistent with the tissues affected by the cancer.[11] Typical signs include a sore or ulcer in the mouth that will not heal (*e.g.*, oral cancer), a sore throat that does not go away (*e.g.*, oropharyngeal cancer), a change or hoarseness in the voice (*e.g.*, cancer of larynx), or a lump in the neck (*e.g.*, lymph node metastasis). Reported symptoms associated with HNC may include unintentional weight loss, fatigue, pain, and difficulty swallowing.[11]

Surgery and radiation therapy are both considered curative treatment options for HNC. Surgery remains a primary therapy for resectable tumors and radiation therapy is a localized treatment modality that is an alternative to invasive surgery for many early stage cancers.[12] For more advanced stage cancers, radiation therapy is usually administered following surgery with or without the addition of concomitant chemotherapy.[11] In many cases, HNC can also be treated with primary chemoradiation that has equivalent survival outcomes while avoiding the cosmetic and functional deficits associated with surgery.[11]

Surgical treatment for HNC most often includes dissection of lymph nodes in the neck, which is used for the purpose of tumor staging and/or for the treatment of lymph node metastases.[13] Several lymph node dissection approaches are used for surgical treatment of the neck in patients with HNC (Table 11-1 and Fig. 11-1).[14]

Table 11-1   CLASSIFICATION OF NECK DISSECTIONS

Type	Features	Lymph Node Levels Dissected
Radical neck dissection (RND)	Sacrifice of SAN, IJV, SCM muscle	Removal of lymph nodes in Levels I to V[15]
Modified radical neck dissection (MRND)	Sparing of one or more of SAN, IJV, SCM: the preserved structure is named	Removal of lymph nodes in Levels I to V[15]
Selective neck dissection (SND)[15]	< I-V lymph node Levels removed Nonlymphatic structures not specified	Lateral: removal of lymph nodes in Levels II to IV[15] Anterolateral (supraomohyoid): removal of lymph nodes in Levels I, II, III, ± IV[15] Posterolateral: removal of lymph nodes in Levels II, III, IV, and V[15] Anterior: removal of lymph nodes in Level VI (pretracheal and paratracheal lymph nodes)[15]
Extended neck dissection	Removal of one or more additional nonlymphatic structures beyond those removed in RND	Any of type of neck dissection[15]

Abbreviations: IJV, internal jugular vein; SAN, spinal accessory nerve; SCM, sternocleidomastoid.

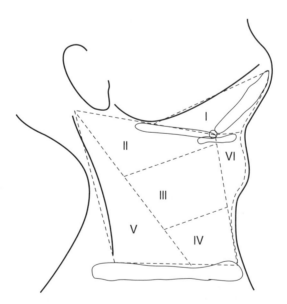

Figure 11-1. Neck dissection is the surgical procedure used to remove contents for the treatment of cervical lymphatic cancers. Neck dissection is classified by six Levels (I-VI), each having specific boundaries and containing specific lymph nodes and anatomical structures. (Reproduced with permission from Lalwani AK, ed. *CURRENT Diagnosis & Treatment in Otolaryngology—Head & Neck Surgery.* 3rd ed. New York, NY: McGraw-Hill; 2012. Figure 28-3.)

Table 11-2   SEQUELAE SPECIFIC TO NECK DISSECTION
Painful incision
Adherent tissue at incision and neck region—development of fibrous cords
Sensory loss in region of head and neck
Discomfort and stiffness in the neck
Cosmetic deficit, if sternocleidomastoid removed
Lymphedema in face and neck
Motor nerve damage (spinal accessory nerve)
Trapezius muscle atrophy: change in contour of neck and shoulder
Discomfort and stiffness in the shoulder
Impaired muscular strength in upper extremity
Functional and activity limitations

Acute sequelae associated with neck dissection include pain, sensory loss, neck and shoulder stiffness, and lymphedema (Table 11-2). The most notable long-term sequelae observed in patients who have undergone neck dissection, however, are related to the removal of, or damage to the spinal accessory nerve (SAN).[14]

The SAN, or cranial nerve XI, functions as a motor nerve for the trapezius and sternocleidomastoid muscles.[16] For the purposes of describing the neck dissection procedure, the neck is divided into six distinct anatomical lymph node levels.[14] Levels II and V are of particular importance in terms of impact on neck and shoulder function.[17] The Level II region includes the upper third of lymph nodes resting along the internal jugular vein and found within the tissue located medial to the sternocleidomastoid muscle.[14] Level V includes lymph nodes contained in the posterior cervical triangle.[14] The spinal accessory nerve passes through Levels II and V and the nerve is in close proximity to lymph nodes in these two levels. When a patient undergoes a neck dissection procedure that includes removal of lymph nodes from either or both of these two levels (even if the nerve is spared during the procedure), the SAN is vulnerable to operative injury.[18] With complete SAN lesions due to sacrifice of the nerve (neurectomy) that occurs with a radical neck dissection, full recovery of trapezius muscle function is unlikely.[18,19] It is estimated that 60% to 100% of these patients will have an ongoing shoulder syndrome (termed a radical neck syndrome) that includes pain and dysfunction in the shoulder region and permanent trapezius muscle denervation.[18-21]

Nerve-sparing procedures such as the modified radical neck dissection (MRND) are used in an attempt to preserve trapezius function and prevent this syndrome.[20] The probability of postoperative trapezius paresis after nerve-sparing procedures is estimated to be between 20% and 60%[18,22,23] because damage to the nerve may still occur due to trauma to the nerve during the dissection procedure.[22,24] In the case of these nerve-sparing neck dissection procedures, the impairment of SAN function is most often transient, with full nerve recovery expected within 12 to 18 months.[18,22] The lateral and anterolateral SND techniques that do not involve dissection of Level V of the neck are associated with less shoulder and neck morbidity when compared to neck dissection techniques that include dissection of level V (*e.g.*, MRND and posterolateral SND).[25,26]

Neck-related impairments following neck dissection include pain or discomfort in the neck region and stiffness with movement. The tightness or stiffness of the neck is often described as a pressing or choking sensation.[27] Some patients describe the tightness as if there is a "tight band or collar around the neck." If the sterno-cleidomastoid is removed during surgery, the patient will have visible depression in the tissues of the neck and movements such as contralateral neck rotation and antigravity neck flexion (*e.g.*, rising from supine) may be compromised.

Initial shoulder impairments following neck dissection surgery include pain, weakness, and limitation in active shoulder movement.[23,28] Although passive shoulder ROM is initially intact, shoulder stiffness may begin to develop within a few weeks after surgery.[29,30] If the SAN has been damaged during the surgical procedure, progressive atrophy of the trapezius muscle will occur over a 6- to 12-week period following surgery. The trapezius muscle is the primary passive support for the shoulder, and consequently, if denervated, the entire shoulder girdle drops downward (depresses) and forward (protracts) and leads to the classic "droop" seen in the shoulder.[18,19,29] The resulting change in the contour of the neckline is often the first sign noticed by the patient. Loss of trapezius function results in weakness in shoulder shrugging, winging of the medial border of the scapula, and limitation in shoulder abduction to 90°.[8,23] Functionally, the impaired ROM at the shoulder causes difficulty in simple tasks such as combing the hair, putting on clothing, and reaching for objects overhead.[28]

Evidence suggests that if signs and symptoms occur after neck dissection, they tend to persist rather than improve and are often *independent* of SAN status.[31] In a recent study of patients undergoing neck dissection, a cluster of signs including shoulder droop and limited active shoulder abduction and flexion ROM at the time of hospital discharge were found to predict mid- to long-term scapular dysfunction.[32] Moreover, the authors found that a separate cluster of symptoms and signs including shoulder pain and limitation in active external rotation were predictive of mid- to long-term glenohumeral joint dysfunction.[32]

Physical Therapy Patient/Client Management

Initial treatment goals in the early days following surgery are focused on mobilizing the patient to prevent postoperative complications.[33] Once the drains have been removed from the surgical site (POD 2-6) or on approval from the surgeon, gentle ROM exercises can be introduced for the neck and shoulder to help minimize pain and prevent stiffness.[11,27,34]

Examination, Evaluation, and Diagnosis

Ideally, the examination of the neck and shoulder should occur preoperatively. Although some deficits may exist prior to surgery due to the individual's age, pre-existing conditions, and the cancer itself, this assessment provides valuable baseline information on which to inform outcomes and follow-up care. Moreover, this session provides the opportunity for education on the importance of postoperative physical

Table 11-3 PATIENT EDUCATION FOCUS	
Education Goals	Education Objectives
• Improve knowledge of sequelae associated with surgery and neck dissection • Increase understanding of the need for and benefit of physical therapy and exercises following surgery • Facilitate ongoing management (including self-management) of sequelae associated with neck dissection	• Have patients understand how to identify sequelae early and when/how to report to the healthcare team • Improve adherence to preventative and maintenance treatment programs and strategies • Reduce secondary complications and overall rehabilitation time

therapy and for teaching postoperative exercises. Table 11-3 outlines the focus of patient education that should ideally occur before the scheduled neck dissection. Even if the patient was provided this education before the surgery, given the volume of information provided preoperatively, the acute care physical therapist should review this education with the patient after the surgery.

Prior to seeing the patient after neck dissection surgery, the physical therapist should obtain detailed information from the medical chart on the type and location of the cancer, the surgery performed including the type of neck dissection, the structures removed and/or preserved during the procedure, and the course of recovery following surgery. Depending on the patient's stage of healing, the physical therapist should perform a thorough examination of general mobility, posture, and cervical spine and shoulder ROM. The assessment should also include measurements of scapular positioning to assess for early signs of trapezius paresis and evaluation of neck and shoulder pain via a numerical rating scale or visual analog scale.

The Neck Dissection Impairment Index (NDII) was developed to measure factors that affect quality of life (QOL) after neck dissection.[35] The NDII is a reliable and valid self-report questionnaire for assessing neck dissection-related impairment. The questionnaire is easy to administer and takes around 5 minutes for the patient to complete. Individual items from the 10-question NDII are scored on a 5-point Likert-type scale with higher scores representing better QOL.[35] The total NDII score is scaled to a 100-point cumulative score. To evaluate changes in the early postoperative period, the NDII can be administered by the physical therapist prior to discharge from the hospital and scores compared to those collected preoperatively.

Plan of Care and Interventions

The physical therapist must provide the patient with specific recommendations regarding positions or activities that should be adopted and avoided. Table 11-4 outlines specific education that should be provided within days after the neck dissection. For this patient, the neck dissection included clearing of lymph nodes in Level II and therefore he is at risk of developing postoperative trapezius paresis.

Table 11-4 EDUCATION FOR THE PATIENT STATUS/POST NECK DISSECTION	
Components	Details
Pathology and consequences of SAN damage	• Understand expected changes in neck and shoulder region that may occur following surgery (*e.g.*, progressive trapezius atrophy may occur over a period of 6-12 weeks following surgery) • Understand length of time needed for full nerve recovery (~12-18 months) • Reinforce the importance of exercises to maintain neck and shoulder ROM • Highlight importance of proper posture and need for reminders to correct positioning
Do's and don'ts	• Encourage supportive positions (*e.g.*, use arm rest, lectern for reading, keep hand on hip or supported in pocket when standing or walking for long periods) • Avoid traction on shoulder complex (*e.g.*, carrying heavy objects) • Avoid prolonged overhead activities. Choose alternate strategies (*e.g.*, place frequently used objects on lower shelves)

In his case, the physical therapist should emphasize the length of time needed for full nerve recovery (~12-18 months) and how the loss of trapezius function (should it occur) may impact his work and lifestyle activities. In the short-term (next 4-6 months), alternatives to running such as cycling on a recumbent bike are recommended to avoid traction on the shoulder complex. When transitioning back to running and sports, he may benefit from a shoulder orthosis to assist in maintaining alignment of the shoulder. In planning return to work, suggestions may include ergonomic evaluation of his desk or work station. Because he is right-hand dominant, an adjustable forearm support may be attached to his desk to reduce the strain on his neck and shoulder when using his computer mouse or keyboard.

The course of recovery following neck dissection surgery can be variable and is best approached in a progressive manner based on the stage of tissue healing. Table 11-5 outlines physical therapy goals and recommended interventions from POD 1 to 1 year after neck dissection.

Recovery is dependent on severity of injury to the SAN. In general, postsurgical recovery can be divided into four phases: acute (~3-6 weeks), subacute (third week to ~3-6 months), nerve recovery (~5-6 months, when early signs of nerve regeneration are evident) and chronic phase (~18 months, when the reinnervation potential of the SAN has peaked). In the acute rehabilitation phase, the main principle of treatment is to protect the shoulder and maintain glenohumeral joint integrity. Goals following hospital discharge (acute and subacute recovery phases) include preventing shoulder droop, reducing or eliminating pain, avoiding pectoralis muscle

Table 11-5   PLAN OF CARE FOR THE SHOULDER AND NECK STATUS/POST NECK DISSECTION

Time Period Relative to Surgery	Aim of Physical Therapy	Suggested Interventions	Special Considerations
Acute: early postoperative phase (POD 1-3, or until drains are removed)	Early general mobilization—prevention of complications (e.g., pneumonia, DVT)	• Gentle active ROM of shoulder with limits in elevation (e.g., to 90°) while drains are in place • Assess mobility • Provide chest physical therapy, ambulation aids as needed	• Approval of surgeon needed • Monitor vitals • Complications: seroma formation, infection • Acute edema in face and neck
Acute: early rehabilitation phase (POD 3-6, or following removal of drains and for the next 3-6 wk)	Optimize healing of incision site and lymphatic vessels Prevention of adhesive capsulitis in shoulder	• Introduction of gentle active ROM exercises for neck and shoulder in supported positions • Active scapular retraction and elevation exercises (no resistance) • Postural correction	• Observe stage of healing (e.g., gentle neck ROM at POD 6, if appropriate) • Provide education and home exercise program • Monitor for signs of trapezius dysfunction and glenohumeral joint restriction • Facilitate referral for outpatient physical therapy
Subacute rehabilitation phase: no signs of active trapezius muscle contraction (weeks 3-16 or longer)	Maintenance of passive glenohumeral ROM Prevention of adaptive muscle tightness (pectorals) Prevention of stretch weakness in compensatory muscles (rhomboids and levator scapula)	• Passive/active assisted glenohumeral ROM • Stretching of pectoralis muscles, serratus anterior, latissmus dorsi, subscapularis • Strengthening of rhomboids, levator scapulae, biceps, triceps, infraspinatus, teres minor in supported positions • Postural education	• Cueing for correct posture often needed • Impaired kinesthetic awareness of the position of scapula • Consider taping or shoulder orthosis if RND or neck dissection includes Level V (posterior triangle)
Nerve recovery phase: signs of active trapezius muscle contraction (weeks 12-52 or longer)	Retraining of trapezius muscle	• Inner range "holds" for movements of scapular elevation and retraction • Bilateral exercises • Modify exercises to emphasize activation of trapezius muscle • Progress to "overhead" movements and functional activities when active abduction ROM is restored	• Start this phase when early signs of active trapezius muscle contraction (e.g., trace contraction) are noted: recovery may be evident as early as 3 months (e.g., after SND that avoids Level V) or be delayed to >12 months (e.g., after MRND that includes Levels II and V) • Limit repetitions: watch for quality of trapezius muscle contraction

contracture, and improving scapular stabilization by strengthening alternative muscles to compensate for the functional loss of the trapezius muscle.[19] For patients with persistent pain, a **shoulder orthosis** that optimizes the alignment of the shoulder and scapula (*e.g.*, Akman-Sari orthosis) may be recommended to support the shoulder complex and minimize the droop.[36]

In the recovery phase when early signs of active trapezius muscle contraction are evident, the focus of exercise is on trapezius muscle retraining and strengthening. Once nerve recovery is complete, or further recovery is not anticipated, ongoing exercise should focus on optimizing scapular positioning and strengthening with movement for return to desired (and, if necessary, modified) leisure and work-related activities.

Published physical therapy treatment regimens vary from simple ROM exercises to programs that include therapeutic exercise, manual therapy, and the use of electrotherapeutic modalities.[19,24,28-30] A recent review of the literature reported that while physical therapy interventions for SAN dysfunction related to HNC surgery were well tolerated, evidence was limited by a lack of research examining interventions in the early postoperative period.[37] However, a study of patients with thyroid cancers provides some evidence in support of early intervention. In this study, **active neck stretching exercises** were introduced on the first day following neck dissection and were found to improve neck symptoms in both the short- and long-term.[27] In the HNC population, **glenohumeral ROM exercises and progressive resistance exercise** training have been shown to be beneficial in improving shoulder pain and dysfunction when carried out in the postsurgical subacute or subsequent recovery phases following surgery.[38,39]

Evidence-Based Clinical Recommendations

SORT: Strength of Recommendation Taxonomy

A: Consistent, good-quality patient-oriented evidence

B: Inconsistent or limited-quality patient-oriented evidence

C: Consensus, disease-oriented evidence, usual practice, expert opinion, or case series

1. A shoulder orthosis that optimizes scapular and shoulder alignment reduces shoulder pain associated with trapezius paresis. **Grade B**

2. Active neck stretching introduced in the early days following neck dissection surgery reduces neck-related symptoms. **Grade B**

3. Shoulder ROM exercises with progressive resistance exercises in the subacute post-neck dissection recovery phase reduce shoulder pain and dysfunction. **Grade B**

COMPREHENSION QUESTIONS

11.1 A physical therapist in the acute care hospital evaluates a patient 10 days following a neck dissection procedure for oropharyngeal cancer. Which of the following is *not* a presentation typically associated with spinal accessory nerve injury?

A. Step deformity

B. Scapular winging

C. Drooping of the shoulder

D. Limited active shoulder abduction range of motion

11.2 A physical therapist has prescribed a home exercise for a patient with right-sided spinal accessory neurapraxia who is being discharged on POD 14 following surgery including a neck dissection procedure. Which of the following is the *most* appropriate focus of shoulder exercises at this time point in recovery?

A. Gentle cervical spine ROM and active shoulder elevation ≤90°

B. Active antigravity shoulder flexion and abduction ROM

C. Gentle exercises to prevent adaptive muscle shortening of pectoral muscles and to maintain glenohumeral joint ROM

D. Active glenohumeral joint abduction against gravity and exercises to improve trapezius muscle strength and restore scapulohumeral rhythm

ANSWERS

11.1 **A.** The classic signs of spinal accessory nerve damage resulting in trapezius paresis include shoulder droop, winging of the scapula, and limited shoulder abduction to ≤ 90°. Other signs include changes in the resting position of scapula (*i.e.*, resting in a downward and protracted position), atrophy of trapezius resulting in a change in contour of the neck line, and symptoms of pain with movement of the shoulder overhead.

11.2 **C.** In the early postoperative period, symptoms of adhesive capsulitis may develop due to lack of movement of the glenohumeral joint and the protective posturing of the head and trunk (forward head posture and rounded shoulders). Initially, the individual may be reluctant to move due to pain and fear of opening the incision. Gentle shoulder ROM with limits in extent of movement (*e.g.*, ≤ 90°) and delayed cervical spine ROM (until drains are removed) are recommended. After hospital discharge, the focus should be on maintaining passive glenohumeral joint movement, preventing secondary changes such as adaptive muscle shortening of the pectorals, and strengthening of alternative muscles to compensate for the functional loss of trapezius. Active abduction against gravity in the coronal plane is ultimately limited by the trapezius muscle paresis (*i.e.*, lack of upward rotation of the scapula) and is dependent on recovery of the spinal accessory nerve. To prevent a secondary impingement syndrome, the movement of abduction against gravity should be avoided until it can be performed with proper scapular motion and no winging.

REFERENCES

1. Argiris A, Eng C. Epidemiology, staging, and screening of head and neck cancer. In: Brockstein B, Masters G, editors. *Head and neck cancer*. New York, NY: Kluwer Academic Publishers; 2003.

2. National Cancer Institute NC. Dictionary of Cancer Terms. http://www.cancer.gov/dictionary. Accessed May 18, 2012.

3. Marur S, D'Souza G, Westra WH, et al. HPV-associated head and neck cancer: a virus-related cancer epidemic. *Lancet Oncol*. 2010;11:781-789.

4. Siegel R, Ward E, Brawley O, et al. Cancer statistics, 2011: the impact of eliminating socioeconomic and racial disparities on premature cancer deaths. *CA Cancer J Clin*. 2011;61:212-236.

5. Mood D. Cancers of the head and neck. In: Varricchio C, ed. A cancer source book for nurses: American Cancer Society Professional Education Publication; 1997:271-272.

6. Hammerlid E, Taft C. Health-related quality of life in long-term head and neck cancer survivors: a comparison with general population norms. *Br J Cancer*. 2001;84:149-156.

7. Clarke LK. Rehabilitation for the head and neck cancer patient. *Oncology*. 1998;12:81-94.

8. Roberts WL. Rehabilitation of the Head and Neck Cancer Patient. In: McGarvey C, ed. *Rehabilitation of the Cancer Patient*. New York: Churchill Livingstone;1990.

9. Masters G, Brockstein B. Overview of Head and Neck Cancer. In: Masters G, Brockstein B, editors. *Head and Neck Cancer*. New York: Kluwar Academic Publishers; 2003.

10. Semple CJ, Sullivan K, Dunwoody L, Kernohan WG. Psychosocial interventions for patients with head and neck cancer. *Cancer Nurs*. 2004;27:434-441.

11. Locati L, Patel S, Pfister DG. Evaluation and treatment of head and neck cancer. In: Stubblefield MD, O'Dell MW, eds. *Cancer rehabilitation: Principles and practice*. New York, NY: Demos Medical; 2009.

12. Hinerman RW, Mendenhall WM, Amdur RJ. Radiation therapy in the management of early-stage head and neck cancer. In: Brockstein B, Masters G, eds. *Head and neck cancer*. New York, NY: Kluwar Academic Publishers; 2003.

13. Nori S, Soo KC, Green RF, et al. Utilization of intraoperative electroneurography to understand the innervation of the trapezius muscle. *Muscle Nerve*. 1997;20:279-285.

14. Medina J. Neck dissection. In: Bailey BJ, ed. *Head and neck surgery—otolaryngology*. Philadelphia, PA: Lippincott Williams and Wilkins; 2006:1595-1610.

15. Medina JE, American Academy of Otolaryngology—Head and Neck Surgery. Selective neck dissections [videorecording]. Washington, DC: American Academy of Otolaryngology—Head and Neck Surgery; 1987.

16. Fehrenbach MJ, Herring SW. *Illustrated anatomy of the head and neck*. 2nd ed. Philadelphia, PA: W.B. Saunders; 2002.

17. Taylor JC, Terrell JE, Ronis DL, et al. University of Michigan Head and Neck Cancer Team. Disability in patients with head and neck cancer. *Arch Otolaryngol Head Neck Surg*. 2004;130:764-769.

18. Remmler D, Byers R, Scheetz J, et al. A prospective study of shoulder disability resulting from radical and modified neck dissections. *Head Neck Surg*. 1986;8:280-286.

19. Villanueva R, Ajmani C. The role of rehabilitation medicine in physical restoration of patients with head and neck cancer. *The Cancer Bulletin*.1977;29:46-54.

20. Hillel A, Patten C. Neck dissection: morbidity and rehabilitation. *Cancer Treat Res*. 1990;52: 133-147.

21. Nahum AM, Mullally W, Marmor L. A syndrome resulting from radical neck dissection. *Arch Otolaryngol*.1961;74:82-86.

22. Koybasioglu A, Tokcaer AB, Uslu S, et al. Accessory nerve function after modified radical and lateral neck dissections. *Laryngoscope*. 2000;110:73-77.

23. Patten C, Hillel AD. The 11th nerve syndrome. Accessory nerve palsy or adhesive capsulitis? *Arch Otolaryngol Head Neck Surg*. 1993;119:215-220.

24. Gordon SL, Graham WP, 3rd, Black JT, et al. Accessory nerve function after surgical procedures in the posterior triangle. *Arch Surg.*1977;112:264-268.

25. Cappiello J, Piazza C, Giudice M, et al. Shoulder disability after different selective neck dissections (levels II-IV versus levels II-V): a comparative study. *Laryngoscope*. 2005;115:259-263.

26. Terrell JE, Welsh DE, Bradford CR, et al. Pain, quality of life, and spinal accessory nerve status after neck dissection. *Laryngoscope*. 2000;110:620-626.

27. Takamura Y, Miyauchi A, Tomoda C, et al. Stretching exercises to reduce symptoms of postoperative neck discomfort after thyroid surgery: prospective randomized study. *World J Surg*. 2005;29:775-779.

28. Herring D, King AI, Connelly M. New rehabilitation concepts in management of radical neck dissection syndrome. A clinical report. *Phys Ther.*1987;67:1095-1099.

29. Saunders WH, Johnson EW. Rehabilitation of the shoulder after radical neck dissection. *Ann Otol Rhinol Laryngol*. 1975;84:812-816.

30. Johnson EW, Aseff JN, Saunders W. Physical treatment of pain and weakness following radical neck dissection. *Ohio State Med J*. 1978;74:711-714.

31. van Wilgen CP, Dijkstra PU, van der Laan BF, et al. Shoulder complaints after neck dissection; is the spinal accessory nerve involved? *Br J Oral Maxillofac Surg*. 2003;41:7-11.

32. Stuiver MM, van Wilgen CP, de Boer EM, et al. Impact of shoulder complaints after neck dissection on shoulder disability and quality of life. *Otolaryngol Head Neck Surg*. 2008;139:32-39.

33. Packel L. Oncological diseases and disorders. In: Malone DJ, Bishop Lindsay KL, eds. *Physical therapy in acute care: A clinician's guide*. Thorofare, NJ: Slack Incorporated; 2006.

34. Tuohy SM, Savodnik A. Postsurgical rehabilitation in cancer. In: Stubblefield MD, O'Dell MW, eds. *Cancer Rehabilitation:Principles and Practice*. New York, NY: Demos Medical; 2009.

35. Taylor RJ, Chepeha JC, Teknos TN, et al. Development and validation of the neck dissection impairment index: a quality of life measure. *Arch Otolaryngol Head Neck Surg*. 2002;128:44-49.

36. Kizilay A, Kalcioglu MT, Saydam L, et al. A new shoulder orthosis for paralysis of the trapezius muscle after radical neck dissection: a preliminary report. *Eur Arch Otorhinolaryngol*. 2006;263:477-480.

37. McGarvey AC, Chiarelli PE, Osmotherly PG, et al. Physiotherapy for accessory nerve shoulder dysfunction following neck dissection surgery: a literature review. *Head Neck*. 2011;33:274-280.

38. McNeely ML, Parliament M, Courneya KS, et al. A pilot study of a randomized controlled trial to evaluate the effects of progressive resistance exercise training on shoulder dysfunction caused by spinal accessory neurapraxia/neurectomy in head and neck cancer survivors. *Head Neck*. 2004;26:518-530.

39. McNeely ML, Parliament MB, Seikaly H, et al. Effect of exercise on upper extremity pain and dysfunction in head and neck cancer survivors: a randomized controlled trial. *Cancer*. 2008;113: 214-222.

Myocardial Infarction

Ronald De Vera Barredo

A 54-year-old office executive went to the emergency department complaining of sudden chest and left arm pain. He is pale, diaphoretic, and reports feeling nauseated. Differential diagnoses include gastric and musculoskeletal etiologies, myocardial infarction, pericarditis, and myocarditis. The 12-lead electrocardiogram readings indicate ST segment elevation in the anterior leads V1-6, I, and aVL, and reciprocal ST segment depression in the inferior leads. Cardiac enzymes reveal elevated levels of creatine kinase-MB (CK-MB) and troponin. Cardiac catheterization revealed an obstruction of the anterior descending branch of the left coronary artery. The patient was immediately scheduled for and underwent coronary artery bypass graft (CABG) surgery without complications. Relevant inpatient medications postsurgery include a statin, β-adrenergic blocker, and an angiotensin-converting enzyme (ACE) inhibitor. After an overnight stay in the critical care unit, the patient was transferred to the acute care ward. He was referred to physical therapy for phase I (inpatient) cardiac rehabilitation with an anticipated hospital discharge within 5 days. The patient lives with his wife and two teenage children. He smokes one pack of cigarettes per day and has elevated blood pressure and cholesterol levels. He also has diabetes mellitus and a history of atherosclerosis and coronary artery disease.

▶ What are the most appropriate examination tests?
▶ What are the examination priorities?
▶ What are the most appropriate physical therapy interventions?
▶ What precautions should be taken during physical therapy examination and/or interventions?
▶ What is his rehabilitation prognosis?

KEY DEFINITIONS

ATHEROSCLEROSIS: Plaque build-up in the arteries

CARDIAC CATHETERIZATION: Medical procedure in which a long, thin, flexible tube is inserted into a blood vessel (usually in the groin) and threaded to the heart vessels; performed to diagnose and/or treat certain cardiac conditions

CORONARY ARTERY BYPASS GRAFT (CABG): Surgical procedure involving removal of a portion of a vein or artery and grafting this vessel onto a blocked coronary artery to re-establish arterial patency

CORONARY ARTERY DISEASE (CAD): Atherosclerosis in the coronary arteries

CREATINE KINASE-MB (CK-MB): Isoenzyme more specific for cardiac muscle; extent of its elevation in serum reflects extent of cardiac muscle infarcted

Objectives

1. Describe the pathophysiology of myocardial infarction.
2. Discuss the role of diagnostic tests in determining the presence of myocardial infarction.
3. Describe the role of medications post-CABG surgery.
4. Explain the multidisciplinary approach to cardiac rehabilitation and the role of physical therapy during phase I cardiac rehabilitation.
5. Describe the utility of activity evaluation, endurance evaluation, and walk tests in early cardiac rehabilitation.
6. Design an appropriate plan of care for the patient in phase I cardiac rehabilitation.

Physical Therapy Considerations

PT considerations during management of the individual status/post myocardial infarction in phase I cardiac rehabilitation:

▸ **General physical therapy plan of care/goals:** Increase exercise tolerance and functional capacity, maximize functional independence and safety while minimizing secondary impairments, manage risk factors associated with the condition

▸ **Physical therapy interventions:** Patient and caregiver education regarding risk factor reduction; range of motion and functional training exercises, endurance training; graded exercise test prior to discharge

▸ **Precautions during physical therapy:** Cardiac precautions; close symptom monitoring; consistent monitoring of vital signs, especially blood pressure (BP); recognize potential adverse drug reactions (ADRs) of cardiac medications

▸ **Complications interfering with physical therapy:** Orthostatic hypotension, abnormal physiologic response to exercise, left ventricular dysfunction, heart failure, ventricular arrhythmias, low functional capacity

Understanding the Health Condition

Atherosclerosis is a disease in which plaque builds up in the arteries.[1] When athero-sclerosis occurs in the coronary arteries, CAD takes place. The plaque build-up from CAD impedes the flow of oxygenated blood to the heart. As the compromised blood flow through the coronary arteries fails to meet the oxygen needs of myocardial tissue, ischemia occurs, resulting in symptoms and signs such as chest pain (angina), diaphoresis, and nausea. In general, this occurs when narrowing of the coronary arteries is greater than 75%.[2] The anterior descending branch of the left coronary artery supplies the left ventricle, the chamber of the heart with the greatest workload. Untreated blockage leads to permanent heart damage, if the individual does not die first, which is why blockage of the anterior descending branch of the left coronary artery is often referred to as the "widow maker."[3]

Patients who experience angina due to CAD may undergo a number of tests. The first step is to rule out a myocardial infarction (heart attack) or some life-threatening condition using tests such as blood enzyme levels, electrocardiogram (ECG), and chest x-ray.[4] Elevation of several enzymes in the serum have traditionally been considered specific to cardiac injury, including CK-MB and cardiac troponins. Cardiac troponin I (TnI) and cardiac troponin T (TnT) are now being used instead of, or along with, the standard markers. TnI is specific for myocardial ischemia and TnT is specific to myo-cardial injury. One of the following numbered criteria satisfies the diagnosis of an acute, evolving, or recent MI: (1) typical rise and gradual fall (troponin) or more rapid rise and fall (CK-MB) of biochemical markers of myocardial necrosis with at least one of the fol-lowing: (a) ischemic symptoms, (b) development of pathologic Q waves on the ECG, (c) ECG changes indicative of ischemia (ST segment elevation or depression), or (d) coronary artery intervention (*e.g.*, coronary angioplasty); (2) pathologic findings of an acute MI.[3,5] Electrocardiography is a painless noninvasive test that assesses the electrical activity of the heart. Cardiac problems can manifest as abnormal rhythms consistent with the condition. For example, in the case study presented, ST segment elevation in the anterior leads V1-6, I and aVL, and reciprocal ST depression in the inferior leads is consistent with acute anterior myocardial infarction.[6]

Cardiac catheterization is a medical procedure used to diagnose and/or treat car-diac certain conditions using a long, thin, flexible tube that is usually inserted into a blood vessel in the groin and threaded to the heart. A special dye that shows up on x-ray can be released from the catheter. As the dye moves through the coronary arteries, the extent or severity of arterial blockage can be determined. This is known as cardiac angiography.[7] Catheterization can allow physicians to improve blood flow by performing a percutaneous transluminal coronary angioplasty (PTCA) in which a balloon catheter is positioned in the area of blockage and inflated so that the plaque is pushed against the arterial wall, increasing the diameter of the vessel. To prevent reblockage of the coronary arteries, stents are used.[8] When the blockage(s) cannot be treated with angioplasty, CABG is another intervention for revascular-ization. CABG surgery is performed to relieve angina in patients who have failed medical therapy and are not good candidates for angioplasty. CABG surgery is ideal for patients with multiple narrowings in multiple coronary artery branches, which is commonly observed in patients with diabetes. CABG surgery has been shown to improve long-term survival in patients with significant narrowing of the left main coronary artery, and in patients with significant narrowing of multiple arteries, especially in those with decreased heart muscle pump function.[9] Also referred to as aorto-coronary bypass (ACG) surgery, CABG uses autogenous saphenous vein or arterial grafts (usually the internal thoracic/mammary artery or occasionally the radial or gastroepiploic artery) to bypass stenotic lesions of the coronary arteries.[10]

After CABG surgery, postoperative medications are given to decrease the workload on the heart. These commonly include: statins to lower blood cholesterol levels, β-blockers to decrease heart rate and blood pressure and decrease the heart's demand for oxygen, and ACE inhibitors to treat high blood pressure. Other medications may be given on a short-term basis to prevent the development of an irregular heart rate (anti-arrhythmics), to manage discomfort associated with healing incisions (analgesics), or to allow for regular bowel movements (laxatives and/or stool softeners).

Patients who have undergone cardiac surgeries such as CABG participate in cardiac rehabilitation as part of their treatment regimen. **Cardiac rehabilitation** is a medically supervised program that helps improve the health and well-being of people who have heart problems including, but not limited to, those who have had: myocardial infarctions, cardiac conditions (*e.g.*, CAD, angina, or heart failure), and cardiac surgeries such as bypass grafts, angioplasties, and stents.[11-13] As a multidisciplinary program to promote physical, social, and psychological function, cardiac rehabilitation is guided by the following four objectives: stratification of risk, improvement of emotional well-being and psychological factors, reduction of CAD risk factors, and minimization of symptoms.[13] Cardiac rehabilitation progresses through three phases. Phase I is the inpatient hospitalization phase consisting of preventative and rehabilitative services to patients after a cardiac event. Phase II is a supervised outpatient exercise program phase generally within the first 3 to 6 months after the event, but continuing for as much as 1 year after the event. Phase III is the maintenance phase that provides longer term delivery of preventative and rehabilitative services for patients in the outpatient/community setting. Depending on the phase, the program may include a medical evaluation, a physical activity evaluation, counseling and education, and/or support and training.[11,12,14]

There are proven beneficial outcomes for cardiac rehabilitation. **Cardiac rehabilitation has been shown to improve exercise tolerance and exercise capacity among men and women regardless of age.** Improvements in lipid and lipoprotein levels, angina, and left ventricular failure have been demonstrated. The multifactorial approach of cardiac rehabilitation programs has exerted a positive effect on body weight management, blood pressure, smoking reduction, stress reduction, and social adjustment and functioning. For those individuals who participate, evidence suggests that cardiac rehabilitation reduces mortality. However, this outcome is not attributable to the exercise alone, but rather to the multifactorial nature of cardiac rehabilitation programs.[11,15]

Physical Therapy Patient/Client Management

After an uncomplicated CABG surgery, patients typically stay in the intensive care unit for 1 to 2 days. The patient is then moved to a step-down unit for 3 to

5 days before going home. While hospitalized, the patient begins inpatient (phase I) cardiac rehabilitation. The primary focus of phase I cardiac rehabilitation is on early mobilization after surgery, progressing to performance of low-level activities as the patient tolerates. Patient and family education is essential during this time, given the presence of comorbidities and lifestyle factors that have contributed to the cardiac event. Inpatient cardiac rehabilitation also includes instruction on self-monitoring of heart rate, perceived exertion, and the signs and symptoms of cardiac distress.

Essential in the management of the patient is the role of the cardiac rehabilitation team, which consists not only of the patient and/or the patient's family, but also includes doctors, nurses, physical and occupational therapists, dieticians, and psychologists or other mental health specialists.[16] If the rehabilitation team determines that a patient is unable to return home upon discharge from the acute care hospital, the patient can be transferred to an inpatient rehabilitation facility where the phase I program is extended (*i.e.*, extended phase I) until functional recovery has occurred to the level at which the patient can safely return home.[17]

Examination, Evaluation, and Diagnosis

Patients recovering from CABG surgery are likely to have impaired function. Factors contributing to this impairment may include: the direct injury to the myocardium; blood loss causing reduced blood volume, hematocrit, and albumin levels; postsurgical movement restrictions, and postoperative infections at the chest and graft donor site surgical incisions. Impairments of the donor limb site may also contribute to impaired function. For example, should the saphenous vein be used during the procedure, the donor limb may have impaired circulation, sensation, and strength. Thus, the physical therapist needs to examine the strength, range of motion, and sensation of the extremities, and the integumentary condition of the surgical and donor incision sites. Since laboratory values for hematology, blood coagulation, and serum chemistry change substantially after uncomplicated CABG with cardiopulmonary bypass, a review of these laboratory values is essential prior to initiating physical therapy.[18,19]

After CABG surgery, the patient is transferred from an intensive care unit to a step-down unit, where he is placed on continuous telemetry monitoring.[20] The therapist should either directly monitor the ECG for arrhythmias when working with the patient or alert the telemetry technician prior to treating the patient so that heart rate (HR) and rhythm can be monitored during physical therapy. The physical therapist must be aware of signs and symptoms of inadequate cardiac output, which may range from tachycardia and poikilothermia of the extremities to diminished peripheral pulses, altered mentation, and hypotension.[20] The therapist should also be cognizant of several cardiac complications. Atrial fibrillation (AF) is a common complication post-CABG surgery and increases the risk of a cerebrovascular accident (stroke) two to five times. If the AF lasts for more than 24 hours, administration of anticoagulation medications may ensue to decrease the likelihood of thrombus and embolus formation. Ventricular arrhythmias can occur any time after CABG surgery, but are more common in the early post-operative period.[21] Although rare, pericardial effusion, which leads to cardiac tamponade, occurs most frequently in the early postoperative stage; however, it can also occur as late as six months postoperatively. The Beck's triad of muffled heart sounds, distended jugular veins, and hypotension is a hallmark of cardiac tamponade. Cardiac tamponade may also present with pulsus paradoxus (> 10 mm Hg drop in systolic blood pressure during inhalation), dyspnea, chest pain, and dizziness.[20,22,23]

The physical therapist should observe for any signs of impairment in the patient's respiratory system. Postoperative pulmonary complications arise from a lack of lung inflation brought about by a number of converging factors, including a change in breathing to a shallow, monotonous breathing pattern without periodic sighs after surgery, prolonged recumbent positioning, and temporary diaphragmatic dysfunction.[24] These, in turn, result in postoperative altered breathing, impaired coughing, and dyspnea. Hypoxemia, which is common after CABG, may be reflected in decreased oxygen saturation on pulse oximetry. Pleural effusion is a common post-operative complication that may result in dyspnea. Effusions can result from bleeding secondary to internal mammary artery harvesting. Whereas smaller effusions can be managed conservatively and resolve spontaneously, larger effusions may require thoracentesis.[20] The physical therapist should assess the patient's breathing status, cough effectiveness, and breath sounds.

Because the primary focus of phase I cardiac rehabilitation is on early mobilization after surgery, the physical therapist should conduct an activity and/or endurance evaluation to assess the patient's physiologic responses to progressively increasing submaximal intensities of activity or aerobic exercise. The assessment usually begins with an activity evaluation in which the patient is progressed from the supine position, to the sitting position, and finally the standing position. During this progression, the patient's HR, ECG, BP, saturation by pulse oximetry (SpO_2), and any signs and symptoms are monitored. If his responses to the changes in position are stable and deemed safe, the patient is asked to perform simple active exercises or some activities of daily living while the therapist continues to monitor his physiologic responses and any signs and symptoms.[25]

If the patient's physiologic responses during the activity evaluation are safe and appropriate, the therapist can perform an endurance evaluation. The patient is instructed to perform progressive ambulation in the hallway for 2 to 3 minutes at a self-selected comfortable and relaxed pace. Immediately afterward, the therapist monitors the patient's vital signs and any signs and symptoms while the patient continues to walk. The patient is also asked about his perceived exertion using a rating of perceived exertion (RPE) scale. If the patient's responses are stable and safe, the patient is asked to increase the intensity of ambulation for another 2 to 3 minutes, at which time the patient's physiologic responses and any signs and symptoms are re-assessed. This procedure is repeated until the patient reports an RPE of "somewhat hard" (13 on a scale of 6-20) or "somewhat strong" (4 on a scale of 1-10), during which time the pace is continued until the patient begins to feel fatigued. At the end of the evaluation, the therapist notes the total exercise time as a baseline measure for endurance.[25]

An alternative to the endurance evaluation is the use of timed walk tests, such as the Six-Minute Walk Test (6MWT). Whereas *time* is the primary outcome in endurance evaluation, *distance* is the outcome of interest with timed walk tests. Patients are instructed to walk at a pace that would allow them to cover as much distance as possible for a specified amount of time over a designated course with or without an assistive device. At the end of the test, BP, HR, SpO_2, RPE, dyspnea, and fatigue levels are recorded. The distance covered during the walk test can be evaluated by estimating energy expenditure by metabolic equivalents of tasks (METs) and/or by comparing the distance to reference values. Walking speed can be used to calculate oxygen consumption and MET values. Alternatively, the distance covered in a walk test can be compared to published norms.[26] The 6MWT is the most extensively researched walk test and is better tolerated by patients with respiratory or cardiovascular disease. Results of the 6MWT correlate strongly with maximum oxygen consumption; it also correlates moderately to strongly with measures of function.[25]

Plan of Care and Interventions

Because of the multidisciplinary nature of cardiac rehabilitation, the physical therapist works closely with the cardiac rehabilitation team in emphasizing the importance of and need for exercise, lifestyle changes, ongoing education, cognitive behavior therapy, and emotional support. If the team determines that a patient is unable to return home upon discharge from the acute care hospital, the patient can be transferred to an inpatient rehabilitation facility where the phase I program is extended (*i.e.*, extended phase I) until functional recovery has occurred to the level at which the patient can safely return home.[27]

Because hospital lengths of stay are increasingly short in duration, phase I programs must provide the patient with detailed education and an exercise prescription before returning home. Phase I programs include a customized exercise program specific to the needs of patient and based on results of his activity and/or endurance assessments. Phase I programs emphasize instruction on self-monitoring of HR, RPE, and signs and symptoms of cardiac distress during and after exercise or physical activity.[17,27] Education is provided regarding activities that can be performed during recovery and those activities that should be avoided or modified. Sternal precautions are an example of movement restrictions given to individuals after cardiac surgeries in which the sternum is cut. **Sternal precautions** are usually focused on restricting movement of the upper extremities and minimizing sternal loading from upper extremity weightbearing. However, recent literature questions the variety, impact, restrictiveness, and effectiveness of these restrictions, given that the basis for these precautions are more theoretical than empirical.[28,29] Table 12-1 presents representative examples of sternal precautions commonly prescribed post-CABG.[13,29]

Lifestyle modification strategies (*e.g.*, smoking cessation, regular exercise, dietary modification) to reduce the risk of future cardiac events are taught and emphasized throughout phase I. Finally, patients are made aware of phase II programs available

Table 12-1 STERNAL PRECAUTIONS	
Precautions Focusing on Restricted Movement of the Upper Extremities	**Precautions Focusing on Minimizing Sternal Loading from the Upper Extremities**
• Do not perform bilateral shoulder flexion above 90° • Do not engage in unilateral or bilateral upper extremity sports • Do not reach behind you when donning upper body clothes • Avoid shoulder horizontal abduction with extreme external rotation	• Do not lift more than 10 lb unilaterally or bilaterally • No driving of motorized vehicles • Do not push or pull with your arms when moving in bed and getting out of bed

in the patient's community.[27] Providing patient education in cardiac care has resulted in measurable improvements in blood pressure, mortality, exercise capacity, and diet. The type of instructional approach (*i.e.*, didactic vs. behavioral) did not influence outcome; however, adherence to educational principles (such as reinforcement, feedback, and individualization) did.[30]

Exercise is an important part of the recovery process post-CABG surgery. Range of motion exercises can begin early in the process within the first 24 to 48 hours, progressing from passive to active assisted, and eventually to active exercises. The physical therapist can prescribe exercises to improve chest expansion and facilitate breathing.[22,31-33] Low-risk patients should be encouraged to perform self-care activities at bedside.[22] When the patient is transferred to a step-down unit, he is expected to perform more functional activities in and out of bed, including walking inside the room and eventually down the hallway. During the performance of exercises or functional activities, the physical therapist should continually monitor the patient's physiologic responses, perceived exertion, and any emergent signs and symptoms. Guidelines that are used to terminate exercise *testing*[31,34,35] may be used to determine when to discontinue an exercise *session* (Table 12-2).

The results of the activity and endurance evaluation conducted prior to the initiation of exercises provides the physical therapist baseline measures regarding positions and functional activities that the patient is able to perform and tolerate. Table 12-3 provides an example of phase I functional activities that demonstrate progression from bed and bedside activities to walking and stair climbing.[36] There are no formalized steps between these activities. Rather, progression is based on the stability of the patient's condition and physiologic responses to the activity and endurance evaluations.

Prior to or shortly after discharge, most patients undergo a low-level graded exercise test to determine not only the MET level above which this patient's activities at home should *not* exceed, but also the maximal METs at which the patient can reasonably work at home when performing exercises or activities of daily living. Almost all activities of daily living can be performed at an energy cost of no more than 4 METs. However, stair climbing requires 5 to 6 METs. After 2 to 6 weeks of recovery at home, the patient is ready to start phase II cardiac rehabilitation.[22,37,38]

Table 12-2   ABSOLUTE AND RELATIVE INDICATIONS FOR DISCONTINUING EXERCISE

Absolute Indications	Relative Indications

Signs and symptoms
• Moderate to severe (grade 3-4) angina
• Cyanosis, pallor, other signs of poor perfusion
• Increasing nervous system signs or symptoms such as ataxia, dizziness, or near-syncope
Physiologic responses
• Drop of > 10 mm Hg in SBP despite increasing workload plus evidence of ischemia
• Abnormal ECG responses
  • Persistent ventricular tachycardia
  • ST elevation ≥ 1.0 mm in leads without diagnostic Q waves (other than V1 or aVR)
Other
• Inability to monitor physiologic responses such as ECG and SBP
• Patient has indicated the desire to stop
	Signs and symptoms
	• Increasing angina
	• Fatigue, dyspnea, muscle pain, leg claudication
	• General appearance such as decrease in skin temperature, cool and light perspiration, peripheral cyanosis
	Physiologic responses
	• Blood pressure changes
	  • Drop of > 10 mm Hg in SBP despite increasing workload without evidence of ischemia
	  • Hypertensive episode (SBP > 250 mm Hg and/or DBP of > 115 mm Hg)
	• Abnormal ECG responses
	  • Abnormal cardiac rhythms other than sustained ventricular tachycardia, such as PVCs, supraventricular tachycardia, heart block, or bradyarrhythmias
	  • ST or QRS changes such as excessive ST depression (> 2 mm of horizontal or downsloping ST segment depression) or marked axis shift
	  • Development of bundle-branch block or intraventricular conduction defect that cannot be distinguished from ventricular tachycardia

Abbreviations: DBP, diastolic blood pressure; ECG, electrocardiogram; PVC, premature ventricular contraction; SBP, systolic blood pressure.

Table 12-3   SAMPLE PROGRESSION IN FUNCTIONAL ACTIVITIES DURING PHASE I CARDIAC REHABILITATION

Functional Activities	Activities in Bed and Bedside	Activities by the Bedside and in Hospital Room	Activities in the Room and in the Hallway	Activities Outside the Room
Bed mobility	Patient sits up in bed with assistance	Patient sits up in bed with assistance as needed	Sit up in bed independently	Ongoing
Standing	Patient stands bedside with assistance	Patient stands with assistance as needed	Patient stands independently	Ongoing
Walking	Not applicable	Patient walks inside the room including the bathroom with assistance	Patient walks down the hall with assistance, 2-3 times per day	Patient walks down the hall with assistance, 3-4 times per day Stair climbing as permitted and tolerated
Self-care	Patient performs self-care in bed or bedside	Perform self-care activities in bathroom	Ongoing	Ongoing

Evidence-Based Clinical Recommendations

SORT: Strength of Recommendation Taxonomy

A: Consistent, good-quality patient-oriented evidence

B: Inconsistent or limited-quality patient-oriented evidence

C: Consensus, disease-oriented evidence, usual practice, expert opinion, or case series

1. Cardiac rehabilitation that includes psychological, educational, and supervised exercise interventions is recommended for all eligible patients after CABG. **Grade A**

2. Cardiac rehabilitation improves exercise tolerance and exercise capacity among men and women regardless of age. **Grade A**

3. Sternal precautions after CABG are effective at reducing the likelihood of abnormal healing post-CABG. **Grade C**

COMPREHENSION QUESTIONS

12.1 Which of the following outcomes demonstrates improving exercise capacity in a patient undergoing cardiac rehabilitation?

    A. Decreasing time to reach the point of fatigue during an endurance evaluation and increasing distance covered during a 6MWT

    B. Increasing time to reach the point of fatigue during an endurance evaluation and decreasing distance covered during a 6MWT

    C. Decreasing time to reach the point of fatigue during an endurance evaluation and decreasing distance covered during a 6MWT

    D. Increasing time to reach the point of fatigue during an endurance evaluation and increasing distance covered during a 6MWT

12.2 When providing patient instruction on exercise performance, the physical therapist should emphasize all of the following instructional variables, *except:*

    A. Reinforcement

    B. Communication medium

    C. Individualization

    D. Feedback

ANSWERS

12.1 **D.** During an endurance evaluation, a patient with increasing exercise capacity is able to walk for a longer period of time before reaching the point of fatigue given the same intensity. The patient is also able to walk a longer *distance* in a 6MWT when compared with baseline measures.

12.2 **B.** Patient education in cardiac care has demonstrated measurable improve-ments in blood pressure, mortality, exercise capacity, and diet. The type of communication medium did not influence outcome; however, adherence to educational principles (such as reinforcement, feedback, and individualization) did.[30]

REFERENCES

1. PubMed Health. http://www.nhlbi.nih.gov/health/health-topics/topics/atherosclerosis/. Accessed November 18, 2011.

2. Mercer University School of Medicine. The Internet Pathology Laboratory for Medical Education. http://library.med.utah.edu/WebPath/TUTORIAL/MYOCARD/MYOCARD.html. Accessed November 20, 2011.

3. Goodman CC, Smirnova IV. Ch 12: The cardiovascular system. In: Goodman CC, Fuller KS. *Pathology—Implications for the Physical Therapist.* 3rd ed. St. Louis, MO: Saunders Elsevier; 2009: 560-561.

4. eMedicineHealth. http://www.emedicinehealth.com/coronary_heart_disease/page5_em.htm. Accessed May 12, 2011.

5. Alpert JS, Thygesen K, Antman E, et al. Myocardial infarction redefined—a consensus document of The Joint European Society of Cardiology/American College of Cardiology Committee for the redefinition of myocardial infarction. *J Am Coll Cardiol.* 2000;36:959-969.

6. ECG Library. http://www.ecglibrary.com/ecghome.html. Accessed November 25, 2011.

7. PubMed Health. http://www.nhlbi.nih.gov/health/health-topics/topics/cath/. Accessed November 25, 2011.

8. WebMD. http://www.webmd.com/heart-disease/treatment-angioplasty-stents. Accessed November 28, 2011.

9. MedicineNet.com. http://www.medicinenet.com/coronary_artery_bypass_graft/page3.htm. Accessed November 28, 2011.

10. Watchie J. *Cardiovascular and pulmonary physical therapy a clinical manual.* 2nd ed. St. Louis, MO: Saunders Elsevier; 2010: 61.

11. eMedicineHealth. http://emedicine.medscape.com/article/319683-overview#aw2aab6b4. Accessed December 7, 2011.

12. American Heart Association. http://www.heart.org/HEARTORG/Conditions/More/CardiacRehab/What-is-Cardiac-Rehabilitation_UCM_307049_Article.jsp. Accessed December 7, 2011.

13. Goodman CC, Smirnova IV. Ch 12: The cardiovascular system. In: Goodman CC, Fuller KS. *Pathology—Implications for the Physical Therapist.* 3rd ed. St. Louis, MO: Saunders Elsevier; 2009: 545.

14. AACVPR/ACC/AHA 2007 Performance Measures on cardiac rehabilitation for referral to and deliv-ery of cardiac rehabilitation/secondary prevention services. *J Am Coll Cardiol.* 2007;50:1400-1433.

15. Wenger NK. Current status of cardiac rehabilitation. *J Am Coll Cardiol.* 2008;51:1619-1631.

16. PubMed Health. http://www.nhlbi.nih.gov/health/health-topics/topics/rehab/. Accessed December 10, 2012.

17. Elrod CS. Patient adherence to self-monitoring recommendations taught in extended phase I cardiac rehabilitation. *Cardiopulm Phys Ther J.* 2007;18:3-14.

18. Wintz G, LaPier TK. Functional status in patients during the first two months following hospital discharge for coronary artery bypass surgery. *Cardiopulm Phys Ther J.* 2007;18:13-20.

19. Möhnle P, Schwann NM, Vaughn WK, et al. Perturbations in laboratory values after coronary artery bypass graft surgery with cardiopulmonary bypass. *J Cardiothorac Vasc Anesth.* 2005;19:19-25.

20. Mullen-Fortino M, O'Brien N. Caring for a Patient after Coronary Artery Bypass Graft. http://www.nursingcenter.com/pdf.asp?AID=819638. Accessed December 15, 2011.

21. Fuster V, et al. ACC/AHA/ESC 2006 guidelines for the management of patients with atrial fibrillation—executive summary: a report of the American College of Cardiology/American Heart Association Task Force on Practice Guidelines and the European Society of Cardiology Committee for Practice Guidelines (Writing committee to revise the 2001 guidelines for the management of patients with atrial fibrillation). *Eur Heart J*. 2006; 27:1979-2030.

22. Medscape. http://emedicine.medscape.com/article/152083-overview. Accessed December 15, 2011.

23. Russo AM, O'Connor WH, Waxman HL. Atypical presentations and echocardiographic findings in patients with cardiac tamponade occurring early and late after cardiac surgery. *Chest*. 1993;104: 71-78.

24. Overend TJ, Anderson CM, Lucy SD, et al. The effect of incentive spirometry on postoperative pulmonary complications: a systematic review. *Chest*. 2001;120:971-978.

25. Watchie J. *Cardiovascular and Pulmonary Physical Therapy—A Clinical Manual*. 2nd ed. St. Louis, MO: Saunders Elsevier; 2010.

26. LaPier TK. Outcome measures in cardiopulmonary physical therapy: focus on walk tests. *Cardiopulm Phys Ther J*. 2004;15:17-21.

27. WebMD. http://www.webmd.com/heart-disease/cardiac-rehab-general-exercise-guidelines-for-phase-i. Accessed December 20, 2011.

28. Tuyl LJ, Mackney JH, Johnston CL. Management of sternal precautions following median sternotomy by physical therapists in Australia: a web-based survey. *Phys Ther*. 2012;92:83-97.

29. Cahalin LP, LaPier TK, Shaw DK. Sternal precautions: is it time for change? Precautions versus restrictions—a review of literature and recommendations for revision. *Cardiopulm Phys Ther J*. 2011;22:5-15.

30. Mullen PD, Mains DA, Velez R. A meta-analysis of controlled trials of cardiac patient education. *Patient Educ Couns*. 1992;9:143-162.

31. Goodman CC, Smirnova IV. Ch 12: The cardiovascular system. In: Goodman CC, Fuller KS. *Pathology—Implications for the Physical Therapist*. 3rd ed. Saunders Elsevier; 2009:546-547.

32. Westerdahl E, Lindmark B, Eriksson T, et al. Deep-breathing exercises reduce atelectasis and improve pulmonary function after coronary artery bypass surgery. *Chest*. 2005;128:3482-3488.

33. Haeffener MP, Ferreira GM, Barreto SS, et al. Incentive spirometry with expiratory positive airway pressure reduces pulmonary complications, improves pulmonary function and 6-minute walk distance in patients undergoing coronary artery bypass graft surgery. *Am Heart J*. 2008;156: e1-e8.

34. Fletcher GF, Balady GJ, Amsterdam EA, et al. Exercise standards for testing and training: a statement for healthcare professionals from the American Heart Association. *Circulation*. 2001;104:1694-1740.

35. Gibbons RJ, et al. ACC/AHA 2002 Guideline update for exercise testing: summary article: a report of the American College of Cardiology/American Heart Association Task Force on Practice Guidelines (Committee to Update the 1997 Exercise Testing Guidelines). *Circulation*. 2002;106: 1883-1892.

36. WebMD. http://www.webmd.com/heart-disease/cardiac-rehab-examples-of-phase-i-exercises-after-a-heart-attack. Accessed December 20, 2011.

37. Phase I Cardiac Rehabilitation. http://jan.ucc.nau.edu/~daa/heartlung/lectures/phase1.html. Accessed December 20, 2011.

38. Garrison SJ. *Handbook of Physical Medicine and Rehabilitation*. 2nd ed. Philadelphia, PA: Lippincott Williams & Wilkins; 2003.

Left Ventricular Assistive Device

Jaime C. Paz

CASE 13

A 59-year-old male was admitted to the hospital 7 days ago because of worsening congestive heart failure (CHF). The patient was initially managed medically with diuretics and positive inotropes but ultimately required left ventricular assist device (LVAD) implantation to achieve hemodynamic stability. During this hospital admission, the patient was placed on the heart transplant list as Status 1B. You are consulted one day status/post LVAD placement for progressive mobility and assistance with discharge planning. The patient's past medical history consists of CHF, hypertension (HTN), Type 2 diabetes mellitus (DM), coronary artery disease (CAD), and asthma. He is married and lives in a single-story home with four steps to enter. His three adult children live nearby and are supportive.

► What are the examination priorities?
► Based on his health condition, what do you anticipate may be the contributors to activity limitations?
► What are possible complications interfering with physical therapy?
► What are the most appropriate physical therapy interventions?
► What precautions should be taken during physical therapy examination and/or interventions?
► Describe a physical therapy plan of care based on each stage of the health condition.

KEY DEFINITIONS

CONGESTIVE HEART FAILURE (CHF): Inability of the left ventricle to effectively pump blood to meet the metabolic demands of the body; as a result, blood pools in the pulmonary vasculature causing congestion and shortness of breath

HEART TRANSPLANT: Replacement of a chronically diseased heart with a donated heart from a recently deceased individual

STATUS 1B: One of several designations defined by the United Network of Organ Sharing, a national nonprofit organ sharing system established by federal United States law in 1984 to classify patients based on different priorities for organ transplantation; patients classified as Status 1B are second in priority for an organ transplant (behind patients classified as Status 1A), have a life expectancy of more than 7 days without heart transplantation, and may have a VAD for more than 30 days or receive continuous intravenous inotropes in a nonintensive care setting

VENTRICULAR ASSIST DEVICE (VAD): Mechanical device that assists the left, right, or both ventricles to improve cardiac output; the pump mechanism of the VAD may be outside or inside the body

Objectives

1. Describe the indications for LVAD implantation.
2. Understand the mechanisms involved with the mechanical circulatory assist provided by LVAD.
3. Identify adverse drug reactions (ADRs) of common heart medications that may affect physical therapy examination and/or interventions.
4. List potential complications for a patient who is status/post LVAD implantation.
5. Outline the physical therapy examination for this patient population.
6. Design a plan of care for the individual with mechanical circulatory support.

Physical Therapy Considerations

PT considerations during management of the individual status/post LVAD implantation:

▶ **General physical therapy plan of care/goals:** Prevent or minimize loss of range of motion (ROM), strength, and functional capacity; maximize functional independence and safety while minimizing secondary impairments; improve quality of life

▶ **Physical therapy interventions:** Patient and caregiver education regarding LVAD precautions, decreasing risk of deep vein thromboses, and decreasing the risk of falls; gait training; caregiver training for safe guarding during ambulation; prescription of a home exercise program; and, if indicated, referral for continued rehabilitation

▶ **Precautions during physical therapy:** LVAD precautions; close physical supervision to decrease risk of falls; consistent monitoring of vital signs and LVAD parameters

▶ **Complications interfering with physical therapy:** Deep vein thrombosis, shortness of breath with or without respiratory distress, infection, falls, LVAD failure

Understanding the Health Condition

Heart failure is a progressive syndrome resulting from several related conditions involving the cardiovascular and pulmonary systems. According to the Centers for Disease Control, the number of non-institutionalized adults with diagnosed heart disease is 26.8 million and approximately 204 people out of 100,000 die with heart disease, including heart failure.[1] In 2009, the National Heart, Lung and Blood Institute reported the prevalence of heart failure in the United States to be 5.7 million.[2]

Hypertension, ischemic heart disease, congenital heart disease, valvular heart disease, and chronic lung disease can all progress to cardiac pump dysfunction. Continued demands on the cardiac system will, over a period of time, lead to failure of the cardiac pump to meet to the metabolic demands of body. Heart failure can occur in the right or left ventricle as well as both ventricles simultaneously.[3] Left-sided heart failure is commonly referred to as CHF because the inability of the left ventricle to pump will lead to pulmonary congestion and shortness of breath.[4]

Medical management of heart failure consists of pharmacological support with various agents aimed at reducing the ventricular workload.[5] Cardiac digitalis glycosides are positive inotropes that improve myocardial contractility to help augment ventricular pump function. The most commonly used cardiac glycoside is digoxin. Positive inotropes may also be prescribed in conjunction with diuretic agents (*e.g.*, Lasix) to further augment ventricular pump effectiveness by decreasing the blood volume, which can reduce cardiac workload. Another class of agents utilized to manage heart failure includes angiotensin converting enzyme (ACE) inhibitors. The ACE inhibitors (*e.g.*, lisinopril, captopril) help reduce cardiac workload by decreasing blood volume and reducing total peripheral resistance. Common adverse drug reactions (ADRs) associated with digoxin and diuretics have significant clinical importance. The ADRs associated with digoxin include cardiac arrhythmias, fatigue, and mental status changes. Unfortunately, these signs and symptoms may be indistinguishable from clinical manifestations of heart failure. Diuretic agents can cause dizziness, weakness, and orthostatic hypotension. Loop diuretics like Lasix may lead to potassium depletion, which can cause muscle cramps and cardiac arrhythmias. Potassium-sparing diuretics or supplemental potassium are alternatives to offset the ADRs associated with non-potassium sparing diuretics. The ACE inhibitors have relatively few ADRs and are less serious than those associated with glycosides or diuretics. Patients may exhibit skin rashes, gastrointestinal discomfort, or dry coughs.[5]

Classification of heart failure is an essential component of disease management in order to achieve optimal control of the disease. The most commonly utilized classification system is the revised New York Heart Association (NYHA)

Table 13-1 AMERICAN COLLEGE OF CARDIOLOGY / AMERICAN HEART ASSOCIATION RECOMMENDED THERAPY FOR HEART FAILURE PATIENTS BY STAGES[7,8]

Stage	Description	Recommended Therapy
A	No structural or functional abnormalities present in cardiac structures but is at high risk for developing heart failure because of associated conditions linked to heart failure	Lifestyle modification (e.g., smoking cessation, increased exercise) Manage hypertension Provide ACE inhibitor or ARB in suitable patients
B	No signs or symptoms of heart failure but has structural changes strongly related to developing heart failure	Similar management to Stage A with the addition of β-blockers in suitable patients
C	Structural heart disease is present with either current or past symptoms of heart failure	Similar management to Stage A with the addition of: • Diuretics if fluid retention is present • ACE inhibitors • β-blockers For certain patients • Hydralazine/nitrates • Digitalis • Biventricular pacing • Implantable defibrillators
D	Specialized management is required as patient is end-stage or refractory to other traditional management	In addition to management for Stages A, B, & C: • Heart transplant • Chronic inotropes for palliation • Mechanical assist devices • Experimental surgery or drugs • Hospice

Abbreviations: ACE, angiotensin-converting enzyme; ARB, angiotensin receptor blocker.

Functional Classification of Heart Disease. The NYHA categorizes heart disease based on four progressive classes from mild disease that does not result in physical activity limitations (Class I) to severe disease that results in signs and symptoms such as fatigue, dyspnea, or angina even at rest (Class IV).[6] While this classification scheme provides good descriptions of a patient's functional capability, management strategies are not offered. Therefore, the American College of Cardiology in conjunction with the American Heart Association devised a four-stage system to help guide management for patients with heart failure (Table 13-1).[7] Patients who have progressed to Classes III to IV (from Revised NYHA Functional Classification) and Stage D (from American College of Cardiology/American Heart Association Stages) are appropriate for LVAD implantation to optimize medical management.[8]

VADs have been in use for the past three decades in patients with advanced heart failure.[8,9] Currently, VADs are used as a bridge to heart transplant (BTT) or as destination therapy (DT) with the goal of partially or completely replacing ventricular function.[10] The patient's native heart is still functioning, albeit inadequately, and VADs can support either the right ventricle (RVAD), left ventricle (LVAD), or both ventricles (BiVAD).[11] Patients who are bridging to transplant with a VAD will remain on mechanical support until a donor heart becomes available. During this timeframe, the VAD may help a patient improve his functional capacity and

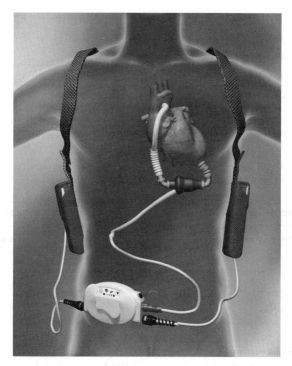

Figure 13-1. Heartmate II LVAD. (Reproduced with permission from Thoratec Corporation.)

endurance, which can lead to a more successful post-transplantation outcome. If a VAD has been implanted for DT, then unfortunately the patient is not a transplant candidate and the VAD is the last treatment option.

These mechanical circulatory assist devices have an external control box connected to a surgically implanted cableline and a pump mechanism. The external control box is typically powered by a battery pack. Synchronization of the VAD pump with the native heart is achieved by the percutaneous lead that is connected to the external system controller.[10] The specific components and mechanisms will vary according to the type of device implanted. Assistance to the ventricle is provided by either bypassing the ventricle(s) via the great vessels or by providing support after blood has left the ventricle. Several companies manufacture VADs that have either a pulsatile or continuous (axial) pump device. Both types of pumps have resulted in improved functional capacity and quality of life in patients with advanced heart failure.[12] The LVAD illustrated in Fig. 13-1 has a continuous pump mechanism and is the Heartmate II by Thoratec Corporation.

Patients with LVAD implantation have demonstrated improvements in quality of life as measured by the Minnesota Living with Heart Failure questionnaire[12,13] and the Kansas City Cardiomyopathy questionnaire.[12] These quality of life improvements have also translated into changes in patients' NYHA classification from Class IV to Class I or II, correlating to improved functional capacity with the LVAD.[12,13] Patients with LVAD implantation have also demonstrated improved aerobic endurance. One to two years after LVAD implantation, patients walked approximately 300 meters on the Six-Minute Walk Test (6MWT), doubling the distance walked prior to LVAD implantation.[12] This post-LVAD functional capacity as measured by the 6MWT is consistent with patients who are categorized as NYHA classes I and II.[12,13]

Complications resulting from LVAD implantation are consistent with cardiac surgical procedures. These include arrhythmias, thromboembolic events, stroke, infection, respiratory failure, gastrointestinal distress, and death.[12,13] Patients with LVAD implantation may also experience mechanical complications such as valve dysfunction in the pump, disconnection of leads and drivelines, and deterioration in the pump mechanism. Mechanical complications may be repaired or may require replacement with another LVAD.[12,13] The prevalence of these complications is variable; patient selection and disease stage at the time of implantation appear to be factors in developing adverse events.[14] Patients who receive VAD implantation for DT may be expected to live 1 to 2 years.[12,14]

Physical Therapy Patient/Client Management

Patients who undergo LVAD implantation have several issues to consider that are similar to those of other patients with chronic heart disease as well as factors that are unique to the mechanical circulatory support. Significant comorbidities will likely be present with concurrent deconditioning resulting from impaired central hemodynamics and disuse muscle atrophy.[10] Understanding the mechanical and safety properties of the LVAD is essential for determining parameters to monitor during functional activity and exercise. Physical therapists need to familiarize themselves with the individual pump characteristics of the specific LVAD device that has been implanted in each patient. In general, LVADs either have stroke volume, cardiac output, or flow to describe the capacity of blood flow from the device. In addition, LVADs have either fixed or adaptive capabilities during exercise.[15] Additional considerations include managing the external pump mechanisms such as the power source and the system controller, which need to be secured in a shoulder holster. To protect the percutaneous lead that exits the patient's body during movement, an abdominal binder must be worn at all times to ensure that no disturbance occurs to this vital link from the control box to the pump.[10]

Patients who undergo LVAD implantation also remain on pharmacological management to help optimize hemodynamic stability while on mechanical circulatory support. Commonly used agents include β-blockers (e.g., carvedilol) and ACE inhibitors or angiotensin receptor blockers. Aspirin therapy is also utilized in all patients who have an implanted HeartMate. This combination of drugs is particularly important for preserving right heart function as well as helping to lessen the deleterious effect of systemic hypertension on long-term LVAD wear.[16]

The primary goal of rehabilitation for the patient with an implanted LVAD is to optimize functional capacity while awaiting a heart transplant (i.e., bridging towards heart transplantation) or for the remainder of his life (i.e., DT). The primary purpose for LVAD implantation (BTT or DT) along with the patient's medical status dictates the length of stay in the acute care setting and subsequent goals that can be achieved.

Examination, Evaluation, and Diagnosis

Prior to seeing the patient, the physical therapist needs to thoroughly review the patient's medical record, including medications, laboratory values, postoperative precautions, and any exercise or mobility restrictions. Implantation of an LVAD typically requires sternotomy and therefore sternal precautions need to be followed.[10,11,17] Critical laboratory values to check include hemoglobin, hematocrit, platelet count, and trends in blood pressure (BP) and flows/cardiac output from the LVAD. Exercise or mobilization should be withheld if hemoglobin, hematocrit, and cell counts are not within safe limits.

Physical therapy examination can generally begin on the **first postoperative day** as long as the patient is hemodynamically stable for mobility.[10] The initial contact with the patient will most likely be in the critical or intensive care setting and may vary according to individual facilities. Thorough review of the medical record and consultation with the medical team helps determine the appropriateness for physical examination to begin.[10,11,17,18] Physical therapy should be terminated and/or withheld and the medical team notified if: the patient is short of breath or reports other symptoms of exercise intolerance (*e.g.*, chest pain or palpitations), systolic BP is less than 80 mm Hg or decreases by more than 20 mm Hg, VAD flow is less than 3 L/min, reduced volumes are detected, the device alarms, or if the therapist notices acute bleeding or neurologic changes.[15]

Similar to other patients who have recently had thoracic surgery, bedside examination includes an assessment of the patient's mental status, integumentary condition, sensation, ROM, strength, and functional mobility.[10] Since these patients are status/post sternotomy, auscultation of lung sounds and cough effectiveness is essential to help prevent pulmonary complications postoperatively. Finally, a scan of the patient's equipment at the bedside is necessary to facilitate functional mobility preparations.[17]

Examination of the patient's pain level is necessary because patients often complain of pain at tubing exit sites in the abdomen or thorax. Patients may have a tendency to splint or favor the side of the exit sites, which can promote a kyphotic or scoliotic position. The ability to maintain an upright posture is critical because a flexed or side-bent posture can lead to pump flow obstructions in the LVAD drivelines, resulting in reduced flow rates to meet metabolic demands.[15,17]

Ongoing evaluation of a patient's **hemodynamic response** is critical during both the initial examination and throughout functional activity and exercise progression. The patient's electrocardiogram (ECG) via telemetry monitors the patient's native heart rate and rhythm. However, given the advanced heart failure of the patient, the primary cardiac output and subsequent BP will be dependent on the LVAD.[17] The power base monitor of the LVAD provides flow rates or cardiac output that can be read on the screen. A flow rate greater than 3-4 L/min is sufficient in most devices in most devices to proceed with mobility.[10,17] If the patient is on a continuous LVAD, such as the Heartmate II, there will be no palpable peripheral pulse because of the axial flow mechanism of this particular pump. Therefore, the ECG is more accurate to determine the heart rate response of the patient to mobilization or exercise.[10] Since the patient will probably be taking β-blockers, the native heart rate response at rest and to exercise will be blunted.

Some LVADs create a *pulsatile* flow, which mimics physiologic systole and diastole. If a patient has an implanted LVAD with a pulsatile mechanism, standard BP measurements with a cuff and stethoscope can be performed. In contrast, the Heartmate II creates a *continuous* flow of blood from the left ventricle to the systemic circulation. Because of this continuous flow, traditional BP with a standard BP cuff is not possible because discernable Korotkoff sounds, which represent systolic and diastolic pressures, will not be present. Since systolic and diastolic pressures cannot be detected, mean arterial pressure (MAP) is measured. The MAP provides a good indication of how well the patient, with LVAD assist, is able to accommodate to functional activity. If the patient is in the intensive care unit, then MAP is monitored invasively. If the patient is not in the intensive care unit, then MAP may be assessed with Doppler ultrasound, which allows sounds to be detected better than via auscultation with a stethoscope. In order to perform this measurement, the therapist utilizes a standard BP cuff with the Doppler ultrasound to listen for the first audible sound upon releasing pressure in the cuff. Since no discernible systolic and diastolic pressures can be heard, the single pressure represents mean arterial pressure.[19] A MAP between 70 and 95 mm Hg at rest and with activity is suitable for most patients, depending on machine capabilities and settings.[10]

To determine the appropriate exercise intensity and response to activity, physical therapists can monitor BP (or MAP), the patient's Rating of Perceived Exertion (RPE) with the Borg Scale, and oxygen saturation as estimated by pulse oximetry. An RPE of 11 to 13 out of 20 is a sufficient intensity level for this patient population to safely exercise and achieve training benefits over a period of time.[17] Regardless of whether the particular LVAD provides a continuous or pulsatile flow, *all* LVADs improve overall cardiac output and blood flow to the periphery. Thus, pulse oximeters can still be used in patients with LVADs to monitor oxygen saturation. Guidelines for monitoring oxygen saturation are similar to other patients without LVADs (e.g., keep above 90% SpO_2).

Outcome measures that have been utilized with patients who have implanted LVADs include the Minnesota Living with Heart Failure questionnaire,[12,13] the Kansas City Cardiomyopathy questionnaires,[12] health-related quality of life via the SF-36,[20] the Functional Independence Measure (FIM)[10] and the **6MWT**.[12] Prognosis depends on several factors including age, number of comorbidities, timing of LVAD implantation, device malfunction, and complications such as infection experienced post-implantation.[14,16,21] For patients who are Status 1B awaiting heart transplant, the median wait time for a donor heart is 78 days.[22] Patients who receive LVADs as DT, as reported above are expected to possibly live 1 to 2 years.[12,14]

Plan of Care and Interventions

Managing a patient with an LVAD is both similar and somewhat different than managing a patient with CHF. Unlike a patient with CHF, a patient with an LVAD rarely has his fluids restricted in order to maintain preload (end diastolic volume), which in many times helps to maintain flow or cardiac output of the mechanical pumps.[10]

However, each patient is unique so confirming any fluid restrictions prior to physical therapy sessions is necessary to ensure safety. Since patients with LVADs have CHF, they respond well to both aerobic and resistance exercise.[23,24] Inpatient physical therapy interventions can include upper and lower extremity range of motion and strengthening exercises, transfer and gait training, energy conservation in activities of daily living, pulmonary hygiene, aerobic conditioning, and patient education for proper care of the external components of the device.[10,17,18] During the initial 8 weeks after surgery, sternal precautions need to be implemented during physical therapy interventions. These precautions are movement restrictions that are designed to allow the sternum to heal from the incision that was required to implant the LVAD. Sternal precautions include lifting no more than 10 lb of weight bilaterally, no bilateral or unilateral upper extremity sports, no driving, no hand over head activities, and no active shoulder flexion or abduction > 90°.[25] Upper extremity ROM and lifting 1 to 3 lb is generally allowable if sternal instability is not detected. Sternal instability may be manifested as movement in the sternum along with pain and cracking or popping sensations. Patients should be instructed to minimize ROM when the onset of sternal instability is noted in the incision site.[25] The presence of pain, tenderness, fever and/or purulent drainage from the incision site may also be indicative of infection.[26]

Patients who exhibit clinical manifestation of orthostatic hypotension or dizziness during interventions should be evaluated promptly because these presentations can be indicative of driveline occlusion or pump malfunction.[17] Prevention of infection at the driveline sites as well as protection via abdominal binders is critical to ensure proper functioning of the mechanical pumps. Patients are restricted from using pools and having tub baths, although they are allowed to shower.[10] A specially designed water kit is available to help protect the VAD system components when showering.[27] Consultation with the nurse or occupational therapist is helpful for this situation.

Patients with LVADs tend to increase functional capacity and aerobic endurance over an 8- to 12-week period.[17,28] Therefore, the focus of the initial intervention plan in the acute care setting is to prevent complications and maximize functional capacity in preparation for endurance training. Discharge planning begins as soon as the patient begins to mobilize and the patient's disposition needs to be considered to help focus the inpatient interventions. For this patient who has been placed on the transplant list as Status 1B, there is a likelihood of him being discharged home to await a suitable organ donor. If the patient requires further inpatient rehabilitation before going home safely, then appropriate referrals need to be made. While awaiting transplantation, aerobic conditioning is essential to facilitate successful outcomes posttransplantation.

Evidence-Based Clinical Recommendations

SORT: Strength of Recommendation Taxonomy

A: Consistent, good-quality patient-oriented evidence
B: Inconsistent or limited-quality patient-oriented evidence
C: Consensus, disease-oriented evidence, usual practice, expert opinion, or case series

1. Individuals with heart disease categorized as NYHA Classes III to IV who are implanted with an LVAD demonstrate improvements in quality of life and functional capacity compared to those patients who are managed only with pharmacologic support. **Grade B**

2. Inpatient physical therapy management of patients with implanted LVADs can be performed safely beginning on the first postoperative day. **Grade C**

3. Hemodynamic monitoring of patients with implanted LVADs should take into account both machine (*e.g.*, pump flows and power [battery] supply) and patient variables (*e.g.*, ECG, subjective complaints of dizziness and pain at access sites, Borg RPE and MAP) to ensure safe mobilization. **Grade C**

4. The 6MWT is an appropriate outcome measure for functional capacity and aerobic endurance in patients with implanted LVADs. **Grade B**

COMPREHENSION QUESTIONS

13.1 Which of the following statements *best* applies to a patient's pharmacologic management status/post LVAD implantation?

A. The mechanical pump will replace both the inotropic and chronotropic support of medications.

B. Cardiac medications are necessary to help augment native cardiac pump function and prevent mechanical pump dysfunction.

C. The LVAD will help strengthen the cardiac muscle so that medications are no longer necessary.

D. Cardiac medications are necessary to help heal cardiac tissue and promote weaning off of the LVAD during destination therapy.

13.2 Which of the following signs or symptoms is essential to monitor to help determine the adequacy of mechanical pump function?

A. Tachycardia

B. Pain

C. Hyperventilation

D. Dizziness

ANSWERS

13.1 **B.** Patients with an LVAD typically require β-blockers, ACE inhibitors, and aspirin therapy to help prevent right ventricular failure as well as systemic hypertension that can overload the mechanical pump. β-Blockers provide chronotropic (heart rate) support while ACE inhibitors can assist with inotropic (contractility) function by maintaining adequate fluid in the circulatory system (option A). While exercise with an LVAD can assist in regaining some cardiac muscle function, pharmacological support will always be necessary to support the chronically diseased heart (option C). The cardiac tissue in the patient with advanced heart failure will not necessarily "heal" as occurs in patients with prolonged myocardial ischemia (option D).

13.2 **D.** Reduced LVAD pump function can result in orthostatic hypotension, manifested as lightheadedness or dizziness. Tachycardia is not likely since the patient will be on β-blockers (option A). Pain can result from many aspects of the surgery and postsurgical healing and therefore is less specific to the mechanical pump (option B). Hyperventilation can result from increased activity or anxiety and is also less specific to the mechanical pump (option C).

REFERENCES

1. Centers for Disease Control. http://www.cdc.gov/nchs/fastats/heart.htm. Accessed August 5, 2011.

2. National Heart, Lung and Blood Institute. http://www.nhlbi.nih.gov/about/factbook/chapter4. htm#4_5. Accessed August 5, 2011.

3. Schoen FJ, Mitchell RN. The heart. In: Kumar V, Abbas AK, Fausto N, Mitchell RN. *Robbins Basic Pathology*. 8th ed. Philadelphia, PA: Saunders Elsevier; 2007:380-381.

4. Collins S. Cardiac system. In: Paz JC, West M. *Acute Care Handbook for Physical Therapists*. 3rd ed. St. Louis, MO: Saunders Elsevier; 2009:23-26.

5. Ciccone CD. *Pharmacology in Rehabilitation*(4th ed.). Philadelphia, PA: FA Davis; 2007: 331-346.

6. Data from the Criteria Committee of the New York Heart Association. *Nomenclature and Criteria for Diagnosis of Diseases of the Heart and Great Vessels* (9th ed.). Boston, MA: Little, Brown & Co; 1994:253-256.

7. Hunt SA, Baker DW, Chin MH, et al. American College of Cardiology/American Heart Association. ACC/AHA guidelines for the evaluation and management of chronic heart failure in the adult: executive summary. A report of the American College of Cardiology/American Heart Association Task Force on Practice Guidelines (Committee to revise Advanced heart failure on maximal medical therapy the 1995 Guidelines for the Evaluation and Management of Heart Failure). *J Am Coll Cardiol*. 2001;38:2101-2113.

8. Russell SD, Miller LW, Pagani FD. Advanced heart failure: a call to action. *Congestive Heart Fail*. 2008;14:316-321.

9. Smedira NG. Implantable left ventricular assist devices. In: Braunwald E, ed. *Harrison's Advances in Cardiology*. New York, NY: McGraw-Hill;2003:538-542.

10. Nissinoff J, Tian F, Therattil M, et al. Acute inpatient rehabilitation after left ventricular assist device implantation for congestive heart failure. *PMR*. 2011;3:586-589.

11. Mulgrew JA. Circulatory assist devices. In: Paz JC, West M. *Acute Care Handbook for Physical Therapists* (3rd ed.). St. Louis, MO: Saunders Elsevier; 2009;479-484.

12. Slaughter MS, Rogers JG, Milano CM, et al. Advanced heart failure treated with continuous-flow left ventricular assist device. *N Engl J Med*. 2009;361:2241-2251.

13. Allen JG, Weiss ES, Schaffer JM, et al. Quality of life and functional status in patients surviving 12 months after left ventricular assist device implantation. *J Heart Lung Transplant*. 2010;29: 278-285.

14. Lietz K, Long JW, Kfoury AG, et al. Outcomes of left ventricular assist device implantation as destination therapy in the post-REMATCH era: implications for patient selection. *Circulation*. 2007;116:497-505.

15. Nicholson C, Paz J. Total artificial heart and physical therapy management. *Cardiopulm Phys Ther*. 2010;21:13-21.

16. Klodell C, Staples ED, Aranda JM Jr, et al. Managing the post-left ventricular assist device patient. *Congestive Heart Fail*. 2006;12:41-45.

17. Humphrey R, Buck L, Cahalin L, et al. Physical therapy assessment and intervention for patients with left ventricular assist devices. *Cardiopulm Phys Ther*. 1998;9:3-7.

18. Sendura M, Mehtap M, Oztekin O. Physical therapy in the Intensive Care Unit in a patient with biventricular assist device. *Cardiopulm Phys Ther*. 2011; 22:31-34.

19. Measuring mean arterial pressure with a Doppler ultrasound. Personal communication with Dr. Therattil, Director, Spinal Cord Injury Medicine & Inpatient Rehabilitation Services Montefiore Medical Center, Asst Prof. Department of Rehabilitation Medicine Albert Einstein College of Medicine, Bronx, NY.

20. Kugler C, Malehsa D, Tegtbur U, et al. Health-related quality of life and exercise tolerance in recipients of heart transplants and left ventricular assist devices: a prospective, comparative study. *J Heart Lung Transplant*. 2011;30:204-210.

21. Schaffer JM, Allen JG, Weiss ES, et al. Infectious complications after pulsatile-flow and continuous-flow left ventricular assist device implantation. *J Heart Lung Transplant*. 2011;30:164-174.

22. Organ Procurement and Transplant Network. Heart Kaplan-Meier Median Waiting Times For Registrations Listed: 1999-2004. Based on OPTN data as of August 19, 2011. http://optn.transplant.hrsa.gov/latestData/rptStrat.asp. Accessed August 29, 2011.

23. Davies EJ, Moxham T, Rees K, et al. Exercise based rehabilitation for heart failure. *Cochrane Database Syst Rev*. 2010;4:CD003331.

24. Haft J, Armstrong W, Dyke DB, et al. Hemodynamic and exercise performance with pulsatile and continuous-flow left ventricular assist devices. *Circulation*. 2007;116:I8-15.

25. Cahalin L, Lapier T, Shaw D. Sternal precautions: is it time for change? Precautions versus restrictions—a review of literature and recommendations for revision. *Cardiopulm Phys Ther*. 2011;22:5-15.

26. Crabtree TD, Codd JE, Fraser VJ, et al. Multivariate analysis of risk factors for deep and superficial sternal infection after coronary artery bypass grafting at a tertiary care medical center. *Sem Thorac Cardiovasc Surg*. 2004;16:53-61.

27. Thoratec Corporation. Frequently Asked Questions. http://www.thoratec.com/patients-caregivers/living-with-vad/faqs.aspx#. Accessed September 12, 2011.

28. de Jonge N, Kirkels H, Lahpor JR, et al. Exercise performance in patients with end-stage heart failure after implantation of a left ventricular assist device and after heart transplantation: an outlook for permanent assisting? *J Am Coll Cardiol*. 2001;37:1794-1799.

Chronic Obstructive Pulmonary Disease

Lawrence P. Cahalin

The patient is a 56-year-old male who was admitted in early December 2011 with a diagnosis of chronic obstructive pulmonary disease (COPD) exacerbation. The patient has a 76 pack-year smoking history (2 packs per day for 38 years). He has a marked barrel-shaped chest and mild paradoxical breathing pattern that worsens with physical activity. His chest radiograph demonstrates markedly enlarged lungs, increased lucency, and numerous bullae (greater in the upper lobes bilaterally), and marked flattening of the diaphragm. The patient has been admitted twice over the past 6 months for similar COPD exacerbations that produced marked dyspnea and fatigue, fever, decreased functional and exercise tolerance, excessive coughing (which made it even more difficult to breathe), and marked anxiety. The patient reports more frequent exacerbations in the winter (especially when family members are ill) and tries to remain indoors throughout most of the season. Six months prior to the current admission, the patient was intubated and received mechanical ventilation for 1 week. However, on the most recent admission 3 months ago, he underwent a trial of bilevel positive airway pressure (BiPAP) noninvasive mechanical ventilation, which prevented the need for him to be intubated and mechanically ventilated. The emergency department admission note for the current hospitalization indicated that the patient demonstrated less of a paradoxical breathing pattern than the last admission and that the patient was posturing himself to facilitate his breathing (sitting with trunk flexion and both forearms resting on his thighs). The patient's pulmonary function test (PFT) results have been stable over the past year (Table 14-1), but his arterial blood gas (ABG) values have been progressively worsening (Table 14-3). The ABG values during this hospitalization reveal a substantially higher level of carbon dioxide and lower level of oxygen. The medical team is contemplating intubation and mechanical ventilation versus a BiPAP trial because of his ABG values, marked dyspnea and fatigue, difficulty breathing, and paradoxical breathing pattern. On the second day after admission, the physical therapist is consulted to examine and treat the patient and to assist the medical team in determining the best treatment plan for the patient (invasive versus noninvasive ventilation).

▶ What examination signs may be associated with this diagnosis?

▶ Based on the patient's diagnosis, what do you anticipate may be the contributing factors to his condition?

▶ What are the most appropriate physical therapy outcome measures for patients hospitalized with an acute exacerbation of COPD?

▶ What is his rehabilitation prognosis?

▶ What are the most appropriate physical therapy interventions?

▶ What precautions should be taken during physical therapy examination and/or interventions?

KEY DEFINITIONS

ARTERIAL BLOOD GASES (ABGs): Blood test at rest or during exercise that measures levels of oxygen (PaO_2), carbon dioxide ($PaCO_2$), and often pH; normal values are 75 to 100 mm Hg for PaO_2 and 35 to 45 mm Hg for $PaCO_2$[1-6]

BILEVEL POSITIVE AIRWAY PRESSURE (BiPAP) NONINVASIVE MECHANICAL VENTILATION: Ventilation administered through either a nasal or nasal and mouth mask that provides two different levels of positive pressure ventilation; higher positive pressure is administered during inhalation and lower positive pressure is administered during exhalation

CONTINUOUS POSITIVE AIRWAY PRESSURE (CPAP) NONINVASIVE MECHANICAL VENTILATION: Ventilation administered through either a nasal mask or nasal and mouth mask that provides one constant level of positive pressure during both inhalation and exhalation

MECHANICAL VENTILATION: Invasive or noninvasive method to assist or completely breathe for a patient unable to adequately breathe independently; factors that typically lead to mechanical ventilation include rising $PaCO_2$, decreasing PaO_2, rapid respiratory rate, ineffective ventilation, and paradoxical breathing pattern

OXYGEN SATURATION (SaO_2): Percentage of oxygen bound to hemoglobin molecules in the blood; 96% to 100% is normal[1-6]

PARADOXICAL BREATHING: Breathing pattern characterized by upward and outward motion of the upper chest and inward motion of the abdominal area during inspiration; believed to be associated with respiratory muscle dysfunction and/or failure

PULMONARY FUNCTION TESTS (PFTs): Breathing tests that provide information about exhalation and inhalation of air from the lungs; body plethysmography or helium dilution techniques measure air volume within lungs; spirometry provides measurements of airflow and volume and is frequently limited to expiratory measurements such as forced expiratory volume at one second (FEV_1) and forced vital capacity (FVC); values are measured in liters or liters/unit of time and normal values depend on sex, age, height, and weight

VENTILATION: Movement of air into and out of the lungs

Objectives

1. Describe COPD and reasons for an acute exacerbation of COPD.
2. Identify several outcome measures to quantify the severity of COPD and factors associated with COPD exacerbations.
3. Describe the manner by which a physical therapist can examine and manage a patient with an acute exacerbation of COPD.

Physical Therapy Considerations

PT considerations during management of the individual with an acute exacerbation of COPD:

▶ **General physical therapy plan of care/goals:** Prevent or minimize loss of range of motion, strength, and aerobic functional capacity; decrease respiratory and peripheral skeletal muscle weakness during mechanical ventilation; improve quality of life

▶ **Physical therapy interventions:** Patient education regarding breathing and mechanical ventilation; respiratory and peripheral skeletal muscle strengthening; functional mobility and exercise training to improve functional status; energy conservation techniques

▶ **Precautions during physical therapy:** Monitor vital signs; oxygen desaturation and rising PCO_2; respiratory muscle weakness, fatigue, and failure

▶ **Complications interfering with physical therapy:** Invasive mechanical ventilation, oxygen desaturation

Understanding the Health Condition

COPD is group of lung disorders including emphysema, bronchitis, and asthma that impair exhalation of air from the lungs. COPD is a major health concern. Approximately 24 million adults in the United States have COPD and it ranks as the fourth leading cause of death. In 2000, COPD was responsible for 8 million outpatient visits, 1.5 million emergency department visits, 726,000 hospitalizations, and 119,000 deaths.[7] Cigarette smoking is the most significant risk factor for the development and progression of COPD. Other major risk factors include air pollution, recurrent respiratory infections, genetic factors, and allergens. The prognosis of patients with COPD is generally poor because diagnosis does not typically occur until patients become symptomatic with moderate to severe COPD. Prognosis is substantially worse if exposure to air pollution or cigarette smoke continues. However, if COPD is diagnosed early and exposure to unfavorable conditions is eliminated, the prognosis is improved.[7] Typically, diagnosis and prognosis of COPD is performed using spirometry. Prognosis can also be predicted using the BODE index. The BODE index is a

Table 14-1 PULMONARY FUNCTION TESTS FOR CASE STUDY PATIENT AND COMPARISON TO PREDICTED NORMS			
	Observed	Predicted	% of Predicted
Spirometry results			
FEV_1 (L)	0.42	2.7	16
FVC (L)	1.11	3.32	33
FEV_1/FVC	35	81	43
Plethysmography results			
Total lung capacity (L)	7.17	4.99	144
Residual volume (L)	6.06	1.78	340

calculation based on four factors that have been shown to predict the risk of death of patients with COPD. The four factors are: body mass index (B), airflow obstruction (O, as measured by FEV_1), dyspnea level (D), and exercise capacity (E, as measured by performance on the Six-Minute Walk Test [6MWT]). The BODE index provides an objective measure, with higher scores associated with poorer survival. The BODE index appears to show good promise in quantifying the disability associated with COPD and prognosis of patients with COPD.[8]

Table 14-1 shows the results from the patient's PFTs that were done prior to his most recent hospital discharge 3 months ago. His values are substantially different than the predicted values for a male of comparable age without COPD.

His FEV_1 was 0.42 L, whereas the predicted value is 2.7 L. Thus, the percentage of the predicted value for FEV_1 was only 16% (0.42/2.7 = 16%). His forced vital capacity (FVC) is similarly decreased at 1.11 L, representing 33% of the predicted percentage, another indication of severe obstructive lung disease. Therefore, the spirometry results indicate that this patient exhales only 16% of what he is expected to exhale at one second of exhalation and only 33% of what he is expected to exhale during a complete untimed forced exhalation. The FEV_1/FVC ratio (0.42/1.11 = 38%) is a useful measurement that helps to categorize the severity of obstructive lung disease.[1,2] An individual without lung disease typically exhales about 75% of the air taken in after a maximal inspiration.[1,2] If an individual has an obstructive lung disease, the amount of air exhaled decreases, yielding an FEV_1/FVC ratio that is less than 75%.[1,2] It can be assumed that the lower the FEV_1/FVC ratio (< 75%), the more severe the obstructive lung disease.[1,2] This patient has very severe obstructive lung disease since his FEV_1/FVC ratio is only 38%. The FEV_1/FVC ratio also distinguishes obstructive from restrictive lung disease—which is associated with an FEV_1/FVC ratio that approaches the value of 1.[1,2] Thus, a patient with restrictive lung disease (such as spinal cord injury or a disease that limits the ability to inhale) will have FEV_1 and FVC values that are very similar.

The American Thoracic Society has published percentage of predicted values of FEV_1, FVC, and the diffusion capacity for carbon monoxide (DLCO) that are associated with mild, moderate, or severe lung disease (Table 14-2).[9]

	Normal	Mild Disease	Moderate Disease	Severe Disease
Test	(% of Predicted)	(% of Predicted)	(% of Predicted)	(% of Predicted)
FVC	≥ 80	60-80	50-60	≤ 50
FEV$_1$	≥ 80	60-80	40-60	≤ 40
DLCO	80	60-80	40-60	≤ 40

Table 14-2 AMERICAN THORACIC SOCIETY CLASSIFICATION OF LUNG DISEASE

Based on spirometry results from 3 months ago, the current patient would be classified as having severe COPD since his percentage of predicted values for FEV$_1$ (16%) and FVC (33%) are less than 40% and 50%, respectively. This patient was unable to hold his breath due to severe dyspnea that prevented the DLCO from being measured. His inability to hold his breath (combined with the poor PFTs) demonstrated his poor respiratory reserve and provides rationale for the frequency of his acute COPD exacerbations.

Inhaled cigarette smoke destroys lung parenchyma and results in severe air trapping due to destruction of alveolar and bronchial tissue without a clear route for inhaled air to be removed.[1,2] Trapped air compresses the airways (and decreases airway diameter so that less air can be exhaled) and presses on thoracic skeletal structures, producing a characteristic barrel-shaped chest.[1,2] The end result of air trapping within the lungs can be better appreciated from the results of body plethysmography, which provides information about the volume of air within the lungs.[1,2] Table 14-1 shows the patient's plethysmograph results prior to discharge from his 9/2011 hospitalization. Marked air trapping is apparent in his total lung capacity (TLC) and residual volume (RV) measurements. His TLC was 7.17 L (144% of predicted) and his RV was 6.06 L (340% of predicted). The RV is the amount of air that remains in the lungs after a maximal exhalation. This patient has such severe air trapping that the RV is far greater than it should be and is responsible for not only his barrel-shaped chest, but also the flattened diaphragm observed on the chest radiograph taken at hospital admission. Suboptimal ventilation combined with trapped air creates an environment in the lungs in which respiratory infections can develop and easily progress to produce an acute COPD exacerbation. The patient's signs and symptoms and an understanding of the mechanisms producing his abnormal PFTs helps the physical therapist grasp the severity of this patient's lung disease and identify specific therapeutic options that might be available to optimize ventilatory capacity and functional outcome.[1,2]

Physical Therapy Patient/Client Management

The management of a patient with an acute exacerbation of COPD requires a team approach in which the physical therapist has an important role.[3,4] The physical therapist's role often includes: (1) examining the patient's breathing pattern, oxygen saturation, symptoms, and vital signs at rest and during functional tasks; (2) examining the effects of body position change, breathing exercises, functional/exercise training, medications, and airway clearance techniques on lung sounds, oxygen saturation, and symptoms; (3) examining respiratory muscle strength and endurance as well as chest wall expansion at rest and during/after functional tasks; and (4) documenting functional status at discharge (and possibly on admission) via a walk test.[3,4]

Examination, Evaluation, and Diagnosis

The current status of the patient with an acute exacerbation of COPD can be better appreciated by reviewing past hospitalizations and therapeutic management strategies previously utilized. Current laboratory values, especially the ABGs, must be reviewed.[3-6] Table 14-3 shows the ABGs from this patient over the previous 6-month period.

The progressive decrease in PaO_2, increase in $PaCO_2$, and decrease in pH (reflecting increased carbon dioxide trapping and decreased ability of the kidneys to buffer the increased acidity) illustrate the worsening status of the patient's condition.

The physical examination of this patient includes: examination of breathing pattern, testing of respiratory muscle strength and endurance, lung auscultation, and a performance of a walk test with vigilant monitoring of oxygen saturation via pulse oximetry. Results of these assessments can provide a more specific physical therapy diagnosis and prognosis and provide evidence-based clinical recommendations.[3-6]

The therapist can examine the breathing pattern visually, via palpation, and/or by using sophisticated devices to examine chest and abdominal motion.[10] At rest, normal breathing is commonly described as a nonlabored process whereby abdominal and upper chest motion are equal and synchronous occurring at a rate of 10 to 12 breaths per minute. Extreme exertion in healthy individuals or in those with lung disease increases the respiratory rate and alters the breathing pattern, resulting in greater use of upper chest motion (i.e., increased accessory muscle use compared to abdominal motion from diaphragm use) to achieve optimal ventilation. Such dependency on upper chest breathing can be seen after extreme exertion in athletes bending forward with hands placed on knees or in patients leaning forward with forearms placed on a cart. Upper chest breathing is accomplished by using the upper extremities as a fulcrum to lift the upper thorax and increase ventilation in this portion of the thorax. Individuals with lung disease rely on upper chest breathing when the diaphragm is impaired due to weakness, fatigue, paralysis, or mimicked paralysis. Mimicked paralysis of the diaphragm is observed in patients with severe hyperinflation of the lungs that places the diaphragm in a severely compromised biomechanical

Table 14-3 CASE STUDY PATIENT'S ABGS DURING HOSPITALIZATIONS FOR ACUTE EXACERBATION OF COPD OVER A 6-MONTH PERIOD			
Date	Admit/Discharge PaO_2	Admit/Discharge $PaCO_2$	Admit/Discharge pH
6/2011	50 mm Hg/70 mm Hg	65 mm Hg/54 mm Hg	7.26/7.38
9/2011	48 mm Hg/68 mm Hg	68 mm Hg/52 mm Hg	7.24/7.38
12/2011	44 mm Hg/68 mm Hg	70 mm Hg/50 mm Hg	7.20/7.37

(shortened-contracted) position. This patient's chest radiograph showed a flattened diaphragm consistent with severe hyperinflation of the lungs indicated by his plethysmography results. This poor biomechanical position impairs diaphragmatic contraction and contributes to the paradoxical breathing pattern noted on his initial admission. The paradoxical breathing pattern is characterized by an upward and outward upper chest motion and inward motion of the abdominal area during inspiration. This motion is paradoxical because it is not the normal synchronous and equal motion of the upper chest and abdominal area.[10]

Examination of the strength and endurance of the respiratory muscles may not be frequently performed in the acute care setting, but often includes an indirect assessment of inspiratory muscle performance via incentive spirometry to examine inspiratory capacity (volume of air inhaled). Because these vital muscles are subject to frequent changes in contractile characteristics due to disease, medications, and other therapeutic modalities such as mechanical ventilation, inspiratory muscle training, and/or exercise training, the examination of both inspiratory and expiratory muscle strength may provide important information to better understand the manifestations of COPD and the effects of therapeutic interventions.[11] Measurement of respiratory muscle strength and endurance should be deferred in patients who are extremely dyspneic and/or demonstrate a marked paradoxical breathing pattern. However, once a patient becomes more comfortable and the breathing pattern normalizes, breathing muscle strength and inspiratory endurance can be measured.[11] Occasionally, tests of respiratory muscle strength will also be performed on patients receiving invasive or noninvasive mechanical ventilation to determine when to terminate mechanical ventilation. To perform these tests, the patient must wear a noseclip and be seated (usually with the trunk supported) with a hip-trunk angle of 90°. Maximal inspiratory pressure (MIP), maximal expiratory pressure (MEP), and inspiratory endurance can be measured with commercially available devices or with a standard sphygmomanometer used to measure blood pressure with the tubing from the manometer attached to a mouthpiece (mm Hg can be converted to cm H_2O by multiplying mm Hg × 1.36). For MIP, the therapist asks the patient to fully exhale (near residual volume). Next, the patient needs to inhale as forcefully as possible. The therapist documents the MIP and has the patient repeat the test until a stable value is achieved. For MEP, the therapist first asks the patient to fully inhale (TLC). Next, the therapist asks the patient to exhale as forcefully as possible. The therapist documents the MEP and asks the patient to repeat the test until a stable value is achieved. The patient's values can then be compared to published norms.[12] For measurement of inspiratory muscle endurance, the patient is asked to inhale at a level that is greater than 50% of MIP with a constant *rate* of inspiration (using a metronome or timer) while monitoring each inspiratory effort. The therapist records the number of inspirations or the amount of time the patient is able to continue inspiring at a level that is greater than 50% of MIP. The endurance test is terminated when the patient is unable to achieve an inspiratory force that is greater than 50% of MIP on two consecutive attempts.[11]

The physical therapist should perform a bedside auscultation of the lungs. Lung auscultation can provide important information about movement of air through the airways, abnormal lung sounds characteristic of particular lung diseases,

Table 14-4 RESULTS FOR 6MWT AT TIME OF DISCHARGE FOR HOSPITALIZATIONS DUE TO ACUTE EXACERBATION OF COPD			
Date	Discharge 6MWT Distance	Discharge SpO$_2$ (Room Air; at End of 6MWT)	Discharge RPE (At End of 6MWT)
6/2011	180 m	88%	8/10
9/2011	178 m	86%	8/10
12/2011	190 m	88%	7/10

and the need for breathing exercises, secretion removal techniques, and coughing exercises.[13] Auscultation can be performed using the diaphragm of the stethoscope and a systematic process assessing the lung fields in the posterior and anterior thorax. Listening to the quality as well as duration of sound in particular areas of the thorax during both inhalation and exhalation helps to differentiate normal from abnormal lung sounds. The presence of a sound not normally heard in any area constitutes an abnormal lung sound and often requires more sophisticated tests to confirm the specific pathology. However, two specific findings worthy of note are: (1) the *absence* of sound when a patient is observed to inhale and exhale (with accompanying chest wall motion); and (2) the *presence* of adventitious lung sounds such as crackles, rhonchi, and wheezing. The absence of sound is suggestive of minimal or no aeration within a particular portion of the lung, while the presence of crackles and rhonchi may indicate the presence of retained pulmonary secretions in need of mobilization.[13] The case study patient demonstrated both of the above findings.

The administration of a standardized walk test such as the 6MWT can provide important information about functional performance, gait, balance, cardiovascular and pulmonary status, symptoms, and response to therapeutic interventions.[14-17] It is critical to measure the patient's perceived exertion and oxygen saturation (estimated via pulse oximetry, SpO$_2$) before, during, and after recovery from the test. If the patient becomes hypoxic (SpO$_2$ < 88%-92%) at any time, supplemental oxygen at rest and during exercise must be provided to maintain safe levels of oxygenation. At the time of this patient's most recent discharge from the hospital, he ambulated only 50% of the predicted distance for his age on the 6MWT.[14-17] He also had an abnormal cardiovascular and pulmonary response to exercise as shown in Table 14-4.

Results from the patient's 6MWT can be used to determine the patient's functional capacity at discharge, provide information about further education needed on energy conservation, exercise training, and whether supplemental oxygen should be recommended to prevent desaturation when the patient is discharged from the hospital. Furthermore, the distance ambulated by the case study patient was at a level that has been observed to be predictive of poorer survival.[17]

Plan of Care and Interventions

Table 14-5 outlines the plan of care and interventions provided to the patient during the current and two previous hospital admissions. Medical care included optimal pharmacologic treatment (oxygen during hypoxemia, inhaled β_2-adrenergic agonists,

Table 14-5   PLAN OF CARE AND INTERVENTIONS ON PREVIOUS AND CURRENT ADMISSIONS

Type of Care	Date (Length of Hospital Stay) 6/2011 (9 Days)	Date (Length of Hospital Stay) 9/2011 (7 Days)	Date (Length of Hospital Stay) 12/2011 (6 Days)
Medical			
Invasive mechanical ventilation	5 d	0 d	0 d
BiPAP	0 d	6 d	5 d
Physical therapy			
Breathing exercises	10 min for 7 d	15 min for 5 d	10 min for 3 d
Inspiratory muscle training (IMT)	—	10 min for 1 d	10 min for 3 d
Cycling (no resistance)	—	3 min for 1 d (40 revolutions/min)	3-5 min for 3 d (50 revolutions/min)
Resistive tubing	—	—	2 d (3-5 repetitions each extremity, every other day)
Hallway ambulation	—	3 d (10-20 ft, 2-3 times/d)	4 d (10-20 ft, 2-3 times/d)
Patient self-care	10 min for 1 d	10 min for 6 d	15 min for 5 d

inhaled anticholinergics, antibiotics, and systemic glucocorticoids, as needed) as well as invasive and noninvasive ventilation. Patient self-care included independent use of the Flutter device (to facilitate mucus clearance, as needed), which the patient had been taught during a previous hospitalization. Physical therapy interventions included postural drainage, chest percussion and vibration, deep breathing, and coughing exercises. Inspiratory muscle training was provided via a Threshold device that requires a specific level of inspiratory pressure be achieved before air moves through the device into the lungs. With the Threshold device, the patient practiced inhaling at 20% of maximal inspiratory pressure for 5 minutes, twice per day. Additional exercise included stationary cycling, seated resistance training for knee extension and shoulder flexion (using yellow Theraband), and hallway ambulation with a front-wheeled walker. Cycling and resistance exercises were performed with BiPAP during the current hospitalization, which enabled greater exercise duration with less dyspnea and fatigue. BiPAP was also used on 3 of the 5 days to assist in recovery from exercise. All exercise was introduced gradually and was performed at a rating of perceived exertion (RPE) of no greater than 4/10.

The primary difference between current and previous hospitalizations was the use of BiPAP during and after functional and exercise training during physical therapy management. In fact, the patient suggested using BiPAP during exercise. He described that using BiPAP at home allowed him to pedal his stationary cycle at a faster cadence and for a longer duration. A stationary cycle was subsequently brought to the patient's room and the patient donned his BiPAP mask and began cycling.

Similar to what he reported at home, the patient was able to cycle faster and longer than during previous hospitalizations. Furthermore, the patient also used BiPAP to recover from exercise and after extensive medical testing was performed on several days. The use of BiPAP also appeared to facilitate inspiratory muscle training, which was previously limited by dyspnea, fatigue, and an apparent lack of motivation.

The evidence supporting the **use of BiPAP or CPAP in patients with an acute exacerbation of COPD at rest** is strong.[18-20] A 2002 meta-analysis of eight studies found that the use of noninvasive positive pressure ventilation (NIPPV) in patients with an acute exacerbation of COPD significantly reduced mortality, need for mechanical ventilation, and length of hospitalization.[19] Although there was a consistent favorable effect with NIPPV in patients with an acute exacerbation of COPD, a more recent meta-analysis of NIPPV in stable patients with severe COPD found a consistent improvement in dyspnea and quality of life, but less consistent improvement in gas exchange, lung hyperinflation, and work of breathing.[20] The case study patient admitted with an acute exacerbation of COPD benefited from NIPPV at rest (*i.e.*, BiPAP) by not requiring intubation and mechanical ventilation, which resulted in a shorter hospitalization than previous admissions.

In patients with COPD, the benefits of **using BiPAP or CPAP during functional and/or exercise training** is also well supported in the literature.[21-25] No study has specifically examined the effects of NIPPV during exercise at the time of an *acute* COPD exacerbation. Nonetheless, a 2002 systematic review of seven studies on the use of NIPPV during exercise in patients with COPD found that NIPPV significantly improved symptoms and exercise duration.[21] Several subsequent studies of NIPPV during exercise in this population found similar results.[22-25] One study found that NIPPV increased exercise duration in patients with severe COPD and this improvement was significantly related to several baseline respiratory parameters including respiratory muscle strength and endurance, ventilation, and ABGs.[22] Patients with poorer MIP and MEP, inspiratory muscle endurance, and ventilation had greater improvements in exercise duration with NIPPV.[22] Bianchi et al.[23] examined the effect of three different modes of NIPPV (CPAP, pressure support ventilation, and proportional assist ventilation) on exercise duration, dyspnea, and supplemental oxygen supply in patients with severe COPD. They found that all modes of NIPPV significantly improved exercise duration and dyspnea and decreased supplemental oxygen requirements, with proportional assist ventilation having the greatest improvement on all of the above variables. A more recent study found that NIPPV (proportional assist ventilation) significantly improved exercise duration, dyspnea, and quality of life for patients with moderate COPD.[24] Finally, in work currently under review, patients who responded favorably to NIPPV tended to have poorer PFTs, greater TLC and residual volume, and poorer exercise tolerance.[25] The case study patient had very poor PFTs, very high residual volume, and poor exercise tolerance at baseline which may have contributed to his success with NIPPV during exercise.

Aerobic exercise or strength training benefits patients with an acute exacerbation of COPD and must be incorporated into the physical therapy plan of care.[26-31] In 2005, a systematic review of six studies examining the effects of respiratory rehabilitation (which included at least some form of physical exercise) in patients with an acute exacerbation of COPD found that respiratory rehabilitation reduced subsequent hospitalizations and mortality and improved quality of life and exercise capacity.[27] However, the time period when exercise was implemented after the acute exacerbation varied and only two of the six studies examined the effects of exercise training during inpatient stays.[27] A subsequent review article on exercise in patients with COPD identified some of these issues and called for a closer examination of exercise in inpatient and outpatient settings with a focus on peripheral muscle training.[28] Previous findings showed that during an acute COPD exacerbation, peripheral skeletal muscle strength deteriorated throughout the hospital stay and only partially recovered by 90 days after hospital discharge.[29] A systematic review of nine studies of peripheral muscle training in patients with COPD revealed that strength training improved upper and lower extremity strength, but did not improve PFTs, psychological status, activity level, or exercise tolerance.[30] One finding was that the decrease in skeletal muscle strength was significantly related to systemic inflammation.[29] Thus, an initial concern for prescribing exercise in patients during hospitalization for COPD exacerbation surfaced because of the possibility that exercise during an acute inflammation could increase the inflammatory response and further worsen skeletal muscle strength.[28-30] However, a study examining the effects of outpatient pulmonary rehabilitation in patients after hospitalization for COPD exacerbation (within 10 days of hospital discharge) found no detrimental effects and patients had improved exercise capacity and health status compared to usual care.[31] The case study patient had poor baseline exercise tolerance that improved during his hospitalization which was likely due to the medical care and gradual progression of low-level exercises that were administered during his hospitalization.

The evidence base for the use of **inspiratory muscle training (IMT)** in patients with COPD is strong.[32-34] However, no study has examined the effects of IMT in patients with an *acute* exacerbation of COPD. Inspiratory muscle training in patients with COPD has been studied extensively resulting in three comprehensive meta-analyses.[32-34] The first meta-analysis in 1992 analyzed 17 studies and only one outcome measure (maximal voluntary ventilation) was significantly improved after IMT.[32] However, subanalysis of these data revealed that in five studies in which the IMT workload was controlled, significantly improved levels of dyspnea and inspiratory muscle strength were observed after IMT.[32] The second meta-analysis in 2002 in which 15 studies (all of which controlled the IMT workload) were analyzed revealed that IMT improved dyspnea as well as inspiratory muscle strength and endurance (with a nearly significant improvement in exercise capacity).[33] The third meta-analysis analyzed 32 studies which revealed that IMT improved inspiratory muscle strength and endurance, dyspnea, walk test distance, and quality of life.[34] An important IMT study in patients with severe COPD that is directly related to patients with an *acute* COPD exacerbation revealed that IMT performed at 60% of MIP for 30 minutes, 6 days per week for 12 months significantly improved dyspnea, MIP, exercise capacity, and quality of life and significantly reduced hospital admissions, number of days hospitalized, and primary care physician utilization.[35] Another noteworthy IMT study in patients with COPD found that IMT resulted in an increase in the proportion of Type I intercostal muscles fibers (by 38%) and hypertrophy of Type II intercostal muscle fibers (by 21%), which was accompanied by significant increases in inspiratory muscle strength and endurance.[36] Although no study has examined the effects of IMT in patients with an acute exacerbation of COPD, the case study patient tolerated IMT without adverse effect. Furthermore, the above literature supports that IMT has the potential to decrease hospital admission for an acute COPD exacerbation.[35]

Breathing exercises and secretion removal techniques include a variety of interventions commonly prescribed to patients to improve oxygenation and expel secretions.[37-42] As a group, the evidence to support their use is fair, with the exception of pursed-lips breathing (PLB) which has a stronger evidence base.[37-41]

A 2002 review found the evidence supporting diaphragmatic breathing in patients with COPD questionable due to poor study design and methods to perform diaphragmatic breathing, and the use of many different outcome measures.[10] The authors suggested that patients with moderate to severe COPD with marked lung hyperinflation without adequate diaphragmatic movement and increase in tidal volume during diaphragmatic breathing may be poor candidates for diaphragmatic breathing. Conversely, patients with COPD who have elevated respiratory rates, low tidal volumes that increase during diaphragmatic breathing, and abnormal ABGs with adequate diaphragmatic movement may benefit from diaphragmatic breathing.[10] The authors of a subsequent review suggested that diaphragmatic breathing should not be performed by patients with COPD due to the fact that any positive effects of diaphragmatic breathing were due primarily to slowing the respiratory rate.[38] Thus, the authors suggested that PLB should be performed by this population to normalize respiratory rates. For the case study patient, PLB was one of the most effective and beneficial forms of breathing retraining.[38] A 2004 review article concluded that PLB is effective and produces more physiologic and efficient ventilation by improving the breathing pattern and respiratory muscle recruitment, tidal volume, gas exchange, and oxygen consumption.[39] Interestingly, this same review questioned the use of PLB to improve dyspnea.[39] However, a classic study by Bianchi et al.[40] found that PLB improved both chest wall motion and dyspnea in patients with moderate to severe COPD. In 2007, another study confirmed that PLB significantly improved dyspnea during functional tasks and provided sustained improvement in exertional dyspnea and physical function in patients with severe COPD.[41]

Surprisingly, the use of secretion removal techniques in patients with COPD has received minimal attention.[37,42] In 1998, a Cochrane Review of seven studies revealed that bronchopulmonary hygiene was effective at clearing sputum in patients with COPD and bronchiectasis, but had no effect on PFTs or other outcome measures.[42] An updated review in 2007 produced no additional studies. However, the authors indicated that a true meta-analysis could not be performed because of different patient groups and outcome measures.[42] In 2000, Bellone et al.[37] examined the effects of three different forms of secretion removal in patients with an acute exacerbation of chronic bronchitis. The secretion removal techniques included postural drainage and percussion, oscillating positive expiratory pressure (via the

Flutter device) in a seated position, and exhalation with an open glottis in a lateral (assumed sidelying, but not specifically stated) body position.[37] All techniques significantly increased sputum production 30 minutes after they were administered, but oscillating positive expiratory pressure and exhalation with an open glottis produced significantly greater sputum quantity than did postural drainage 60 minutes after the techniques were administered.[37] The patient in this case had been previously provided a Flutter device and he found it useful during acute COPD exacerbations. The patient also used the Flutter device at home for 5 to 10 minutes, twice per day (typically in the morning after waking and in the evening before going to bed) to help clear retained secretions.

More research in patients with an acute exacerbation of COPD is warranted. A comprehensive overview of the physical therapy management of patients with lung disorders (in which patients with an acute exacerbation of COPD are included) has been published by the British Thoracic Society and Chartered Society of Physiotherapy and may serve as a useful resource.[18]

Evidence-Based Clinical Recommendations

SORT: Strength of Recommendation Taxonomy

A: Consistent, good-quality patient-oriented evidence

B: Inconsistent or limited-quality patient-oriented evidence

C: Consensus, disease-oriented evidence, usual practice, expert opinion, or case series

1. BiPAP or CPAP noninvasive mechanical ventilation decreases mortality, need for mechanical ventilation, and length of hospitalization in patients with an acute exacerbation of COPD. **Grade A**

2. Use of BiPAP or CPAP during functional activities and/or exercise training significantly improves symptoms, exercise duration, dyspnea, and quality of life in individuals with COPD. **Grade A**

3. Aerobic exercise or strength training reduces subsequent hospitalizations and mortality and improves quality of life, exercise capacity, and upper and lower extremity strength in individuals with COPD. **Grade B**

4. In individuals with COPD, inspiratory muscle training (IMT) improves maximal voluntary ventilation, dyspnea, inspiratory muscle strength and endurance, exercise capacity, walk test distance, and quality of life and reduces hospital admissions, number of days hospitalized, and primary care physician utilization. **Grade A**

5. Breathing exercises, breathing retraining, PLB, and secretion removal techniques improve breathing pattern and respiratory muscle recruitment, tidal volume, gas exchange, oxygen consumption, and sputum production in individuals with COPD. **Grade B, except for pursed-lips breathing, which is Grade A**

COMPREHENSION QUESTIONS

14.1 Diaphragmatic breathing exercises for the case study patient:
   A. Should not be performed
   B. Should be performed carefully while examining chest and abdominal motion
   C. Should be performed without concern for chest and abdominal motion
   D. Should be performed several times per day

14.2 The use of noninvasive positive pressure ventilation (NIPPV) by the case study patient during exercise *most* likely:
   A. Rested the respiratory muscles during exercise and worsened oxygenation
   B. Exercised the respiratory muscles during exercise and worsened oxygenation
   C. Rested the respiratory muscles during exercise and improved oxygenation
   D. Exercised the respiratory muscles during exercise and improved oxygenation

ANSWERS

14.1 **A.** The patient in this case has a diaphragm that is in a poor biomechanical position (noted on the chest x-ray) due to severe hyperinflation of the lungs (as shown by plethysmograph results) that contributed to a paradoxical breathing pattern noted at rest on admission and worsened with most functional tasks (both on admission and discharge from the hospital). Patients with moderate to severe COPD and marked hyperinflation of the lungs without adequate diaphragmatic movement because of compromised biomechanical position may be poor candidates for diaphragmatic breathing. PLB may be the most useful form of breathing for the case study patient.[10,38]

14.2 **C.** A 2002 systematic review of seven studies on the use of NIPPV during exercise in patients with COPD found that NIPPV significantly improved symptoms and exercise duration.[21] Several subsequent studies of NIPPV during exercise in patients with COPD found similar results as well as several important findings relevant to the case study patient.[22-25] One study found that NIPPV improved the exercise duration of patients with severe COPD and the improvement in exercise duration was significantly related to several baseline respiratory parameters including respiratory muscle strength and endurance, ventilation, and ABGs.[22] Patients with poorer maximal inspiratory and expiratory pressure, inspiratory muscle endurance, and ventilation had greater improvements in exercise duration with NIPPV.[22] Another study examined three different modes of NIPPV (CPAP, pressure support ventilation, and proportional assist ventilation) on exercise duration, dyspnea, and supplemental oxygen supply in patients with severe COPD and found all modes of NIPPV significantly improved exercise duration, dyspnea, and decreased supplemental oxygen requirements.[23] These studies demonstrate that NIPPV assists ventilation, which decreases the work of the respiratory muscles (thus resting them) and by doing so has the potential to improve oxygenation by decreasing oxygen demand because the muscles work more efficiently.

REFERENCES

1. West JB. *Respiratory Physiology—The Essentials*. 5th ed. Baltimore, MD: Williams & Wilkins; 1995.

2. West JB. *Pulmonary Pathophysiology—The Essentials*. 4th ed. Baltimore, MD: Williams & Wilkins; 1992.

3. American Association of Cardiovascular and Pulmonary Rehabilitation. *Guidelines for Pulmonary Rehabilitation Programs*. 4th ed. Champaign, IL: Human Kinetics Publishers; 2011.

4. Ries AL, Bauldoff GS, Carlin BW, et al. Pulmonary rehabilitation: Joint ACCP/AACVPR evidence-based clinical practice guidelines. *Chest*. 2007;131:4S-42S.

5. McCrory DC, Brown C, Gelfand SE, et al. Management of acute exacerbations of COPD: a summary and appraisal of published evidence. *Chest*. 2001;119:1190-1209.

6. Rabe KF, Hurd S, Anzueto A, et al. Global strategy for the diagnosis, management, and prevention of chronic obstructive pulmonary disease: GOLD executive summary. *Am J Respir Crit Care Med*. 2007;176:532-555.

7. Chronic Obstructive Pulmonary Disease Surveillance—United States, 1971-2000. http://www.cdc.gov/mmwr/preview/mmwrhtml/ss5106a1.htm. Accessed May 22, 2012.

8. Celli BR, Cote CG, Marin JM, et al. The body-mass index, airflow obstruction, dyspnea, and exercise capacity index in chronic obstructive pulmonary disease. *N Eng J Med*. 2004;350:1005-1012.

9. Pellegrino R, Viegi G, Brusasco V, et al. Interpretive strategies for lung function tests. *Eur Respir J*. 2005;26:948-968.

10. Cahalin LP, Braga M, Matsuo Y, et al. Efficacy of diaphragmatic breathing in persons with chronic obstructive pulmonary disease: a review of the literature. *J Cariopulm Rehabil*. 2002;22:7-21.

11. Reid WD, Dechman G. Considerations when testing and training the respiratory muscles. *Phys Ther*. 1995;75:971-982.

12. Black LF, Hyatt RE. Maximal respiratory pressures: normal values and relationship to age and sex. *Am Rev Respir Dis*. 1969;99:696-702.

13. Karnath B, Boyars MC. Pulmonary Auscultation. *Hospital Physician*. 2002;38:22-26 http://www.turner-white.com/pdf/hp_jan02_pulmonary.pdf. Accessed May 22, 2012.

14. Enright PL, Sherrill DL. Reference equations for the six-minute walk test in healthy adults. *Am J Resp Crit Care Méd*. 1998;158:1384-1387.

15. Cahalin L, Pappagianopoulos P, Prevost S, et al. The relationship of the 6-min walk test ot maximal oxygen consumption in transplant candidates with end-stage lung disease. *Chest*. 1995;108: 452-459.

16. Solway S, Brooks D, Lacasse Y, et al. A qualitative systematic overview of the measurement properties of functional walk tests used in the cardiorespiratory domain. *Chest*. 2001;119:256-270.

17. Pinto-Plata VM, Cote C, Cabral H, et al. The 6-min walk test distance: change over time and value as a predictor of survival in severe COPD. *Eur Respir J*. 2004;23:28-33.

18. Bott J, Blumenthal S, Buxton M, et al. Guidelines for the physiotherapy management of the adult, medical, spontaneously breathing patient. *Thorax*. 2009;64(Suppl 1):1-51.

19. Peter JV, Moran JL, Phillips-Hughes J, et al. Noninvasive ventilation in acute respiratory failure—a meta-analysis update. *Crit Care Méd*. 2002;30:555-562.

20. Kolodziej MA, Jensen L, Rowe B, et al. Systematic review of noninvasive positive pressure ventilation in severe stable COPD. *Eur Resp J*. 2007;30:293-306.

21. van't Hul A, Kwakkel G, Gosselink R. The acute effects of noninvasive ventilatory support during exercise on exercise endurance and dyspnea in patients with chronic obstructive pulmonary disease: a systematic review. *J Cardiopulm Rehabil.* 2002;22: 290-297.

22. van't Hul A, Gosselink R, Hollander P, et al. Acute effects of inspiratory pressure support during during exercise in patients with COPD. *Eur Resp J.* 2004;23:34-40.

23. Bianchi L, Foglio K, Pagani M, et al. Effects of proportional assist ventilation on exercise tolerance in COPD patients with chronic hypercapnia. *Eur Resp J.* 1998;11:422-427.

24. Barakat S, Michele G, Nesme P, et al. Effect of a noninvasive ventilatory support during exercise of a program in pulmonary rehabilitation in patients with COPD. *Int J Chron Obstruct Pulmon Dis.* 2007;2:585-591.

25. Cahalin LP, Kacmarek R, Wain J, et al. Exercise performance during assisted noninvasive ventilation with bi-level positive airway pressure (BiPAP) in patients with end-stage obstructive lung disease awaiting lung transplantation: results of a clinical pilot trial. Manuscript in review.

26. Troosters T. Rehabilitation and acute exacerbations in chronic obstructive pulmonary disease. *Advanced Med Technologies,* Business Briefing: Global Healthcare, 2004:1-5 www.touchbriefings. com/pdf/950/troosters.pdf. Accessed May 22, 2012.

27. Puhan MA, Scharplatz M, Troosters T, et al. Respiratory rehabilitation after acute exacerbation of COPD may reduce risk for readmission and mortality—a systematic review. *Resp Res.* 2005;6:54.

28. Morgan MD. Peripheral muscle training in COPD: still much to learn. *Thorax.* 2005;60:359-360.

29. Spruit MA, Gosselink R, Troosters T, et al. Muscle force during an acute exacerbation in hospitalised patients with COPD and its relationship with CXCL8 and IGF-I. *Thorax.* 2003;58:752-756.

30. O'Shea SD, Taylor NF, Paratz J. Peripheral muscle strength training in COPD: a systematic review. *Chest* 2004;126:903-914.

31. Man WD, Polkey MI, Donaldson N, et al. Community pulmonary rehabilitation after hospitalisation for acute exacerbations of chronic obstructive pulmonary disease: randomised controlled study. *BMJ.* 2004;329:1209.

32. Smith K, Cook D, Guyatt GH, et al. Respiratory muscle training in chronic airflow limitation: a meta-analysis. *Am Rev Respir Dis.* 1992;145:533-539.

33. Lotters F, van Tol B, Kwakkel G, et al. Effects of controlled inspiratory muscle training in patients with COPD: a meta-analysis. *Eur Resp J.* 2002;20:570-576.

34. Gosselink R, De Vos J, van den Heuvel SP, et al. Impact of inspiratory muscle training in patients with COPD: what is the evidence? *Eur Resp J.* 2011;37:416-425.

35. Beckerman M, Magadle R, Weiner M, et al. The effects of 1 year of specific inspiratory muscle training in patients with COPD. *Chest.* 2005;128:3177-3182.

36. Ramirez-Sarmiento A, Orozco-Levi M, Guell R, et al. Inspiratory muscle training in patients with chronic obstructive pulmonary disease: structural adaptation and physiologic outcomes. *Am J Respir Crit Care Med.* 2002;166:1491-1497.

37. Bellone A, Lascioli R, Raschi S, et al. Chest physical therapy in patients with acute exacerbation of chronic bronchitis: effectiveness of three methods. *Arch Phys Med Rehabil.* 2000;81:558-560.

38. Dechman G Wilson CR. Evidence underlying breathing retraining in people with stable chronic obstructive pulmonary disease. *Phys Ther.* 2004;84:1189-1197.

39. Fregonezi GA de F, Resqueti VR, Guell Rous R. Pursed lips breathing. *Arch Bronconeumol.* 2004;40:279-282.

40. Bianchi R, Gigliotti F, Romagnoli I, et al. Chest wall kinematics and breathlessness during pursed-lip breathing in patients with COPD. *Chest.* 2004;125:459-465.

41. Nield MA, Soo Hoo GW, Roper JM, et al. Efficacy of pursed-lips breathing: a breathing pattern retraining strategy for dyspnea reduction. *J Cardiopulm Rehabil Prev.* 2007;27:237-244.

42. Jones AP, Rowe BH. Bronchopulmonary hygiene physical therapy for chronic obstructive pulmonary disease and bronchiectasis. *Cochrane Database Syst Rev.* 2000;(2):CD000045.

Lung Cancer Status/Post Lobe Resection

Lindsey M. Montana

A 57-year-old female presented to her primary physician's office with complaints of generalized fatigue and a persistent dry cough for the past month. Further diagnostic work-up revealed a localized mass in her left upper lung field that was identified as stage I non–small cell lung cancer (NSCLC). The patient was admitted to the hospital 2 weeks later for a planned flexible bronchoscopy and left posterolateral thoracotomy with left upper lobe lobectomy. Her past medical history is significant for paroxysmal atrial fibrillation, hyperlipidemia, and a 30 pack-year smoking history. The patient is referred for a physical therapy evaluation on postoperative day 1 (POD 1) for left lower lobe atelectasis and poor cough effect. The patient is a newly retired electrician who is actively involved in her community bowling league. She lives with her husband and teenage grandson in a two-story home. She is expected to be discharged home on POD 5.

▶ Based on her health condition, what do you anticipate may be the contributors to activity limitations?
▶ What are possible complications interfering with physical therapy?
▶ What are the most appropriate physical therapy interventions?
▶ What is her rehabilitation prognosis?
▶ Identify referrals to other medical team members.

KEY DEFINITIONS

ATELECTASIS: Collapse and airlessness of lung tissue

BRONCHOSCOPY: Internal inspection of the tracheobronchial tree with the use of a bronchoscope (flexible or rigid viewing instrument)

HEMOPTYSIS: Expectoration of blood from the lungs due to pulmonary or bronchial hemorrhage

PNEUMOTHORAX: Presence of air within the pleural space

SUBCUTANEOUS EMPHYSEMA: Presence of free air in the subcutaneous tissues (typically in skin over the chest, neck, or face), resulting from an air-leak in the lungs

Objectives

1. Understand the incidence, prevalence, and risk factors for NSCLC.

2. Describe two standard surgical procedures for the excision of early stage lung cancer.

3. Identify possible complications of thoracic surgery that may extend hospital stay and/or interfere with physical therapy interventions.

4. Describe the key elements of physical therapy examination, evaluation, and diagnosis in a patient status/post lung surgery.

5. Design an appropriate physical therapy plan of care for a patient status/post lung surgery based upon the goals, interventions, and considerations discussed in this case.

Physical Therapy Considerations

PT considerations during management of the individual status/post lobectomy due to lung cancer:

▶ **General physical therapy plan of care/goals:** Prevent or minimize loss of range of motion (ROM), strength, aerobic functional capacity, and risk of postoperative complications; optimize lung volumes, oxygen transport, ventilation–perfusion matching, and airway clearance; maximize quality of life through restoring physical endurance and functional independence

▶ **Physical therapy interventions:** Patient and family/caregiver education regarding benefits of early and frequent mobility after lung surgery; decrease risk of postoperative pneumonia and atelectasis through deep breathing activities and effective airway clearance techniques (ACTs), upper extremity and chest wall ROM exercises, gait and stair training, prescription of home exercise program focused on safe progression of exercise/activity and discharge planning

▶ **Precautions during physical therapy:** Consistent monitoring of vital signs, laboratory values, chest x-rays; close physical supervision to decrease risk of falls; management of multiple tubes and lines

▶ **Complications interfering with physical therapy:** Atelectasis, pneumothorax, pneumonia, subcutaneous emphysema, atrial fibrillation, hypoxemia, deep vein thromboses, pulmonary emboli, acute lung injury, respiratory failure

Understanding the Health Condition

Lung cancer is the second most common cancer in both men and women.[1] With greater than 220,000 new diagnoses and almost 157,000 lung cancer-related deaths each year, it is estimated that 400,000 people were alive in the United States with lung cancer in 2011.[1] NSCLCs account for 85% to 90% of all lung cancer diagnoses, and may be divided into three subtypes: squamous cell carcinoma, adenocarcinoma, and large cell carcinoma.[1] **Cigarette smoking** is the number one risk factor for developing lung cancer, followed by environmental factors (exposure to asbestos, radiation, arsenic, air pollution), and personal or familial history of the disease.[1] While signs and symptoms do not always present in the early stages of disease, they may include: persistent cough, hemoptysis, pleuritic chest pain, shortness of breath, generalized fatigue, weight loss, and recurrent pulmonary infections such as bronchitis or pneumonia.[1] Treatments for NSCLC are usually multifaceted and consist of any one or combination of surgery, chemotherapy, or radiation therapy.

Surgical resection is the treatment of choice for early-stage, localized lung cancers.[2] Lung resections may be accomplished with a variety of basic to complex thoracic surgical techniques, and are named according to the portion of lung tissue excised (Table 15-1).[3]

The posterolateral thoracotomy is the most common surgical approach for resection of lung tumors.[2] Access to the thoracic cavity is classically achieved via a rib-spreading incision at the intercostal space most convenient to the location of the lesion.[2] Surgical division of the serratus anterior, intercostal muscles, latissimus dorsi, trapezius, and/or rhomboid muscles may occur.[2,4] At the conclusion of the procedure, two chest tubes are generally placed to evacuate serosanguinous fluid and air from the pleural space during the postoperative period.[3,4] Chest tube collection

Table 15-1 COMMON LUNG RESECTION TECHNIQUES	
Resection Technique	**Portion of Lung Removed**
Wedge resection	Small sample or wedge
Segmentectomy	Entire bronchopulmonary segment
Lobectomy	Entire lobe
Bronchoplastic/sleeve resection	Entire lobe and a portion of the mainstem bronchus
Pneumonectomy	Entire lung, which may or may not include the surrounding pleura

Reproduced with permission from Watchie J. Cardiovascular and Pulmonary Physical Therapy. 2nd ed. St. Louis, MO: Saunders Elsevier; 2010.

systems may be connected to underwater seal or low wall suction to properly facilitate drainage, restore negative intrapleural pressure, and verify if air leaks are present.[3,4] Whenever possible, less invasive surgical techniques (such as video-assisted thoracic surgery [VATS] or muscle-sparing approaches) are utilized to reduce trauma and risk of complications following surgery.[5]

VATS is a minimally invasive surgical technique for the excision of early-stage, well-defined NSCLC.[6] VATS procedures are generally performed with robotic assistance, entailing three small, non–rib-spreading incisions.[5,6] Advantages to VATS include shorter hospital stay, decreased acute postoperative pain, and fewer and less severe postoperative complications when compared to open thoracotomy.[5] Disadvantages include video imaging rather than direct visualization of the thoracic cavity, and limitations of instrument maneuverability and tactile feedback through the small incisions.[6]

Clinically significant pulmonary complications occur postoperatively in 10% to 20% of all patients status/post thoracic surgery for lung resection.[7] These complications include atelectasis, pneumonia, pneumothorax, acute lung injury, and acute respiratory distress syndrome.[7] Severe postoperative cardiac complications, such as acute coronary syndromes and heart failure, occur in only 2% to 4% of this population.[7] Ten to fifteen percent of patients experience atrial fibrillation, a less severe but still clinically significant cardiac complication, and 5% to 6% of patients experience subcutaneous emphysema or pulmonary embolus.[8,9] Patients with significant preoperative comorbidities that cause reduced lung diffusing capacity of carbon monoxide (DLCO) to < 70% of predicted and patients who receive preoperative chemotherapy treatments are independently at higher risk for postoperative pulmonary complications.[7]

The most important prognostic factors for patients with NSCLC are the primary cell type, aggressiveness of the disease, and staging at the time of diagnosis.[1] Other determinants in survival are responsiveness of the cancer to treatment, as well as the patient's overall health and comorbid factors.[1] Five-year survival rates for stage I NSCLC at time of diagnosis range from 45% to 49%, while 5-year survival for stage IV is reduced to only 1%.[1]

Physical Therapy Patient/Client Management

In the acute care setting, the physical therapist coordinates care with other members of the multidisciplinary team, and consults new services as needed. Team members involved in the management of patients status/post lung surgery include: the thoracic-oncology surgical team, pathology, nursing, physical therapy, respiratory therapy, occupational therapy, case management, and social work. Additional services may also include: cardiology, pulmonary medicine, integrative medicine, nutrition services, smoking cessation, and a patient representative. As a physical therapist bringing value to the care delivered for patients, it is important to identify when a patient may benefit from referral to additional services and discuss these recommendations with the medical team.

The primary role of physical therapy in patients acutely status/post lung surgery is to restore or optimize the patient's functional and endurance capacity, prevent postoperative complications through provision of patient education and skilled interventions, and establish appropriate discharge recommendations.[4] Treatment interventions may vary based upon the patient's overall presentation, type of surgical approach, and amount of lung tissue resected.

Examination, Evaluation, and Diagnosis

Prior to seeing the patient, the physical therapist must complete a thorough chart review including: past medical history, history of present illness, operative note, medications, lab values, postoperative precautions, heart rate and blood pressure parameters, and the most recent postoperative chest imaging. Critical laboratory values to review include: hemoglobin (Hgb), hematocrit (Hct), platelet count (Plt), prothrombin time (PT), international normalized ratio (INR), and white blood cell count (WBC). Review of the patient's hospital course with the primary nurse is recommended prior to the start of physical therapy. Absolute contraindications to physical therapy include: hemodynamic instability, uncontrolled cardiac arrhythmia, pending imaging for ruling out pulmonary embolus, Hgb < 7.0 g/dL, Plt < 10,000, and INR > 3.0.[10] Laboratory value parameters and specific contraindication guidelines may vary among institutions and patient populations. The physical therapist must be knowledgeable and respectful of institutional guidelines at all times. The physical therapist should notify the surgical team and withhold therapy if any contraindications to exercise are identified in the chart review process.

During patient observation, the physical therapist needs to note the locations of the patient's medical attachments, incisions, and dressings.[4] Immediately after surgery, patients may have multiple tubes and lines including: central or peripheral intravenous (IV) access, an epidural or IV patient controlled analgesia (PCA) pump, one or more chest tubes, Foley catheter, supplemental oxygen, telemetry, and a pulse oximetry monitoring device. Figure 15-1 shows a typical posterolateral thoracotomy incision utilized for lung resection, a single chest tube inserted on the left side of the patient's thorax, and an epidural insertion and dressing to the right of the spine. Figure 15-2 shows a chest tube drainage collection system (Fig. 15-2A), PCA pump (Fig. 15-2B), and a portable suction unit with canister (Fig. 15-2C) to provide suction during ambulation for patients receiving low wall suction at the bedside. It is important for all attachments to be identified and secured for patient safety prior to mobilization.

The physical therapist obtains a detailed patient history and functional assessment to formulate a complete pre- and postoperative comparison for the identification of new impairments. Dyspnea, pain, and vital signs are monitored before, during, and after functional activities to assess for patient tolerance. A Six-Minute Walk Test (6MWT) may be employed for objective evaluation of functional exercise capacity.[11] Administration of the 6MWT is practical for patients status/post lung surgery in the acute care setting as it only requires a 100-foot hallway and 6 minutes to complete.[11] Assistive devices and supplemental oxygen may be utilized by the patient during the test as needed.[11] The 6MWT may be performed on initial evaluation and as a repeated measure to assess patient progress and treatment effectiveness over a period of time. Dose and timing of medications, such as bronchodilators, administered before the test are documented because they may impact patient performance.[11]

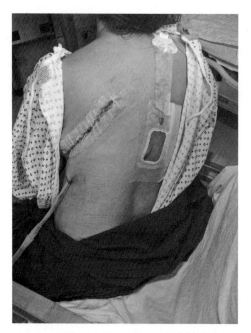

Figure 15-1. Patient sitting at edge of bed on POD 2 after posterolateral thoracotomy. Note the incision utilized for lung resection on the left upper back and flank, a single chest tube on the left side of the patient's thorax, and an epidural insertion and dressing to the right of the spine.

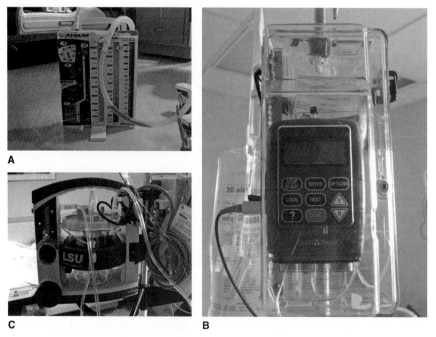

Figure 15-2. Typical equipment attached to patient after thoracotomy. **A.** Chest tube drainage collection system. **B.** PCA pump. **C.** Portable suction unit with canister.

The physical therapist is responsible for examining chest expansion and posture. The resting and dynamic chest is observed and palpated for symmetry, configuration, diameter, excursion, breathing pattern, and muscle activation.[2,3] Posture and positioning of the thoracic spine, shoulder girdles, and rib cage are inspected. Patients with posterolateral thoracotomy incisions may display increased muscle tone in the ipsilateral thorax due to pain and inflammation. If these changes are present, decreased chest wall compliance may contribute to decreased lung volumes and increased work of breathing during the postoperative recovery period.[2] Use of accessory muscles of breathing (vs. diaphragmatic activation) and upper extremity ROM and quality of movement must be noted by the physical therapist.[2]

Auscultation of the lungs is performed in a systematic fashion comparing each bronchopulmonary segment to the corresponding segment on the contralateral side, working in the craniocaudal direction.[2-4] The diaphragm of the stethoscope is placed directly against the patient's skin, and the patient instructed to inhale and exhale deeply through an open mouth. Seated positioning of the patient during auscultation is most favorable, as it allows for best access to the entire lung space including anterior, posterior, and lateral aspects of the chest wall.[2-4] Diminished breath sounds are the most common finding after lung surgery; however, adventitious sounds may be present if the patient has consolidation or atelectasis.[2]

Finally, a patient's cough must be examined for strength and effectiveness. Due to the nature of thoracic incisions and chest tube placements, coughing may be quite painful and difficult for patients in the acute phase status/post lung surgery. Adequate inspiratory volume, glottal closure, expiratory force, and expiratory flow are all considered components of an effective cough maneuver.[3,4] If any of these components are deficient, the patient may not be able to clear secretions efficiently and may be at elevated risk for postoperative pulmonary complications. A minimum threshold of forced expiratory volume in 1 second (FEV_1) ≥ 60% of a patient's actual vital capacity indicates adequate muscle strength for expulsion of secretions.[4] The main question the physical therapist must answer *clinically* is whether the patient's cough is effective enough to clear secretions. To do so, cough is assessed by the presence of spontaneous, deep inspiration, a complete breath hold separating peak inspiration and expulsion (evidence of glottal closure), active contraction of intercostal and abdominal muscle groups, and forceful expulsion resulting in mobilization of air and/ or secretions.[4] Secretions expectorated are examined for quantity, color, viscosity, and odor.[2-4] Concerning changes in sputum must be documented and reported to the surgical team.

Plan of Care and Interventions

Plan of care and treatment interventions for patients acutely status/post lung surgery are selected based upon impairments identified during physical therapy examination, evaluation, and diagnosis. Goals of care in this setting are focused to optimize patient function, prevent postoperative complications, and prepare the patient for hospital discharge. Education is provided on safe and effective exercise technique, as well as on the benefits of each intervention to increase patient participation and program adherence.

Therapeutic exercise interventions begin on POD 1 and are targeted primarily at increasing lung volumes, thoracic expansion, chest wall mobility, and shoulder ROM. Deep breathing activities, inspiratory muscle training, and incentive spirometry have demonstrated reductions in postoperative atelectasis, pneumonias, and length of hospital stay when compared to control groups.[12,13] Patients are encouraged to perform 10 repetitions of at least one deep breathing activity hourly during the daytime. Examples of deep breathing activities may include: incentive spirometry, pursed lip breathing, diaphragmatic breathing, segmental breathing, and sniffing exercises. **Thoracic cage and shoulder range of motion activities** have been associated with less shoulder pain, less total pain at hospital discharge, and improved postoperative physical function.[14] Active and active assisted ROM activities for the thoracic cage and shoulder may be employed on POD 1. Light resistance with elastic resistance bands (*e.g.*, Thera-Band) may be added as early as POD 3.[15]

To provide the patient with independent strategies for airway clearance, the physical therapist needs to review splinted and self-assisted cough techniques and positioning on POD 1. Nurses, respiratory therapists, and physical therapists reinforce these techniques throughout the patient's hospital stay. Additional ACTs including manual percussion, vibration, postural drainage, and active cycle breathing are utilized on an as-needed basis. Manual ACTs are selected when clearly indicated by patient presentation, and are only utilized when benefits of intervention outweigh possible risks. Positioning on the ipsilateral side of the surgical incision and chest tube insertions is not contraindicated, but rather encouraged, because it is essential for the patient to change positions frequently for improved oxygen transport, ventilation-perfusion matching, and adequate postural drainage.[3,4] Care is taken to ensure that the chest tubes do not become kinked, blocked, or elevated higher than the level of the chest during positioning efforts.[3,4]

Chest physical therapy (CPT) is a broad term that may refer to any of several ACTs.[2-4] Evidence (even of poor quality) examining the effectiveness of CPT status/post lung surgery is largely under-represented and inconclusive in the current literature. It is usual practice that CPT interventions are used in *combination* for optimal airway clearance and patient outcome. For example, a manual ACT such as a percussion may be coupled with postural drainage, in addition to the patient's deep breathing and coughing program. Success is further increased with a regular ambulation schedule, increased time spent out of bed, and diligent positioning efforts. Possible indications, specific interventions, precautions, and contraindications for various treatment techniques that physical therapists may utilize to facilitate airway clearance are listed in Table 15-2. While ACTs are an important part of rehabilitation status/post lung surgery, the application, appropriateness, and contradictory evidence surrounding individual ACTs is beyond the scope of this case.

In addition to therapeutic exercise and ACTs, it is important to encourage the patient to remain out of bed and to ambulate with assistance as much as possible during the daytime to decrease the risks of postoperative immobility and bedrest, including infection, pneumonia, deep vein thrombosis, pulmonary embolus, and hypoxemia.[4] Oxygen therapy may be utilized as prescribed by the physician for patients who experience decreased peripheral oxygen saturation upon exertion. Physical therapy treatments may be coordinated with pain medications and respiratory therapy treatments

Table 15-2 AIRWAY CLEARANCE TECHNIQUES: INDICATIONS, INTERVENTIONS, PRECAUTIONS, CONTRAINDICATIONS			
Possible Indications	**Possible Interventions**	**Relative Precautions to Manual Techniques (Percussion/Vibration/ Shaking)**	**Relative Contraindications to Manual Techniques (Percussion/Vibration/ Shaking)**
Impaired mucociliary clearance	Postural drainage positioning	Osteoporosis	Rib fractures
Impaired ventilation	Percussion	Osteolytic spine metastasis	Osteolytic rib metastasis
Atelectasis	Vibration	History of cardiac instability	Recent skin graft or myocutaneous flap to chest wall
Consolidation	Shaking	Incision and chest tube locations	Subcutaneous emphysema
V/Q mismatching	Deep breathing activities	Implanted chest wall devices (*e.g.,* PICC line, Mediport catheter, pacemaker, automatic implantable cardioverter defibrillator)	Pulmonary blebs
Impaired cage mobility	Incentive spirometry	Active confusion/ agitation	Elevated INR (> 3.0)
Ineffective cough	Manual techniques (*e.g.,* rib mobilization, myofascial release)	Pulmonary embolus	Low platelets (< 20,000)
Respiratory muscle weakness	Manual-assisted/ self-assisted cough techniques	Low platelets (< 50,000)	Active cardiac instability
	Huffing	Place tube feeds on hold/ ensure patient has not eaten for at least 45 min prior to treatment	Uncontrolled hypertension
	Active cycle breathing		Active bleeding
	Autogenic drainage		
	Ambulation		
	Suctioning		

Abbreviation: PICC, peripherally inserted central catheter.

for optimal patient comfort and benefit. It is recommended that inhaled bronchodilators be administered prior to physical therapy for decreased airway resistance and improved secretion mobilization, while inhaled antibiotics (if prescribed) are given after secretion removal for optimal absorbtion.[4] Energy conservation techniques may be implemented to combat postoperative fatigue and assist patients in remaining active throughout the day.[3,4] Written education materials outlining the patient's exercise prescription, goals, home exercise program, and postsurgical precautions are highly encouraged for reinforcement and continuity of care between providers.

Evidence-Based Clinical Recommendations

SORT: Strength of Recommendation Taxonomy

A: Consistent, good-quality patient-oriented evidence

B: Inconsistent or limited-quality patient-oriented evidence

C: Consensus, disease-oriented evidence, usual practice, expert opinion, or case series

1. Cigarette smoking increases the risk of lung cancer. **Grade A**

2. Thoracic cage and shoulder range of motion exercises performed immediately after lung surgery reduce shoulder pain and total pain at hospital discharge. **Grade B**

3. Manual chest physical therapy interventions (percussion, vibration, shaking, etc.) decrease the incidence of postoperative atelectasis status/post lung surgery. **Grade C**

COMPREHENSION QUESTIONS

15.1 A 66-year-old male is referred to physical therapy on POD 1 status/post right posterolateral thoracotomy for a right total pneumonectomy. What portion of this patient's right lung was resected?

    A. A complete bronchopulmonary segment

    B. One entire lobe

    C. A small sample or wedge

    D. The entire right lung

15.2 A physical therapist is completing a chart review for an 87-year-old female status/post left VATS with left upper lobe wedge resections × 3. Which of the following is a contraindication to physical therapy evaluation?

    A. Controlled atrial fibrillation with a ventricular rate of 91 beats per minute

    B. Hemoglobin level of 13.1 g/dL

    C. Pending computerized tomography angiogram to rule out a pulmonary embolus

    D. Platelet count of 170,000

15.3 A physical therapist is providing education on postoperative positioning and airway clearance to a 74-year-old female status/post right posterolateral thoracotomy with right lower lobe lobectomy. Which of the following statements is the *most* appropriate?

A. Avoid positioning on the ipsilateral side of the incision and chest tube

B. Avoid practicing deep breaths to minimize postoperative pain

C. Change positions frequently to optimize postural drainage

D. Minimize coughing attempts to prevent stressing the surgical incision

ANSWERS

15.1 **D.** The term pneumonectomy refers to the excision of an entire lung.[3] A segmentectomy is removal of an entire bronchopulmonary segment (option A). Removal of one lobe is a lobectomy (option B) and removal of a small sample or wedge is a wedge resection (option C).

15.2 **C.** Physical therapy is contraindicated in patients awaiting imaging to rule out a pulmonary embolus. Pulmonary embolism is a potentially fatal postoperative complication that must either be ruled out or appropriately treated prior to the initiation of physical therapy.[2] Hemoglobin and platelets are within normal limits (options B and D). Controlled atrial fibrillation (option A) is not a contraindication to physical therapy.

15.3 **C.** Patients status/post lung surgery are encouraged to change positions frequently to optimize postural drainage, ventilation–perfusion matching, and oxygen transport.[3,4] Patients are also encouraged to incorporate positioning on the ipsilateral side of the incision and chest tube into their positioning schedule, as well as to perform deep breathing activities and effective coughing maneuvers.[3,4]

REFERENCES

1. American Cancer Society Website. http://www.cancer.org. Accessed November 26, 2011.

2. Hillegass EA, Sadowsky HS. *Essentials of Cardiopulmonary Physical Therapy.* 2nd ed. Philadelphia, PA: WB Saunders Co.; 2001.

3. Watchie J. *Cardiovascular and Pulmonary Physical Therapy.* 2nd ed. St. Louis, MO: Saunders Elsevier; 2010.

4. Frownfelter D, Dean E. *Cardiovascular and Pulmonary Physical Therapy.* 4th ed. St. Louis, MO: Mosby Elsevier; 2006.

5. Cattaneo SM, Park BJ, Wilton AS, et al. Use of video-assisted thoracic surgery for lobectomy in the elderly results in fewer complications. *Ann Thorac Surg.* 2008;85:231-236.

6. Park BJ, Flores RM, Rusch VW. Robotic assistance for video-assisted thoracic surgical lobectomy: technique and initial results. *J Thorac Cardiovasc Surg.* 2006;131:54-59.

7. Amar D, Munoz D, Shi W, et al. A clinical prediction rule for pulmonary complications after thoracic surgery for primary lung cancer. *Anesth Analg.* 2010;110:1343-1348.

8. Whitson BA, Andrade RS, Boettcher A, et al. Video-assisted thorascopic surgery is more favorable than thoracotomy for resection of clinical stage I non-small cell lung cancer. *Ann Thorac Surg.* 2007;83:1965-1970.

9. Cerfolio RJ, Bryant AS, Maniscalco LM. Management of subcutaneous emphysema after pulmonary resection. *Ann Thorac Surg.* 2008;85:1759-1765.

10. Memorial Sloan-Kettering Cancer Center. *Institutional Policy on Safe Activity Guidelines for Patients Receiving Oncology Rehabilitation.* New York, NY. Accessed November 2011.

11. American Thoracic Society. ATS statement: guidelines for the six-minute walk test. *Am J Respir Crit Care Med.* 2002;166:111-117.

12. Shannon VR. Role of pulmonary rehabilitation in the management of patients with lung cancer. *Curr Opin Pulm Med.* 2010;16:334-339.

13. Weiner P, Man A, Weiner M, et al. The effect of incentive spirometry and inspiratory muscle training on pulmonary function after lung resection. *J Thorac Cardiovasc Surg.* 1997;113:552-557.

14. Reeve J, Stiller K, Nicol K, et al. A postoperative shoulder exercise program improves function and decreases pain following open thoracotomy: a randomised trial. *J Physiother.* 2010;56:245-252.

15. Memorial Sloan-Kettering Cancer Center. *Post-Operative Pulmonary Program for Patients Receiving Thoracic Surgery.* New York, NY. Accessed November 2011.

Cystic Fibrosis

John D. Lowman
Anne K. Swisher

CASE 16

The patient is a 25-year-old third-year graduate student working on her PhD in bio-chemistry. She was diagnosed with cystic fibrosis (CF; $\Delta F508/\Delta F508$) during newborn screening. Relevant medical history includes two hospitalizations for acute CF exac-erbations (at age 17 and 19 years), and a diagnosis of CF-related diabetes 1 year ago. She has "moderate" CF lung disease (forced expiratory volume in one second [FEV_1] 62% on last clinic visit).[1] Her last sputum cultures were positive for *Pseudomonas aeru-ginosa* and methicillin-resistant *Staphylococcus aureus*, but not for *Burkholderia cepacia*. At baseline, she produces approximately 30 mL/day of greenish yellow sputum using a combination of high-frequency chest wall oscillation (The Vest) and vibratory posi-tive expiratory pressure (PEP; acapella) 1 to 2 times per day each. She walks to school each day, including six blocks uphill on the way home, takes the stairs at school (her lab is on the fifth floor), and plays intramural soccer. However, for the past several weeks, her daily mucous production has increased (to ~100 mL), the color changed to green-ish brown, and it has been thicker and more difficult to expectorate. She initiated an inhaled antibiotic (Tobi) and increased her airway clearance frequency. She also reports general malaise, decreased appetite, and increased dyspnea and leg fatigue after climb-ing the stairs/walking uphill. As a result of these symptoms, she has been driving to school, taking the elevator, and ceased any form of exercise. Yesterday, she came to the emergency department after several episodes of frank hemoptysis (~250 mL in < 24 hours), increased shortness of breath at rest, and new onset right-sided chest pain. She was diagnosed with a CF pulmonary exacerbation and a spontaneous right upper lobe pneumothorax and admitted to the pulmonary step-down unit. The physical therapist is asked to evaluate and treat her on the second day of hospital admission.

▶ Based on her health condition, what do you anticipate will be the contributors to activity limitations?
▶ What are the examination priorities?
▶ What are the most appropriate tests and measures?
▶ What are the most appropriate physical therapy interventions?
▶ What precautions should be taken during physical therapy interventions?

KEY DEFINITIONS

HEMOPTYSIS: Coughing up blood or bloody mucous; can range from scant (< 5 mL) blood-streaked mucous to massive (> 240 mL) amounts of pure bright red blood; treatment can range from monitoring at home to hospital admission for bronchial artery embolization

PNEUMOTHORAX: Collection of air in the pleural space, leading to a collapsed lung; occurs "spontaneously" in CF; can be treated with observation, needle aspiration, or insertion of a chest tube, depending on the severity

PULMONARY EXACERBATION: Acute worsening of respiratory symptoms, including increased cough and sputum production, shortness of breath, chest pain, loss of appetite, weight loss, decreased exercise tolerance and decline in lung function; typically requires treatment with intravenous antibiotics in a hospital setting

Objectives

1. Describe the multisystem involvement of CF.

2. Describe and recognize common pulmonary complications associated with a CF pulmonary exacerbation.

3. List common medications used for the acute and chronic management of CF and describe potential adverse drug reactions (ADRs) of these medications and how they may impact physical therapy management.

4. Develop an examination strategy to assess the common physical therapy-related patient-identified problems in an individual with a CF pulmonary exacerbation.

5. Select appropriate outcome measures to assess effectiveness of interventions.

6. Design an appropriate plan of care for the anticipated cardiopulmonary and musculoskeletal impairments expected for an individual with a CF pulmonary exacerbation.

Physical Therapy Considerations

PT considerations during management of the individual with CF pulmonary exacerbation:

▶ **General physical therapy plan of care:** Improve airway clearance; decrease resting and exertional dyspnea; improve aerobic and anaerobic exercise tolerance; improve posture, flexibility, and thoracic mobility; screen for urinary stress incontinence

▶ **Physical therapy interventions:** Patient and caregiver education regarding alternative airway clearance techniques (ACTs) and importance of aerobic and resistance exercise training; ACTs; therapeutic exercise (aerobic, resistance, flexibility, and breathing strategies); manual therapy; supplemental oxygen; if indicated, referral for outpatient PT to further advance independent home exercise routine and/or management of urinary stress incontinence

▶ **Precautions during physical therapy:** Consistent monitoring of vital signs, including pulse oximetry (SpO_2) and perceived dyspnea; recognize potential ADRs

▶ **Complications interfering with physical therapy:** Moderate to massive hemoptysis, pneumothorax, respiratory failure (hypoxemia and/or hypercapnia), hyperglycemia and hypoglycemia

Understanding the Health Condition

Cystic fibrosis is an inherited autosomal recessive disease and is the most common lethal genetic disease among Caucasians.[2] Currently, the disease is typically diagnosed with newborn screening. CF has historically been considered a pediatric disease. However, CF is no longer a disease of just children—over 90% of people with CF born after 1986 survive into adulthood (≥ 18 years old) and the median age of survival for individuals with CF has increased from 27 years in 1986 to over 38 years in 2010.[3]

CF is caused by a mutation in the cystic fibrosis transmembrane conductance regulator (CFTR) gene.[2] CFTR is responsible for conducting chloride across the apical membrane in epithelial cells of exocrine glands. In the lungs, the inability of chloride to enter epithelial cells through the CFTR channel concurrent with sodium transport through the sodium channel results in deficient fluid secretion from the epithelial cells and a loss of airway-surface liquid volume. This depleted airway-surface liquid results in hyperviscous secretions and mucosal obstruction in the lung. Thick secretions and obstructions also occur in all other exocrine glands (*e.g.*, pancreas, liver, vas deferens, skin).[4] Consequently, in addition to pulmonary involvement, CF results in gastrointestinal abnormalities,[5] sterility,[6] and heat intolerance.[7]

Pulmonary involvement typically includes mucous plugging of distal airways and related bronchiectasis. Bronchiectasis is an irreversible destruction of the bronchi due to inflammation and repeated infection. The bronchi become dilated, thinner, and easily collapsible. As bronchiectasis worsens, it can involve bronchial arteries and result in hemoptysis.[8] Typically, the hemoptysis is mild and indicated by blood-streaked sputum or small amounts of bright red blood. Massive hemoptysis is defined as acute bleeding > 240 mL in a 24-hour period or recurrent bleeding > 100 mL/day over several days.[8] Management of significant hemoptysis includes hospitalization with intravenous antibiotics, discontinuation of nonsteroidal anti-inflammatories (which act to inhibit platelet function), chest computed tomography (CT) scan, bronchoscopy, and bronchial artery embolization if the patient is clinically unstable.[9]

Pneumothorax is a common complication in patients with CF. There is no conclusive explanation for the pathogenesis of spontaneous pneumothorax in CF, but hypotheses include the rupture of an emphysematous cyst or subpleural blebs, as well as increased alveolar pressure and volume due to mucous plugging that could drive air into the mediastinum, resulting in pleural rupture.[10] Approximately 1 in 5 adults with CF will experience a pneumothorax. Most individuals that develop a pneumothorax have moderate to severe lung disease. Hemoptysis is often present (~20% of time) with a pneumothorax. The most common presenting symptom is acute onset dyspnea (65%) and chest pain (50%).[10] Management of a pneumothorax in CF includes placement of a chest tube if the pneumothorax is large or if the patient is clinically unstable. If it is a recurrent pneumothorax, pleurodesis may be performed. This procedure involves insertion of a substance between the pleura to cause them to fuse together. Procedures and interventions that increase intrapulmonary pressure should be temporarily discontinued, including spirometry, bilevel positive airway pressure (BiPAP), PEP therapies, intrapulmonary percussive ventilation (IPV), flying on a plane, and weightlifting (due to risk of Valsalva maneuver).[9]

Although pulmonary involvement (including bronchiectasis) is almost universal in CF, it is a multisystem disease, with many nonpulmonary complications relevant to the physical therapist.[11] Pancreatic insufficiency often occurs in young children, but CF-related diabetes (CFRD) typically occurs in adults. CFRD is similar to but not the same as either Type 1 or Type 2 diabetes mellitus (DM). Individuals with CFRD have both insulin deficiency as well as insulin resistance, but less pronounced than in Type 1 or Type 2 DM.[12] The prevalence of CFRD in patients over age 20 years is almost 50%, and many more are glucose intolerant. Not only does CFRD require additional self-monitoring and medication, but it is also associated with lower body weight, decreased pulmonary function, and increased mortality.[12] CFRD is treated with insulin; during pulmonary exacerbations, increased insulin dosing is typically required. Because of less predictable glucose metabolism during a pulmonary exacerbation, blood glucose should be monitored prior to exercise interventions that may result in hypoglycemia.

CF-related bone disease (CFRBD) is another relevant, nonpulmonary complication. Due to nutritional factors, glucocorticoid use, and perhaps decreased physical activity, virtually everyone with CF is at risk for skeletal demineralization.[13] Approximately 20% of adults with CF have CFRBD, and virtually all patients referred for lung transplantation have CFRBD.[12] Fracture rates due to CFRBD are high, especially in the hands, forearms, ribs, and vertebrae. Almost 50% of patients on the lung transplant list have vertebral fractures, which also results in significant kyphosis.[12] While regular weightbearing exercise is advocated for the prevention and treatment of CFRBD,[12] precautions should be taken to avoid activities that place excessive compressive forces on the spine, especially for individuals with overt osteoporosis. Other CF-related musculoskeletal disabilities that should be evaluated by the physical therapist include impaired posture and back pain,[14] impaired muscle performance,[15] and urinary stress incontinence.[16]

Originally called "cystic fibrosis of the pancreas,"[17] CF is now known more for the pulmonary involvement of the disease. Lung pathology is the primary contributor to mortality in patients with CF,[4] and often leads to hospitalization for a "pulmonary exacerbation."[18] Although there is no standard definition of a CF pulmonary exacerbation, the signs and symptoms include: increased cough, increased sputum production, decreased exercise tolerance, decline in weight-for-age percentile, reduced appetite, hemoptysis, fever, and new adventitious breath sounds.[18] Pulmonary exacerbations become more frequent and severe as the disease progresses and are associated with increased morbidity and mortality.[18] The vast majority of adults with CF require treatment of a pulmonary exacerbation at least once per year.[19] Treatment of a CF pulmonary exacerbation typically involves a hospital admission for intravenous administration of multiple classes of antibiotics, an increased dosage of airway clearance therapies, and a continuation of chronic maintenance therapies.[20] Maintenance therapies for the pulmonary treatment of CF usually include daily inhaled medications such as hypertonic saline and dornase alfa (a mucolytic), intermittent inhaled tobramycin (an antibiotic), and physical therapy interventions (ACTs and exercise).[2]

Physical Therapy Patient/Client Management

Management of patients with CF requires a multidisciplinary team. Almost all patients with CF are cared for at Cystic Fibrosis Foundation accredited "CF Care Centers" that include access to pulmonary physicians that specialize in CF, clinical nurse specialists, respiratory therapists, physical therapists, dieticians, social workers, psychologists, and clinical pharmacists.[11,21] There are currently 115 accredited CF care centers nationwide, including 95 adult programs.[22] Patients are seen by the CF care team on an outpatient quarterly basis. They are also managed by an interdisciplinary team if and when they are admitted to the hospital for a pulmonary exacerbation.

Examination, Evaluation, and Diagnosis

Based on the diagnosis and typical physical therapy problem list for patients with CF, the initial data collection (including chart review and patient interview) is hypothesis-driven.[23] Medications, clinical laboratory studies, arterial blood gas (ABG) results, pulmonary function test results, and chest radiograph reports must be reviewed.

Medications and when they are administered will clue the therapist in to potential ADRs and help schedule the ideal time to provide interventions. Table 16-1 presents frequently prescribed medications and their main actions for individuals with CF. Common medications for a hospitalized patient with a CF pulmonary exacerbation may include: inhaled Pulmozyme (dornase alfa), Tobi (tobramycin), Combivent (albuterol and ipratropium), and hypertonic saline; intravenous tobramycin (aminoglycoside antibiotic), ceftazidime (β-lactam antibiotic), and prednisolone (glucocorticoid); subcutaneous insulin; and oral pancrelipase. Frequently, adult patients have a peripherally inserted central catheter (PICC line) or Port-a-cath (a more permanent central line) placed due to frequent intravenous therapy.

Although some clinicians suggest that Pulmozyme be given prior to ACTs, there is no strong support to be rigid in the timing or sequence of these multiple interventions.[24] Patient preference with respect to timing of therapy interventions should also be considered with hypertonic saline inhalation.[25] However, for patients responsive to bronchodilators (e.g., Combivent), it is probably beneficial to schedule airway clearance and exercise interventions after administration of these drugs. For patients on intravenous medications, exercise sessions should ideally be scheduled

Table 16-1   COMMONLY USED MEDICATIONS FOR CF[11]

Category and Delivery Mode	Common Name (Trade Name)	Main Action	Comments
Mucolytic (inhaled)	Dornase alfa (Pulmozyme)	Thins mucous to make it easier to cough out	Improve lung function, reduce exacerbations
Antibiotic (intravenous)		Fight bacterial infection	Antimicrobial resistance may occur
Antibiotic (oral)	Azithromycin (Zithromax)	Fight bacterial infection and anti-inflammatory agent	Antimicrobial resistance may occur; azithromycin improves lung function and reduces exacerbations
Antibiotic (inhaled)	Tobramycin (Tobi) Colistin (Coly-Mycin) Gentamicin Ceftazidime	Fight bacterial infection	Antimicrobial resistance may occur; Tobi shown to improve lung function; bronchospasm may occur with colistin
Hypertonic saline (inhaled)	Hyper-Sal	Increase hydration of airway surface liquid	Improve lung function, reduce exacerbations
Nonsteroidal anti-inflammatory drugs (NSAIDs, oral)	Ibuprofen	Decrease airway inflammation	Slows loss of lung function
Glucocorticoids (oral or intravenous)	Prednisone Prednisolone	Decrease airway inflammation	Often used for acute exacerbations. ADRs include glucose intolerance, bone loss, and myopathy
Beta$_2$ adrenergic receptor agonists (inhaled)	Albuterol Salmeterol	Relaxes airway smooth muscle	Improve lung function. ADRs include tachycardia and tremor
Antimuscarinic agents (inhaled)	Ipratropium (Atrovent)	Relaxes airway smooth muscle	Improve lung function
Pancreatic enzyme replacement (oral)	Pancrelipase	Helps digest carbohydrate, protein and fat	Improves nutrient digestion and absorption, and weight gain

Adapted with permission from Swisher AK, Downs AM, Dekerlegand RL. CF 101 for the Physical Therapist. Cystic Fibrosis Foundation; 2010.

when patients are not getting an infusion so that they can be more mobile. The catabolic effects of glucocorticoids (given to decrease airway inflammation associated with CF exacerbations) on both muscle and bone can be attenuated with weightbearing exercise and resistance training,[26,27] so it is important to notice that this patient is receiving intravenous glucocorticoid (prednisolone). Blood glucose should be monitored prior to exercise to prevent hypoglycemic episodes in patients on insulin therapy for either CFRD or prednisolone-induced hyperglycemia.

Clinical laboratory studies and ABG data also provide important initial data to help formulate an examination strategy and plan of care. A basic metabolic panel and complete blood count (CBC) can assist the therapist in predicting a patient's potential response to physical activity. Patients with a high white blood cell count (*i.e.*, leukocytosis) or a low hemoglobin and hematocrit (*i.e.*, anemia) will likely feel fatigued, if not at rest, then with physical activity. Anemia can be a particular concern for patients who have had significant hemoptysis. Sputum culture results give the therapist an indication of the variety of organisms and severity of lung disease. The majority of adult patients with CF are chronically infected with *Pseudomonas aeruginosa*. Other typical infectious agents include *Staphylococcus aureus*, *Haemophilus influenzae*, and *Burkholderia cepacia*.[28] While all of these organisms are easily transmitted, *B. cepacia* is particularly contagious and results in increased morbidity and mortality post–lung transplant;[28] thus, extra precautions should be taken to prevent transmission between patients. ABG results are not routinely performed during admission for a pulmonary exacerbation, unless the patient is critically ill. If available, then ABG results provide important data on a patient's ventilation (ability to get rid of CO_2) and oxygenation status (ability to get oxygen into the blood). Patients with end-stage CF may develop acute or chronic respiratory failure (hypoxemia and/or hypercapnia; PaO_2 < 80 mm Hg and $PaCO_2$ > 45 mm Hg, respectively).

The FEV_1 is one of several pulmonary function tests that can be used to classify patients with CF as having normal (≥ 90% predicted) lung function, or mild (70%-89% predicted), moderate (40%-69% predicted), or severe (< 40% predicted) lung disease.[29] Knowing the severity of a patient's lung disease can help the therapist anticipate her physical activity limitations and assist in setting realistic goals. The chest radiograph or chest CT often indicates the presence of an acute localized infection; this information can help the therapist determine the most important postural drainage positions to use.

Based on data obtained from the medical record, the interview should be hypothesis-driven, and should elicit the patient's identified problems. Hypothesized problems for patients with CF include: (1) difficulty clearing secretions, (2) shortness of breath, (3) fatigue, (4) decrease endurance/poor exercise tolerance, (5) back pain, and (6) urinary stress incontinence. The interview and systems review, including resting vital signs, should screen for these common complaints. Then, based on the patient-identified problem list and the initial data collected, an examination strategy is formulated.

Specific physical therapy tests and measures are used to further assess the specific problems common to patients with CF. These include measures of ventilation and respiration/gas exchange, airway clearance, aerobic capacity, muscle performance, posture, and pain.[11,30]

Important measures in the assessment of ventilation and respiration/gas exchange include a physical examination of the chest, pulse oximetry, and dyspnea rating. Auscultation of lung sounds can give the physical therapist an idea of the severity of lung disease as well as response to treatment. Crackles are quite common in patients with CF, occurring in over 25% of adults during routine "well" clinic visits, compared to wheezes that are present in only 5% of adults with CF.[31] During a pulmonary exacerbation, crackles are much more common. These adventitious breath

Table 16-2	MRC DYSPNEA/BREATHLESSNESS SCALE
Grade	Degree of Breathlessness Related to Activities
1	Not troubled by breathlessness except on strenuous exertion
2	Short of breath when hurrying on the level or walking up a slight hill
3	Walks slower than contemporaries on level ground because of breathlessness, or has to stop for breath after ~1 mile (or after 15 min) when walking at own pace
4	Stops for breath after walking about 100 yd (or after a few minutes) on level ground
5	Too breathless to leave the house, or breathless after dressing or undressing

Reproduced with permission from Fletcher CM, Elmes PC, Fairbairn AS, Wood CH. Significance of Respiratory Symptoms and the Diagnosis of Chronic Bronchitis in a Working Population. Br Med J. 1959;2:257-266.

sounds typically decrease over the hospitalization, and may improve immediately following physical therapy interventions as secretions are cleared.

Dyspnea, occurring at rest and/or with exertion, is one of the most common complaints by patients with CF,[32] and can be difficult to assess due to its qualitative and quantitative components.[33] The Medical Research Council (MRC) dyspnea scale is a simple, self-administered, reliable, and valid measure (Table 16-2).[34] The MRC dyspnea/breathlessness scale does not quantify dyspnea, but rather it describes dyspnea that occurs when it should not (Grades 1 and 2) or it rates the associated activity limitation (Grades 3–5).[35]

The most common measures used to quantify dyspnea, especially during exercise are the Borg CR10 Scale[36,37] and a visual analog scale (VAS).[38] The Borg CR10 Scale is a reliable and valid measure that uses a 0 to 10 category-ratio scale;[39] it is not linear in nature, so it allows more specificity in quantifying dyspnea beyond "moderate" severity, and is used more often in pulmonary rehabilitation than the VAS.[37,40] The VAS for dyspnea consists of a vertical or horizontal line 100 mm in length with anchors at either extreme (*i.e.*, "Not breathless at all" to "Extremely breathless"), and the patient places a mark on the line to denote her dyspnea level. The minimal clinically important difference (MCID) is 1 unit for the Borg CR10 Scale and 10-20 mm for the VAS.[41] Correct usage of the Borg CR10 Scale is important. For further information regarding its use for training and rehabilitation, refer to the text *Borg's Perceived Exertion and Pain Scales*.[39]

Gas exchange is best assessed via an ABG sample, but oxygen saturation by pulse oximetry (SpO_2) is much less invasive, cheaper, and can be used during physical activity. Signal accuracy of pulse oximeters decreases with hypoxemia (< 70%), dark skin pigment, motion artifact (*e.g.*, walking), and poor peripheral circulation. Ideally, SpO_2 should remain stable during exercise, but a drop in SpO_2 with activity or exercise, indicating a gas exchange impairment, is often seen in patients with CF. The degree and timing of any drop should be documented along with the level of activity which resulted in the drop. Safe SpO_2 values for activity are typically considered to be > 88% to 90%,[42,43] but during an initial assessment it may be acceptable to allow someone to temporarily drop as low as 80% to 85%.

A further assessment of airway clearance includes a specific history of the patient's currently used ACTs and observation to ensure each technique is performed appropriately. In addition, the therapist should assess the patient's cough effectiveness as well as the sputum quantity and quality (color, viscosity, odor).[11,30]

Aerobic capacity/endurance can be considered a "vital sign" for CF, since peak oxygen consumption (VO_2) is one of the factors most closely correlated to survival in CF.[44] However, it is rare to measure peak VO_2 during a hospitalization. Instead, field tests are used as surrogate markers for peak VO_2.[45] These tests are cheaper, more convenient, and can be used to guide exercise prescription. The three most commonly used tests in the CF population are the 3-Minute Step Test (3MST), 6-Minute Walk Test (6MWT), and Modified Shuttle Test (MST).[11] The 3MST requires a 15-cm step and a metronome (120 beats/min); the patient steps up and down at a rate of 30 steps/min and the typical outcome measures are change in heart rate (HR), SpO_2, and dyspnea.[46] The 3MST does not predict peak VO_2, but it does identify people who may not desaturate walking on level ground (e.g., 6MWT).[11]

The 6MWT should be performed in a standardized manner (consistent with American Thoracic Society guidelines),[47] including a $\geq$ 30 m (100 ft) hallway (shorter courses slow down times due to increased number of turns), standardized encouragement (every 60 seconds), and, ideally, at least one practice walk.[48] The primary outcome of the 6MWT is distance walked, although change in HR, SpO_2, and dyspnea, distance saturation product,[49] and 6-minute walk work[50,51] are other potential outcomes. The 6MWT is commonly performed pre- and post-lung transplantation.[52,53] However, unless a patient has end-stage pulmonary disease, the 6MWT is likely a submaximal test, since many patients are able to jog or run.

The MST is a progressive, incremental test that may be maximal for many patients, especially those in the hospital with a pulmonary exacerbation. The MST requires two cones and an audio recording of the "bleep" (available from Dr. Sally Singh[54]). Patients begin walking around a 10-m oval course with two cones set 9 m apart (one "shuttle" = 10 m). Each minute, the rate of the "bleeps" increases and patients are required to get to the next cone before the "bleep." A maximal test takes 15 minutes to complete and the last few stages often require a jogging/running pace. The MST has been validated in both children and adults with CF,[55,56] can be used to estimate peak VO_2,[55] and has been used in hospitalized patients.[57,58] The primary outcome measure is distance (number of laps until the patient can no longer maintain the required pace), as well as change in HR, SpO_2, and dyspnea.

Muscle performance is often impaired in patients with CF,[15] but frequently overlooked as a potential target for intervention. Although manual muscle testing for strength may be relatively normal (4+ to 5/5), this does not mean that muscle power and endurance are not impaired. Vertical jump height,[59-61] timed repetitions of push-ups and sit-ups,[61] and isometric plank hold time[62] can provide objective measures of lower extremity, upper extremity, and core muscle performance with minimal equipment. In addition, inspiratory muscle performance is another area for assessment and intervention,[63] but is probably best initiated in an outpatient setting rather than in acute care.

Poor posture and back pain are common impairments in patients with CF.[64] Postural alignment should be observed for exaggerated spinal curves, forward head, and scapular elevation and protraction, and, if indicated, joint mobility of the spine, ribs, and shoulders can be assessed.[65] Lateral side bending distance (assessment of lateral trunk flexion), shoulder flexion ROM (gross measure of combined thoracic extension, scapula mobility, and glenohumeral mobility), and acromial angle distance are all simple, objective tests that can be used as outcome measures for postural and flexibility interventions.[60,65] Acromial angle distance is measured as the distance from the acromial angle to the wall in standing, which is a gross measure of thoracic kyphosis, scapular mobility, and pectoralis tightness.

Based on the patient-identified problems from the interview, additional nonpatient-identified problems discovered during the examination, and anticipated problems, a refined problem list is developed and hypotheses generated to explain why the problems exist (or are likely to occur). For both inpatients and outpatients, this list may be quite similar and include: (1) airway clearance dysfunction, (2) impaired endurance, (3) impaired peripheral and ventilatory muscle performance, (4) impaired posture and musculoskeletal pain, and (5) urinary stress incontinence.

Plan of Care and Interventions

A plan of care is developed from this problem list, including establishing goals, testing criteria, and intervention strategies and tactics (Table 16-3).

Since CF is a chronic health condition, the ability of the patient and family to manage the disease is critical to outcome. In the early years of the child with CF, the health literacy of the parents is an important consideration in structuring instruction and education sessions that meet their needs. In adulthood, the patient's own health literacy level must be assessed and strategies implemented to ensure that health literacy is not a barrier to effective self-management. Quality, tailored patient/client-related instruction geared toward promoting independence, health, and overall fitness should form the backbone of all of the therapist's procedural interventions.

ACTs improve secretion clearance, enhance ventilation/gas exchange, and can improve respiratory symptoms and exercise tolerance.[66] According to recent clinical practice guidelines, ACTs "should be performed on a regular basis in all patients" with CF.[67] Traditional "chest PT" (typically defined as postural drainage, percussion, and vibration/shaking) has been a mainstay of treatment for patients with CF. Although there is no robust scientific evidence to support chest PT,[68] it is considered a standard of care and is the standard ACT against which all newer therapies are compared. These "newer" techniques include: (1) high frequency chest wall oscillation (HFCWO), (2) IPV, (3) PEP, (4) active cycle of breathing technique, (5) autogenic drainage, and (6) exercise.

High-frequency chest wall oscillation (e.g., The Vest, SmartVest) involves the patient wearing an inflatable belt or vest around the chest; air is pumped in and out of the device at high frequencies that vibrate the chest from the outside in (much like manual vibration) to loosen and mobilize secretions.[11] It has been found to be as effective as chest PT, but can be self-administered.[69] IPV works on a similar principle of high frequency oscillating airflow, except it is delivered via a mouthpiece. IPV is more novel and much less common, but a small pilot study found it to be as effective as traditional chest PT.[70]

Problems	Goals	Testing Criteria	Intervention Strategies	Intervention Tactics
Airway clearance dysfunction	Patient perceives that sputum is easier to expectorate	Independently and correctly performs a non-PEP alternative airway clearance technique	Airway clearance techniques	*Mode:* Active cycle of breathing technique *Duration:* 10-15 min *Frequency:* 4 times per day while in hospital
Shortness of breath	Dyspnea at rest of 1 on Borg CR10 Scale	Resting respiratory rate decreases	Breathing strategies	Pursed-lips breathing Relaxed breathing
	Dyspnea with exertion of ≤5 on Borg CR10 Scale	Respiratory rate at relative, sub-maximal activity is decreased	See strategies below for Problem: "Walking long distances"	
Walking long distances and running	Walk ≥ 600 m (~2,000 ft) in 6 min (with or without supplemental oxygen)	Ventilatory response to sub-maximal exercise is decreased (lower respiratory rate, decreased dyspnea, higher SpO_2 for a given FiO_2)	Breathing strategies	Pursed-lips breathing with exertion Paced breathing (*e.g.*, inhale for two steps, exhale for four steps)
			Aerobic exercise training	*Mode:* Treadmill walking *Intensity:* ~80% of baseline 6MWT velocity *Frequency:* daily *Duration:* Initially, three 5- to 10-min sessions, progressing to one ≥ 30-min session by discharge
				Patient encouraged to independently ambulate on hospital ward 2-3 times per day at comfortable pace (using supplemental oxygen)
			Resistance exercise training	See tactics below for Problem: "Climbing stairs and hills"
			Supplemental oxygen	Oxygen flow rate with standard nasal cannula titrated to keep SpO_2 ≥ 90% with exercise

(Continued)

Table 16-3   SAMPLE PLAN OF CARE FOR TYPICAL IDENTIFIED OR ANTICIPATED PROBLEMS IN PATIENTS WITH CF (CONTINUED)

Problems	Goals	Testing Criteria	Intervention Strategies	Intervention Tactics
Climbing stairs and hills	Climb 1 flight of stairs in 20 sec without handrail (with supplemental oxygen, if indicted)	20 repetitions of sit-to-stand in 30 sec	Resistance exercise training	3 sets of 10 repetitions of maximal "squat jumps" every other day
				10 repetitions of sit-to-stand-to sit each time she gets out of bed, chair, and toilet
		5/5 bilateral knee extensor strength		Climb 10-12 stairs in the therapy gym before and after treadmill training
Urinary stress incontinence	Over the next year, patient will not report any episodes of urinary stress incontinence	Patient is independent in pelvic floor muscle exercises and understands when stress incontinence is likely	Resistance exercise	Teach pelvic floor muscle exercises
			Referral	Arrange follow-up with the Women's Health PT Clinic for further consultation

PEP devices ideally produce an expiratory pressure of 10-20 cm H_2O. This pressure during expiration is theorized to help mobilize secretions by splinting open distal airways, promoting collateral ventilation, and prolonging expiration. PEP can also include vibratory or oscillatory PEP (*e.g.*, acapella and Flutter). PEP therapy is not more effective than other ACTs, but is relatively inexpensive compared to HFCWO and IPV, and some patients prefer PEP over manual chest PT.[71]

The active cycle of breathing technique (ACBT) and autogenic drainage are breathing techniques that the patient can do independently and require no equipment. ACBT is easy to learn and teach. It involves repeated cycles of (1) breathing control (relaxed tidal breathing), (2) thoracic expansion (full, vital capacity breaths with a maximal inspiratory hold), and (3) forced expiratory technique (FET; a forced sigh or "huff"). ACBT can be performed in sitting or in various postural drainage positions. The therapist can also provide percussion and/or vibration during the thoracic expansion phase.[11] The **active cycle of breathing technique is as effective as other ACTs and may be preferred over traditional chest PT.**[72,73] Autogenic drainage is more difficult to master, requires a knowledgeable therapist and a motivated patient, and therefore, the acute care setting may not be the ideal location to teach this technique.

One of the many benefits of exercise is that it improves secretion clearance, especially exercise that requires deep breathing and involves chest "vibration" (*e.g.*, running, walking, jumping jacks, small trampolines[74,75]). Although aerobic exercise should *not* be the sole method of airway clearance, it is an important adjunct and also has additional health benefits beyond airway clearance.[67]

Patients with hemoptysis and pneumothorax require special precautions.[9] In cases of massive hemoptysis, all ACTs should be stopped. Clot formation could be impaired with the vibration, oscillation, and shear stresses from ACTs. For patients with mild to moderate hemoptysis, a conversation with the pulmonologist should occur before proceeding with, perhaps, less vigorous airway clearance. In the case of scant hemoptysis (< 5 mL), cautious, usual airway clearance therapy can continue.[9]

For patients with an acute or recent pneumothorax, regardless of size, IPV or PEP therapies should not be used, and exercise should be held if the patient has a large pneumothorax. Other ACTs may be appropriate and cautiously used. For a small pneumothorax, or if a chest tube is in place, ACTs should continue with caution.[9] If a chest tube is in place, patients often have pain with HFCWO and chest PT. Therefore, ACBT may be the most appropriate ACT under these circumstances.

The reader can refer to recent CF clinical practice guidelines[11,67] and/or cardiopulmonary texts[30,76] for more specifics regarding the evidence and application of each of these ACTs.

Therapeutic exercise is a mainstay of physical therapy, and this is no different when it comes to patients with CF.[77] In fact, the phrase "Exercise is Medicine"[78] is frequently used with regard to CF.[79,80] Important aspects of therapeutic exercise for the patient with a CF pulmonary exacerbation include: (1) aerobic capacity/endurance training, (2) strength, power, and endurance training for skeletal muscles (including pelvic floor muscles), (3) flexibility exercises, and (4) breathing strategies.

Aerobic exercise has been a cornerstone of the recommendations for patients with CF. No different than with any other population, the principles include mode, intensity, frequency, and duration.[81] The *mode* of aerobic exercise in the hospital typically involves walking in the hallways, but if available, can include treadmill walking, stationary cycling, and/or circuit training. As a patient's condition improves, stair climbing and stepping machines can be utilized. Jumping jacks and jumping rope are other aerobic activities that can be performed in relatively small spaces.

Exercise *intensity* is measured by monitoring HR and dyspnea rating. Because there is a relatively linear increase in HR with increasing work rate and VO_2, HR is the most common method used to measure intensity. The target HR can be determined via several methods. For example, adverse signs or symptoms such as oxygen desaturation or severe dyspnea requiring the patient to stop walking during an initial exercise test typically occur at a reproducible HR; the target HR for exercise prescription could then be set ~5 beats per minute below that point.[81] In patients with moderate to severe CF, peak HR during the 6MWT or MST may well represent maximal HR (HRmax) and can be used to calculate target HR for exercise prescription. If a maximal test is not available, HRmax can be estimated based on age. Although the equation HRmax = 220 − age is familiar to most physical therapists, it overestimates HRmax for patients under age 40 years. A revised age-predicted maximal heart rate equation HRmax = 208 − 0.7 × age is a more accurate estimate.[82] Once HRmax is determined (either directly or estimated), a percentage of HRmax can be used to set exercise intensity, typically 70% to 85% of HRmax or 60% to 80% of HR reserve (HRR = HRmax − HRrest; target HR range = ([HRR × percent intensity] + HRrest) is considered "moderate" to "strong" intensity.[81] Patients can be taught to monitor their own HR or use commercially available HR monitors. Since dyspnea rating is also correlated with VO_2,[83] it can be used to prescribe exercise. A Borg CR10 dyspnea rating of 3 to 5 is often used for "moderate" to "strong" aerobic exercise intensity, but some recommendations include higher intensity exercise (4 to 6).[84] However, a dyspnea rating of 6 is likely near the anaerobic threshold,[85] and typically cannot be sustained for more than a few minutes. Therefore, a rating of 3 to 4 should be used if endurance is the primary goal, while 5 to 6 can be used with interval training or if the goal is to increase aerobic work capacity.

Consistent with guidelines for healthy adults,[81] the typical *frequency* of outpatient pulmonary rehabilitation programs is 3 to 5 days per week, with the goal for exercise to "become part of a daily routine."[86] For patients in the hospital with an acute exacerbation, multiple sessions of shorter *duration* exercise may be indicated, perhaps more intense and monitored aerobic exercise daily with the physical therapist and a low to moderate intensity walking exercise bout to be performed independently. For example, acutely ill patients could perform bouts of short-duration exercise followed by brief rest periods (*e.g.*, 2 to 4 repetitions of 5-minute walk, interspersed with a 2-minute rest), with the goal of being able to perform moderate or higher intensity exercise for 20 to 30 minutes continuously by discharge.[81,87] Interval training can also be an effective alternative to typical endurance training for very debilitated patients or those with severe dyspnea on exertion. Shorter exercise intervals allow patients to reach a beneficial (moderate to high) training intensity if only for a brief period.[88]

Although some reports suggest that it takes about 8 weeks of training for patients to achieve meaningful improvements in symptoms, exercise tolerance, and quality of life,[89] others report significant increases in endurance and peak VO_2 with aerobic training during hospitalization for a CF pulmonary exacerbation above and beyond the improvement from pharmacologic and airway clearance therapies.[90,91]

Peripheral muscle resistance exercise training has not been studied as much as aerobic exercise training.[92] Resistance training during an inpatient hospital stay for a CF pulmonary exacerbation has been found to be effective at improving not only strength, but also muscle mass.[90,91] There are no specific resistance training guidelines for individuals with CF, so resistance training programs can be designed based on evidence from healthy populations that address the goals of improving muscle strength, power, and hypertrophy and increasing bone density. Indirect evidence from other populations suggests that resistance exercise increases bone density and helps control blood glucose.[93]

The *mode* of resistance training may include free weights or machines, if available, as well as resistance bands/tubing and calisthenics (especially where patients are not allowed to leave their hospital room due to concerns about infection control). Hand-held weights, bands/tubing, and calisthenics have the advantage that these exercises can also be performed at home. Whatever the mode, the exercise should feel comfortable throughout the range of motion and should engage key upper extremity, lower extremity, and core muscle groups.[94] Table 16-4 provides a sample of exercises that can be performed in a hospital room or at home.

Intensity and number of quality repetitions that can be performed are inversely related, so the number of repetitions of an exercise can be used to estimate intensity. The intensity should be high enough so that the last repetition is "difficult, if not impossible, while maintaining good form."[94] Repetitions of 3 to 15 have been shown to increase muscle strength, power, and hypertrophy. However, exercises that can be performed for 3 to 10 repetitions significantly improve bone density compared to higher repetitions. The patient should maintain consistent form throughout the *duration* of the repetition (during the concentric and eccentric phases). With regard to the number of sets, 1 to 3 is commonly used, but there does not appear to be a benefit with regards to strength or hypertrophy beyond one well-performed set. Most resistance training studies suggest a frequency of 2 to 3 times per week (every other day) when training for hypertrophy, strength, and power.[94] Breathing control during resistance training and avoidance of the Valsalva maneuver is important. Ideally, this includes inhalation during the concentric phase or with trunk flexion motions and exhalation during the eccentric phase or with trunk extension motions.[95]

Table 16-4 SAMPLE RESISTANCE EXERCISES		
Lower Extremities	**Core**	**Upper Extremities**
Squats	Sit-ups	Push-ups
Lunges	Crunches	Bicep curls
Squat jumps	Superman	Tricep dips
Bunny hops	Plank hold	Military press

Although likely not an initial patient-identified problem, screening for **urinary stress incontinence** reveals a high proportion of individuals with CF that frequently leak urine, especially during coughing episodes. Once identified, an individualized program of pelvic floor muscle exercises can improve muscle performance and reduce urine leakage.[96] Although improvements in muscle performance may take weeks, the acute care therapist can initiate an exercise program, suggest some simple techniques to help reduce urine leakage and make referrals to appropriate outpatient therapy clinics for further management of urinary stress incontinence. One technique that has been recommended to be taught to all patients with CF is "the knack," an active pelvic floor muscle contraction (similar to stopping urine stream) prior to anticipated coughing.[97] In addition, tips such as emptying the bladder prior to performing ACTs and performing ACTs in proper postures can be quite useful.

For both aerobic and resistance exercise programs, a proper warm-up and cool-down including low-intensity aerobic exercise and flexibility exercises are appropriate to help reduce the risk of musculoskeletal injury. Unfortunately, the intensity of aerobic and resistance exercise training often falls below the threshold required to achieve clinically meaningful results for the patient. Therefore, regular re-examination is required to ensure proper progression of exercise at a level above the intensity thresholds required for a continued therapeutic benefit.[98]

Flexibility in individuals with CF declines with age and is more pronounced than in healthy controls.[59] Massery[65,99] has highlighted the interconnectedness of the musculoskeletal, neuromuscular, and respiratory systems and describes the success of a home-based program to improve posture, flexibility, and motor control in a 9-year-old with moderate CF. A 6-week comprehensive outpatient physical therapy program including aerobic exercise, ACBT, and posture exercises resulted in improvements in thoracic mobility (i.e., maximal chest circumference at three levels) and trunk flexibility (i.e., forward bending, lateral flexion, trunk rotation, and trunk hyperextension) in kids with CF.[100] In another outpatient study, the sit and reach test (assessing hamstring and lower back flexibility) improved in children after a static and dynamic flexibility exercise program.[59] Even during a 7- to 10-day hospital stay for a pulmonary exacerbation, improvements in posture and flexibility were achieved with an every other day static and dynamic stretching and postural awareness interventions.[91] Yoga or Pilates typically include whole body flexibility exercises, but the therapist may need to include stretching of specific muscle groups that were identified as tight during physical examination (e.g., neck flexors, pectoral muscles, lateral trunk flexors, low back extensors, and hip flexors).[11,65]

Specific controlled-breathing tactics to help relieve dyspnea in patients with obstructive lung disease include pursed-lips breathing (PLB), diaphragmatic breathing, relaxation, and paced breathing (altering the "duty cycle" of inspiration and expiration).[101] The bulk of the evidence is with PLB.[102] To our knowledge, there has been only one study investigating breathing strategies in patients with CF, which found that biofeedback-assisted breathing retraining (including diaphragmatic and PLB) improved FEV_1 and forced vital capacity and decreased respiratory rate and accessory muscle use.[103]

Many patients with obstructive lung disease (which includes CF) learn to do PLB on their own. PLB acutely decreases respiratory rate, minute ventilation, $PaCO_2$, and dyspnea, while increasing SpO_2 and tidal volume.[104,105] When respiratory rate slows, there is a longer expiratory time, which reduces dyspnea by preventing or minimizing dynamic hyperinflation (a slow increase in functional residual capacity during exercise caused by air trapping). As respiratory rate decreases, the rate of work of breathing is also reduced,[106] which likely also explains the faster post-exercise recovery when patients employ PLB.[107] PLB is typically easy to teach and quick to learn. However, PLB is not a tactic that should be pursued if patients do not learn it relatively quickly or if dyspnea is not improved.[108] Diaphragmatic breathing may take a little longer to learn for those accustomed to a dysfunctional breathing pattern. Diaphragmatic breathing is an important part of learning to relax and breathe effectively (reducing the work of breathing). It is an important adjunct to perform along with airway clearance therapies.[95]

Manual therapy, including spinal and intercostal joint mobilization and soft tissue mobilization, has also been shown to reduce pain and dyspnea in both out-patients and during hospitalization for a pulmonary exacerbation.[109] In particular, rib mobilization and thoracic extension and rotation mobilizations can help restore chest wall mobility. Caution should be used in patients with a history of vertebral wedging due to CF-related osteoporosis.[11]

Although "room air" at most habituated altitudes contains sufficient oxygen for normal life, patients with CF during a pulmonary exacerbation often require supplemental oxygen to compensate for hypoxemia. Many consider desaturation ($SpO_2 \leq 88\%$) with sleep or activity an indication for "intermittent oxygen use."[110] Indeed, nocturnal and exercise desaturation are of particular concern for patients with CF, and **supplemental oxygen during sleep and exercise** can prevent desaturation, increase sleep quality, and improve exercise tolerance.[111] Often the physical therapist is the first member of the interdisciplinary team to measure a patient's oxygen desaturation when evaluating a patient's activity limitation and complaints of dyspnea. Even when patients are on supplemental oxygen at rest, this resting oxygen "dose" may not be sufficient for exercise or even performing activities of daily living. While oxygen therapy improves exercise SpO_2 and exercise performance, it may result in a mild, and likely clinically insignificant, increase in CO_2 retention.[111,112] Since medical oxygen is considered a "prescription drug," any application, discontinuation, or changes in the mode of delivery or dose of oxygen requires a physician's prescription.[42] An APTA document titled "Oxygen Administration During Physical Therapy" notes that physicians may prescribe a resting or exercise dose in a manner designed to keep SpO_2 greater than a certain threshold (e.g., "titrate FiO_2 to keep $SpO_2 > 88\%$").[113] This type of prescription allows the physical therapist to increase the flow rate of the nasal cannula, or even change to an alternative device (e.g., Venturi mask or partial- or non-rebreather mask) to ensure adequate oxygenation with activity.[42,114] If there is any uncertainty about the prescription or if it needs to be altered for physical activity/exercise, the therapist should communicate with the physician.[42] Also, because not all devices are equivalent, especially portable and oxygen-conserving devices, pulse oximetry monitoring and titration of oxygen during exercise should be done "employing the device the patient will be using."[114]

In addition to producing the tangible and immediate benefits to aerobic capacity, muscle performance, flexibility and posture,[90,91] the in-hospital exercise program for individuals with CF models the appropriate physical activity that should be encouraged when they leave the hospital. Empowering patients/clients to be independent outside of physical therapy sessions should be our ultimate goal. Jerry Cahill, an adult with CF, has an informative exercise-related website with additional ideas for individuals with CF on the entire range of topics covered in this intervention section.[115]

Evidence-Based Clinical Recommendations

SORT: Strength of Recommendation Taxonomy

A: Consistent, good-quality patient-oriented evidence
B: Inconsistent or limited-quality patient-oriented evidence
C: Consensus, disease-oriented evidence, usual practice, expert opinion, or case series

1. The timing of dornase alfa (Pulmozyme) inhalation does not impact the timing of airway clearance interventions for individuals with cystic fibrosis (CF). **Grade A**

2. The active cycle of breathing technique is an appropriate substitute for other ACTs (traditional chest physical therapy, high frequency chest wall oscillation, and oscillating PEP) in individuals with CF. **Grade B**

3. Exercise training for individuals with CF has short and long-term benefits. **Grade B**

4. It is important to screen for urinary stress incontinence in individuals with CF because it is frequently underreported, yet can be successfully treated. **Grade B**

5. Supplemental oxygen during sleep and exercise can prevent arterial oxygen desaturation, increase sleep quality, and improve exercise tolerance in individuals with CF. **Grade A**

COMPREHENSION QUESTIONS

16.1 A 30-year-old male was admitted to the hospital with mild hemoptysis and a mild left upper lobe pneumothorax. He is being treated with intravenous antibiotics for an acute CF pulmonary exacerbation and is on supplemental oxygen at a rate of 2 L/min at rest, but there is a standing order to titrate the flow rate to keep SpO_2 > 90%. His MST distance during the initial physical therapy examination was 460 m (level 7) using supplemental oxygen. Which of the following ACTs would be *most* appropriate?

  A. Active cycle of breathing technique

  B. Intrapulmonary percussive ventilation

  C. Oscillating positive expiratory pressure

  D. Postural drainage with manual percussion and vibration

16.2 After walking on the treadmill at a 5% incline and speed of 2.75 mph for 5 minutes during a treatment session, the patient in Question 16.1 rates his dyspnea level as 6/10 on the Borg CR10 Scale and his SpO_2 is 86%. What is the *most* appropriate action for the physical therapist to take?

  A. Decrease the speed of the treadmill

  B. Decrease the incline of the treadmill

  C. Increase the oxygen flow rate

  D. Terminate the exercise session

16.3 Using the Borg CR10 Scale to grade intensity, which of the following ranges of perceived dyspnea would be *most* appropriate for a 20-minute continuous aerobic exercise program on a stationary cycle?

  A. 1 to 2

  B. 3 to 4

  C. 5 to 6

  D. 7 to 8

ANSWERS

16.1 **A.** The active cycle of breathing technique and autogenic drainage (AD) are appropriate techniques for patients with less than massive hemoptysis. In addition, ACBT and AD do not include high levels of positive expiratory pressure. Intrapulmonary percussive ventilation (option B) and oscillating positive expiratory pressure (option C) both provide high levels of positive pressure for the lungs. In patients with a current or recent pneumothorax, this positive pressure should be avoided (as it could cause air to leak out into the pleural space). There is still concern in patients with mild to moderate hemoptysis that manual percussion and vibration (option D) could impair clot formation.

16.2 **C.** Decreasing the speed (option A) or incline (option B) of the treadmill would be appropriate if supplemental oxygen were *not* available or if there was not an order in the chart to titrate his oxygen with activity. Either of these options would decrease the exercise intensity and likely improve his oxygenation and decrease his breathlessness. However, increasing the oxygen flow rate (option C) to, perhaps, 4 L/min, would improve his oxygenation and likely decrease his breathlessness and allow him to continue the exercise session. A Borg CR10 dyspnea rating of 6 and a SpO_2 of 86% are not "dangerous" levels, so there is no need to terminate the exercise session (option D), unless he did not respond to increased supplemental oxygen and continued to desaturate and complain of increasing breathlessness.

16.3 **B.** A Borg CR10 dyspnea rating of 3 to 5 is often used for "moderate" to "strong" aerobic exercise intensity. During a 20-minute continuous aerobic session, endurance is likely the primary goal for this session. A rating of 3 to 4 is appropriate if endurance is the primary goal. A rating of 1 to 2 (option A) would not be at sufficient intensity to achieve aerobic benefits. A rating of 5 to 6 (option C) could be used with interval training (but not for a continuous 20-min exercise bout) and a rating of 7 to 8 (option D) would be too high to maintain for even a few minutes.

REFERENCES

1. Schluchter MD, Konstan MW, Drumm ML, et al. Classifying severity of cystic fibrosis lung disease using longitudinal pulmonary function data. *Am J Respir Crit Care Med.* 2006;174:780-786.

2. O'Sullivan BP, Freedman SD. Cystic fibrosis. *Lancet.* 2009;373:1891-1904.

3. Cystic Fibrosis Foundation. *Cystic Fibrosis Foundation Patient Registry 2010 Annual Data Report.* Bethesda, MD; 2011.

4. Rowe SM, Miller S, Sorscher EJ. Cystic fibrosis. *N Engl J Med.* 2005;352:1992-2001.

5. Stallings VA, Stark LJ, Robinson KA, et al. Evidence-based practice recommendations for nutrition-related management of children and adults with cystic fibrosis and pancreatic insufficiency: results of a systematic review. *J Am Diet Assoc.* 2008;108:832-839.

6. Harris A, Coleman L. Ductal epithelial cells cultured from human foetal epididymis and vas deferens: relevance to sterility in cystic fibrosis. *J Cell Sci.* 1989;92:687-690.

7. Bar-Or O, Hay JA, Ward DS, et al. Voluntary dehydration and heat intolerance in cystic fibrosis. *Lancet.* 1992;339:696-699.

8. Flume PA, Yankaskas JR, Ebeling M, et al. Massive hemoptysis in cystic fibrosis. *Chest.* 2005;128:729-738.

9. Flume PA, Mogayzel PJ, Robinson KA, et al. Cystic fibrosis pulmonary guidelines: pulmonary complications: hemoptysis and pneumothorax. *Am J Respir Crit Care Med.* 2010;182:298-306.

10. Flume PA. Pneumothorax in cystic fibrosis. *Chest.* 2003;123:217-221.

11. Swisher AK, Downs AM, Dekerlegand RL. *CF 101 for the Physical Therapist.* Cystic Fibrosis Foundation; 2010.

12. Curran DR, McArdle JR, Talwalkar JS. Diabetes mellitus and bone disease in cystic fibrosis. *Semin Respir Crit Care Med.* 2009;30:514-530.

13. Conway SP, Morton AM, Oldroyd B, et al. Osteoporosis and osteopenia in adults and adolescents with cystic fibrosis: prevalence and associated factors. *Thorax.* 2000;55:798-804.

14. Tattersall R, Walshaw MJ. Posture and cystic fibrosis. *J R Soc Med.* 2003;96(Suppl 43):18-22.

15. Swisher A. Not just a lung disease: peripheral muscle abnormalities in cystic fibrosis and the role of exercise to address them. *Cardiopulm Phys Ther J.* 2006;17:9-14.

16. Nankivell G, Caldwell P, Follett J. Urinary incontinence in adolescent females with cystic fibrosis. *Paediatr Respir Rev.* 2010;11:95-99.

17. Anderson DH. Cystic fibrosis of the pancreas and its relation to celiac disease: a clinical and patho-logic study. *Am J Dis Child.* 1938;56:344-399.

18. Ferkol T, Rosenfeld M, Milla CE. Cystic fibrosis pulmonary exacerbations. *J Pediatr.* 2006;148:259-264.

19. Rabin HR, Butler SM, Wohl ME, et al. Pulmonary exacerbations in cystic fibrosis. *Pediatr Pulmonol.* 2004;37:400-406.

20. Flume PA, Mogayzel PJ, Robinson KA, et al. Cystic fibrosis pulmonary guidelines: treatment of pulmonary exacerbations. *Am J Respir Crit Care Med.* 2009;180:802-808.

21. Kerem E, Conway S, Elborn S, et al. Standards of care for patients with cystic fibrosis: a European consensus. *J Cyst Fibros.* 2005;4:7-26.

22. Cystic Fibrosis Foundation. Locations, Locations, Locations. Available from: http://www.cff.org/aboutCFFoundation/Locations/FindACareCenter/. Accessed February 5, 2012.

23. Rothstein JM, Echternach JL, Riddle DL. The Hypothesis-Oriented Algorithm for Clinicians II (HOAC II): a guide for patient management. *Phys Ther.* 2003;83:455-470.

24. Dentice R, Elkins M. Timing of dornase alfa inhalation for cystic fibrosis. *Cochrane Database Syst Rev.* 2011(5):CD007923.

25. Dentice R, Elkins M, Bye P. A randomized trial of the effect of timing of hypertonic saline inhala-tion in relation to airway clearance physiotherapy in adults with cystic fibrosis. *Pediatric Pulmonology.* 2010;45(S33):384.

26. LaPier TK. Glucocorticoid-induced muscle atrophy: the role of exercise in treatment and preven-tion. *J Cardiopulm Rehabil.* 1997;17:76-84.

27. Braith RW, Conner JA, Fulton MN, et al. Comparison of alendronate vs alendronate plus mechanical loading as prophylaxis for osteoporosis in lung transplant recipients: a pilot study. *J Heart Lung Transplant.* 2007;26:132-137.

28. Chaparro C, Maurer J, Gutierrez C, et al. Infection with Burkholderia cepacia in cystic fibrosis: outcome following lung transplantation. *Am J Respir Crit Care Med.* 2001;163:43-48.

29. Flume PA, O'Sullivan BP, Robinson KA, et al. Cystic fibrosis pulmonary guidelines: chronic medi-cations for maintenance of lung health *Am J Respir Crit Care Med.* 2007;176:957-969.

30. Mejia-Downs A, Bishop KL. Physical therapy associated with airway clearance dysfunction. In: DeTurk WE, Cahalin LP, eds. *Cardiovascular and pulmonary physical therapy: an evidence-based approach.* 2nd ed. New York, NY: McGraw-Hill Medical; 2011:xi, 778 p.

31. VanDevanter DR, Rasouliyan L, Murphy TM, et al. Trends in the clinical characteristics of the U.S. cystic fibrosis patient population from 1995 to 2005. *Pediatr Pulmonol.* 2008;43:739-744.

32. Leroy S, Perez T, Neviere R, et al. Determinants of dyspnea and alveolar hypoventilation during exercise in cystic fibrosis: impact of inspiratory muscle endurance. *J Cyst Fibros.* 2011;10:159-165.

33. American Thoracic Society. Dyspnea. Mechanisms, assessment, and management: a consensus statement. American Thoracic Society. *Am J Respir Criti Care Med.* 1999;159:321-340.

34. Darbee J, Ohtake P. Outcome measures in cardiopulmonary physical therapy: Medical Research Council (MRC) dyspnea scale. *Cardiopulm Phys Ther J.* 2006;17:29-37.

35. Stenton C. The MRC breathlessness scale. *Occup Med (Lond).* 2008;58:226-227.

36. Burdon JG, Juniper EF, Killian KJ, et al. The perception of breathlessness in asthma. *Am Rev Respir Dis.* 1982;126:825-828.

37. Kendrick KR, Baxi SC, Smith RM. Usefulness of the modified 0-10 Borg scale in assessing the degree of dyspnea in patients with COPD and asthma. *J Emerg Nurs.* 2000;26:216-222.

38. Mahler DA. The measurement of dyspnea during exercise in patients with lung disease. *Chest.* 1992;101(5 Suppl):242S-247S.

39. Borg G. *Borg's Perceived Exertion and Pain Scales.* Champaign, IL: Human Kinetics; 1998.

40. Mador MJ, Rodis A, Magalang UJ. Reproducibility of Borg scale measurements of dyspnea during exercise in patients with COPD. *Chest.* 1995;107:1590-1597.

41. Ries AL. Minimally clinically important difference for the UCSD Shortness of Breath Questionnaire, Borg scale, and visual analog scale. *COPD.* 2005;2:105-110.

42. Crouch R. Oxygen use in physical therapy practice. *Cardiopulm Phys Ther J.* 2008;19:49-52.

43. McDonald CF, Crockett AJ, Young IH. Adult domiciliary oxygen therapy. Position statement of the Thoracic Society of Australia and New Zealand. *Med J Aust.* 2005;182:621-626.

44. Nixon PA, Orenstein DM, Kelsey SF, et al. The prognostic value of exercise testing in patients with cystic fibrosis. *N Engl J Med.* 1992;327:1785-1788.

45. Noonan V, Dean E. Submaximal exercise testing: clinical application and interpretation. *Phys Ther.* 2000;80:782-807.

46. Narang I, Pike S, Rosenthal M, et al. Three-minute step test to assess exercise capacity in children with cystic fibrosis with mild lung disease. *Pediatr Pulmonol.* 2003;35:108-113.

47. ATS. ATS Statement: Guidelines for the Six-Minute Walk Test. *Am J Respir Crit Care Med.* 2002;166:111-117.

48. Troosters T, Gosselink R, Decramer M. Six minute walking distance in healthy elderly subjects. *Eur Respir J.* 1999;14:270-274.

49. Lettieri CJ, Nathan SD, Browning RF, et al. The distance-saturation product predicts mortality in idiopathic pulmonary fibrosis. *Respir Med.* 2006;100:1734-141.

50. Carter R, Holiday DB, Nwasuruba C, et al. 6-minute walk work for assessment of functional capacity in patients with COPD. *Chest.* 2003;123:1408-1415.

51. Cunha MT, Rozov T, de Oliveira RC, et al. Six-minute walk test in children and adolescents with cystic fibrosis. *Pediatr Pulmonol.* 2006;41:618-622.

52. Kadikar A, Maurer J, Kesten S. The six-minute walk test: a guide to assessment for lung transplantation. *J Heart Lung Transplant.* 1997;16:313-319.

53. Tuppin MP, Paratz JD, Chang AT, et al. Predictive utility of the 6-minute walk distance on survival in patients awaiting lung transplantation. *J Heart Lung Transplant.* 2008;27:729-734.

54. Singh SJ. Modified Shuttle Test. Dept. of Respiratory Medicine, Glenfield Hospital NHS Trust; contact: leslie.shortt@uhl-tr.nhs.uk.

55. Bradley J, Howard J, Wallace E, Elborn S. Validity of a modified shuttle test in adult cystic fibrosis. *Thorax.* 1999;54:437-439.

56. Selvadurai HC, Cooper PJ, Meyers N, et al. Validation of shuttle tests in children with cystic fibrosis. *Pediatr Pulmonol.* 2003;35:133-138.

57. Cox NS, Follett J, McKay KO. Modified shuttle test performance in hospitalized children and adolescents with cystic fibrosis. *J Cyst Fibros.* 2006;5:165-170.

58. Phillips A, Lee L, Britton L, et al. The efficacy of a standardized exercise protocol in inpatient care of patients with cystic fibrosis. *Pediatr Pulmonol.* 2008;43(S31):385.

59. Gruber W, Orenstein DM, Braumann KM, et al. Health-related fitness and trainability in children with cystic fibrosis. *Pediatr Pulmonol.* 2008;43:953-964.

60. Lowman J, Moore K, Peeples A, et al. Reliability of musculoskeletal outcome measures. *Pediatr Pulmonol.* 2010;45(S33):387.

61. Sahlberg M, Svantesson U, Magnusson Thomas E, et al. Muscular strength after different types of training in physically active patients with cystic fibrosis. *Scand J Med Sci Sports.* 2008;18:756-764.

62. Christiansen J, Thompson L, McNamara J, et al. Cystic fibrosis core strengthening and respiratory exercise program (CSREP). *Pediatr Pulmonol.* 2010;45(S33):387.

63. Enright S, Chatham K, Ionescu AA, et al. Inspiratory muscle training improves lung function and exercise capacity in adults with cystic fibrosis. *Chest.* 2004;126:405-411.

64. Parasa RB, Maffulli N. Musculoskeletal involvement in cystic fibrosis. *Bull Hosp Jt Dis.* 1999;58: 37-44.

65. Massery M. Musculoskeletal and neuromuscular interventions: a physical approach to cystic fibrosis. *J R Soc Med.* 2005;98 Suppl 45:55-66.

66. Murray MP, Pentland JL, Hill AT. A randomised crossover trial of chest physiotherapy in non-cystic fibrosis bronchiectasis. *Eur Respir J.* 2009;34:1086-1092.

67. Flume PA, Robinson KA, O'Sullivan BP, et al. Cystic fibrosis pulmonary guidelines: airway clearance therapies. *Respir Care.* 2009;54:522-537.

68. van der Schans C, Prasad A, Main E. Chest physiotherapy compared to no chest physiotherapy for cystic fibrosis. *Cochrane Database Syst Rev.* 2000(2):CD001401.

69. Scherer TA, Barandun J, Martinez E, et al. Effect of high-frequency oral airway and chest wall oscillation and conventional chest physical therapy on expectoration in patients with stable cystic fibrosis. *Chest.* 1998;113:1019-1027.

70. Marks JH, Hare KL, Saunders RA, et al. Pulmonary function and sputum production in patients with cystic fibrosis: a pilot study comparing the PercussiveTech HF device and standard chest physiotherapy. *Chest.* 2004;125:1507-1511.

71. Elkins MR, Jones A, van der Schans C. Positive expiratory pressure physiotherapy for airway clearance in people with cystic fibrosis. *Cochrane Database Syst Rev.* 2006(2):CD003147.

72. Robinson KA, McKoy N, Saldanha I, et al. Active cycle of breathing technique for cystic fibrosis. *Cochrane Database Syst Rev.* 2010(11):CD007862.

73. Syed N, Maiya AG, Siva Kumar T. Active Cycles of Breathing Technique (ACBT) versus conventional chest physical therapy on airway clearance in bronchiectasis—a crossover trial. *Advances in Physiotherapy.* 2009;11:193-198.

74. Sahlberg M, Strandvik B. Trampolines are useful in the treatment of cystic fibrosis patients. *Pediatr Pulmonol.* 2005;40:464.

75. Currant J, Mahony M. Trampolining as an adjunct to regular physiotherapy in children with cystic fibrosis. *Ir Med J.* 2008;101:188.

76. Downs A. Airway clearance interventions. In: Frownfelter DL, Dean E, eds. *Cardiovascular and Pulmonary Physical Therapy Evidence and Practice.* 5th ed. St. Louis, MO: Mosby; 2013.

77. Bradley J, Moran F. Physical training for cystic fibrosis. *Cochrane Database Syst Rev.* 2008(1): CD002768.

78. American College of Sports Medicine. Exercise is Medicine. 2008; Avaialable from: http://exerciseismedicine.org/. Accessed February 2, 2012.

79. Exercise is Medicine. Exercising with Cystic Fibrosis. Available from: http://www.exerciseismedicine.org/documents/YPH_CysticFibrosis.pdf. Accessed February 8, 2012.

80. Wheatley CM, Wilkins BW, Snyder EM. Exercise is medicine in cystic fibrosis. *Exerc Sport Sci Rev.* 2011;39:155-160.

81. American College of Sports Medicine., Thompson WR, Gordon NF, Pescatello LS. *ACSM's Guidelines for Exercise Testing and Prescription.* 8th ed. Philadelphia, PA: Lippincott Williams & Wilkins; 2010.

82. Tanaka H, Monahan KD, Seals DR. Age-predicted maximal heart rate revisited. *J Am Coll Cardiol.* 2001;37:153-156.

83. Mejia R, Ward J, Lentine T, et al. Target dyspnea ratings predict expected oxygen consumption as well as target heart rate values. *Am J Respir Crit Care Med.* 1999;159:1485-1489.

84. Nici L, Donner C, Wouters E, et al. American thoracic society/european respiratory society statement on pulmonary rehabilitation. *Am J Respir Crit Care Med.* 2006;173:1390-1413.

85. Horowitz MB, Mahler DA. Dyspnea ratings for prescription of cross-modal exercise in patients with COPD. *Chest.* 1998;113:60-64.

86. Mahler DA. Pulmonary rehabilitation. *Chest.* 1998;113(4 Supplement):263S-268S.

87. Ries AL, Bauldoff GS, Carlin BW, et al. Pulmonary rehabilitation: Joint ACCP/AACVPR evidence-based clinical practic guidelines. *Chest.* 2007;131:4S-42S.

88. Langer D, Hendriks E, Burtin C, et al. A clinical practice guideline for physiotherapists treating patients with chronic obstructive pulmonary disease based on a systematic review of available evidence. *Clin Rehabil.* 2009;23:445-462.

89. Troosters T, Casaburi R, Gosselink R, et al. Pulmonary rehabilitation in chronic obstructive pulmonary disease. *Am J Respir Crit Care Med.* 2005;172:19-38.

90. Selvadurai HC, Blimkie CJ, Meyers N, et al. Randomized controlled study of in-hospital exercise training programs in children with cystic fibrosis. *Pediatr Pulmonol.* 2002;33:194-200.

91. Lee L, Phillips A, Britton L, et al. Combined aerobic and resistance exercise training for inpatients with cystic fibrosis. *Cardiopulm Phys Ther J.* 2008;19:139-140.

92. Shoemaker MJ, Hurt H, Arndt L. The evidence regarding exercise training in the management of cystic fibrosis: a systematic review. *Cardiopulm Phys Ther J.* 2008;19:75-83.

93. Dwyer TJ, Elkins MR, Bye PT. The role of exercise in maintaining health in cystic fibrosis. *Curr Opin Pulm Med.* 2011;17:455-460.

94. Carpinelli RN, Otto RM, Winett RA. A critical analysis of the ACSM position stand on resistance training: Insufficient evidence to support recommended training protocols. *JEPonline.* 2004;7:1-60.

95. Frownfelter D, Massery M. Facilitating ventilation patterns and breathing strategies. In: Frownfelter D, Dean E, eds. *Cardiovascular and Pulmonary Physical Therapy.* St. Louis, MO: Mosby; 2013.

96. McVean RJ, Orr A, Webb AK, et al. Treatment of urinary incontinence in cystic fibrosis. *J Cyst Fibros.* 2003;2:171-176.

97. Button B, Holland A. Physiotherapy for cystic fibrosis in Australia: a consensus statement. Available from: http://www.thoracic.org.au/physiotherapyforcf.pdf. Accessed February 22, 2012.

98. Avers D, Brown M. White paper: strength training for the older adult. *J Geriatr Phys Ther.* 2009;32:148-158.

99. Massery M. Refered by the cystic fibrosis clinic's PT: Treatment of posture and pain. *Pediatr Pulmonol.* 2008;43(S31):112-114.

100. Elbasan B, Tunali N, Duzgun I, et al. Effects of chest physiotherapy and aerobic exercise training on physical fitness in young children with cystic fibrosis. *Ital J Pediatr.* 2012;38:2.

101. Gosselink R. Controlled breathing and dyspnea in patients with chronic obstructive pulmonary disease (COPD). *J Rehabil Res Dev.* 2003;40:25-33.

102. Hillegass E. Breathing retraining for individuals with chronic obstructive pulmonary disease—a role for clinicians. *Chron Respir Dis.* 2009;6:43-44.

103. Delk KK, Gevirtz R, Hicks DA, et al. The effects of biofeedback assisted breathing retraining on lung functions in patients with cystic fibrosis. *Chest.* 1994;105:23-28.

104. Mueller RE, Petty TL, Filley GF. Ventilation and arterial blood gas changes induced by pursed lips breathing. *J Appl Physiol.* 1970;28:784-789.

105. Tiep BL, Burns M, Kao D, et al. Pursed lips breathing training using ear oximetry. *Chest.* 1986;90:218-221.

106. Lowman JD, Jr. Breathing exercises for patients with COPD: To teach or not to teach. *Phys Ther.* 2003;83:948-951.

107. Garrodl R, Dallimore K, Cook J, et al. An evaluation of the acute impact of pursed lips breathing on walking distance in nonspontaneous pursed lips breathing chronic obstructive pulmonary disease patients. *Chron Respir Dis.* 2005;2:67-72.

108. Dechman G, Wilson CR. Evidence underlying breathing retraining in people with stable chronic obstructive pulmonary disease. *Phys Ther.* 2004;84:1189-1197.

109. Lee A, Holdsworth M, Holland A, et al. The immediate effect of musculoskeletal physiotherapy techniques and massage on pain and ease of breathing in adults with cystic fibrosis. *J Cyst Fibros.* 2009;8:79-81.

110. Stoller JK, Panos RJ, Krachman S, et al. Oxygen therapy for patients with COPD: current evidence and the long-term oxygen treatment trial. *Chest.* 2010;138:179-187.

111. Elphick HE, Mallory G. Oxygen therapy for cystic fibrosis. *Cochrane Database Syst Rev.* 2009(1): CD003884.

112. Coates AL. Oxygen therapy, exercise, and cystic fibrosis. *Chest.* 1992;101:2-4.

113. APTA. Oxygen Administration During Physical Therapy. 2011; Available from: http://www.apta.org/OxygenAdministration/. Accessed February 2, 2012.

114. Casaburi R. Long-term oxygen therapy: state of the art. *Pneumonol Alergol Pol.* 2009;77:196-199.

115. Cahill J. CF Wind Sprints. 2011; Available from: http://www.cfwindsprints.com/. Accessed May 22, 2012.

Liver Transplant

David W. Mandel

Case 17

A 56-year-old male just received a liver transplant for end-stage liver cirrhosis after being on the transplant wait list for 11 months. He was removed from mechanical ventilation 12 hours after surgery and is breathing normally on 2 L/min O_2 by nasal cannula. A central venous catheter has been placed in the left internal jugular vein for intravenous fluids and medications; two Jackson-Pratt drains are emerging from his large abdominal incision, and a Foley urinary catheter is in place. Prior to surgery, significant protein malnutrition (muscle wasting), fatigue, ascites, and hepatic encephalopathy limited his mobility and quality of life. Postoperatively, the ascites and encephalopathy are slowly resolving, but lower extremity and scrotal edema persists. Relevant medications for immunosuppression include: Prograf (tacrolimus), prednisolone, and cyclosporine. The transplant surgeon has asked the physical therapist to perform an evaluation and treatment today on postoperative day 1 (POD 1). In addition, there are orders for the patient to be out of bed beginning POD 1.

▶ Based on his health condition, what do you anticipate may be the contributors to activity limitations?
▶ What are possible complications interfering with physical therapy?
▶ What precautions should be taken during physical therapy examination and/or interventions?
▶ What is his rehabilitation prognosis?

KEY DEFINITIONS

ASCITES: Accumulation of fluid in the peritoneal cavity surrounding the intestines; associated with scrotal and bipedal edema

CIRRHOSIS: Progressive replacement of normal hepatocytes with fibrotic nodular tissue that impairs liver function

ESOPHAGEAL VARICES: Extremely dilated submucosal veins in the esophagus due to portal vein hypertension

HEPATIC ENCEPHALOPATHY: Confusion and decreased level of consciousness due to factors resulting from chronic liver disease

PORTAL VEIN HYPERTENSION: Increased pressure at the portal vein (carries venous blood to the liver from stomach, intestines, pancreas, and spleen) due to scarring of liver tissue and thrombosis

VALSALVA MANUEVER: Sudden increase in intra-abdominal pressure due to attempted forceful exhalation with a closed airway

Objectives

1. Describe protein energy malnutrition that occurs as a result of liver cirrhosis.
2. Identify outcome measures of functional strength and performance in the patient post-liver transplant with protein energy malnutrition.
3. Identify critical laboratory values that should be checked prior to treating the patient.
4. Understand the precautions associated with treating this patient population.
5. Prescribe a program of resistance exercise to assist in the reversal or mitigation of muscle wasting.

Physical Therapy Considerations

PT considerations during management of the individual status/post liver transplant due to chronic liver cirrhosis:

▸ **General physical therapy plan of care/goals:** Prevent or minimize skin breakdown, loss of range of motion, and the risk of atelectasis, pneumonia, and infection; maximize functional mobility and improve quality of life

▸ **Physical therapy interventions:** Bed mobility and transfer training, ambulation and gait training, posture training, breathing exercises, endurance activities, muscle strengthening

▸ **Precautions during physical therapy:** Avoid Valsalva maneuver to prevent risk of bleeding from esophageal varices and injury to abdominal surgical site; monitor vitals for orthostatic hypotension; lifting restrictions (≤ 20 lb) for 6 weeks to prevent surgical incision dehiscence; emphasize handwashing and clean equipment to minimize infection due to patient's pharmacological immunosuppression; close supervision with mobility and exercise intervention due to encephalopathy

▶ **Complications interfering with physical therapy:** Ascites, lower extremity and scrotal edema, infection, pneumonia, incisional dehiscence, hematemesis from esophageal varices, hepatic vein thrombosis, falls

Understanding the Health Condition

As there is no cure for liver cirrhosis, transplantation has become a major treatment modality to prolong survival and improve quality of life. Transplantation is performed for patients with primary biliary cirrhosis, primary sclerosing cholangitis, biliary atresia, alpha-1-antitrypsin disease, Laennec's (alcohol-related) cirrhosis, hepatitis B virus (HBV) and hepatitis C virus (HCV) cirrhosis, cryptogenic cirrhosis, and fulminant hepatic failure.[1] Advanced cirrhosis secondary to HCV is the most common indication for liver transplantation in the United States. Based on data from the Organ Procurement and Transplantation Network (a branch of the United States Department of Health and Human Services), the current 1-year survival rate after liver transplantation is 81% for hepatitis related necrosis, 89% for cholestatic liver disease, and 86% for biliary cirrhosis.

Liver cirrhosis is a catabolic disease leading to profound muscle wasting.[2] The prevalence of severe muscle wasting (cachexia) or protein-energy malnutrition approaches 80% of individuals with cirrhosis.[2,3] However, patient perception of muscle wasting is much lower because the loss of lean tissue is masked by the weight gain due to ascitic fluid collection that results from the impaired liver's inability to regulate fluid balance.[2] Additional factors that contribute to protein-energy malnutrition include: decreased dietary protein intake, malabsorption, decreased activity, and increased resting energy expenditure.[2,4-6] Clinically, the loss of muscle tissue is more important than the loss of body fat in individuals with liver cirrhosis and it is associated with poorer prognosis.[3,7] Chronic liver disease preferentially alters phasic, fast twitch type II fibers and these changes may persist as long as 9 months post-transplant.[8-10]

The surgical procedure for liver transplantation stimulates the inflammatory process and increases cytokine production, resulting in further depletion of body mass that includes all the metabolically active cellular tissue (muscle, organ, intracellular and extracellular water, and bone) in the body. Serum albumin and serum protein levels decline postoperatively. Total body fat loss has been observed to be as much as 200 g (0.44 lb) during the first 7 days after hepatic surgery.[11] During the first 2 weeks after liver transplant, individuals can lose an additional 10% of their body protein stores.[12] Elevated resting energy expenditures and increased fuel metabolism result in impaired protein storage post-transplant.[12] Therefore, due to the continued loss and limited restoration of muscle mass, individuals have prolonged impairments in strength, activity performance, and quality of life after receiving a new liver.

During the surgery, a large abdominal incision and significant retraction of the rib cage is required to access the abdominal cavity. Frequently, individuals complain of significant musculoskeletal pain at the surgical site for several weeks to months post-liver transplant. There are many arteries and veins that are reconnected during surgery. The hepatic artery that supplies oxygenated blood to the liver is at risk for thrombosis, which would result in organ rejection. The new liver is denervated. Therefore, instead of direct neural control, the central nervous system signals the release of hormones into the blood to communicate with the liver for proper glucose regulation.[13]

Post-transplantation patients are on high doses of many different medications, which individually or in combination can impair muscle strength and cardiovascular function. The pharmacopoeia post-liver transplantation usually includes immuno-suppressants, antifungals, antivirals, antibiotics, antihypertensives, glucose regulators, antidepressants, and/or anti-osteoporotics.[14] Glucocorticoids, a common class of immunosuppressant drugs, have been linked with muscle weakness.[15] The immu-nosuppressant cyclosporine can affect the sympathetic nervous system, resulting in decreased heart rate and decreased mitochondrial skeletal muscle respiration.[16] Postoperative medications also complicate the results of exercise testing because many blunt heart rate response to exercise and impair muscle contractility and the muscles' ability to utilize ATP.[14,16,17] Therefore, medications taken by individuals post-liver transplantation can impair strength and function and limit tolerance to exercise during rehabilitation.

Physical Therapy Patient/Client Management

Post liver transplant, patients typically spend the first 24 to 48 hours in the inten-sive care unit (ICU). Patients are weaned off ventilator support within 24 hours and permitted out of bed with assistance on POD 1. Patients are then transferred to the medical/surgical floor for approximately five to six more days. Physical thera-pists work with the transplant team (surgeons, nurse coordinators, hepatologists, and dieticians) in developing functional goals and determining safety of interven-tions and how quickly to progress the patient. Immunosuppression for prevention of organ rejection places the patients at a very high risk for nosocomial infection. To decrease the risk, the transplant team aims to discharge the patient home as soon as he is medically stable. Individuals with chronic liver disease have progressively declined in muscle strength and functional performance while awaiting transplant surgery. The primary goal of physical therapy immediately after liver transplant is to improve functional mobility enough to allow a safe return home. The second physical therapy goal is to prescribe patients a home exercise program aimed at improving muscle strength, endurance, and functional mobility to improve quality of life and return to prior employment.

Examination, Evaluation, and Diagnosis

Prior to seeing the patient, the physical therapist needs to acquire information from the medical chart, including laboratory values, postoperative precautions, and any exercise or mobility restrictions from the surgeons. Critical laboratory values to check that are indicative of liver function and anemia include albumin, total bilirubin, International Normalized Ratio (INR), hemoglobin, and hematocrit. Patients are not typically placed on anticoagulants (e.g., Coumadin) post-liver transplant unless the surgeon feels the patient is at high risk for hepatic artery thrombosis. If the patient is taking Coumadin, the INR level should be elevated for therapeutic anticoagulation. Elevated liver enzymes indicative of liver damage that need to be monitored are alkaline phosphatase (ALP), alanine amino transferase (ALT), and aspartate amino transferase (AST). After liver transplant, all of these laboratory values should return to normal levels. However, individuals with hepatitis C typically continue to have elevated values for their lifetime. As with all postsurgical patients, electrolytes such as sodium, potassium, and calcium should be monitored because alterations from normal values may increase risk for muscle weakness, sensory impairments, cognitive impairments, cardiac arrhythmias, and seizures. If laboratory values are abnormal, the physical therapist should communicate with the patient's transplant nurse coordinator prior to any therapy intervention.

A thorough skin inspection must be performed to assess for areas of pressure because the patient has decreased strength and mobility and he has been supine during the lengthy surgical procedure and in the ICU bed on ventilator support. Surgical incisions, intravenous lines, and drain sites should be monitored for signs of infection.

Pneumonia is one of the leading causes of sepsis and mortality after liver transplantation.[18] Lung auscultation, cough evaluation, vital capacity, and maximal inspiratory pressure assessments must be performed by the physical therapist upon initial evaluation and frequently reassessed. These measures are easily completed at bedside and should be performed when the patient is supine, sitting, and standing.

After liver transplantation, individuals are deconditioned from both the surgical procedure and their chronic progressive decline in muscle strength and function. Simple functional strength assessments such as **bridging, standing (single or double) heel-rise test, and the 30-second chair stand test** can be performed at the bedside. Currently, there is little published evidence on these measures in the post-liver transplant population. Plantar flexor strength has been assessed using the standing heel-rise test in patients awaiting liver transplant.[19,20] Though no norms for this population exist, 25 repetitions for the single limb heel-rise test has been proposed as normal strength for healthy adults.[20] The 30-second chair stand test was observed to have good test-retest reliability (ICC = 0.84) in a similar population of renal transplant candidates.[21] Once the patient reaches the subacute phase of recovery (approximately 2 weeks post-transplant), the Six-Minute Walk Test (6MWT) is a measure that can be performed in a minimum 100 ft hallway to assess functional performance and aerobic capacity.[22,23] The 6MWT has primarily been used to predict the mortality of liver transplant candidates; however, there are several studies using the 6MWT to assess functional performance and quality of life in individuals after liver transplant.[24-27]

Plan of Care and Interventions

In addition to addressing specific findings from the examination, physical therapy interventions should include patient education regarding nutrition, especially protein supplementation needed for muscle strengthening, a home exercise program of progressive resistance exercises (PRE) for the lower extremities (to begin immediately) and for the upper extremities and core musculature (to begin 6 weeks post-transplant surgery). The staggered PRE program is due to the lifting restrictions placed on individuals after all types of abdominal surgery.[28] There are no evidence-based guidelines supporting the prescription of **lifting restrictions** for the first 6 weeks post-abdominal surgery. However, surgeons still place these conservative restrictions to decrease the likelihood of herniation and dehiscence at the surgical site. In this population, it is especially important to follow these restrictions to prevent any damage or rejection to the newly transplanted liver.

To decrease the likelihood of atelectasis and pneumonia, the patient should be instructed in the proper splinting technique of his abdominal incision for an effective cough. Diaphragmatic breathing exercises and incentive spirometry should be performed for 10 breaths every hour for the first week after surgery. Segmental breathing should be instructed based on the auscultation findings during the examination. For example, if the patient was observed during lung auscultation to have decreased breath sounds in the lateral basilar segment of the right lower lobe, the therapist can place his or her hand over that segment to provide tactile cueing and ask the patient to take a slow, deep breath into that area.

To decrease pain and discomfort with bed mobility, the patient should be instructed to "log-roll"—that is, the hips and shoulders should move at the same time to prevent tension on the abdominal incision. Abdominal incision pain and the large abdomen due to ascites may initially prevent prone activities. Donning undergarments such as mesh briefs or a diaper prior to mobility provides support and comfort for the patient's edematous scrotum during mobility.

Post-transplant medications are administered to inhibit the immune system in order to prevent organ rejection. Even though it is standard precautions, the therapist must be vigilant in proper hand washing and frequent cleaning of all equipment brought into the patient's room for mobility training and exercise (*e.g.*, gait belt and assistive devices).

Prior to all mobility, the patient's drains and Foley catheter should be emptied to decrease the risk of pulling the patient's tissues, causing pain, and spillage. The intravenous lines need to be placed on slack and the intravenous pump(s) need to be unplugged to permit mobilization of the patient out of bed and ambulation.

Postsurgically, the patient may have low blood volume and could develop orthostatic hypotension upon initial sitting and standing. Blood pressure, heart rate, and pulse oximetry (SpO_2) should be monitored before, during, and after interventions.

Altered mental status from hepatic encephalopathy progressively resolves after surgery. Commands and instructions for the patient must be simple to ensure the patient's safety and proper performance of mobility and exercise. The patient and caregivers must be educated that all mobility and exercise must be performed with supervision and/or assistance at all times, in order to prevent injury and complications until the patient's cognition and safety awareness improve.

Aerobic exercise such as walking and cycling is very beneficial in improving function and endurance in individuals with chronic liver disease and it does not harm the liver.[29] However, aerobic walking exercise is not enough to improve muscle strength.[30,31] Targeted **progressive resistance exercise** is required to stimulate protein synthesis and help reverse catabolic muscle wasting impairments.[32] Although lifting restrictions of ≤ 20 lb for 6 weeks are imposed to prevent dehiscence of the surgical incision,[28] progressive resistance exercises can initially target the lower extremities because no restrictions have been documented on lower extremity exercise in this population or in any related abdominal surgery population. Prescription of exercise intensity and duration should follow the American College of Sports Medicines guidelines: exercising 3 to 4 days per week with a day of recovery between each day of exercise.[33] The physical therapist should direct the patient to emphasize the eccentric lowering portion of the contraction to further stimulate muscle protein synthesis.[34] Patients with a history of liver disease related coagulopathy and esophageal varices must be educated on proper breathing techniques to prevent performing the Valsalva maneuver during resistance exercises. Teaching a patient to count out loud each repetition or timing for the hold of a contraction prevents the closed glottis and Valsalva maneuver. Teaming with a dietician is ideal for appropriate prescription of protein supplementation to the patient's diet. The addition of protein is essential to prevent catabolically consuming the newly acquired muscle mass for energy during the training.[35]

Evidence-Based Clinical Recommendations

SORT: Strength of Recommendation Taxonomy

A: Consistent, good-quality patient-oriented evidence
B: Inconsistent or limited-quality patient-oriented evidence
C: Consensus, disease-oriented evidence, usual practice, expert opinion, or case series

1. Physical therapists can use bridging, 6MWT, heel-rise test, and the 30-second chair stand test to assess functional strength and performance in individuals post-liver transplant. **Grade B**

2. Following "lifting restrictions" after abdominal surgery decreases risk of abdominal incision dehiscence. **Grade C**

3. Progressive resistance exercise improves muscle strength in patients post-liver transplant for chronic liver disease. **Grade B**

COMPREHENSION QUESTIONS

17.1 Protein energy malnutrition significantly impacts muscle strength and functional mobility in individuals with chronic liver disease. Which other complication of chronic liver disease has the greatest impact on functional performance?

   A. Hepatic encephalopathy

   B. Pruritis

   C. Jaundice

   D. Ascites

17.2 During resistance exercise, the patient's SpO_2 drops to 87%. The patient reports slight fatigue, but is willing to continue. Which of the following actions is appropriate for the physical therapist to perform at this point?

A. Stop exercise immediately, place the patient on hold for therapy, and call the transplant surgeon.

B. Educate the patient not to perform a Valsalva maneuver during the resistance exercise.

C. Teach the patient an effective cough using a pillow for splinting.

D. Instruct the patient on inspiratory muscle training.

ANSWERS

17.1 **D.** Although encephalopathy, pruritus, and jaundice (options A, B, and C) each pose significant impacts on the patient's quality of life, ascites impacts functional performance the most. The large bloated abdomen of fluid in the peritoneal space affects rolling and positioning in bed. The body's center of mass has shifted forward, which impacts transfers and balance. To compensate for the change in center of mass position, the patient must widen his stance, flex his knees, and shift the upper trunk backward. These changes from normal standing posture and walking biomechanics increase energy demands and fatigue. In addition, the large volume of fluid in the abdomen prevents the diaphragm from descending, drastically limiting respiratory function and lung volume. Gas exchange becomes limited, decreasing oxygen availability for the muscle tissue. Movement efficiency is reduced, which further impacts energy expenditure and limits functional performance and quality of life.

17.2 **B, C, D.** There are many reasons for declining SpO_2. Exercise or therapy should not be immediately stopped (option A) before some problem-solving is attempted. During resistance exercise, most patients frequently hold their breath and bear down, essentially performing a Valsalva maneuver. This causes oxygen saturation to drop and is contraindicated in this population due to the increased risk of esophageal varice bleeding and injury to the abdominal incision (option B). After abdominal surgery, most patients do not take deep breaths or cough effectively due to abdominal pain. Instructing the patient to properly splint the abdominal incision with a pillow or blanket often decreases the pain enough to allow deeper inspirations, allowing for a more effective cough. Clearing the airway improves oxygen saturation (option C). The respiratory musculature is just as susceptible to catabolic wasting as extremity musculature. Respiratory muscle strength can be targeted with resistance exercise using an inspiratory muscle-training device. The physical therapist initially measures the patient's maximal inspiratory pressure (MIP). For respiratory muscle strength training, the therapist initially sets the resistance level on the inspiratory muscle training (IMT) device to 30% of the patient's measured MIP. If this resistance level is too difficult for the patient, then the resistance level is reduced (e.g., 10% of the MIP) until the patient can reach the 30% MIP goal. If the patient's SpO_2 drops *every* time the physical therapist performs an intervention, then the transplant nursing coordinator should be notified.

REFERENCES

1. Killenberg PG, Clavien PA. *Medical Care of the Liver Transplant Patient: Total Pre-, Intra-, and Post-operative Management*. 3rd ed. Oxford: Blackwell Science; 2006.

2. Vintro AQ, Krasnoff JB, Painter P. Roles of nutrition and physical activity in musculoskeletal complications before and after liver transplantation. *AACN Clin Issues*. 2002;13:333-347.

3. Plauth M, Schutz ET. Cachexia in liver cirrhosis. *Int J Cardiol*. 2002;85:83-87.

4. Greco AV, Mingrone G, Benedetti G, Capristo E, Tataranni PA, Gasbarrini G. Daily energy and substrate metabolism in patients with cirrhosis. *Hepatology*. 1998;27:346-350.

5. Yamanaka H, Genjida K, Yokota K, et al. Daily pattern of energy metabolism in cirrhosis. *Nutrition*. 1999;15:749-754.

6. Muller MJ, Bottcher J, Selberg O, et al. Hypermetabolism in clinically stable patients with liver cirrhosis. *Am J Clin Nutr*. 1999;69:1194-1201.

7. Pasini E, Aquilani R, Dioguardi FS. Amino acids: chemistry and metabolism in normal and hypercatabolic states. *Am J Cardiol*. 2004;93(8A):3A-5A.

8. Hussaini SH, Soo S, Stewart SP, et al. Risk factors for loss of lean body mass after liver transplantation. *Appl Radiat Isot*. 1998;49:663-664.

9. Rothstein JM. Muscle biology. Clinical considerations. *Phys Ther*. 1982;62(12):1823-1830.

10. Franssen FM, Wouters EF, Schols AM. The contribution of starvation, deconditioning and ageing to the observed alterations in peripheral skeletal muscle in chronic organ diseases. *Clin Nutr*. 2002;21:1-14.

11. Gupta R, Thurairaja R, Johnson CD, Primrose JN. Body composition, muscle function and psychological changes in patients undergoing operation for hepatic or pancreatic disease. *Pancreatology*. 2001;1:90-95.

12. Plank LD, Metzger DJ, McCall JL, et al. Sequential changes in the metabolic response to orthotopic liver transplantation during the first year after surgery. *Ann Surg*. 2001;234:245-255.

13. Perseghin G, Regalia E, Battezzati A, et al. Regulation of glucose homeostasis in humans with denervated livers. *J Clin Invest*. 1997;100:931-941.

14. Krasnoff JB. Liver disease, transplant, and exercise. *Clin Exercise Physiol*. 2001;3:27-37.

15. Horber FF, Scheidegger JR, Grunig BE, Frey FJ. Thigh muscle mass and function in patients treated with glucocorticoids. *Eur J Clin Invest*. 1985;15:302-307.

16. Beyer N, Aadahl M, Strange B, et al. Improved physical performance after orthotopic liver transplantation. *Liver Transpl Surg*. 1999;5:301-309.

17. Torregrosa M, Aguade S, Dos L, et al. Cardiac alterations in cirrhosis: reversibility after liver transplantation. *J Hepatol*. 2005;42:68-74.

18. Weiss E, Dahmani S, Bert F, et al. Early-onset pneumonia after liver transplantation: microbiological findings and therapeutic consequences. *Liver Transpl*. 2010;16:1178-1185.

19. Leitao AV, Castro CL, Basile TM, Souza TH, Braulio VB. Evaluation of the nutritional status and physical performance in candidates to liver transplantation. *Rev Assoc Med Bras*. 2003;49: 424-428.

20. Lunsford BR, Perry J. The standing heel-rise test for ankle plantar flexion: criterion for normal. *Phys Ther*. 1995;75:694-698.

21. Bohannon RW, Smith J, Hull D, Palmeri D, Barnhard R. Deficits in lower extremity muscle and gait performance among renal transplant candidates. *Arch Phys Med Rehabil*. 1995;76:547-551.

22. Alameri HF, Sanai FM, Al Dukhayil M, et al. Six Minute Walk Test to assess functional capacity in chronic liver disease patients. *World J Gastroenterol*. 2007;13:3996-4001.

23. Mandel D. Comparison of targeted resistance exercise with usual care progressive ambulation post-liver transplantation. *J Acute Care Phys Ther*. Fall 2010;1:31-32.

24. Jonsson BI, Overend TJ, Kramer JF. Functional measures following liver transplantation. *Physiotherapy Canada*. 1998;50:141-146.

25. van Ginneken BT, van den Berg-Emons RJ, Kazemier G, Metselaar HJ, Tilanus HW, Stam HJ. Physical fitness, fatigue, and quality of life after liver transplantation. *Eur J Appl Physiol.* 2007;100:345-353.

26. Foroncewicz B, Mucha K, Szparaga B, et al. Rehabilitation and 6-minute walk test after liver transplantation. *Transplant Proc.* 2011;43:3021-3024.

27. Beyer N, Aadahl M, Strange B, et al. Improved physical performance after orthotopic liver transplantation. *Liver Transpl Surg.* 1999;5:301-309.

28. Gerten KA, Richter HE, Wheeler TL II, et al. Intraabdominal pressure changes associated with lifting: implications for postoperative activity restrictions. *Am J Obstet Gynecol.* 2008;198:306.e1-e5.

29. Ritland S, Foss NE, Gjone E. Physical activity in liver disease and liver function in sportsmen. *Scand J Soc Med Suppl.* 1982;29:221-226.

30. Sarsan A, Ardic F, Ozgen M, Topuz O, Sermez Y. The effects of aerobic and resistance exercises in obese women. *Clin Rehabil.* 2006;20:773-782.

31. Rooks DS, Kiel DP, Parsons C, Hayes WC. Self-paced resistance training and walking exercise in community-dwelling older adults: effects on neuromotor performance. *J Gerontol A Biol Sci Med Sci.* 1997;52:M161-M168.

32. Roubenoff R, Wilson IB. Effect of resistance training on self-reported physical functioning in HIV infection. *Med Sci Sports Exerc.* 2001;33:1811-1817.

33. American College of Sports Medicine Position Stand. The recommended quantity and quality of exercise for developing and maintaining cardiorespiratory and muscular fitness, and flexibility in healthy adults. *Med Sci Sports Exerc.* 1998;30:975-991.

34. Evans WJ. Protein nutrition, exercise and aging. *J Am Coll Nutr.* 2004;23(6 Suppl):601S-609S.

35. Agin D, Gallagher D, Wang J, Heymsfield SB, Pierson RN Jr, Kotler DP. Effects of whey protein and resistance exercise on body cell mass, muscle strength, and quality of life in women with HIV. *AIDS.* 2001;15:2431-2440.

Gastric Bypass Surgery

Erin E. Jobst

CASE 18

A 43-year-old African American female with a body mass index (BMI) of 49 was admitted to the hospital yesterday for elective bariatric surgery. She was scheduled to have a laparoscopic Roux-en-Y gastric bypass, but the surgical procedure was changed to an open Roux-en-Y during the operation due to her large abdominal pannus. Notable medical history includes hypertension, obstructive sleep apnea, bilateral knee osteoarthritis, diabetes mellitus, and gastroesophageal reflux disease (GERD). Preoperative medications included nonsteroidal anti-inflammatory drugs, metformin, and insulin. Prior to admission, the patient was able to walk limited community distances without an assistive device. She was limited by bilateral knee pain. She has been using a continuous positive airway pressure (CPAP) device for approximately 4 years for treatment of obstructive sleep apnea. She has brought her CPAP device with her to use at night during her hospital stay. The physical therapist is asked to evaluate and treat the patient before she is discharged to her single-level home, where she lives alone. The bariatric surgeon stated that she must follow "abdominal precautions" and wear an abdominal binder whenever she is out of bed.

▶ What are the examination priorities?
▶ What are the most appropriate physical therapy interventions?
▶ What are possible complications interfering with physical therapy?
▶ What is her rehabilitation prognosis?

KEY DEFINITIONS

ABDOMINAL PANNUS (PANNICULUS): "Apron" of excess skin and subcutaneous fat in the lower abdominal area of morbidly obese individuals

BARIATRICS: Branch of medicine specialized in providing healthcare for individuals with excess weight, variously defined as those with: body mass index > 30 kg/m^2, body weight > 300 lb, or overweight by more than 100 to 200 lb

BODY MASS INDEX (BMI): Weight in relation to height (weight/height^2); common clinical measurement that has been adopted as a valid proxy for body fat

CONTINUOUS POSITIVE AIRWAY PRESSURE (CPAP) DEVICE: Machine that provides compressed air into a mask over the nose or nose and mouth in order to keep the airway open and prevent sleep apnea

LAPAROSCOPIC SURGICAL PROCEDURE: Surgeon makes several small incisions and uses small instruments and a camera to guide the surgery

OBSTRUCTIVE SLEEP APNEA (OSA): Repetitive lapses in breathing during sleep caused by obstruction of the upper airway; risk factors include older age, male sex, obesity, and increased neck circumference

OPEN SURGICAL PROCEDURE: Surgeon makes large incisions that enable direct access and visualization of the structures involved

Objectives

1. Identify classifications of obesity and the guidelines for choosing eligible bariatric surgery candidates.

2. Understand the two broad categories of bariatric surgical procedures (restrictive and/or malabsorptive) and recommended postoperative dietary and exercise guidelines.

3. Define abdominal precautions given to patients after open abdominal surgery.

4. Identify short-term (*e.g.*, vomiting) and long-term (*e.g.*, weight regain, nonadherence to diet and exercise) complications after bariatric surgery and strategies to mitigate these problems.

5. List the long-term benefits of bariatric surgery.

6. Prescribe an appropriate intensity aerobic and resistance exercise program for the individual status/post gastric bypass surgery.

7. List common barriers to regular exercise after bariatric surgery and potential solutions to each.

Physical Therapy Considerations

PT considerations during management of the individual status/post open gastric bypass surgery for morbid obesity:

▶ **General physical therapy plan of care/goals:** Prevent or minimize loss of range of motion, strength, and aerobic functional capacity; decrease risk of deep vein thromboses; improve quality of life

▶ **Physical therapy interventions:** Patient education regarding abdominal precautions, decreasing risk of deep vein thromboses and pulmonary complications; gait training; prescription of home exercise program to facilitate maintenance of weight loss and prevention of strength loss due to loss of lean muscle mass; referral to outpatient exercise facilities/programs and bariatric surgery support groups

▶ **Precautions during physical therapy:** Abdominal precautions; monitor vital signs; keep head of bed elevated approximately 25°

▶ **Complications interfering with physical therapy:** Vomiting, dumping syndrome, upper extremity peripheral nerve injuries, abdominal incisional hernia

Understanding the Health Condition

Overweight and obesity are defined as excessive fat accumulation that may impair health.[1] While there are several tools used in research settings to accurately determine body fat percentage (*e.g.*, dual-energy x-ray absorptiometry, air displacement plethysmography), BMI and waist circumference are two frequently used clinical measurements of body fat. In most individuals, BMI and waist circumference are closely correlated with body fat.[2,3] Currently, 66% of American adults are considered overweight (BMI 25-29.9) or obese (BMI ≥ 30)[2] and more than one-third are obese.[4,5] The World Health Organization lists three classifications of obesity based on increasing BMI: Class I: 30.0-34.9; Class II: 35.0-39.9; and, Class III: ≥ 40.[6] Table 18-1 lists the confusing and sometimes overlapping terminology that has been used to describe different classes of obesity.

The prevalence of obesity varies by racial and ethnic group. During the 10-year period from 1999 to 2008, the age-adjusted overall prevalence of obesity for American women was 35.5%. However, for non-Hispanic black women, the obesity rate was 49.6%, compared to 33% for non-Hispanic white women.[5,11] The rate of

Table 18-1 CLINICAL DESCRIPTIONS USED FOR OBESITY CLASSES	
Classes of Obesity	Definition
Extreme	BMI ≥ 35 (Class II and III)
Morbid	BMI ≥ 40 (Class III); corresponding to ~100 lb (45 kg) over ideal weight
Severe	BMI ≥ 35[7] or ≥ 40[8]
Super	BMI ≥ 50[9]
Super-super	BMI ≥ 60[10]

class III obesity among non-Hispanic black women is increasing as well. For non-Hispanic black women between the ages of 40 to 59 years of age, almost 18% have a BMI ≥ 40,[5] up from 10% reported for that same group in 2001.

Obesity affects every organ system. Common obesity-related comorbidities include type 2 diabetes, cardiovascular disease (*e.g.*, deep vein thromboses, hypertension, hyperlipidemia), hypoventilation syndrome, asthma, obstructive sleep apnea (OSA), osteoarthritis, GERD, depression, several types of cancer, and even shortened life expectancy.[12-15] Even in obese individuals, weight loss of as little as 5% to 10% of initial body weight results in clinically significant metabolic and cardiac health benefits.[14,16-19] However, there has been only one clinical trial demonstrating the effectiveness of a diet and exercise intervention in adults with BMIs ≥ 35.[7] In this single-blind randomized trial, 101 severely obese adults lost 8% to 10% of their initial body weight and showed corresponding decreases in blood pressure, waist circumference, and insulin resistance during a 1-year lifestyle intervention.[7] Thus, for the majority of the millions of obese American adults, lifestyle and pharmacological (*e.g.*, sibutramine, orlistat) interventions have not been successful weight-loss strategies.[20,21]

Bariatric surgery has emerged as the most effective weight loss and maintenance intervention in individuals with class III obesity.[22-24] In 1991, the National Institutes of Health established consensus guidelines for choosing eligible bariatric surgery candidates. These included individuals who are morbidly obese (BMI > 40 kg/m^2) or have a BMI > 35 kg/m^2 with life-threatening or disabling obesity-related comorbidities. In addition, candidates must have failed nonsurgical weight-loss efforts, be free from medical and psychological contraindications to surgery, and be motivated and well informed. [25] Since 1991, surgeons have performed bariatric procedures on individuals outside of these criteria. New criteria that expand the ranges of BMI, age, and comorbidity severity have been proposed.[26] If widely accepted, the eligible pool of bariatric surgery candidates can be expected to dramatically increase.

How weight loss is reported in the bariatric literature is confusing.[27-29] In published trials of nonsurgical interventions, weight loss is described in terms of the percentage of initial body weight. In contrast, the most common method used to report weight loss after bariatric surgery is percentage of excess weight loss. Percentage of excess weight loss (%EWL) is usually defined by the formula: [(weight loss/excess weight) × 100], where excess weight = presurgical weight − "ideal weight."[24,27] An obvious problem with this definition is how "ideal weight" is defined. In fact, variability in "ideal weight" used in the equation has led to variability in %EWL across different studies.[30] A successful weight-loss outcome after bariatric surgery has been defined as a loss of at least 50% of excess weight[25] or greater than 50% EWL that is maintained for at least 5 years after surgery.[31] In a systematic review of over 10,000 bariatric surgery outcomes, the mean %EWL for all types of bariatric surgical procedures was 61%. The %EWL varied from 40% after simple bariatric procedures (primarily restrictive, *e.g.*, gastric banding) to > 70% after more complex procedures (restrictive/malabsorptive, *e.g.*, duodenal switch).[24] Excess weight loss usually peaks 12 to 18 months after bariatric surgery and %EWL of 50% has been reported by about two-thirds of patients for 7 to 10 years after certain procedures.[23,32]

The benefits of bariatric surgery extend beyond weight loss. Several (though not all) bariatric procedures result in improved or resolved comorbidities such as diabetes,

OSA, hypertension, hyperlipidemia, and GERD in 75% to 100% of patients.[10,22,24] Long-term studies have shown that bariatric surgery also reduces mortality; risk of death over time was roughly 35% lower among extremely obese patients who had bariatric surgery compared to those who did not.[33,34]

Bariatric surgical procedures are broadly classified into categories based on whether they restrict food intake, cause malabsorption, or produce a combination of both. Choice of particular procedure is based on BMI, patient-related factors, medical and psychological comorbidities, and previous surgeries.[10] Understanding whether a procedure is primarily restrictive, primarily malabsorptive, or mixed restrictive/malabsorptive is important in the clinical management and prevention of postoperative complications. Primarily restrictive procedures (*e.g.*, adjustable gastric banding and vertical banded gastroplasty) decrease the size of the stomach, but allow nutrients to complete their normal passage through the small intestine. The Roux-en-Y gastric bypass (RYGB) is a restrictive and malabsorptive procedure that has been considered the gold standard weight loss procedure, accounting for > 80% of all bariatric surgical procedures performed in the United States.[35] In the RYGB, a large portion of the stomach and the duodenum are "bypassed" (Fig. 18-1). First, a small stomach pouch is created by partitioning away the upper part of the stomach from the remainder of the stomach (using staples and reinforced with stitches).

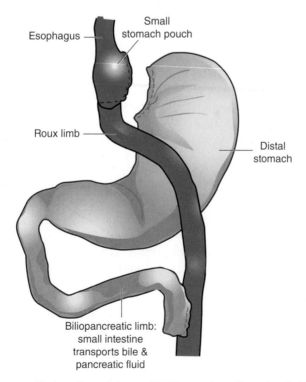

Figure 18-1. Diagram of Roux-en-Y gastric bypass (RYGB) procedure. (Reproduced with permission from Greenberger NJ, Blumberg RS, Burakoff R. *CURRENT Diagnosis & Treatment: Gastroenterology, Hepatology, & Endoscopy.* 2nd ed. Copyright © The McGraw-Hill Companies, Inc. All rights reserved. Figure 19-1.)

This decreases the stomach from the size of a football to roughly the size of a golf ball (≤ 10-30 mL).[36] Next, the jejunum is cut and the upper (or middle) part of the jejunum is brought up to connect to the new stomach pouch. This part of the small intestine that is attached to the newly created stomach pouch is called the Roux limb; it connects to the pouch via a small outlet. Last, the stomach remnant, duodenum, and disconnected length of proximal jejunum (referred to as the biliopancreatic limb) is anastomosed to the ileum. This creates a common intestinal limb of variable length in which digestive enzymes and acid from the stomach, liver, and pancreas join with ingested food entering from the Roux limb. After the RYGB procedure, food enters the mouth, descends the esophagus and enters the small stomach pouch, goes through the first anastomosis into the Roux limb and eventually into the common limb (via the distal anastomosis) to mix with acid and digestive enzymes from the biliopancreatic limb. The RYGB procedure is *restrictive* because the stomach pouch dramatically restricts the food volume that can be contained and it is *malabsorptive* because food bypasses the majority of the stomach and the duodenum, substantially reducing the absorption of several nutrients and calories. Thus, less food can be eaten and fewer calories can be absorbed. Other less common bariatric restrictive/malabsorptive surgical procedures include the duodenal switch, biliopancreatic diversion, and the very, very long-limb RYGB. Patients who have undergone laparoscopic RYGB experience %EWL loss of 60% to 70%, and roughly 75% of individuals have resolved or improved comorbidities.[25,37] In contrast, the primarily restrictive banding procedures result in %EWL of only 45% to 50% with less predictable improvement of comorbidities.[24]

The number of bariatric procedures has increased considerably in the past decade. In 1998, roughly 13,000 people in the United States elected to have bariatric surgery.[35] In 2008, over 220,000 people had a bariatric surgical procedure.[36] The overall risk of death and acute postoperative adverse events is relatively low. In a multicenter study of 4776 adults undergoing procedures at 10 clinical sites from 2005 to 2007, the 30-day death rate among patients who had an RYGB or laparoscopic adjustable gastric banding was 0.3%; only 4.3% had at least one major adverse outcome.[38] Deep vein thrombosis (or venous thromboembolism) or abdominal operative reintervention occurred in 0.4% and 2.6% of the cases, respectively.[38] While the relative frequency is low, the *absolute* number of adverse events can be expected to increase as the number of bariatric surgical procedures increases. Clinicians involved in the care of these patients should be cognizant of procedural and patient profiles that increase the likelihood of postoperative complications. Surgical procedure and patient characteristics that have been associated with an increased likelihood of adverse outcomes include: open and laparoscopic RYGB (as compared to laparoscopic adjustable gastric banding),[38] extremely high BMI (> 50 kg/m^2),[38,39] inability to walk 200 ft,[38] history of deep vein thrombosis or venous thromboembolism,[38,39] unrecognized or untreated OSA,[38,39] male sex,[39-41] patients older than 45 years,[39-41] high blood pressure,[39-41] diabetes mellitus,[39-41] and asthma.[39-41]

Minimally invasive laparoscopic approaches, which have lower morbidity and mortality rates compared to open procedures, have contributed to the significant increase in the number of bariatric procedures performed. In 2009, the average length of stay for laparoscopically performed bariatric procedures was approximately

3 days.[32,42] Compared to open RYGB, laparoscopic RYGB decreases blood loss, opioid requirements, hospital length of stay, and wound complications.[43-45] In a 3-year follow-up of 155 patients randomly assigned to either laparoscopic or open RYGB, fewer abdominal incisional hernias occurred after the laparoscopic procedure (5%) compared to the open procedure (39%).[46] Despite the significant reduction in postsurgical hernias, laparoscopic RYGB may not be possible for patients with very large ventral hernias, high BMI with central obesity, severe intra-abdominal adhesions, or a larger liver.[10]

Physical Therapy Patient/Client Management

To maximize the patient's potential for a successful outcome, the physical therapist must be knowledgeable about the potential short-term and long-term complications associated with bariatric surgical procedures as well as the postsurgical dietary progression and exercise recommendations. Many hospitals where bariatric surgeries are frequently performed have a comprehensive multidisciplinary team that provides both pre- and postoperative care for the bariatric surgery candidate. Prospective surgical candidates usually complete 6 to 12 months of counseling with a psychologist or nurse counselor, social worker, dietitian, and surgeon.[47] Ideal preoperative programs include medical, nutritional, and psychological evaluations, an exercise assessment, and an evaluation of the patient's understanding of the surgery.[48] These programs include extensive education about the surgery and the required lifetime commitment to follow-up care and recommended postsurgical behavioral changes—including compliance with nutritional guidelines and regular exercise.[49-51]

After bariatric surgery, patients must follow a specific dietary regimen for about 12 weeks. Patients may not be allowed to eat for 1 to 2 days[52] and then they typically start with a clear liquid diet and progress to full liquids.[53] Patients usually receive a pureed diet for at least 1 day before hospital discharge.[54] For the next 3 months, patients are advised to eat multiple small meals, progressing from pureed to soft foods. At the 3-month surgical follow-up, patients are advised to advance to a regular diet, though meal size must be limited to 1 to 1.5 cups of food due to the smaller stomach capacity.[53] In the first 6 months after surgery, eating too much or too quickly may cause vomiting or intense pain under the sternum.[52] Long-term vitamin and mineral supplementation is usually recommended for all patients after bariatric surgery. Those who have had malabsorptive procedures (e.g., RYGB) require more extensive replacement supplementation (e.g., iron, vitamin B$_{12}$, calcium, vitamin D) to prevent nutritional deficiencies.[55,56] It is also recommended that patients eat 60 to 120 g of protein daily to help maintain lean body mass during weight loss and for long-term weight maintenance.[55]

The role of the physical therapist during management of the patient status/post bariatric surgery is twofold. The first role is similar to that for any postoperative patient: decrease the likelihood of immediate postoperative complications (e.g., thromboembolisms, pulmonary complications, incisional hernia), teach modified mobility following surgeon-prescribed restrictions (e.g., log-rolling, use of abdominal binder), and assess the patient's ability to safely return home. Therapists should also be aware of two common post-bariatric surgery complications: vomiting and dumping syndrome. One-third to two-thirds of patients report postoperative vomiting.[57] It is thought that vomiting is due to the limited volume capacity of the new small gastric pouch. To limit postoperative vomiting, patients should be encouraged to sip 1 to 2 fluid ounces throughout the day.[53] Dumping syndrome, caused by consuming refined sugar or energy-dense foods, is initially experienced by approximately 75% of patients who have a RYGB.[23,58] Signs and symptoms include abdominal cramping and pain, tachycardia, nausea, tremor, flushing, lightheadedness, syncope, and diarrhea. Dumping syndrome is thought to be due to peptides released by the gut when food bypasses the stomach and enters the small intestine.[59] For some patients, this unpleasant dumping syndrome may aid weight loss by conditioning them to avoid eating calorically dense liquids or sugary foods.[53,55] Although patients should only be consuming small amounts of liquids during the acute hospital admission, it is possible for patients to drink too much fruit juice (or soda) and experience signs and symptoms of dumping syndrome. The physical therapist should be aware of this not infrequent occurrence. Dietary adjustment is the first line of therapy for dumping syndrome.

The second role for the physical therapist in treating this patient population is to provide the education and encouragement necessary to reduce the probability of long-term complications and to improve the patient's ability to achieve and maintain long-term weight loss and health benefits after bariatric surgery. Weight regain after bariatric surgery is common. In 2010, an Endocrine Society Clinical Practice Guideline reported that it can be expected that 20% to 25% of lost weight after bariatric surgery will be regained over a period of 10 years.[55] In general, restrictive procedures are more commonly associated with weight regain than procedures with a malabsorptive component. If weight regain occurs, it typically begins 18 to 24 months after surgery.[53] Physical therapists can help patients understand the self-management that is required after bariatric surgery through education. The documented **predictors of successful maintenance of weight loss** include preoperative realistic expectations,[55] adherence to scheduled postoperative visits,[60] compliance with nutritional recommendations, regular physical activity of at least 150 minutes per week,[61] and periodic assessment to prevent and treat eating or other psychiatric disorders.[60,62] In general, patients report greater physical activity over the long-term compared with the pre-bariatric surgery period.[22] However, of all the postsurgical recommendations, exercise has the highest rate of non-adherence at 12-month surgical follow-up.[49] Thus, it is incumbent upon the inpatient physical therapist to provide, remind, and reinforce specific exercise guidelines throughout the patient's length of stay to enable her to maximize her long-term weight loss and fitness success.

Examination, Evaluation, and Diagnosis

Upon admission of a bariatric patient (often defined as weight > 350 lb), many hospitals initiate multidisciplinary protocols or guidelines for the most effective, safe, and dignified care of this patient population.[63,64] These guidelines typically specify weight-rated and sized equipment that must be made available (*e.g.*, bed, mechanical lift, trapeze bar for over the bed, commode, wheelchair, slide sheets) as well as safe bariatric patient handling programs. In addition, bariatric patients admitted for elective procedures are often encouraged to bring their own clothing to the hospital to avoid the indignity of potentially having to wear two gowns when moving around the hospital.

Prior to seeing this patient, the physical therapist acquires pertinent information from her chart, including laboratory values, postoperative mobility restrictions, and whether the surgeon has advised the patient to wear an abdominal binder when she is out of bed. Critical laboratory values to check before seeing any postsurgical patient include hemoglobin, hematocrit, white blood cell count, and platelet count. Exercise or mobilization should be withheld if these values are not within safe limits. Caring for bariatric patients should include a thoughtful plan to create a patient-friendly environment. Before initiating the examination, the physical therapist should bring to the patient's room (or ensure there is ready access to): a bariatric blood pressure cuff, an extended-size gown (or two), large pants and/or robe, and a bariatric wheeled walker. It is the responsibility of the physical therapist to ensure that the weight capacity of any physical device used to help mobilize the bariatric patient meets the needs of the individual patient. For example, the weight capacity of a standard facility wheeled walker may be 250 lb, whereas the weight capacity of most standard facility bariatric walkers is 350 lb. In preparation for assessing the patient's ambulation capacity, the therapist should position a chair without armrests (or a large wheelchair) in the hallway that will allow the patient to comfortably sit down. If the surgeon requires that the patient wear an abdominal binder for out-of-bed mobility, a large enough binder must be obtained. Sometimes, two binders may need to be secured together to construct a comfortable and secure binder.

During the patient interview, the therapist should ask the patient whether she had any presurgical mobility restrictions as well as what type of activities she will need to do after hospital discharge, and if anyone will be able to assist her. The physical therapist evaluates the patient's pain level before, during, and after the therapy session. Multimodal postoperative analgesia (*e.g.*, local anesthetics in the wound, nonsteroidal anti-inflammatory drugs, modest doses of opioids, and continuous epidural analgesia) promotes early mobilization and minimizes respiratory depression.[54,65] The majority of adults admitted for elective bariatric surgery are independent in bed mobility, transfers, and ambulation of limited distances with or without an assistive device prior to hospital admission.[66] Patients are usually encouraged to get out of bed and walk on either the day of surgery or the following day. If patients need physical assistance with bed mobility or functional transfers, physical therapists should be especially careful to plan ahead to avoid the potential for injury. Patient handling algorithms (for transfers, repositioning, and toileting) are available that provide a sequential guide to asking questions relating to a patient's physical and cognitive capabilities.[67] The answers then guide the healthcare provider in choosing the safest patient handing technique. Ensuring that the activity is safe for both the patient and the therapist may include using mechanical lifts and/or extra personnel.

When the physical therapist entered the room, the patient in this case was recumbent with the head of the bed raised approximately 30°. This head-up position has been shown to be associated with greater lung volumes, decreased incidence of atelectasis, and increases in mean arterial oxygen saturations in severely obese adults.[68] Therefore, the traditional supine-to-sit transfer should incorporate at least this degree of head-up position. The patient was wearing an abdominal binder over the incision, and the physical therapist ensured that it was secure before the patient initiated the first transfer out of bed. The patient was able to independently log roll from this position to sitting at the edge of the bed. A brief systems review and strength testing of the upper and lower extremities can be performed in this position. The physical therapist should also assess for the presence of ulnar neuropathies and/or brachial plexus stretch injuries because these injuries are more common in hospitalized patients with higher BMIs.[54] This may be the consequence of ulnar nerve compression due to excessive arm abduction, inadequate support of out-stretched arms, or prolonged elbow flexion positioning that occurs during surgery. Ulnar neuropathies may also result from sustained compression on the nerve in the ulnar groove that can occur when larger patients rest their arms on the bedrails (especially if they are not in extended-width beds) or on their chest or abdomen. Patients should be educated to avoid these positions to minimize this risk.

The therapist should observe how the patient is sitting at the edge of the bed and ensure that she can sit independently prior to asking her to stand. When working with bariatric patients, the therapist must appreciate the different biomechanical patterns that obese individuals demonstrate during transfers and ambulation compared to individuals of normal weight. For example, therapists often cue patients to lean their trunks forward to initiate a sit-to-stand transfer. However, obese individuals tend to have limited trunk flexion and move their feet backwards from the initial sitting position to perform this task.[69] This patient also had a large abdominal pannus, which necessitated her hips to be significantly abducted prior to initiating the sit-to-stand transfer. At this point, the therapist must determine whether the patient can stand independently (or with minimal assistance) or whether a mechanical lift is indicated. If the patient requires more than minimal assistance, both patient and therapist are at risk of injury due to the large size of the patient. **Dionne's Egress Test** is a simple three-part functional test designed to simulate the components of a bed-to-chair transfer, without leaving the safety of the patient's bedside.[70,71] Before initiating Dionne's Egress Test, the patient should be sitting near a locked and upright bedrail for upper extremity weightbearing and/or balance support, if needed. First, the patient is asked to perform 3 repetitions of a sit-to-stand transfer at the edge of the bed. The first repetition consists of only a 1 to 2 inch lift of the buttocks from the surface of the bed in order to test the patient's ability to bear full body weight on the lower extremities. On the second and third repetitions, the therapist asks the patient to stand fully upright. Upon standing after the third repetition, the therapist asks the patient to march in place (with a self-selected stance width) 3 times. The patient must clear the stepping foot from the ground each time. In the last stage of Dionne's Egress Test, the patient takes one step forward and away from the bed, which requires shifting body weight onto the stepping foot, and then returns the foot back to the starting position. If the bariatric patient cannot successfully complete any segment of the test (e.g., buckling of the stance extremity, loss of balance), or requires more than minimal assistance, Dionne recommends a mechanical lift for out-of-bed mobilization. In a pilot study with 15 bariatric patients admitted to a community hospital, Dionne's Egress Test was shown to have moderate inter-rater reliability ($K = 0.659$) among three physical therapists experienced in the test administration and 15 nurses newly trained in its administration.[71] The validity of Dionne's Egress Test (*i.e.*, if passing or failing the test relates to whether a patient falls) has not yet been tested. However, its simplicity and reliability suggest that it may be a useful addition to the screening algorithms for mobilizing bariatric patients.

Plan of Care and Interventions

Early mobilization after surgery is indicated for the individual after gastric bypass. This patient's only mobility restrictions are abdominal precautions. While specific restrictions may vary by institution and/or by surgeon, abdominal precautions typically include: (1) no lifting > 10 lb; (2) no bending more than 90° at the hips; (3) no Valsalva maneuvers; and (4) use of a velcro-fastened elasticized soft abdominal binder. The primary intent of these precautions is to protect the incision and reduce the likelihood of an incisional herniation by decreasing intra-abdominal pressure and use of the abdominal muscles. Patients are generally advised to follow these precautions for 4 to 8 weeks, depending on the extent of the incision(s), surgeon's preference, and patient's size. To get out of bed, patients are advised to "log roll" from supine (with hips and knees in hooklying position) to sidelying to limit abdominal contractions. Next, the patient can use her upper extremities to assist in transitioning from sidelying to sitting; this transition generally causes the most pain the patient will experience during mobility in the inpatient setting. To decrease the pain during transfers and to facilitate the patient's ability to take deeper breaths, the therapist can advise the patient to provide counterpressure over the incision site with a pillow. Some surgeons advise that patients wear an abdominal binder after *any* abdominal surgical procedure. Incisional hernias are much less common after laparoscopic than after open bariatric procedures (0.45% vs. 9%-20%).[53,72] Preventing incisional hernias is always a priority because abdominal obesity in conjunction with the early rapid weight loss and malnutrition induced by bariatric surgery requires that most incisional hernias be surgically repaired. There is no evidence that abdominal binders decrease the likelihood of incisional hernias; however, **wearing an abdominal binder** decreases pain and improves postsurgical walking distance. In a randomized controlled trial of 75 adults undergoing major abdominal surgery, subjects who wore an elasticized abdominal binder starting on the first postoperative day reported unchanged pain levels after surgery, in contrast to those in the control group (no binder) for whom pain measures were significantly higher throughout the entire inpatient hospital stay. Subjects who wore the abdominal binder (applied before getting out of bed and worn at all times out of bed) walked an average of 45% of their preoperative levels by the fifth postoperative day, whereas subjects who did not wear the binder walked an average of only 33% of their preoperative levels.[73]

After the first postsurgical day, most patients are nearly independent in bed mobility, transfers, and hallway ambulation without an assistive device. Most individuals return to their normal activities in 3 to 5 weeks and return to work approximately 1 month after surgery. During the inpatient hospital days, the physical therapist serves as the primary educator regarding exercise recommendations post-bariatric surgery. The therapist should recognize that many bariatric patients struggle with the demands of changing their behavior, eating differently, and/or the uncertainty that weight loss brings after gastric bypass. In addition, therapists should be cognizant of the fact that long-term successful outcomes after gastric bypass depend in part on routine physical exercise; however, 1 year after surgery, 41% do not exercise.[50] Thus, the therapist should approach this time as an opportunity to empower the patient and provide her tools to succeed in the lifestyle challenges ahead.

The large-scale weight loss after gastric bypass results in significant decreases in muscle strength and no improvement in exercise capacity.[74,75] Carey et al.[75] showed that 30% to 35% of the weight loss in the first 6 months after Roux-en-Y gastric bypass was a loss in fat-free mass. This skeletal muscle atrophy is accompanied by a decrease in muscle strength. Stegen et al.[74] evaluated muscle strength and aerobic capacity in 15 morbidly obese adults 4 months after gastric bypass. Eight subjects participated in a 12-week aerobic and strength training program (75-minute training sessions, 3 times per week); seven subjects served as untrained controls. Both groups experienced similar weight loss in fat mass and fat-free mass. However, while the untrained subjects lost 16% of their quadriceps strength, and more than one-third of their biceps and triceps strength, the trained group experienced no loss in arm strength and had a 72% *improvement* in their quadriceps strength. The 12-week training program also improved the subjects' functional capacity as measured by the number of sit-to-stand repetitions in 30 seconds and the distance walked in the Six-Minute Walk Test.

The aim of exercise regimens is to offset any negative skeletal effects from rapid weight loss and to improve physical fitness. There have been no randomized controlled trials comparing different physical activity protocols after bariatric surgery. Protocols are derived from experience with this patient population and represent expert opinions. The American Society for Metabolic and Bariatric Surgery recommends that all patients initiate walking on the first day after bariatric surgery.[76] Most bariatric surgical patients continue to choose walking as their aerobic activity of choice.[53] An appropriate baseline to start may be 3 to 5 minutes of walking.[53] The expectation is that patients will be able to gradually increase both the duration and intensity of their walking program.[66] The physical therapist can provide helpful objective guidelines for the patient to advance her walking program. During the first week postoperatively, a baseline for total distance walked can be calculated using a pedometer. During the second week, the patient should walk the average daily number of steps that she did during the first week. From the third week until the eighth week postsurgery, the patient should increase her daily minimum step count by 250 to 500 steps each week until reaching the goal of 10,000 steps per day.[76] Adherence is usually more effective with accumulated activity throughout the day than with single bouts of exercise.[53] The therapist should initiate a discussion with the patient regarding the best way to incorporate walking throughout her day, which allows the patient to be an active collaborator in her own care. Strength training to preserve lean muscle mass must be incorporated, although the ideal timing of its initiation has not been established. In the inpatient setting after surgery, isometrics or limb-weight resistance is often encouraged (*e.g.*, standing or sidelying single limb hip abduction or standing double-leg squats). Stegen et al.[74] showed dramatic strength improvements and no adverse effects with a weight-training program (60%-75% of 1 repetition maximum values) initiated in adults only 1 month after gastric bypass surgery. Resistance exercises should focus on major muscle groups in the trunk and upper and lower extremities. Appropriate dosing includes 1 set of 12 to 15 repetitions to near exhaustion for each major muscle group performed 2 to 3 times weekly.

The current patient was able to walk 275 ft in the hospital hallway without an assistive device. The limiting factor for distance ambulated was bilateral knee pain. Osteoarthritis of the knee is one of the biggest musculoskeletal problems for obese patients, and the effect of increased BMI on osteoarthritis risk is greater in women than in men.[77] During the stance phase of the gait cycle, 60% to 80% of the greatest forces in the lower extremities are across the medial knee joint.[78] Body weight increases this compressive load; for each pound of additional weight, compressive forces across the medial knee compartment increase by 4 lb.[79] After bariatric surgery, the frequency of knee pain can drop from 57% to 14%.[80] The therapist provided encouragement to the patient that her knee pain would likely improve with the anticipated weight loss. Since weightbearing exercise was currently too painful, the therapist suggested that the patient try a recumbent stationary bicycle in the inpatient gym. The patient found this exercise boring, though not painful. The therapist collaborated with her regarding the development of a daily exercise program that would be relatively pain-free, convenient, and enjoyable. The patient said that if she had her music playing, she would be able to enjoy the bicycling activity. The therapist referred the patient to the Arthritis Foundation website and was able to locate both land and water exercise programs that would be appropriate for obese clients.[81] The therapist prescribed strengthening exercises for the quadriceps (quad sets) and gluteus medius (sidelying hip abduction) because strengthening these muscles can improve pain and function in patients with knee osteoarthritis[82] and decrease forces across the knee.[83] Last, the therapist provided guidelines to the patient to indicate if her exercise routine was too intense. Exercise intensity may be too high if more than mild dyspnea occurs, heavy perspiration occurs, muscles feel weak or burn immediately after exercise, or if exercised muscle groups are sore the next day.[76]

To prevent weight regain after bariatric surgery, patients must follow advice regarding diet and exercise. For exercise, it is recommended that patients participate in at least 150 minutes of moderate (or higher) intensity physical activity per week.[61] Among the recommended behavioral modifications after bariatric surgery, adherence to exercise is particularly low. In a study of 100 patients, non-adherence to recommendations was 2% for drinking soda, 37% for snacking, and 41% for not exercising.[49] Table 18-2 presents common barriers to regular activity and potential solutions that the inpatient physical therapist may be able to initiate with patients. Therapists should inform patients about postoperative bariatric support groups and be aware of any programs their facility offers or hosts. Attendance and participation in support groups improves postoperative results and helps prevent and treat weight regain.[84]

Table 18-2 COMMON BARRIERS TO REGULAR EXERCISE AND POTENTIAL SOLUTIONS

Exercise Barrier	Potential Solutions
Frustrations with recommendations to exercise	• Reinforce benefits of exercise: maintenance of weight loss, increased functional capacity, decreased joint pain, increased strength[61,74,75,79,82] • Give precise recommendations for aerobic and strength training (e.g., number of minutes or steps per day, specific dosing for strength training)
Reluctance to exercise in public places	• Home exercise programs • Exercise programs specifically designed for overweight/obese individuals[82]
Lack of time	• Incorporate activities throughout the day
Joint pain	• Encourage RICE—rest, ice, compression, elevation of painful joints • No heels—even 1.5-in heels increase knee joint torque[85] • Referral to physical therapists that specialize in obese clients, aquatic therapy, and/or orthotics (e.g., many obese individuals have pes planus, which would benefit from arch supports) • Referral to primary care physician for advice on analgesic medications (patients usually need to avoid nonsteroidal anti-inflammatory drugs due to increased risk of gastrointestinal bleeding after surgery)[53,77]
Lack of interest or motivation	• Choose exercises that are practical, enjoyable, and easily integrated into daily lifestyle • Referral to professionally supervised bariatric support groups, which is recommended for all patients for at least 6 months after bariatric surgery[53] ° ASMBS Web site,[36] hospital-based support groups

Evidence-Based Clinical Recommendations

SORT: Strength of Recommendation Taxonomy

A: Consistent, good-quality patient-oriented evidence
B: Inconsistent or limited-quality patient-oriented evidence
C: Consensus, disease-oriented evidence, usual practice, expert opinion, or case series

1. Predictors of successful maintenance of weight loss after bariatric surgery include preoperative realistic expectations, adherence to scheduled postoperative visits, compliance with nutritional recommendations, regular physical activity of at least 150 minutes per week, and periodic assessment to prevent and treat eating or other psychiatric disorders. **Grade A**

2. Dionne's Egress Test, which simulates the components of a bed-to-chair transfer, is a reliable test that is useful as a screening algorithm for mobilizing bariatric patients. **Grade C**

3. Elasticized abdominal binders worn after major abdominal surgery decreases pain and improves postsurgical walking distance. **Grade B**

COMPREHENSION QUESTIONS

18.1 Which of the following individuals is *most* likely to have postsurgical complications after a bariatric procedure?

A. 42-year-old female with knee osteoarthritis and a BMI of 40 kg/m^2

B. 58-year-old male with a BMI of 52 kg/m^2, obstructive sleep apnea, and history of deep vein thromboses

C. 45-year-old male with a BMI of 42 kg/m^2 and gastroesophageal reflux disease

D. 55-year-old female with BMI of 42 kg/m^2 and knee osteoarthritis

18.2 A physical therapist is walking in the hall with a patient who had a laparoscopic Roux-en-Y gastric bypass 3 days ago. The patient suddenly complains of abdominal cramps and pain and lightheadedness. These findings are *most* indicative of:

A. Orthostatic hypotension

B. Incisional hernia

C. Dumping syndrome

D. Knee osteoarthritis

ANSWERS

18.1 **B.** The overall rate of postoperative complications for bariatric surgical procedures is low. However, as the number of bariatric surgical procedures increases, the absolute number of adverse events can be expected to increase. Clinicians should be cognizant of procedural and patient profiles that increase the likelihood of postoperative complications. Surgical procedure and patient characteristics associated with increased likelihood of adverse outcomes include extremely high BMI (> 50 kg/m^2),[38,39] inability to walk 200 ft,[38] history of deep vein thrombosis or venous thromboembolism,[38,39] unrecognized or untreated OSA,[38,39] male sex,[39-41] patients older than 45 years,[39-41] high blood pressure,[39-41] diabetes mellitus,[39-41] and asthma.[39-41]

18.2 **C.** Dumping syndrome, caused by consuming refined sugar or energy-dense foods, is initially experienced by approximately 75% of patients who have an RYGB.[23,58] Signs and symptoms include abdominal cramping and pain, tachycardia, nausea, tremor, flushing, lightheadedness, syncope, and diarrhea. Although patients should only be consuming small amounts of liquids during the acute hospital admission, it is possible for patients to drink too much fruit juice and experience signs and symptoms of dumping syndrome. While light-headedness is a symptom of orthostatic hypotension, orthostatic hypotension typically occurs during initial postural transitions (*e.g.*, sitting to standing) and does not present with abdominal pain (option A). Incisional hernias are uncommon after laparoscopic bariatric procedures (0.45%)[53] and would be more likely to occur during times of increased intra-abdominal pressure such as when lifting, performing a Valsalva maneuver, or twisting (option B). While knee osteoarthritis is common in obese individuals, the symptoms are knee pain and stiffness (option D).

REFERENCES

1. World Health Organization. Obesity and overweight fact sheet. No. 311. Available at: http://www.who.int/mediacentre/factsheets/fs311/en/index.html. Accessed May 2, 2012.

2. WIN-Weight-control Information Network. An information service of the NIDDK. Available at: http://win.niddk.nih.gov/publications/tools.htm. Accessed May 1, 2012.

3. Flegal KM, Shephard JA, Looker AC, et al. Comparisons of percentage body fat, body mass index, waist circumference, and waist-stature ratio in adults. Am J Clin Nutr. 2009;89:500-508.

4. Adult Obesity Facts. Centers for Disease Control and Prevention. Available at: http://www.cdc.gov/obesity/data/adult.html. Accessed May 2, 2012.

5. Flegal KM, Carroll MD, Ogden CL, Curtin LR. Prevalence and trends in obesity among US adults, 1999-2008. JAMA. 2010;303:235-241.

6. Global Database on Body Mass Index. World Health Organization. Available at: http://apps.who.int/bmi/index.jsp?introPage=intro_3.html. Accessed May 2, 2012.

7. Goodpaster BH, Delany JP, Otto AD, et al. Effects of diet and physical activity interventions on weight loss and cardiometabolic risk factors in severely obese adults: a randomized trial. JAMA. 2010;304:1795-1802.

8. Samaha FF, Iqbal N, Seshadri P, et al. A low-carbohydrate as compared with a low-fat diet in severe obesity. N Engl J Med. 2003;348:2074-2081.

9. Sturm R. Increases in morbid obesity in the USA: 2000-2005. Public Health. 2007;121:492-496.

10. Farrell TM, Haggerty SP, Overby DW, Kohn GP, Richardson WS, Fanelli RD. Clinical application of laparoscopic bariatric surgery: an evidence-based review. Surg Endosc. 2009;23:930-949.

11. Overweight and Obesity Statistics. WIN-Weight-control Information Network. Available at: http://win.niddk.nih.gov/publications/PDFs/stat904z.pdf. Accessed May 2, 2012.

12. Must A, Spadano J, Coakley EH, Field AE, Colditz G, Dietz WH. The disease burden associated with overweight and obesity. JAMA. 1999;282:1523-1529.

13. Overweight, obesity, and health risk. National Task Force on the Prevention and Treatment of Obesity. Arch Intern Med. 2000;160:898-904.

14. Clinical Guidelines on the Identification, Evaluation, and Treatment of Overweight and Obesity in Adults: The Evidence Report. NIH publication 98–4083. Available at: www.nhlbi.nih.gov/guidelines/obesity/ob_gdlns.pdf. Accessed May 2, 2012.

15. Mizuno T, Shu IW, Makimura H, Mobbs C. Obesity over the life course. *Sci Aging Knowledge Environ.* 2004(24):re4.

16. Yanovski SZ, Yanovski JA. Obesity. *N Engl J Med.* 2002;346:591-602.

17. Dixon JB, Anderson M, Cameron-Smith D, O'Brien PE. Sustained weight loss in obese subjects has benefits that are independent of attained weight. *Obes Res.* 2004;12:1895-1902.

18. Tuomilehto J, Lindstrom J, Eriksson JG, et al; Finnish Diabetes Prevention Study Group. Prevention of type 2 diabetes mellitus by changes in lifestyle among subjects with impaired glucose tolerance. *N Engl J Med.* 2001;344:1343-1350.

19. Gregg EW, Gerzoff RB, Thompson TJ, Williamson DF. Intentional weight loss and death in overweight and obese U.S. adults 35 years of age and older. *Ann Intern Med.* 2003;138:383-389.

20. Goodrick GK, Poston WS II, Foreyt JP. Methods for voluntary weight loss and control: update 1996. *Nutrition.* 1996;12:672-676.

21. Wing RR. Behavioral approaches to the treatment of obesity. In: Bray GA, Bouchard C, James WPT, eds. *Handbook of Obesity.* New York: Marcel Dekker, Inc.; 1998:855-873.

22. Sjöström L, Lindroos AK, Peltonen M, et al; Swedish Obese Subjects Study Scientific Group. Lifestyle, diabetes, and cardiovascular risk factors 10 years after bariatric surgery. *N Engl J Med.* 2004;351:2683-2693.

23. Pories WJ, Swanson MS, MacDonald KG, et al. Who would have thought it? An operation proves to be the most effective therapy for adult-onset diabetes mellitus. *Ann Surg.* 1995;222: 339-350.

24. Buchwald H, Avidor Y, Braunwald E, et al. Bariatric surgery: a systematic review and meta-analysis. *JAMA.* 2004;292:1724-1737.

25. NIH conference Gastrointestinal surgery for severe obesity. Consensus Development Conference Panel. *Ann Intern Med.* 1991;115:956-961.

26. Yermilov I, McGory ML, Shekelle PW, Ko CY, Maggard MA. Appropriateness criteria for bariatric surgery: beyond the NIH guidelines. *Obesity.* 2009;17:1521-1527.

27. Dixon JB, McPhail T, O'Brien PE. Minimal reporting requirements for weight loss: current methods not ideal. *Obes Surg.* 2005;15:1034-1039.

28. Bray GA, Bouchard C, Church TS, et al. Is it time to change the way we report and discuss weight loss? *Obesity.* 2009;17:619-621.

29. Sharma AM, Karmali S, Birch DW. Reporting weight loss: is simple better? *Obesity.* 2010;18:219.

30. Montero PN, Stefanidis D, Norton HJ, Gersin K, Kuwada T. Reported excess weight loss after bariatric surgery could vary significantly depending on calculation method: a plea for standardization. *Surg Obes Relat Dis.* 2011;7:531-534.

31. Fobi MA. Surgical treatment of obesity: a review. *J Natl Med Assoc.* 2004;96:61-75.

32. Picot J, Jones J, Colquitt JL, et al. The clinical effectiveness and cost-effectiveness of bariatric (weight loss) surgery for obesity: a systematic review and economic evaluation. *Health Technol Assess.* 2009;13:215-357.

33. Sjöström L, Narbro K, Sjöström CD, et al. Swedish Obese Subjects Study. Effects of bariatric surgery on mortality in Swedish obese subjects. *N Engl J Med.* 2007;357:741-752.

34. Adams TD, Gress RE, Smith SC, et al. Long-term mortality after gastric bypass surgery. *N Engl J Med.* 2007;357:753-761.

35. Santry HP, Gillen DL, Lauderdale DS. Trends in bariatric surgical procedures. *JAMA.* 2005;294: 1909-1917.

36. American Society of Metabolic and Bariatric Surgery. Available at: http://asmbs.org. Accessed May 4, 2012.

37. Colquitt J, Clegg A, Loveman E, Royle P, Sidhu MK. Surgery for morbid obesity. *Cochrane Database Syst Rev.* 2005;4:CD003641.

38. Flum DR, Belle SH, King WC, et al; Longitudinal Assessment of Bariatric Surgery (LABS) Consortium. Perioperative safety in the longitudinal assessment of bariatric surgery. *N Engl J Med.* 2009;361:445-454.

39. Ballantyne GH, Svahn J, Capella RF, et al. Predictors of prolonged hospital stay following open and laparoscopic gastric bypass for morbid obesity: body mass index, length of surgery, sleep apnea, asthma, and the metabolic syndrome. *Obes Surg.* 2004;14:1042-1050.

40. Dallal RM, Mattar SG, Lord JL, et al. Results of laparoscopic gastric bypass in patients with cirrhosis. *Obes Surg.* 2004;14:47-53.

41. Cooney RN, Haluck RS, Ku J, et al. Analysis of cost outliers after gastric bypass surgery: what can we learn? *Obes Surg.* 2003;13:29-36.

42. Agency for Healthcare Research and Quality. Healthcare Cost and Utilization Project (HCUP). Available at: http://hcupnet.ahrq.gov/HCUPnet.jsp. Accessed May 14, 2012.

43. Nguyen NT, Goldman C, Rosenquist CJ, et al. Laparoscopic versus open gastric bypass: a randomized study of outcomes, quality of life, and costs. *Ann Surg.* 2001;234:279-291.

44. Westling A, Gustavsson S. Laparoscopic vs open Roux-en-Y gastric bypass: a prospective, randomized trial. *Obes Surg.* 2001;11:284-292.

45. Lujan JA, Frutos MD, Hernandez Q, et al. Laparoscopic versus open gastric bypass in the treatment of morbid obesity: a randomized prospective study. *Ann Surg.* 2004;239:433-437.

46. Puzziferri N, Austrheim-Smith IT, Wolfe FM, Wilson SE, Nguyen NT. Three-year follow-up of a prospective randomized trial comparing laparoscopic versus open gastric bypass. *Ann Surg.* 2006;243:181-188.

47. Sammons DE. Roux-en-Y gastric bypass: a surgical treatment for morbid obesity. *Am J Nurs.* 2002;102:24A-D.

48. Korenkov M, Sauerland S, Junginger T. Surgery for obesity. *Curr Opin Gastroenterol.* 2005;21:679-683.

49. Elkins G, Whitfield P, Marcus J, Symmonds R, Rodriguez J, Cook T. Noncompliance with behavioral recommendations following bariatric surgery. *Obes Surg.* 2005;15:546-551.

50. Evans RK, Bond DS, Demaria EJ, Wolfe LG, Meador JG, Kellum JM. Initiation and progression of physical activity after laparoscopic and open gastric bypass surgery. *Surg Innov.* 2004;11:235-239.

51. Hochwalt C, Anderson R. Laparoscopic Roux-en-Y bariatric gastric bypass in an adolescent. *JAAPA.* 2009;22:27-30.

52. Mayo Clinic. Gastric bypass surgery. What you can expect. Available at: http://www.mayoclinic.com/health/gastric-bypass/MY00825/DSECTION=what-you-can-expect. Accessed May 14, 2012.

53. McMahon MM, Sarr MG, Clark MM, et al. Clinical management after bariatric surgery: value of a multidisciplinary approach. *Mayo Clin Proc.* 2006;81:S34-S45.

54. McGlinch BP, Que FG, Nelson JL, Wrobleski DM, Grant JE, Collazo-Clavell ML. Perioperative care of patients undergoing bariatric surgery. *Mayo Clin Proc.* 2006;81:S25-S33.

55. Heber D, Greenway FL, Kaplan LM, Livingston E, Salvador J, Still C. Endocrine and nutritional management of the post-bariatric surgery patient: an Endocrine Society Clinical Practice Guideline. *J Clin Endocrinol Metab.* 2010;95:4823-4843.

56. Shikora SA, Kim JJ, Tarnoff ME. Nutrition and gastrointestinal complications of bariatric surgery. *Nutr Clin Pract.* 2007;22:29-40.

57. Mitchell JE, Lancaster KL, Burgard MA, et al. Long-term follow-up of patients' status after gastric bypass. *Obes Surg.* 2001;11:464-468.

58. Monteforte MJ, Turkelson CM. Bariatric surgery for morbid obesity. *Obes Surg.* 2000;10:150-154.

59. Ukleja A. dumping syndrome: pathophysiology and treatment. *Nutr Clin Pract.* 2005;20:517-525.

60. Pontiroli AE, Fossati A, Vedani P, et al. Post-surgery adherence to scheduled visits and compliance, more than personality disorders, predicts outcome of bariatric restrictive surgery in morbidly obese patients. *Obes Surg.* 2007;17:1492-1497.

61. Evans RK, Bond DS, Wolfe LG, et al. Participation in 150 min/wk of moderate or higher intensity physical activity yields greater weight loss after gastric bypass surgery. *Surg Obes Relat Dis.* 2007;3:526-530.

62. van Hout GC, Verschure SK, van Heck GL. Psychosocial predictors of success following bariatric surgery. *Obes Surg.* 2005;15:552-560.

63. Muir M, Archer-Heese G. Essentials of a bariatric patient handling program. *Online Journal of Issues in Nursing.* 2009;14: Manuscript 5.

64. SafeLiftingPortal. Available at: http://www.safeliftingportal.com/. Accessed May 14, 2012.

65. Chand B, Gugliotti D, Schauer P, Steckner K. Perioperative management of the bariatric surgery patient: focus on cardiac and anesthesia considerations. *Clev Clin J Med.* 2006;73:S51-S56.

66. Collazo-Clavell ML, Clark MM, McAlpine DE, Jensen MD. Assessment and preparation of patients for bariatric surgery. *Mayo Clin Proc.* 2006;81:S11-S17.

67. Patient Care Ergonomics Resource Guide: Safe Patient Handling and Movement. Developed by the Patient Safety Center of Inquiry (Tampa, FL), Veterans Health Administration and Department of Defense. October 2001. Available at: www.visn8.va.gov/patientsafetycenter/resguide/ErgoGuidePt One.pdf. Accessed May 14, 2012.

68. Dixon BJ, Dixon JB, Carden JR, et al. Preoxygenation is more effective in the 25 degrees head-up position than in the supine position in severely obese patients: a randomized controlled study. *Anesthesiology.* 2005;102:1110-1115.

69. Sibella F, Galli M, Romei M, Montesano A, Crivellini M. Biomechanical analysis of sit-to-stand movement in normal and obese subjects. *Clin Biomech.* 2003;18:745-750.

70. Dionne's Safe Patient Handling and Bariatric Rehabilitation. Choice Physical Therapy, Inc. 5233 Indian Circle, Gainesville, GA 30506. Seminar presented April 8, 2011 in Portland, OR.

71. Smith BK. A pilot study evaluating physical therapist-nurse inter-rater reliability of Dionne's Egress Test in morbidly obese patients. *Acute Care Perspectives.* 2008 Available at: http://www.thefreelibrary.com/A+pilot+study+evaluating+physical+therapist-nurse+inter-rater...-a 0200409972. Accessed May 15, 2012.

72. Podnos YD, Jimenez JC, Wilson SE, Stevens CM, Nguyen NT. Complications after laparoscopic gastric bypass: a review of 3464 cases. *Arch Surg.* 2003;138:957-961.

73. Cheifetz O, Lucy SD, Overend TJ, Crowe J. The effect of abdominal support on functional outcomes in patients following major abdominal surgery: a randomized controlled trial. *Physiother Can.* 2010;62:242-253.

74. Stegen S, Derave W, Calders P, Van Laethem C, Pattyn P. Physical fitness in morbidly obese patients: effect of gastric bypass surgery and exercise training. *Obes Surg.* 2011;21:61-70.

75. Carey DG, Pliego GJ, Raymond RL, Skau KB. Body composition and metabolic changes following bariatric surgery: effects on fat mass, lean mass and basal metabolic rate. *Obes Surg.* 2006;16:469-77.

76. Petering R, Webb CW. Exercise, fluid, and nutrition recommendations for the postgastric bypass exerciser. *Curr Sports Med Rep.* 2009;8:92-97.

77. Hooper MM. Tending to the musculoskeletal problems of obesity. *Cleve Clin J Med.* 2006;73: 839-845.

78. Baliunas AJ, Hurwitz DE, Ryals AB, et al. Increased knee joint loads during walking are present in subjects with knee osteoarthritis. *Osteoarthritis Cartilage.* 2002;10:573-579.

79. Messier SP, Gutenkunst DJ, Davis C, DeVita P. Weight loss reduces knee-joint loads in overweight and obese older adults with knee osteoarthritis. *Arthritis Rheum.* 2005;52:2026-2032.

80. McGoey BV, Deitel M, Saplys RJ, Kliman ME. Effect of weight loss on musculoskeletal pain in the morbidly obese. *J Bone Joint Surg Br.* 1990;72:322-333.

81. Arthritis Foundation—Programs for better living. Available at: http://www.arthritis.org/programs.php. Accessed May 14, 2012.

82. Fransen M, Crosbie J, Edmonds J. Physical therapy is effective for patients with osteoarthritis of the knee: a randomized controlled clinical trial. *J Rheumatol.* 2001;28:156-164.

83. Chang A, Hayes K, Dunlop D, et al. Hip abduction moment and protection against medial tibio-femoral osteoarthritis progression. *Arthritis Rheum.* 2005;52:3515-3519.

84. Orth WS, Madan AK, Taddeucci RJ, Coday M, Tichansky DS. Support group meeting attendance is associated with better weight loss. *Obes Surg.* 2008;18:391-394.

85. Kerrigan DC, Johansson JL, Bryant MG, Boxer JA, Della Croce U, Riley PO. Moderate-heeled shoes and knee joint torques relevant to the development and progression of knee osteoarthritis. *Arch Phys Med Rehabil.* 2005;86:871-875.

Low Back Pain in the Emergency Department

Jeff Hartman

A 30-year-old male presented to the Fast Track component of an inner city emergency department (ED) as a level IV trauma. The patient reported a 6-month history of back pain and was initially evaluated by a nurse practitioner. The practitioner's evaluation demonstrated no evidence of trauma. The patient's pain was in the low back with radiation into the posterior aspect of both lower extremities extending to the knees. The patient denied any nausea, vomiting, or fever and reported no changes in his bowel and bladder habits. Over the past few months, he has had multiple visits to the ED for the same problem and he reports the only management of his symptoms to date has been prescribed opiates for pain. The patient has not worked in the past 2 years and he has no medical insurance. The physical therapist is consulted in the evaluation and treatment of this patient in the ED.

▶ What are the most appropriate examination tests?
▶ How would this individual's contextual factors influence or change your patient/client management?
▶ What are possible complications that may limit the effectiveness of physical therapy?
▶ What are the most appropriate physical therapy interventions?
▶ Identify the psychological (or psychosocial) factors apparent in this case.
▶ What relevant questions about the patient remain unanswered?

KEY DEFINITIONS

DISC EXTRUSION: When the nucleus pulposus of the intervertebral disc has ruptured through the annulus fibrosus, causing a wide range of signs and symptoms depending on the tissues impinged

FAST TRACK: A fast track service within the ED allows patients with acute but non-life-threatening conditions to be treated more quickly and then released; this system is designed to improve the efficiency and decrease the patient's wait time in the ED[1]

LEVEL IV TRAUMA: Many EDs in the United States triage patients into different levels of trauma based on severity of their condition; the triage system usually places patients on a scale of I-V, with a level I trauma patient being a life-threatening injury and levels IV and V being non-life-threatening and requiring fewer diagnostic needs

Objectives

1. Describe the differences between a patient evaluation performed by a physical therapist (PT) and an evaluation performed by a medical doctor (MD) and nurse practitioner (NP) in the ED.

2. Explain how a physical therapist may contribute to the management of a patient in the ED.

3. Describe the types of patients managed by PTs in the ED and how their examination and treatment approach differs from that of other healthcare providers.

Physical Therapy Considerations

PT considerations during management of the individual presenting in the ED with low back pain:

▶ **General physical therapy plan of care/goals:** Pain relief and increased function; self-management and prevention strategies; patient understanding of current condition and prognosis; individualized follow-up plan

▶ **Physical therapy interventions:** Manual techniques, modalities, and therapeutic exercise for pain relief and functional improvement; patient education regarding diagnosis and prognosis; advice about self-management of the condition, options for further management and treatment after discharge; home exercise program

▶ **Differential diagnoses:** Degenerative or traumatic disc pathology (*e.g.*, protrusion, extrusion, or sequestration), progressive congenital or traumatic spondylolisthesis, local infection or inflammatory pathology (*e.g.*, discitis, abscess), neoplasm

▶ **Complications interfering with physical therapy:** Lack of interprofessional understanding and respect for the physical therapist's potential contributions to patient management; differentiating between objective findings and secondary gains; limited options for treatment in a single visit; psychosocial barriers (*e.g.,* limited insurance, employment, intrinsic patient motivation)

Understanding the Health Condition

Emergency departments around the country are facing many challenges such as increasing number of patients and long wait times,[2] poor patient satisfaction and high costs,[3] and a decreasing ability to provide safe care.[4] They are continually evaluating operations and looking for new ways to become more efficient and effective. To aid in the provision of healthcare services, many departments around the country are utilizing nurse practitioners (NPs) and physician assistants (PAs) as physician extenders and they are expanding their use of physical therapists. In 1998, Carondelet St. Joseph's Hospital in Tuscon, AZ was the first hospital in the United States to staff a full-time physical therapist in the ED. Since then, it has served as a model for other programs around the country. Leaders of the Emergency Department Special Interest Group (ED SIG) of the American Physical Therapy Association (APTA) now estimate that 15 to 20 emergency departments in the United States staff part-time or full-time physical therapists, and more departments are in the early stages of program development.

The physical therapy profession has been rapidly advancing with increased entry-level education and physical therapist-driven research. Currently, 96% of entry-level physical therapy programs offer a clinical doctorate degree in physical therapy (DPT),[5] making the DPT the entry-level degree of choice for the profession. The primary content areas in the DPT curriculum include anatomy, physiology, biomechanics, neuroscience, orthopaedics, pharmacology, radiology, pathology, behavioral sciences, clinical reasoning, and evidence-based practice. Graduates of accredited DPT programs are trained in critical and integrative thinking and medical screening for non-musculoskeletal pathology. Physical therapists provide a wide variety of educational and physical interventions, enabling them to practice in many different settings, including the ED. In fact, studies have demonstrated that physical therapists are effective and safe in collaborating with other professionals in diagnosing and managing musculoskeletal and neuromuscular disorders.[6] As a result of utilizing **physical therapists in the ED,** hospitals have experienced decreased wait times to see a practitioner, decreased through time (*i.e.,* total time spent in the ED),[7] and increased patient satisfaction.[7,8] In addition, physical therapists facilitate more efficient follow-up to outpatient services including outpatient physical therapy.[7] Anecdotally, facilities utilizing physical therapists have reported higher quality of care and improved patient outcomes, decreased costs and increased income, and decreased medical errors.

More than 80% of the patients seen in emergency departments around the country have non-life-threatening conditions, many of these involving chronic pain.[9] While physicians and NPs in the ED are well-trained to diagnose medical conditions, they are limited primarily to pharmacological treatment and referral options for these conditions. As a result, physical therapists are consulted for assistance in the diagnosis and treatment of a wide variety of conditions such as acute and chronic spinal and extremity injuries, wounds, and positional vertigo as well as splinting of fractures and dislocations in both emergent and non-emergent situations.[10] Physical therapists also assist the medical team in discharge planning by performing balance and functional assessments and offering recommendations for appropriate work modifications. Finally, physical therapists assist the medical team in screening patients who may have secondary gains such as drug-seeking behavior or litigious interests. What physical therapists bring to the ED setting is an advanced level of knowledge and skill to appropriately treat many conditions and the ability to perform additional tests and measures to confirm the medical diagnosis or aid in the ongoing diagnostic and discharge planning process.

Compared to other healthcare providers in the ED, **physical therapists are able to spend more time with patients.** When patients are seen by a physical therapist in the ED, they spend 36% of their total visit time interacting with the therapist, compared to 20% and 19% with the physician and NP, respectively.[8] As a result of additional direct patient interaction, therapists may have more time to thoroughly explain the diagnosis and educate the patient about current prognosis and plan for future management. This extra time with a healthcare professional may reduce anxiety, stress, and pain, and can often empower the patient. This can go a long way in maximizing the patient's progress and recovery and minimize the risk of complications. With this additional time spent providing patient education, physical therapists often help prevent frequent and expensive return visits to the ED.[11] In addition, many patients evaluated in the urban ED lack insurance and often are unable to pay the cost of the services that they are provided. Thus, the ability to prevent return visits is a financial benefit for hospitals that employ physical therapists in the ED.

Physical Therapy Patient/Client Management

This patient was evaluated in the Fast Track by an NP and given a diagnosis of mechanical low back pain. The patient was not given any medications at that time due to the concern of drug-seeking behavior since the patient had made multiple trips to EDs in the area, each time receiving opiates for his pain. Because the patient was diagnosed with chronic mechanical LBP, the physical therapist was contacted to see if this patient was appropriate for consultation. During the electronic chart review, the PT noticed that the patient had never been evaluated or treated by a PT and did not appear to have a pattern of repeated ED visits for other conditions. The therapist felt the patient deserved a thorough evaluation and accepted the referral.

Examination, Evaluation, and Diagnosis

The information gathered from the NP's evaluation demonstrated a young male in acute pain of insidious onset for the past 6 months. The patient had been seen in the ED three previous times and was given pain medications that provided no lasting relief. The NP's examination demonstrated no midline tenderness but did note increased "tone and spasm" in the low back musculature and decreased spinal range of motion (ROM) limited by pain. There were no signs of foot drop and no gait abnormality noted. Patellar reflexes were symmetrical and intact and strength was grossly rated 5/5 on the right lower extremity and 4/5 on the left. The patient had a positive straight leg raise (SLR) on the left with pain noted on the right side of the low back and sensation was grossly intact. The formal diagnosis given was sciatica and the NP determined that there was no need for diagnostic imaging. The NP documented that the total time spent with the patient was 10 minutes.

During the physical therapy evaluation, the patient revealed an acute onset of pain while playing a pick-up game of basketball 6 months ago. Because of the severity of his pain, he was unable to finish the game and went to the ED the next morning. He was given pain medications (opiates) and sent home. When the physical therapist asked the patient to be more specific in the description of his symptoms, the patient explained that the pain was initially constant and sharp only in his back and then the pain went down both of his legs to the back of his knees and calves. At the time of the evaluation, he described his symptoms as a constant tightness and soreness in his low back and hamstrings with intermittent "stabbing" and shooting pain. He admitted that he would rate his pain as a 7 or 8 on a 10-point visual analog scale and not a 10 as he reported to the NP; he stated that he was trying to "prove" a point that he was really "hurting." For a couple of days after the initial incident he had some urinary incontinence, but this quickly resolved. He did not feel the need to report this to the NP because he did not think this was related to his back and leg pain. The patient appeared very frustrated with the lack of attention to his injury and subsequent symptoms and said he appreciated the therapist's time spent investigating the problem.

Upon observation in standing, the patient presented with decreased lumbar lordosis and paraspinal guarding. A possible "step" was palpated at L4/5, indicating a concern for a spondylolisthesis. Active trunk ROM was very limited, with flexion limited to the ability to reach his knees and extension limited to just slightly past neutral. Bilaterally, the patient's hip flexors were guarded, even in the supine position.

The neurologic examination revealed significant findings. The patient had bilateral four-beat clonus that could be indicative of an upper motor neuron lesion. He had a positive SLR at 35° bilaterally and a positive slump test (*i.e.*, patient's pain was reproduced with sitting in a forward flexed position with knee extension). Both the SLR and slump tests are neurodynamic mobility tests that increase the mechanical stress on neural structures by placing the patient in various positions. These tests are designed to determine whether neural structures are inflamed or adaptively shortened. In particular, the SLR and slump tests evaluate the lumbosacral plexus by placing stress on the sciatic nerve. In patients with lumbar disc herniations, the slump test was found to be more sensitive (84%) than the SLR (52%). However, the SLR was found to be slightly more specific (89%) than the slump test (83%). Thus, the slump test might be used more frequently as a sensitive physical examination tool in patients with symptoms of lumbar disc herniations to rule out this condition, if the test is negative. In contrast, owing to its higher specificity, a positive SLR test may especially help identify patients who have herniations with root compression requiring surgery.[12] Myotomal testing demonstrated weakness in L4/5 and S1 regions bilaterally. On a scale from 0 to 4+, patellar reflexes tested 3+ and Achilles reflexes 4+ bilaterally. Hoffman's sign was negative.

Because of the significant neurologic findings, the evaluation process was terminated earlier than usual and elements of a complete physical therapy evaluation such as manual muscle testing, flexibility testing, and joint play assessment were not performed. The physical therapist discussed the findings with the NP. Based on the mechanism of injury, presence of significant upper motor neuron findings, possible L4/5 step sign, previous urinary incontinence, and repeated trips to the ED, the physical therapist strongly recommended a magnetic resonance imaging (MRI) scan of the lumbar spine and further consultation, depending on the results. At this point, the NP and physical therapist discussed several differential diagnoses. First, there could be discogenic involvement such as disc herniation, extrusion, or possibly sequestration that initially put pressure on the spinal cord and may be continuing to cause problems such as central canal stenosis. Second, because of the possible step palpated in standing, there was concern for vertebral instability such as a spondylolisthesis due to a traumatic fracture or a congenital malformation. Less probable, but of potential concern, was pathologies such as a tumor, bone cancer, or an abscess around the spine or intra-abdominal region putting pressure on the spinal cord, cauda equina, or peripheral nerves. The attending physician was consulted and the medical team agreed that an MRI scan was indicated and was ordered by the attending MD. The detailed impression from the MRI findings were: (1) L4/5 central disc protrusion causing moderate to severe spinal canal stenosis and moderate foraminal stenosis bilaterally, with the left being worse than the right. (2) L5/S1 central disc extrusion with cranial migration. The thecal sac was completely effaced with severe spinal canal stenosis. The herniated disc extended to the subarticular recess with the right side being worse than the left. Moderate bilateral foraminal stenosis was noted with facet and ligamentum flavum hypertrophy.

In 2007, Ball et al.[13] explored practice trends among physical therapists, physicians, and NPs in the ED and noted several significant differences among the practitioners in written instructions to patients, referral trends, and structural support. They noted that **instructions given by physical therapists** were typically more detailed and patient satisfaction was higher for advice and information given, explanation of the results, what would happen next, and the overall care given. Murphy et al.[14] noted a difference in the quality of exercise instruction between physicians and physical therapists. They noted physicians often limited their instruction to verbal encouragement such as "walk more," and "be more active," while physical therapists are uniquely qualified to be more specific and directly address barriers that prevent patients from exercising. Williams et al.[15] noted that 43% of 165 American ED physicians surveyed did not feel prepared to prescribe proper exercises. Based on these studies and anecdotal evidence, one could hypothesize that if the physical therapist was not a member of the ED staff, this patient would likely have been sent home with a general description of "sciatica" and a generic set of back exercises. Depending on the provider, he may have received another prescription for opiates for his pain and possibly an anti-inflammatory medication. In addition, he may have been labeled a "drug-seeker" in his chart, which could potentially influence any future visits to the ED. This is an all too common scenario in EDs around the country and may be avoided or minimized with the inclusion of physical therapy in the ED.

Plan of Care and Interventions

Once the MRI findings were discussed and the neurosurgeons concluded that surgery was not indicated, the physical therapist returned and spent time educating the patient on the MRI findings and his prognosis. It was explained that because there did not appear to be a regression in neurologic function and no current signs of spinal cord compression (saddle anesthesia, progressive weakness and incontinence), conservative treatment was the treatment of choice. The therapist instructed the patient to monitor his symptoms for cord compression and to return to the ED if these symptoms occurred. He was given a good prognosis if he remained patient and compliant with the recommendations given by the medical team.

The patient was encouraged by the fact that he had a "reason" for his pain and he reported that this information reduced his anxiety. He also said he understood the magnitude of the spinal problem which allowed him to accept the pain for the time being. He said it was going to be difficult but the fact that he has some control over the situation and a plan gave him hope and provided him with improved coping strategies.

After the initial discussion of his situation, the evaluation process continued and included joint play assessment, ROM and flexibility testing of the peripheral joints, and gross flexibility and passive accessory movement of the spine. Significant findings were bilateral: hip flexion to 110° (limited by tight posterior hip capsules), hip extension to 10° (limited by tight hip flexors), and hamstring tightness. The patient also presented with mild hypomobility in the lower thoracic and upper lumbar spine from T8-L2 and he was unable to engage his transversus abdominis and multifidi muscles. Formal manual muscle testing was not performed at this time.

Treatment focused on gaining more spinal mobility and functional ability with various manual techniques and exercises. The physical therapist performed grade III and IV anterior, inferior, and posterior hip joint mobilization techniques in both supine and prone positions along with stretching of the hip flexors and hamstrings. In addition to the stretching and mobilization techniques, similar grade passive intervertebral mobilization and stretching of the thoracic spine was performed. The patient noted an increase in mobility and a decrease in his pain to 4/10 afterward. Manual and positional lumbar traction and neural mobilization techniques were attempted but none of these techniques was successful in reducing his symptoms.

Since the manual and stretching techniques demonstrated benefit, the patient was prescribed self-mobilization and stretching exercises to perform at home and core stabilization exercises that focused on co-contraction of the multifidi and transversus abdominis as described by Richardson and Jull.[16] The patient was instructed on how to progress these exercises in terms of repetitions and difficulty as he gained improved strength and control in the future. The physical therapist spent time discussing and practicing the "neutral spine" position and how to use his hips and legs for bending and lifting. The physical therapist discussed the utilization of heat for muscle tightness and stiffness, ice for acute flare-ups, and use of the medications as prescribed by the NP. The physical therapist also emphasized that time was a significant factor in his healing and that he was going to need patience during this process.

Typically, the NP or physician would recommend that the patient follow-up with his primary care doctor and would give the patient a referral to the local spine surgeon for a follow-up appointment. In this case, the patient did not have a primary care doctor and financial limitations prevented him from seeing a specialist unless it was absolutely necessary. Because of the patient's situation, the physical therapist contacted a case manager who provided the patient with a list of local free or reduced cost healthcare clinics as well as insurance programs for which he would qualify.

Evidence-Based Clinical Recommendations

SORT: Strength of Recommendation Taxonomy

A: Consistent, good-quality patient-oriented evidence
B: Inconsistent or limited-quality patient-oriented evidence
C: Consensus, disease-oriented evidence, usual practice, expert opinion, or case series

1. The inclusion of physical therapists as part of the medical team in hospital emergency departments decreases wait and through times, increases patient satisfaction, provides more efficient follow-up to outpatient services, and decreases frequency of return visits to the ED. **Grade B**

2. In the ED, physical therapists often spend more time with patients compared to physicians and nurse practitioners. **Grade B**

3. Physical therapists in primary care settings such as the ED typically provide more detailed instructions, especially with regards to exercise implementation, compared to those provided by physicians and nurse practitioners. **Grade C**

COMPREHENSION QUESTIONS

19.1 Which of the following is not a reason why physical therapists are an instrumental part of the healthcare team in the emergency department?

    A. Physical therapists typically have more interaction time with the patient than physicians and nurse practitioners.

    B. Physical therapists are effective and safe in collaborating with other professionals in diagnosing and managing musculoskeletal and neuromuscular disorders.

    C. Physical therapists can often provide more treatment options for common musculoskeletal conditions.

    D. Physical therapists are better trained in diagnosing musculoskeletal disorders.

19.2   The use of physical therapists in hospital emergency departments in the United States has been associated with all of the following benefits *except*:

A.   Decreased wait times

B.   Increased patient satisfaction

C.   Decrease in the number of outpatient referrals

D.   Decreased costs

ANSWERS

19.1   **D.** Physical therapists are not better trained in diagnosing musculoskeletal disorders, but they have a skill set in which they complement the medical team to assist in the diagnosis and treatment of many conditions.

19.2   **C.** Physical therapists play a significant role in the discharge planning and recommendations for the patient in the ED. Physical therapists facilitate referrals to a variety medical professionals including primary care physicians, specialists, and outpatient physical therapists. Thus, physical therapists can help *increase* the number outpatient referrals.

REFERENCES

1.   Wiler JL, Gentle C, Halfpenny JM, et al. Optimizing emergency department front-end operations. *Ann Emerg Med*. 2010;55:142-160.

2.   United States Government Accountability Office Report to the Chairman, Committee on Finance, U.S. Senate. Hospital Emergency Departments: Crowding Continues to Occur, and Some Patients Wait Longer than Recommended Time Frames. April 2009. Available at: www.gao.gov/new.items/d09347.pdf. Accessed May 23, 2012.

3.   The American College of Emergency Physicians. Available at: http://www.acep.org/content.aspx?id=25908. Accessed May 23, 2012.

4.   Magid DJ, Sullivan AF, Cleary PD, et al. The safety of emergency care systems: results of a survey of clinicians in 65 US emergency departments. *Ann Emerg Med*. 2009;53:715-723.

5.   The American Physical Therapy Association. Available at: http://www.apta.org/PTEducation/Overview/. Accessed May 23, 2012.

6.   Daker-White G, Carr AJ, Harvey I, et al. A randomized controlled trial: shifting boundaries of doctors and physiotherapists in orthopaedic outpatient departments. *J Epidemionl Community Health*. 1999;53:643-650.

7.   Lebec MT, Jogodka CE. The physical therapist as a musculoskeletal specialist in the emergency department. *J Orthop Sports Phys Ther*. 2009;39:221-229.

8.   McClellen CM, Greenwood R, Benger JR. Effect of an extended scope physiotherapy service on patient satisfaction and the outcome of soft tissue injuries in an adult emergency department. *Emerg Med J*. 2006;23:384-387.

9.   Wilsey BL, Fishman SM, Ogden C, Tsodikov A, Bertakis KD. Chronic pain management in the emergency department: a survey of attitudes and beliefs. *Pain Med*. 2008;9:1073-1080.

10.   Lebec MT, Cernohous S, Tenbarge L, Gest C, Severson K, Howard S. Emergency department physical therapist service: a pilot study examining physician perceptions. *IJAHSP*. 2010;8:1-12. Available at: http://ijahsp.nova.edu. Accessed May 23, 2012.

11. Richardson B, Shepstone L, Poland F, et al. Randomised controlled trial and cost consequences study comparing initial physiotherapy assessment and management with routine practice for selected patients in an accident and emergency department of an acute hospital. *Emerg Med J*. 2005;22:87-92.

12. Majlesi J, Togay H, Unalan H, Toprak S. The sensitivity and specificity of the Slump and the Straight Leg Raising tests in patients with lumbar disc herniation. *J Clin Rheumatol*. 2008;14:87-91.

13. Ball ST, Walton K, Hawes S. Do emergency department physiotherapy practitioner's, emergency nurse practitioners and doctors investigate, treat and refer patients with closed musculoskeletal injuries differently? *Emerg Med J*. 2007;24:185-188.

14. Murphy BP, Greathouse D, Matsui I. Primary care physical therapy practice models. *J Orthop Sports Phys Ther*. 2005;35:699-707

15. Williams JM, Chinnis AC, Gutman D. Health promotion practices of emergency physicians. *Am J Emerg Med*. 2000;18:17-21.

16. Richardson CA, Jull GA. Muscle control-pain control. What exercises would you prescribe? *Man Ther*. 1995;1:2-10.

Electrotherapy in Pain Management

Joyce M. Campbell

A 60-year-old male was admitted to the hospital 5 days ago after a fall while playing tennis. Radiographs revealed two nondisplaced pelvic fractures on the right and magnetic resonance imaging (MRI) revealed internal derangement of his right knee as well as mild to moderate degenerative changes in the lumbar and sacral spine. Two days ago, his right knee was surgically repaired. There is mild swelling in the right lower limb and he reports mild to moderate pain in his surgical knee. He is medically cleared to begin walking with toe-touch weightbearing (TTWB) on the right lower extremity. He is limited by pain in the low back, perineum, left hip, and posterior left leg and sole of the foot. He can walk 20 ft with a front-wheeled walker with TTWB on the right. Walking is limited by pain and an inability to maintain *left* knee extension in stance. He was receiving fentanyl (intramuscular) until today when his pain medication was changed to oxycodone (oral) in preparation for discharge from the hospital. A review of his prior medical records reveals that the patient was seen in outpatient physical therapy 2 years ago for hip and low back pain (left side greater than right). At that time, he demonstrated muscle weakness in the hip extensors, plantar flexors, ankle evertors, and toe extensors. He improved over a 4-week course of physical therapy and upon re-evaluation 6 months later, his lower limb muscle strength had returned to normal (5/5 on Manual Muscle Test). Back then, his x-ray and MRI studies had already demonstrated mild to moderate degenerative changes in the lumbar spine. One month ago, he was seen in the emergency department for a sudden onset of severe low back pain that occurred when he was working out at the gym. He was discharged with pain medication and a recommendation for bedrest. He is to be discharged home in 2 to 4 days. He lives alone in a multilevel house. He is an investment broker who drives to work, where he has to walk approximately one block from the parking structure to his office. In recent years, he has played tennis at least two to three times each week. On the second postoperative day (POD 2), the physical therapist is asked to evaluate and treat this patient and make recommendations for further rehabilitation.

▶ Based upon his health condition, what do you anticipate will be the contributors to activity limitations?

▶ What are the examination priorities?

▶ What precautions should be taken during the physical therapy evaluation?

▶ What are the most appropriate physical therapy interventions at this time?

KEY DEFINITIONS

CHRONIC PAIN: Pain that outlasts normal tissue healing time, is greater than would be expected from the extent of injury, and occurs in the absence of identifiable tissue damage[1]

DERMATOME: Area of skin supplied by cutaneous branches from a single spinal nerve

ELECTRONEUROMYOGRAPHY (ENMG): Electrodiagnostic studies done with cutaneous electrodes (strength-duration tests, motor and sensory evoked potential studies), intramuscular electrodes (diagnostic intramuscular electromyographic [EMG] studies), or fine wire electrodes (kinesiological EMG studies)

FIBRILLATION POTENTIALS: Spontaneous electrical potentials generated by single muscle fibers that are no longer innervated; observable only with intramuscular EMG electrodes[2-4]

LARGE–GIANT MOTOR UNIT ACTION POTENTIAL (MUAP): Electrical potential (observable only with intramuscular EMG electrodes) generated by a single motor unit that has acquired more muscle fibers than in the original innervation ratio; additional muscle fibers in the motor unit produce a higher amplitude[2-4]

MOTOR UNIT ACTION POTENTIAL (MUAP): Action potential reflecting electrical activity of the part of a single anatomical motor unit that is within the recording range of an intramuscular electrode [2-4]

MYOTOME: Muscles receiving innervation from an individual spinal nerve or motor segment (*e.g.*, S1 myotome may be assessed by manually muscle testing gluteus maximus [L5, S1, S2], soleus [S1, S2], fibularis longus [L5, S1] and extensor hallucis [L5, S1]); if intramuscular EMG testing is available, the S1 myotome can be thoroughly assessed by testing these same muscles and adding long head of biceps femoris (S1, S2), short head of biceps femoris (L5, S1), medial gastrocnemius (S1, S2), lateral gastrocnemius (L5, S1), and spinal extensor muscles for S1 spinal segment[2-6]

NEUROPRAXIA: Block in nerve conduction

PARTIAL DENERVATION OF MUSCLE (or PARTIAL AXONOTMESIS OF NERVE): Loss of nerve supply to a portion of the muscle fibers within a muscle; could be due to a partial peripheral nerve injury or loss of a spinal segment (anterior horn cell, motor rootlets or spinal nerve); reinnervation of muscle fibers may occur by axonal regrowth (1-3 mm/day) or by terminal sprouting of remaining motor axons within original motor unit territory (completion expected about 6 months after injury)[3,7,8]

PERIPHERAL NERVE: Includes motor anterior horn cells, motor rootlets, spinal nerve, dorsal and anterior rami, plexus pathway, branches into specific nerves, afferent sensory fibers, sensory cell bodies, and sensory fibers supplying the dorsal horn of the spinal cord. Pathology of anterior horn cells, rootlets, and/or the spinal nerve results in muscle weakness in a myotomal pattern (*e.g.*, S1). Pathology of an individual peripheral nerve, such as the tibial nerve, results in weakness within the distribution of that nerve. If the pathology of the sensory fibers is at the spinal nerve, sensory cell bodies, and/or central sensory fibers, the sensory abnormalities will be dermatomal. If the sensory compromise is located distally (*e.g.*, sural nerve), the sensory abnormalities will be in the distribution of the sensory nerve.

STRENGTH DURATION CURVE: Electrodiagnostic test used to screen for partial or complete muscle denervation; pulse duration is varied from 300 to 0.01 ms and the intensity (mA) required to produce a small muscle contraction is plotted against the pulse durations; individual pulses (instant rise time, unidirectional current) are applied with skin electrodes; a smooth curve with chronaxie less than 1.0 ms is considered normal.[9,10]

TRANSCUTANEOUS ELECTRICAL NERVE STIMULATION (TENS): Use of electrical stimulation for the purpose of pain modulation

WALLERIAN DEGENERATION: Disintegration of the axon and breakdown of its myelin sheath distal to the point of severance or death of the axon[3,7,8]

Objectives

1. Identify potential adverse drug reactions (ADRs) of opioid analgesics that may affect physical therapy examination or interventions and describe possible therapy solutions.

2. Describe examination procedures for the physical therapy assessment of a patient with recent trauma and a history of low back and hip pain.

3. Recognize patterns of peripheral nerve pain and muscle weakness.

4. Discuss the use of electrical stimulation to modulate pain.

5. Identify when and why a referral for an ENMG study is appropriate.

6. Describe appropriate ENMG examinations that a patient could be referred to have (by a physical therapist electroneuromyographer or by a physician) to determine if he is a current or potential future candidate to become pain-free, strengthen weak muscles, discontinue any orthoses provided during rehabilitation, and/or return to recreational sports.

7. Define the ENMG assessment milestones that will guide the progression of the patient's physical therapy interventions throughout the course of rehabilitation.

8. Describe appropriate patient education and home instructions at the time of discharge as well as for the entire period of rehabilitation.

9. Describe an appropriate physical therapy plan of care after discharge from the acute care setting.

Physical Therapy Considerations

PT considerations during management of the individual with peripheral neuropathy, pain, and muscle weakness due to trauma and/or degenerative joint disease:

▶ **General physical therapy plan of care/goals:** Prevent or minimize risk of deep venous thrombosis (DVT); modulate pain; minimize fall risk and maximize functional independence and safety while walking with a walker and toe-touch weightbearing (TTWB) on postsurgical lower extremity

▶ **Physical therapy interventions:** Patient education related to decreasing risk of DVT and risk of falls; provision of ankle-foot orthosis (AFO) to stabilize the knee during ambulation with a walker; gait and stair training; electrical stimulation to modulate pain; prescription of home exercise program; referral for ENMG examination; referral for outpatient physical therapy for postsurgical rehabilitation of right knee and strengthening of left lower extremity

▶ **Precautions during physical therapy:** Immobilization and TTWB of postsurgical knee; left AFO to decrease risk of falling and allow increased functional walking distance

▶ **Complications interfering with physical therapy:** Right knee immobilization and weightbearing precautions; postsurgical pain in right knee; perineal and left hip, leg, and foot pain; collapse of left knee in stance associated with left calf weakness

Understanding the Health Condition

Electrical stimulation (ES) has been employed to manage pain in a variety of conditions since the 1960s. The use of both cutaneous and implanted ES systems was originally based on neurophysiological evidence referred to as the "gate-control" theory of Melzack and Wall, first published in 1965.[11-13] The gate-control theory postulates that activity in the large, fast-conducting, primary somatosensory nerve fibers modulates the activity of neurons in the dorsal horns that are responsible for transmitting noxious information to the brain. When afferent activity in the large sensory nerve fibers is increased by sensory input (or by electrical stimulation), the activity in noxious pathways is reduced, resulting in diminished pain perception. A few years later, it was demonstrated that ES over certain peripheral areas also results in the release of endorphins from the pituitary gland. Endorphins suppress pain by reducing ascending pain impulses from the periphery to the brain.[13] In the 1970s, it was hypothesized that intense ES over peripheral nerves (at acupuncture sites) was required for endorphin release.[14] Subsequent investigators have demonstrated that comfortable ES over the limbs, and not necessarily over peripheral nerves, still resulted in endorphin release.[15] Regardless of the physiological mechanisms, it appears that ES can stimulate the body's endogenous pain suppression mechanisms.

While extensive research has been done to understand the mechanisms of endogenous and electrically-stimulated pain modulation, the **efficacy of ES**

for pain control in clinical trials is unclear.[16,17] Confounding factors in studies designed to assess the ability of ES to modulate pain include lack of homogeneity among subjects, variability in ES parameters and protocols (including amount of time/day when ES was available to subjects), and habituation of the nervous system when ES is relied upon over an extended period of time. One of the key concerns in these studies is that subjects did not have constant, ready access to ES; in order for ES to suppress pain, the patient must have access to ES, as needed, on a 24-hour basis. Although there may be one to several hours of effective and continuous pain modulation after ES, pain has not been shown to be reduced on a 24-hour per day basis.[18-20] Cutaneous ES (*i.e.*, TENS) for pain modulation in patients with low back and lower extremity pain may be a useful adjunct to treat pain in the acute phase (1-2 months after pain onset), but it has not been shown to be effective over a prolonged period in patients with chronic low back pain.[21] Despite significant investigative effort, no single profile of ES (*e.g.*, waveform, pulse repetition rate, intensity, modulation or placement of electrodes) has been shown to provide *optimal* pain relief. Proposed physiologic mechanisms underlying TENS interventions for pain control include spinal cord gating, descending pain inhibition, release of endogenous opioids, and activation of serotonin, norepinephrine and muscarinic receptors.[22] Cutaneous electrodes should be placed near the site of injury or pain, or over the nerve pathway to the brain in order to affect the fields of the sensitized neurons.[22] An inexpensive ES device ($65-$100) can be made available and used as needed by the patient 24 hours per day while the patient is awaiting diagnosis of the primary cause of his pain. A comfortable waveform (300 microseconds balanced biphasic) in combination with a well-tolerated pulse repetition rate (40-100 pulses per second) should be used.[23]

If it is possible to identify the exact location and inciting cause of the pain, appropriate measures should be instituted to remove or mitigate the cause, and the patient's pain should be minimized or resolved. In the absence of such problem-solving and positive results, the patient is generally labeled a "chronic pain" patient. Chronic pain is referred to as non-protective and it serves no biological purpose. Pain may be considered chronic if the pain is present after normal tissue healing time, is greater than expected from the extent of the injury and occurs in the absence of identifiable tissue change.[1,22] Physical therapists have the skills required to identify patterns of nerve involvement. Accurate identification of nerve involvement can set the stage in the acute care setting and for the entire rehabilitation period. Specific manual muscle tests, assessment of sensation, and observational gait analysis may reveal the need for further evaluation to identify the source of the patient's pain. Because physical therapists in the acute care setting already perform these assessments, little to no extra time is required for this type of problem solving. For example, this patient presents with pain in the perineum, hip, and posterior leg and foot on the *non-operative* side. This is a common pain pattern when the S1 spinal nerve or sensory rootlets are compromised. It is important to recognize that pain in the hip may be referred from pathology in the S1 spinal nerve as well.[2,3,8,24,25] Inadequate tibial control in stance with collapse of the knee is expected because of the large contribution of the S1 segment to the soleus muscle and other plantar flexors. If assessment of the gluteus maximus and other muscles receiving S1 innervation revealed weakness, it would help confirm the suspicion of an S1 problem because the gluteus maximus receives at least 50% of its nerve supply from the S1 spinal segment.[5,6,24,26,27]

Assessment of myotomal weakness is often misunderstood in the literature and in clinical assessment scales. It is common to find instructions to test one muscle to represent a myotome. For example, the reader may be instructed that if the fibularis longus and brevis muscles are weak, the patient has a problem with the S1 myotome.[28] Alternatively, a different source suggests testing the soleus to determine if there is an S1 myotomal deficit.[29] However, testing only one muscle restricts the conclusion to the strength of that muscle and its particular nerve supply. In other words, testing one (or two) representative muscles does not reflect the intactness of an entire myotome. Appropriate assessment of the S1 myotome *mandates* testing of muscles containing a significant S1 contribution (equal to or more than 50%), but supplied by different peripheral nerves. Weakness in the soleus (S1 and S2 myotomes; posterior tibial nerve), fibularis longus (L5 and S1 myotomes; superficial fibular nerve,), extensor hallucis longus (L5 and S1 myotomes; deep fibular nerve) and gluteus maximus (L5, S1, and S2 myotomes; inferior gluteal nerve) in the absence of weakness in muscles that do not receive S1 innervation would strongly suggest an S1 myotomal problem. Some orthopaedic textbooks suggest using the "strength" of a joint motion to assess myotomal integrity. For example, ankle dorsiflexion has been suggested to reflect the L4 myotome.[30] However, the muscles causing ankle dorsiflexion have significant contribution from L4, L5, and S1 myotomes, so weak ankle dorsiflexion would not sufficiently rule in the hypothesis of an L4 myotomal deficit.[2,6,31]

When clinical assessments (sensory testing, manual muscle testing, gait analysis) reveal a potential nerve dysfunction,[6,27] the physical therapist may screen for muscle denervation with a traditional electrodiagnostic test such as the strength-duration (SD) curve prior to referral for further ENMG evaluation (intramuscular electromyography as well as motor and sensory evoked potential studies). The strength-duration test is performed with skin electrodes. It is easy, quick to perform, and is within the scope of entry-level practice for physical therapists. If partial denervation of the weak muscles exists, prolonged chronaxie and plateaus in the SD curve would be evident.[9]

The absence of partial denervation findings in electrodiagnostic studies does not rule out a problem with the S1 myotome. It is possible that compromise of the S1 sensory fibers along with neuropraxia of the S1 motor fibers could explain the patient's pain and weakness. If the motor involvement is more severe, it is possible that there is some denervation of deeper muscle fibers that was not detected by the SD curve screening. It is also possible that the patient's prior problems (up to 2 years ago as indicated in his medical history) resulted in partial denervation with re-innervation of the orphaned muscle fibers by terminal sprouting, which would result in fewer large motor units.[2-4,7] Although each motor unit has the capacity to adopt four to five times the number of muscle fibers in its original territory,[32,33] there are penalties for this extensive terminal sprouting. For example, the re-innervated muscle will be weaker than the original and fatigue more rapidly than in the normal motor unit configuration (as expected in the post-polio condition). Axonotmesis of the S1 motor fibers at the spinal nerve will result in axonal re-growth at a rate of 1 to

3 mm/day from the point of injury in the peripheral nerve. The distance from the S1 spinal nerve to the leg and foot would require 1.5 to 2 years for the axons to re-grow and innervate the orphaned muscle fibers. Simultaneously, terminal sprouting in the motor unit territories of healthy axons begins. This latter process will win the race to re-innervate muscle fibers in approximately 6 months.[3,4,7,8] To thoroughly document the nature and severity of the S1 spinal nerve problem, **ENMG studies** (including intramuscular EMG, motor evoked potential studies of the tibial and deep fibular nerves with F-waves, and an H-reflex study of the tibial nerve) are required. It would not be uncommon for medical caregivers and third party payers to defer ENMG assessment for this patient until he is discharged from the hospital. However, early ENMG assessment may lead to resolution of his pain now, improved walking and function, improved rehabilitation of his postsurgical knee and realistic planning for strengthening of his weak muscles as well as prediction of future orthotic needs. For example, if the ENMG testing determined that conduction in the S1 spinal nerve on the patient's non-operative side was blocked and/or some of the muscle fibers innervated by S1 have lost their nerve supply, it cannot be expected that the strength, work capacity, or resistance to fatigue of these muscles will improve at this time. In fact, overuse of the partially denervated muscles by volitional exercise or by electrical stimulation may inhibit the motor axons' ability to reconnect with the denervated muscle fibers.[31,34-35] Terminal sprouting within the partially dener-vated muscles can be expected to be complete in 6 months if the cause of nerve compromise is resolved. At that time, there will be a window of opportunity for improvement in muscle performance, although the strength and work capacity in these muscles may never return to the pre-injury level and fatigue will be more rapid after the formation of large to giant motor units. Once the cause of the nerve com-promise is remedied, the pain associated with the compromise should be markedly improved. If Wallerian degeneration is still in progress (during the month following axonotmesis), burning pain within the involved muscles may persist. Once the axonal degeneration is complete, the patient should have minimal to no pain in the S1 distribution.

Physical Therapy Patient/Client Management

While this patient may appear to be an "orthopaedic" patient with a treatment team including nurses, physical therapists, orthopaedic surgeon, and a pain management physician, the role of the physical therapist in the postoperative phase includes performing a thorough examination of the etiology of his pain and weakness pat-terns with any necessary referrals to other professionals such as an orthotist, electro-neuromyographer, and neurologist. Specific roles of the physical therapist include anticipating possible ADRs and modifying evaluation and intervention appropri-ately; preventing or minimizing postoperative complications; assessing range of motion, sensation, pain, muscle strength, gait and ability to perform functional tasks within postoperative precautions; providing intervention for pain modulation that can be used 24 hours per day; providing necessary equipment and training for safe mobility; educating the patient regarding postoperative precautions for the postsurgical knee, signs and symptoms of DVT and pulmonary embolism that would require immediate emergency medical care; evaluating candidacy for walking brace-free and returning to recreational sports; referring for electrodiagnostic assessment in the very near future; and, referring to outpatient physical therapy for specific impairment consideration during the full rehabilitation period.

Examination, Evaluation, and Diagnosis

Prior to seeing the patient, the physical therapist needs to acquire information from his chart, including: past medical history, medications, lab values, postoperative precautions, and any exercise or mobility restrictions. For the immediate post-operative patient, it is important to check hemoglobin, hematocrit, platelet count, blood pressure, heart rate, and respiratory rate.[36,37]

When a review of the patient's medication list reveals administration of opioid analgesics such as oxycodone, therapy should be scheduled to take advantage of maximum pain modulation effectiveness and potential ADRs must be recognized. It would be appropriate to schedule physical therapy one to three hours after administration of oxycodone, since peak effectiveness is generally 60 minutes after intake and the duration of action is three to four hours. Assessment of patient alertness and dizziness when coming to sitting and standing are of particular importance because of the potential for drowsiness, mental slowing, and orthostatic hypotension. Nausea and vomiting may occur, along with respiratory depression in some cases.[38,39]

During introductions, the physical therapist assesses the patient's level of alertness and orientation. Specific questions should be asked regarding the patient's prior level of function, including back and left leg pain, and current status since surgery. Screening for DVT, sensation testing, and joint range of motion are most easily performed with the patient supine. Pain distribution and intensity may be documented supine, during bed mobility, and preparation for transfer out of bed. Manual muscle testing may be modified to accommodate the patient's precautions and pain tolerance. Testing of specific muscles is essential to the process of recognizing nerve patterns (myotomal versus individual peripheral nerves). It is possible to perform an examination that takes approximately the same amount of time as a "gross muscle test," but allows the physical therapist to acquire information about myotomes, key plexus components, and peripheral nerves. This author has developed a Pocket Guide to Manual Muscle Testing to allow physical therapists to perform a screening manual muscle test (MMT) that allows one to distinguish weakness patterns due to myotomal, plexus, or individual peripheral nerve(s) dysfunction (Fig. 20-1). The therapist begins muscle testing with the muscle at the top of the list and proceeds to test each of the specified muscles (within the patient's medical clearance for movement and weightbearing). After noting the weak muscles, the therapist follows the arrows to determine if there is a specific nerve pattern (listed on the right side of the column) or a spinal segmental pattern (listed on the left side of the column). When the examination is complete and muscle weakness is identified, the physical therapist may conclude that there is a weakness pattern representing a myotome, a portion of

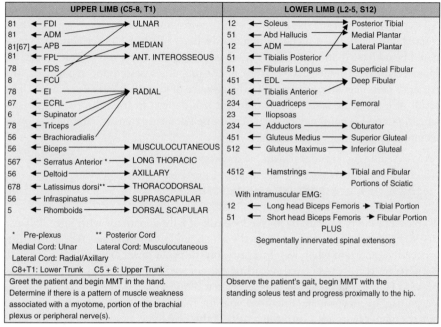

UPPER LIMB (C5-8, T1)		LOWER LIMB (L2-5, S12)	
81	← FDI ──────→ ULNAR	12	← Soleus ──────→ Posterior Tibial
81	← ADM	51	← Abd Hallucis ──→ Medial Plantar
81[67]	← APB ──────→ MEDIAN	12	← ADM ──────→ Lateral Plantar
81	← FPL ──────→ ANT. INTEROSSEOUS	51	← Tibialis Posterior
78	← FDS	51	← Fibularis Longus ──→ Superficial Fibular
8	← FCU	451	← EDL ──────→ Deep Fibular
78	← EI ──────→ RADIAL	45	← Tibialis Anterior
67	← ECRL	234	← Quadriceps ──→ Femoral
6	← Supinator	23	← Iliopsoas
78	← Triceps	234	← Adductors ──→ Obturator
56	← Brachioradialis	451	← Gluteus Medius ──→ Superior Gluteal
56	← Biceps ──────→ MUSCULOCUTANEOUS	512	← Gluteus Maximus ──→ Inferior Gluteal
567	← Serratus Anterior * ──→ LONG THORACIC	4512	← Hamstrings ──→ Tibial and Fibular Portions of Sciatic
56	← Deltoid ──────→ AXILLARY		
678	← Latissimus dorsi** ──→ THORACODORSAL	With intramuscular EMG:	
56	← Infraspinatus ──────→ SUPRASCAPULAR	12	← Long head Biceps Femoris → Tibial Portion
5	← Rhomboids ──────→ DORSAL SCAPULAR	51	← Short head Biceps Femoris → Fibular Portion
* Pre-plexus ** Posterior Cord		PLUS	
Medial Cord: Ulnar Lateral Cord: Musculocutaneous		Segmentally innervated spinal extensors	
Lateral Cord: Radial/Axillary			
C8+T1: Lower Trunk C5 + 6: Upper Trunk			
Greet the patient and begin MMT in the hand. Determine if there is a pattern of muscle weakness associated with a myotome, portion of the brachial plexus or peripheral nerve(s).		Observe the patient's gait, begin MMT with the standing soleus test and progress proximally to the hip.	

Abbreviations: FDI, first dorsal interosseous; ADM, abductor digiti minimi; APB, abductor pollicis brevis; FPL, flexor pollicis longus; FCU, flexor carpi ulnaris; EI, extensor indicis; ECRL, extensor carpi radialis longus; EDL, extensor digitorum longus.

Figure 20-1. Pocket Guide to Manual Muscle Testing: quick and easy approach to distinguish weakness patterns due to myotomal, plexus, or individual peripheral nerve(s) dysfunction.

a plexus, one or more peripheral nerves, or that there is no specific nerve pattern. As an example, if a patient demonstrates muscle weakness only in the soleus, abductor hallucis, abductor digiti minimi and tibialis posterior, it would be reasonable to conclude that there is a problem with the posterior tibial nerve. On the other hand, if the patient demonstrates weakness in these muscles as well as in the fibularis longus and gluteus maximus, it would be appropriate to question if the patient had an S1 spinal nerve dysfunction.

It is important to remember that if a nerve pattern of weakness is identified, those muscles that test 4/5 rather than 5/5 in the MMT position have lost at least 50% of force generation capability.[6,26,27] The natural companion assessment to upright manual muscle testing for key muscles like the soleus is observational gait analysis: stability of the patient's hip, knee, and ankle in the stance phase and flexion for limb advancement at each joint in the swing phase. Such observations are compromised when the patient is using an ambulatory aid, but obvious joint instability deserves intervention for safety in walking. Documentation of walking ability while maintaining TTWB, including the maximum distance walked, is essential.

In this patient with acute trauma and a history of low back pain, his current pain in the perineal area, hip, leg, and sole of the foot could be interpreted by the healthcare team as greater than expected from the pelvic fractures and recent contralateral knee surgery and lasting longer than expected. If the physical therapist recognizes an S1 spinal nerve pattern (both motor and sensory) and if ENMG assessment is performed, the cause of the pain—which may be due to S1 spinal nerve compression—could be addressed and potentially resolved during the acute rehabilitation period. However, if the spinal nerve pattern is not properly assessed and recognized, the patient's pain may be considered "in the absence of identifiable tissue change." The result of inadequate assessment would put this patient in the "chronic pain" classification and his pain may be treated as a disease, rather than as a manifestation of a curable condition.[1,22]

Plan of Care and Interventions

To promote safety in walking and reduce risk of falling, patients with knee collapse due to calf weakness can be stabilized with an ankle-foot orthosis (AFO).[27] This is especially important when weightbearing on the other lower extremity is restricted. Patients need to be educated regarding the importance of using the AFO to help prevent falls and improve endurance when walking with a walker. Muscle strengthening may or may not be a realistic goal for the patient with current or previous peripheral nerve injury. Until the results of the ENMG assessment are known, continued use of the AFO will be required.

Referral for ENMG assessment should be considered an important part of acute care intervention for the patient with pain that exceeds the expected location and/or severity, especially in the presence of a nerve pattern of muscle weakness (such as the S1 myotomal pattern observed in this patient). The referral should request specific tests and intramuscular diagnostic EMG examination of the weak functional muscles (based upon MMT and gait analysis). The physical therapist must obtain **information from the ENMG studies** to allow appropriate goal setting for improving muscle performance and to allow prediction of future orthotic needs. From the EMG studies, it is important to learn about the presence of fibrillations at rest, the amplitude and firing rate of the first recruited motor unit potentials, the motor unit recruitment strategy employed to increase force production, and the ability to recruit a sufficient pool of motor units with increased effort.[2-4,8] The patient should be educated about the implications of such findings for management of his pain and muscle weakness in the present and in the future. It is critical to differentiate pain that can be addressed now (*e.g.*, by surgical decompression of a spinal nerve) from a pattern of chronic pain that will lead to a different medical diagnosis and rehabilitation pathway.[1] Table 20-1 outlines potential findings from the current patient's ENMG studies, expected outcomes and timeframes, as well as physical therapy implications.

The patient with pelvic fractures and surgical repair of the knee is commonly referred to outpatient physical therapy by the surgeon. It is appropriate for the acute care physical therapist to make a referral to outpatient physical therapy as well. Documentation of the physical therapy evaluation findings and evidence of referrals made set the stage for appropriate intervention at the optimal time during the full rehabilitation period.

Table 20-1	PHYSICAL THERAPY IMPLICATIONS OF POTENTIAL ENMG FINDINGS FOR THIS PATIENT AND BASIS FOR PATIENT EDUCATION DURING ACUTE AND OUTPATIENT REHABILITATION		
ENMG Findings	**Expected Outcome with Intervention**	**Estimated Time**	**Physical Therapy Implications**
S1 sensory compromise	Pain resolution	Immediately following medical/surgical intervention	Improved ease of bed mobility, transfers, walking
S1 neuropraxia (or neuropraxic contribution to weakness)	Improvement in muscle strength	Immediately following medical/surgical intervention	If neuropraxia is responsible for muscle weakness: return to 5/5 strength on MMT If neuropraxia is *partially* responsible for weakness: improvement in muscle strength Evaluate for discontinuation of AFO
S1 axonotmesis with partial denervation of muscles receiving S1 innervation	Terminal sprouting will result in reinnervation, resulting in some improvement in muscle strength.	Approximately 6 months after medical/surgical intervention	There will be a window of opportunity to strengthen muscles when reinnervation is complete. May achieve 4/5 or 5/5 strength on MMT, but expect earlier fatigue than before injury. Evaluate for discontinuation of AFO.
Prior S1 axonotmesis with terminal sprouting (6 mo or more prior to current injury)	Do not expect change in muscle performance.	Once formed, large fast-firing motor units are permanent.	Muscle strengthening cannot be expected. Expect early fatigue. AFO may continue to be required.

Evidence-Based Clinical Recommendations

SORT: Strength of Recommendation Taxonomy

A: Consistent, good-quality patient-oriented evidence

B: Inconsistent or limited-quality patient-oriented evidence

C: Consensus, disease-oriented evidence, usual practice, expert opinion, or case series

1. Electrical stimulation may effectively modulate pain during the acute rehabilitation period. **Grade B**

2. Intramuscular electromyography and motor evoked potential studies from ENMG studies are the only clinical tools to identify nerve conduction block as well as current and/or past partial muscle denervation. **Grade A**

3. ENMG findings provide an objective basis for expected improvement in muscle performance, force generation, and fatigue resistance. **Grade C**

COMPREHENSION QUESTIONS

20.1 A 65-year-old patient who just had surgery on his knee and has non-weightbearing precautions on the surgical limb, complains of 7-9/10 pain in the *contralateral* (non-surgical) hip and leg during bed mobility, transfers and walking with a walker. He is taking opioid analgesic medication and pain on the non-surgical side is still interfering with transfers and ambulation. What is the *most* appropriate course of action for the physical therapist to take?

A. Ask the nurses to authorize additional pain medication around-the-clock.

B. Ask (in a team conference) if he might be a "chronic pain" patient.

C. Contact the surgeon and ask for an evaluation of his nonsurgical hip to see if it could be the source of the patient's pain complaints and if ENMG referral is indicated to determine if his pain is coming from an S1 spinal nerve problem.

D. Assume that this pain pattern is typical for an elderly person.

20.2 Electrical stimulation for pain modulation can be expected to be *most* successful:

A. When a paired monophasic spike (high-volt) current is used.

B. When cutaneous electrodes are placed near the injury or source of pain, or proximally along the nerve pathway and electrical stimulation is available 24 hours per day, as needed.

C. When electrical stimulation is used once per day for 20 minutes.

D. When cutaneous electrodes are placed bilaterally over the proximal cervical spine.

20.3 A patient walks in knee flexion and is at risk of falling because of knee "buckling" after walking a short distance. What is the *most* reasonable course of action for the physical therapist to take?

A. It would be reasonable to prescribe knee extension strengthening exercises.

B. In order to demonstrate an S1 problem, it would be necessary to perform manual muscle testing of the gluteus maximus, soleus, fibularis longus and extensor hallucis in the initial evaluation.

C. In order to demonstrate an S1 problem, it would be necessary to perform manual muscle testing of the gluteus medius, tibialis anterior, gastrocnemius and hamstrings in the initial evaluation.

D. It would be necessary to include manual muscle testing of the knee extensors.

20.4 An individual in the acute care setting demonstrates 3+ to 4/5 MMT grades in muscles supplied by the S1 spinal segment. It is *most* reasonable for the physical therapist to:

A. Ask if this is a recent nerve pattern and/or 6 months or more since onset.

B. Consider if this patient is a candidate for improving muscle strength and fatigue resistance now or at any time in the future, or whether he requires an AFO and ambulatory aid for safe walking.

C. Refer this patient immediately for ENMG assessment with request for specific information to justify physical therapy intervention and patient education.

D. All of the above.

ANSWERS

20.1 **C.** The patient's pain is more severe than anticipated and in a distribution that would not be expected after knee surgery and might lead to a medical diagnosis of "chronic pain syndrome." It is important to rule out referred pain in the S1 distribution from hip pathology. If the hip, perineal, and limb pain are secondary to a verifiable S1 spinal nerve problem, surgical intervention can be directed to resolution of the S1 spinal nerve. If there is no S1 spinal nerve pattern and there is unilateral evidence of hip degeneration on the painful side, surgical attention to the hip is appropriate. In the absence of ENMG assessment, patients with hip pain may undergo hip arthroplasty and experience no relief of their pain. With adequate ENMG assessment, the etiology of the pain could be narrowed to S1 spinal nerve compromise. Although older individuals often have degenerative changes in their hips, their pain may be coming from an S1 nerve compromise and not from degenerative hip pathology.

20.2 **B.** Electrical stimulation for pain modulation has been successful with a variety of different waveforms. It is reasonable to place cutaneous electrodes near the source of pain or proximally along the nerve pathway in order to affect the neurons supplying the structures in the area of injury (skin, muscle, and joint). Although there may be a 1- to 2-hour period of carry-over in pain relief, ES must be available to the patient around the clock for optimal pain modulation.

20.3 **B.** The patient who walks on a flexed knee can only do so with strong quadriceps because of the increased demands on the knee extensors with maintained knee flexion in the closed kinetic chain (options A and D). Significant weakness of the soleus and other calf muscles results in inadequate tibial control in single limb support. In the presence of calf weakness, it is essential to perform strength testing on other muscles in the S1 myotome, including one muscle from different proximal and distal peripheral nerves.

20.4 **D.** Now is the time for the acute care therapist to document the potential S1 spinal nerve pattern and to refer for ENMG assessment with a request for specific information to justify physical therapy intervention (now and in the future). The acute care therapist sets the stage for intervention throughout the rehabilitation period. Acute inpatient hospital stays do not permit complete patient assessment for rehabilitation, but accurate screening and referral may be critical to patient success in the long term.

REFERENCES

1. Merskey H, Bogduk N. *Classification of Chronic Pain: Description of Chronic Pain Syndromes and Definition of Pain Terms.* Seattle: IASP Press; 1994.

2. Chu-Andrews J, Johnson RJ. *Electrodiagnosis: An Anatomical and Clinical Approach.* Philadelphia: JB Lippincott; 1986.

3. Dumitru D, Amato AA, Zwarts MJ. *Electrodiagnostic Medicine.* 2nd ed. Philadelphia: Hanley & Belfus, Inc.; 2002.

4. Johnson E, Pease JW, eds. *Practical Electromyography.* 3rd ed. Baltimore: Williams & Wilkins; 1997.

5. Kendall HO, Kendall FP, Wadsworth GE. *Muscles, Testing and Function.* 2nd ed. Baltimore: Williams & Wilkins; 1971.

6. Hislop JH, Montgomery J. *Daniels and Worthingham's Muscle Testing: Techniques of Manual Examination.* 8th ed. St. Louis: Saunders Elsevier; 2007.

7. Sumner AJ. *The Physiology of Peripheral Nerve Disease.* Philadelphia: WB Saunders, 1980.

8. Sunderland SS. *Nerves and Nerve Injuries.* Edinburgh: Churchill Livingstone; 1978.

9. Haymaker W, Woodhall B. *Peripheral Nerve Injuries: Principles of Diagnosis.* Philadelphia: WB Saunders; 1953.

10. Johnson EW, ed. *Practical Electromyography.* Baltimore: Williams & Wilkins; 1980.

11. Melzack R, Wall PD. Pain mechanisms: a new theory. *Science.* 1965;150:971-978.

12. Wall PD, Sweet WH. Temporary abolition of pain in man. *Science.* 1967;155:108-109.

13. Fields HL, Basbaum AI. Central nervous system mechanisms of pain modulation. In: Wall PD, Melzack R, eds. *Textbook of Pain.* 3rd ed. New York: Churchill Livingstone; 1999:243-257.

14. Chapman CR, Wilson ME, Gehrig JD. Comparative effects of acupuncture and transcutaneous stimulation on the perception of painful dental stimuli. *Pain.* 1976;2:265-283.

15. Salar G, Job I, Mingrino S, Bosio A, Trabucchi M. Effect of transcutaneous electrotherapy on CSF beta-endorphin content in patients without pain problems. *Pain.* 1981;10:169-172.

16. McMahon SB, Koltzenberg M. *Textbook of Pain.* 5th ed. Edinburgh: Churchill Livingstone; 2006.

17. Loeser JD, Butler SHC, Chapman R, Turk DC. *Bonica's Management of Pain.* Philadelphia: Lippincott Williams & Wilkins; 2001.

18. Deyo RA, Walsh NE, Martin DC, Schoenfeld LS, Ramamurthy S. A controlled trial of transcutaneous electrical nerve stimulation (TENS) and exercise for chronic low back pain. *N Eng J Med.* 1990;322:1627-1634.

19. Grimmer KA. A controlled double blind study comparing the effects of strong burse mode TENS and high rate TENS on painful osteoarthritic knees. *Austral J Physiother.* 1992;48:49-56.

20. Johnson MI, Ashton CH, Thrompson JW. An in-depth study of long-term users of transcutaneous electrical nerve stimulation (TENS): implications for clinical use of TENS. *Pain.* 1991;44: 221-229.

21. Khadilkar A, Odebiyi DO, Brosseau L, Wells GA. Transcutaneous electrical nerve stimulation (TENS) versus placebo for chronic low-back pain. *Cochrane Database Syst Rev.* 2008;4:CD003008.

22. Robinson AJ, Snyder-Mackler L. *Clinical Electrophysiology*. 3rd ed. Baltimore, MD: Lippincott Williams & Wilkins; 2008.

23. Bowman BR, Baker LL. Effects of waveform parameters on comfort during transcutaneous neuromuscular electrical stimulation. *Ann Biomed Eng*. 1985;13:59-74.

24. Liveson JA, Spielholz NI. *Peripheral Neurology: Case Studies in Electrodiagnosis*. Philadelphia: FA Davis Company; 1979.

25. Goodman CC, Snyder TEK. *Differential Diagnosis for Physical Therapists: Screening for Referral*. St. Louis: Saunders Elsevier; 2007.

26. Sharrard WJ. The distribution of the permanent paralysis in the lower limb in poliomyelitis: a clinical and pathological study. *J Bone Joint Surg Br*. 1955;37B:540-548.

27. Perry J, Burnfield JM. *Gait Analysis: Normal and Pathological Function*. 2nd ed. Thorofare, NJ, Slack Inc.; 2010.

28. Hoppenfeld S. *Physical Examination of the Spine and Extremities*. New York: Appleton-Century-Crofts; 1976.

29. Maynard FM Jr, Bracken MB, Creasey G, et al. International standards for neurological and functional classification of spinal cord injury. *Spinal Cord*. 1997;35:266-274.

30. Magee DJ. *Orthopedic Physical Assessment*. 5th ed. St. Louis: Saunders Elsevier; 2008.

31. Herbison GJ, Jaweed MM, Ditunno JF Jr. Exercise therapies in peripheral neuropathies. *Arch Phys Med Rehabil*. 1983;64:201-205.

32. Thompson W, Jansen JK. The extent of sprouting of remaining motor units in partly denervated immature and adult rat soleus muscle. *Neuroscience*. 1977;2:523-535.

33. Desmedt JE, ed. Motor unit types, recruitment and plasticity in health and disease. *Progress in Clinical Neurophysiology*. Volume 9. Basel: S. Karger; 1981.

34. Lieber RL. *Skeletal Muscle Structure, Function & Plasticity: The Physiological Basis of Rehabilitation*. 2nd ed. Philadelphia: Lippincott Williams & Wilkins; 2002.

35. Sanes JR. Axon guidance during reinnervation of skeletal muscle. *Trends in Neurosci*. 1985;8:523-528.

36. Paz JC, West MP. *Acute Care Handbook For Physical Therapists*. 2nd ed. Boston: Butterworth Heinemann; 2002.

37. Goodman CC, Fuller KS. *Pathology–Implications for the Physical Therapist*. 3rd ed. St. Louis: Saunders Elsevier; 2009.

38. Panus PC, Katzung B, Jobst EE, Tinsley SL, Masters SB, Trevor AJ. *Pharmacology for the Physical Therapist*. New York, McGraw Hill Medical; 2009.

39. Ciccone CD. *Pharmacology in Rehabilitation*. 3rd ed. Philadelphia: F.A. Davis; 2002.

Vertebral Compression Fracture

Karen Kemmis

CASE 21

A 72-year-old Caucasian female was admitted to the hospital 4 days ago with complaints of severe back pain. The pain developed suddenly after lifting her 1-year-old granddaughter (21 lb) over her head. Radiographs show acute, moderate vertebral compression fracture at T7 and minor compression fractures at T6 and T8, which do not appear to be acute. Previous medical history includes hysterectomy with oophorectomy at age 43 years, left wrist fracture 20 years ago following a fall when she tripped on a broken sidewalk, right hip and lumbar pain due to osteoarthritis, and hyperlipidemia controlled with atorvastatin (20 mg daily). She had been managing pain in her back and hip with ibuprofen (400 mg taken on an as needed basis). She has never had an evaluation for osteoporosis or a bone density test by dual x-ray absorptiometry. After her discharge home from the hospital, she consults an endocrinologist for an osteoporosis evaluation. The physical therapist is asked to evaluate and treat the patient before discharge in 2 days, when she returns to her two-level home where she lives with her husband. The orthopaedic surgeon did not provide any precautions to movement and she is permitted to ambulate within pain tolerance. She currently reports a pain level of 7/10 on the numerical rating scale (NRS) in the region of T7. She also reports pain in her right hip when weightbearing (2/10). Upon admission, she was placed on morphine using a patient-controlled analgesia (PCA) pump. She experienced adverse drug reactions (ADRs) including lightheadedness, a feeling of being off-balance, nausea, and constipation. She requested to stop the "strong" pain medications in favor of other medications and non-pharmacological pain management. Prior to this incident, she was very active, participating in water aerobics twice weekly and playing doubles tennis once weekly.

▶ What are the examination priorities?
▶ What are the most appropriate physical therapy outcome measures for anthropometrics, posture, gait, and balance?
▶ What are the most appropriate physical therapy interventions?
▶ What precautions should be taken during the physical therapy examination and interventions?

► What are possible complications interfering with physical therapy?

► How would this individual's contextual factors influence or change your patient/client management?

► Based on her health condition, what do you anticipate will be the contributors to activity limitations?

KEY DEFINITIONS

DUAL X-RAY ABSORPTIOMETRY (DXA): Imaging technique for measuring bone mineral density; gold standard and most commonly used technique for the diagnosis of osteoporosis

HYSTERECTOMY WITH OOPHERECTOMY: Surgical removal of the uterus and ovaries

OSTEOPOROSIS: Disease in which there is porous bone, low bone mass, and disruption of bone architecture and strength that leads to an increased risk of fractures

VERTEBRAL COMPRESSION FRACTURE: Broken bone in the spine; common site of fracture in individuals with osteoporosis; the fracture may be clinical or morphometric (identified by a change in shape of a bone rather than from pain or other symptoms)

Objectives

1. Identify risk factors for osteoporosis.

2. Select key tests and measures to be included in the examination of a person with osteoporosis and acute vertebral compression fracture.

3. Describe movement precautions for a person with osteoporosis and vertebral fracture(s).

4. Identify interventions to address impairments and functional limitations for a person with osteoporosis and vertebral fracture.

5. Prescribe an appropriate home exercise program for a person with osteoporosis.

Physical Therapy Considerations

PT considerations during management of the individual with osteoporosis and vertebral fracture:

► **General physical therapy plan of care/goals:** Decrease pain; improve gait and balance to decrease the risk of falls; improve postural control and body mechanics to decrease the risk of subsequent vertebral fractures; maximize safe return to previous activities including exercise programs; improve quality of life

▶ **Physical therapy interventions:** Patient education regarding osteoporosis, risk of fractures and complications; posture and body mechanics instruction to decrease the risk of vertebral fractures; initiate a safe and effective exercise program

▶ **Precautions during physical therapy:** Spinal movement precautions, supervision to decrease risk of falls

▶ **Complications interfering with physical therapy:** Pain, balance dysfunction, ADRs of medications

Understanding the Health Condition

Osteoporosis is a disease characterized by low bone mass, deterioration of bone tissue, and disruption of bone architecture leading to decreased bone strength and an increased risk of fracture. The World Health Organization (WHO) defines osteoporosis in terms of bone mineral density (BMD) measured by DXA at the hip or spine that is ≥ 2.5 standard deviations below the young normal mean reference population (healthy 30-year-old). A DXA measurement of 1 to 2.5 standard deviations below the reference mean is considered low bone density or osteopenia. Osteoporosis can be assumed clinically if a person sustains a low-trauma fracture (considered a fracture sustained from standing height or less). An estimated 10 million Americans have osteoporosis and 33.6 million have low BMD, placing them at risk of developing osteoporosis. Over the age of 50 years, the risk of osteoporosis-related fracture is approximately one out of two and one out of five for Caucasian women and men, respectively. The most common sites of osteoporotic fracture are the vertebrae, hip, and distal forearm.[1]

There are many **risk factors** for osteoporosis and osteoporotic fractures including lifestyle factors such as low calcium and vitamin D intake, inadequate physical activity, excessive alcohol intake, smoking, and falling. Other risks include endocrine disorders and gastrointestinal disorders (causing malabsorption of vitamins and minerals); family history of hip fracture; and use of certain medications (e.g., glucocorticoids, anticonvulsants, anticoagulants, and chemotherapeutic drugs).[1] A person's risk of fracture can be estimated by using FRAX, a tool developed by the WHO that integrates known risk factors and bone density of the femoral neck by DXA to determine an individual's 10-year probability of a hip or major osteoporotic fracture (http://www.shef.ac.uk/FRAX/). When using FRAX, it is important to choose the appropriate geographic region of residence and ethnic background of the individual (when available) for the most accurate estimation of fracture risk. Significant risk factors used in the algorithm include age (risk increases with age), sex (females have greater risk across the lifespan), weight and height (low body mass index increases risk), previous fracture (including morphometric vertebral fracture), parental history of a fractured hip, current smoking, glucocorticoid use (ever used ≥ 5 mg/day of oral prednisone for ≥ 3 months), rheumatoid arthritis, secondary osteoporosis, alcohol intake of three or more drinks per day, and low femoral neck bone density.[2] Increasing thoracic kyphosis has also been shown to be an independent risk factor for future fractures. A prospective study of community-dwelling women, aged 47 to 92 years, showed that an increasing thoracic kyphosis was associated with future fractures (spine or extremity) even after controlling for low BMD and history of fracture.[3]

Vertebral fractures have many consequences including loss of height and an increased thoracic kyphosis that can worsen over time; breathing difficulties, abdominal pains and digestive discomfort; decreased quality of life, mobility, and energy; pain and deterioration of physical function; and increased long-term morbidity and mortality.[4-9] Many vertebral fractures are asymptomatic—more than two-thirds of vertebral compression fractures are not detected by the individual.[10] In the year following a vertebral fracture, almost 20% of women experience another vertebral fracture.[11] Women with osteoporosis and thoracic hyperkyphosis have reduced muscle strength and increased body sway, gait unsteadiness, and increased risk of falls.[12] Katzman et al.[13] found that increasing thoracic kyphosis in community-dwelling elderly women was associated with worsening mobility, demonstrated by slower performance on the Timed Up and Go test. The majority of research on vertebral fractures has been done with women; however, it is likely that similar results would be found in men.

While several risks for osteoporosis are not modifiable (*e.g.*, sex, age, personal and family history), it is still possible to reduce the risk of osteoporosis and fracture. Primary prevention can be achieved by determining an individual's risk of osteoporosis and fracture and improving bone health with adequate calcium and vitamin D, weightbearing and muscle-strengthening exercises, avoidance of tobacco use and excessive alcohol intake, and treatment of other specific risk factors for falls and fracture. A wrist fracture is often the first indication that a person has osteoporosis.[1] Unfortunately, the majority of individuals who sustain a wrist fracture are not educated about osteoporosis and do not receive a BMD evaluation or initiate treatment for osteoporosis. The American Academy of Orthopaedic Surgeons and the National Osteoporosis Foundation have teamed up for a campaign to increase awareness and improve early diagnosis and education on decreasing osteoporosis progression and fracture risk reduction. Physical therapists can facilitate this process through patient education. Once an individual has been diagnosed with osteoporosis, she is advised to start or continue preventative lifestyle changes and consider pharmacological interventions. Since **most osteoporotic fractures are the result of a fall,** fall prevention strategies should be included for all individuals with osteoporosis.[1]

Physical Therapy Patient/Client Management

There are several appropriate interventions for an individual with osteoporosis and acute vertebral fracture. A comprehensive examination and evaluation guides the chosen interventions. Possible treatments include modalities to manage pain, therapeutic exercise, functional training (while maintaining a neutral spine) and prescription of an assistive device to decrease stress on the spine and the risk of falls. The patient may benefit from consultation with an orthopaedic surgeon or interventional radiologist for surgical intervention (kyphoplasty or vertebroplasty), an endocrinologist or other physician who specializes in osteoporosis to initiate the medical work-up to determine whether the patient has primary or secondary osteoporosis, and an occupational therapist to prescribe devices to aid in activities of daily living (including dressing and toileting). The patient may also benefit from psychological support to manage pain and decreased function and to help deal with the diagnosis of this disease. Prior to discharge, the patient should be able to demonstrate safe movements that decrease the likelihood of future fractures. She should be able to verbalize or demonstrate safe exercises for posture, body mechanics, improved bone health, and to maximize return to her activities of daily living and recreational activities.

Examination, Evaluation, and Diagnosis

The physical therapist should conduct a chart review prior to the examination. Important information includes medical and surgical history, medications, movement or exercise precautions, living environment, and prior functional status in self-care, home activities, and job and leisure activities. Prior to the examination, the therapist should assess the patient's pain level, any reports of lightheadedness or dizziness, and understanding of movement precautions. Vital signs (blood pressure, heart rate, respiratory rate) should be evaluated at rest and as indicated during the examination and interventions. Pain can be assessed using a NRS by asking the patient to report her level of pain from 0 (no pain) to 10 (the worst pain imaginable).

The extent of the examination is based on the patient's tolerance to activity. Bed mobility, the need for an assistive device, and pain must be addressed. Further examination of this patient could include an accurate height measurement, kyphotic index (KI) using a surveyor's flexible ruler, gait, balance, and body mechanics.

Non-invasive techniques such as height and the kyphotic index can help the physical therapist to determine whether an individual has a new vertebral compression fracture or clinical kyphosis. Height should be measured using a wall-mounted stadiometer, which has been shown to be accurate for serial height measurements. A stadiometer consists of a vertical ruler with an attached rod that rests on the top of the head. A height loss of > 2.0 cm *suggests* a new vertebral compression fracture in those at risk of fractures. This patient should have her height measured routinely to monitor any change warranting a vertebral radiograph to detect a new fracture.[4] The KI is a measurement of the degree of thoracic kyphosis that can be repeated to determine an improvement or worsening of the kyphosis over time. It can be measured using a flexible ruler (available at an art supply store), a washable marker, and graph paper. The patient stands in her best upright posture as the ruler is molded to the spine from the seventh cervical vertebrae to the lumbosacral junction (both of which have been marked with the marker). The therapist places the molded ruler on graph paper, traces the curve, and calculates the thoracic height and width. An instructional video is available from the American Physical Therapy Association Section on Geriatrics.[14] The KI is equal to thoracic width divided by thoracic length multiplied by 100. A clinical kyphosis is defined as a KI ≥ 13.[15] To allow for this measurement, the patient would need to be able to tolerate 5 to 10 minutes of upright standing, though some amount of upper extremity support can be provided (*e.g.*, holding onto the sink or counter in the hospital room).

Gait can be evaluated with the Timed Up and Go (TUG) test. This test is quick, easy to perform, functional, reliable, can be performed with an assistive device, and correlates well with the Berg Balance Scale. Normal values for older adults without disability for the 3-m TUG have been determined by a meta-analysis. The reference values are 8.1, 9.2, and 11.3 seconds for those aged 60 to 69, 70 to 79, and 80 to 99 years, respectively.[16] In addition, the physical therapist can calculate the patient's gait speed.

Since many osteoporotic fractures are the direct result of a fall, static and dynamic balance should be assessed when possible. In the acute care setting, especially if the patient has substantial pain, extensive testing may not be feasible. Static balance can be assessed with a single limb stance test. The test is done with the patient in bare feet. The patient is instructed to stand on one foot for as long as possible. The test is stopped if the standing foot is displaced, the elevated foot touches the ground, or the elevated lower extremity braces the standing leg. Community-dwelling adults (≥ 50 years of age) who had fallen in the previous year had a stance time of 9.6 seconds, compared to 31.3 seconds in those who had not fallen.[17] In a meta-analysis, normal single leg stance times were 27.0, 17.2, and 8.5 seconds in people aged 60 to 69, 70 to 79, and 80 to 89, respectively.[18] Due to high levels of pain (7/10 on NRS), this patient would likely not tolerate dynamic balance testing (i.e., Berg Balance Scale and Dynamic Gait Index) at this time, but these would be beneficial tests in the future.

Body mechanics can be examined through observation of common tasks. Activities may include bed mobility, transfers, ambulation, self-care (donning and doffing pants, undergarments, socks, and shoes), and simulations of home management (e.g., leaning as if reaching into a car trunk, oven, clothes dryer, or dishwasher) and community activities (e.g., twisting while sitting as if backing out of a parking space or driveway in the car). Since this patient sustained a vertebral fracture playing with her granddaughter, simulated childcare activities could also be examined.

Once the appropriate tests and measures are performed in the examination, the physical therapist can move onto evaluation, diagnosis, and prognosis. Some considerations for this patient are her high levels of pain, results of the tests and measures, and the impact of a new diagnosis of osteoporosis. The physical therapy diagnosis for this patient, according to the *Guide to Physical Therapist Practice*, may include impairment associated with fracture, impairment associated with a spinal disorder, and/or risk reduction for skeletal demineralization based on the pathological fracture and/or impaired posture due to an acquired kyphosis or kyphoscoliosis.[19] Her prognosis is good given her prior activity level and the expectation that the acute pain from the vertebral fracture usually resolves within 6 to 12 weeks.[20] Minimizing complications during the first several weeks and providing education for safe movement and continued exercise improves the prognosis.

Plan of Care and Interventions

In a recent systematic review on conservative care for osteoporotic vertebral fractures over the past 45 years, there is a consensus for the following interventions:

short period of bedrest, pain medication, bracing, and physical therapy.[20] Specific physical therapy interventions include early mobilization, education in safe movements, posture exercises to decrease thoracic kyphosis, strengthening to improve spinal alignment, and fall prevention strategies. There is controversy over the use of vertebral augmentation techniques such as kyphoplasty and vertebroplasty.[20]

For pain management, acetaminophen or salicylates and nonsteroidal anti-inflammatory drugs (NSAIDs) are preferred over the use of opiate medications that have many ADRs including constipation, urinary retention, respiratory dysfunction, as well as cognitive deficits and balance dysfunction that can increase the risk of falls. Muscle relaxants may provide benefit, but drowsiness and dizziness should be monitored to prevent imbalance and falls. Some osteoporosis-specific medications, including calcitonin, teriparatide, and bisphosphonates, may also be beneficial for pain relief.[20] Options for non-pharmacological interventions for pain management include modalities provided by the physical therapist. There is no evidence to directly support the use of heat, ice, transcutaneous electrical nerve stimulation (TENS) or interferential stimulation to manage pain from a vertebral compression fracture specifically. However, the physical therapist can initiate a trial of a selected modality and assess the patient's pain to determine its efficacy.

Some physicians recommend and prescribe a back brace for the individual with an acute vertebral compression fracture. Back braces (orthoses) can inhibit movement of the spine to help manage acute pain and provide support to decrease fatigue of the back muscles. Use of a brace for the initial 6 to 8 weeks may improve the patient's ability to be more active with less pain medication. The brace should be comfortable, easy to don and doff, lightweight, and allow for normal breathing. Common thoracolumbar orthoses (TLO) are often named for the companies that manufacture them. They include the Jewett, the cruciform anterior spinal hyperextension (CASH), the Cheneau thermoplastic brace, the Taylor brace, the Knight-Taylor brace, or a custom-made TLO. The brace for the patient with a thoracic compression fracture should place the patient in a position of thoracic hyperextension and prevent spinal flexion.[20] Use of a rolling walker may also help the patient by providing support to the thoracic spine through the upper extremities. The physical therapist should instruct the patient in proper upright posture while walking and to avoid lifting the walker, which would place increased stress on the spine. The patient should also be taught to carry items closer to her chest or abdomen, which decreases stress on the spine. Although "lifting precautions" (avoiding lifting > 5-10 lb) are frequently given to individuals with compression fractures, there is no evidence to support that this recommendation decreases the risk of future vertebral compression fractures.

It is important to facilitate early mobilization of the patient while minimizing spinal pain. Instruction in core control exercises can help promote proper contraction of the spine stabilizers. Hodges and Richardson[21,22] have demonstrated that in adults without back pain, the multifidii and abdominal muscles contract prior to upper extremity and lower extremity movement. However, in those with low back pain, there is dysfunctional motor control of the deep spinal stabilizers (*i.e.*, transversus abdominis).[21] Specific stabilizing exercises have been shown to decrease the rate of recurrence of low back pain.[23] Though this work was performed on individuals with lumbar pain, the same principles could be applied to this patient with acute onset thoracic pain. She could be taught to initiate gentle spine stabilization/core control exercises in a comfortable position (*e.g.*, supine hooklying) while maintaining a neutral spine. The therapist could then instruct her how to perform bed mobility, transfers, and ambulation utilizing the core stabilizers to support the spine (with or without a brace).

Education in safe movements—with maintenance of a *neutral spine*—is essential during the acute phase to prepare the patient for a safe hospital discharge. Here, the neutral spine refers to maintaining the natural cervical lordosis, thoracic kyphosis, and lumbar lordosis in an attempt to avoid excessive compression on the vertebral bodies that could contribute to future compression fractures. The therapist examines body mechanics through observation of typical activities for the patient. There is evidence that **spine flexion, rather than extension, is associated with a significantly increased risk of new vertebral compression fractures** in post-menopausal women with osteoporosis. Women who performed seated trunk flexion stretches and abdominal sit-up strengthening exercises for rehabilitation of low back pain had significantly more subsequent vertebral compression fractures (89% with new fractures) compared to those who were prescribed prone back extension and seated scapular retraction exercises (16% with new fractures).[24] Biomechanical evidence has shown that increased thoracic kyphosis, trunk flexion during activities, and holding weights in front of the body place increased stress on the spine.[25,26] The patient should be encouraged to maintain the normal curves of the spine, avoid increases in spinal flexion, hinge and pivot at the hips rather than through the spine, and avoid reaching forward while holding objects. The patient may lack sufficient strength or range of motion in the extremities to allow proper movements, necessitating specific interventions to address these deficits.

Exercises to promote best posture should be initiated as soon as the patient is able to perform them. In a small randomized, single-blind controlled trial, Bennell et al.[27] demonstrated that daily home exercise, manual therapy, and education aimed at improving posture decreased back pain and improved health-related quality of life and physical function in men and women with painful osteoporotic vertebral fracture. Exercises focused on posture correction through stretching the anterior shoulder region and strengthening cervical, upper back, core, and lower extremity musculature. Manual therapy interventions included postural taping, postero-anterior vertebral mobilizations and soft tissue massage to the erector spinae, rhomboids, and upper trapezeii. Though the participants had sustained vertebral fractures 3 months to 5 years previously, suitable techniques could be initiated for this patient based on her tolerance. Having osteoporosis and thoracic hyperkyphosis may decrease balance and increase mobility dysfunction and risk of falls.[12,13] Therefore, fall prevention programs addressing impaired balance, decreased muscle strength, increased thoracic kyphosis, and reduced proprioception should be initiated with this patient when she can tolerate the exercises.

Possible equipment needs at hospital discharge may include a portable TENS unit, rolling walker, shower chair (and grab bars if she is not able to stand without support), raised toilet seat if she is unable to perform sit to stand with neutral spine, and adaptive equipment (e.g., sock aid, long-handled sponge, reacher, toilet aid, and long-handled shoe horn). If the patient has a back brace that is donned in a supine position, her husband may need training to assist her. To allow a safe transfer home, the patient should be instructed in how to perform car transfers with limited spinal flexion and rotation. In some hospital gyms, a car transfer simulator can be used to practice getting in and out of a car seat on either the passenger's side or driver's side. Alternatively, the therapist can use the hospital's drop-off area to practice getting in and out of a car.

Upon discharge, this patient would benefit from a referral for home or out-patient physical therapy to modify and advance a safe exercise progression, pain management strategies, and continuation of fall risk reduction implementation within her home and community. The multicomponent exercise program should focus on impairments, functional limitations, and disabilities associated with the vertebral compression fracture. In general, interventions should include strengthening and stretching to address postural faults, promote safe body mechanics and prevent future vertebral fractures; strength training and weightbearing exercises to maximize bone density at the hip and spine; exercises to improve balance and decrease the risk of falls; and interventions to improve function and quality of life. Home-based exercises focused on strengthening the spine extensor muscles have been shown to prevent the progression of hyperkyphosis in middle-aged women.[28] A community-based, physical therapist-led, group exercise program focused on posture correction exercises resulted in decreased kyphosis and increased spine extensor muscle strength, range of motion, and physical performance in women (age 72.0 ± 4.2 years) with hyperkyphosis.[29] **Progressive back-strengthening exercises** (prone trunk extension with weights on the upper back) performed in post-menopausal women resulted in increased back extensor muscle strength, increased bone density, and decreased incidence of future vertebral compression fractures.[30]

High-intensity exercises (e.g., resistance machines for lateral pulldown, hip extension, knee extension, and trunk strengthening) can improve bone density, balance, muscle mass, and strength in post-menopausal women.[31] In a 2011 Cochrane Review of randomized controlled trials, it was determined that the most effective exercises to attenuate post-menopausal bone density loss at the hip are non-weightbearing progressive resistance strength training; for the spine, combination programs of strength training and weightbearing exercises are the most effective.[32] Once the vertebral fracture has healed and there is minimal to no spine pain, the patient's exercise program should include strength training and weightbearing activities.

A multidimensional home-based exercise program can also improve quality of life measures in older women with osteoporotic vertebral fractures.[33] A 10-week community program including exercises for improving balance and muscle strength (including spine stabilization) decreased pain and the use of analgesic medications and improved function, quality of life, balance, and strength in post-menopausal women with a history of vertebral compression fracture.[34]

Following return home, if this patient's pain persists, she may opt for a vertebral augmentation technique such as kyphoplasty or vertebroplasty. These procedures have been shown to be effective in reducing pain but have associated risks including the possibility of a new fracture in adjacent vertebrae. If the patient does have one of these procedures, she should be encouraged to be vigilant about proper posture and body mechanics and to engage in an exercise program to reduce the risks of future problems.

Evidence-Based Clinical Recommendations

SORT: Strength of Recommendation Taxonomy

A: Consistent, good-quality patient-oriented evidence
B: Inconsistent or limited-quality patient-oriented evidence
C: Consensus, disease-oriented evidence, usual practice, expert opinion, or case series

1. There are several identifiable risk factors to determine a person's risk for osteoporotic fracture. **Grade A**

2. Many osteoporotic fractures of the vertebrae and hip are the direct result of a fall. **Grade A**

3. Physical therapists can use non-invasive techniques (*e.g.*, accurate height measurements and kyphosis index) to identify a possible new vertebral compression fracture or clinical kyphosis. **Grade B**

4. Spine flexion increases the risk of vertebral compression fractures. **Grade C**

5. Exercise helps prevent vertebral compression fractures. **Grade B**

COMPREHENSION QUESTIONS

21.1 Which of the following statements is *not* true about vertebral compression fractures?

   A. A height loss of > 2.0 cm suggests a new vertebral compression fracture in a person at risk of fracture.

   B. A clinical or morphometric vertebral fracture is a clinical indication of osteoporosis.

   C. There is always pain at the initial onset of a vertebral compression fracture.

   D. Vertebral compression fractures increase mortality.

21.2   A physical therapist in the acute care setting receives a referral to see a patient with a new vertebral compression fracture. The patient has moderate levels of pain (5/10) during bed mobility, transfers, and ambulation without an assistive device. Appropriate interventions at this time would include all of the following *except*:

   A.   Instruction in and performance of activities using a neutral spine, including hinging at the hips instead of flexing the spine during activities of daily living

   B.   Gait training with a rolling walker to provide support through the upper extremities for the spine

   C.   Education in the importance of proper posture, body mechanics, and fall prevention strategies to prevent future fractures

   D.   Core strengthening with spine flexion, such as abdominal curl-up exercises to promote spinal stability

ANSWERS

21.1   **C.** The majority of vertebral compression fractures are silent with no symptoms experienced by the patient. Because of this, it is important for a person to understand her risk for osteoporosis and to have annual height assessments to determine a loss of height that indicates the possibility of a new vertebral fracture. If the person has substantial decrease in height, a radiographic examination may be indicated to diagnose vertebral fracture(s). If a person is at risk for osteoporosis, she should take steps to promote bone health and decrease the risk of fracture including lifestyle changes and safe movements during activities and exercise.

21.2   **D.** Activities should be done with the spine in a neutral position to avoid compression on vertebral bodies. Gentle core stability exercises may be indicated for this patient but should be done with the spine in a neutral position. This is typically achieved with the patient in supine with knees flexed, on a comfortable surface. Flexion movements of the spine such as abdominal curl-ups are associated with an increased risk of future vertebral compression fractures.[23]

REFERENCES

1.   National Osteoporosis Foundation. Clinician's Guide to Prevention and Treatment of Osteoporosis. Available at: http://www.nof.org/professionals/clinical-guidelines. Accessed May 24, 2012.

2.   FRAX® WHO Fracture Risk Assessment Tool. Available at: http://www.shef.ac.uk/FRAX/. Accessed December 14, 2011.

3.   Huang MH, Barrett-Connor E, Greendale GA, Kado DM. Hyperkyphotic posture and risk of future osteoporotic fractures: the Rancho Bernardo study. *J Bone Miner Res.* 2006;21:419-423.

4.   Siminoski K, Jiang G, Adachi JD, et al. Accuracy of height loss during prospective monitoring for detection of incident vertebral fractures. *Osteoporos Int.* 2005;16:403-410.

5. Cortet B, Roches E, Logier R, et al. Evaluation of spinal curvatures after a recent osteoporotic vertebral fracture. *Joint Bone Spine.* 2002;69:201-208.

6. Fechtenbaum J, Cropet C, Kolta S, Horlait S, Orcel P, Roux C. The severity of vertebral fractures and health-related quality of life in osteoporotic postmenopausal women. *Osteoporos Int.* 2005;16:2175-2179.

7. Cortet B, Houvenagel E, Puisieux F, Roches E, Garnier P, Delcambre B. Spinal curvatures and quality of life in women with vertebral fractures secondary to osteoporosis. *Spine.* 1999;24:1921-1925.

8. Oleksik AM, Ewing S, Shen W, van Schoor NM, Lips P. Impact of incident vertebral fractures on health related quality of life (HRQOL) in postmenopausal women with prevalent vertebral fractures. *Osteoporos Int.* 2005;16:861-870.

9. Hasserius R, Karlsson MK, Jonsson B, Redlund-Johnell I, Johnell O. Long-term morbidity and mortality after a clinically diagnosed vertebral fracture in the elderly—a 12- and 22-year follow-up of 257 patients. *Calcif Tissue Int.* 2005;76:235-242.

10. Cummings SR, Melton LJ. Epidemiology and outcomes of osteoporotic fractures. *Lancet.* 2002;359: 1761-1767.

11. Lindsay R, Silverman SL, Cooper C, et al. Risk of new vertebral fracture in the year following a fracture. *JAMA.* 2001;285:320-323.

12. Sinaki M, Brey RH, Hughes CA, Larson DR, Kaufman KR. Balance disorder and increased risk of falls in osteoporosis and kyphosis: significance of kyphotic posture and muscle strength. *Osteoporos Int.* 2005;16:1004-1010.

13. Katzman WB, Vittinghoff E, Ensrud K, Black DM, Kado DM. Increasing kyphosis predicts worsening mobility in older community-dwelling women: a prospective cohort study. *J Am Geriatr Soc.* 2011;59:96-100.

14. APTA Section on Geriatrics Instructional Video: Kypholordosis Measurement Using a Flexible Curve. Available at: http://www.geriatricspt.org/store/index.cfm?carttoken=0&action=ViewDetails&itemid=13709. Accessed December 28, 2011.

15. Chow RK, Harrison JE. Relationship of kyphosis to physical fitness and bone mass on postmenopausal women. *Am J Phys Med.* 1987;66:219-227.

16. Bohannon RW. Reference values for the Timed Up and Go Test: a descriptive meta-analysis. *J Geriatr Phys Ther.* 2006;29:64-68.

17. Hurvitz EA, Richardson JK, Werner RA, Ruhl AM, Dixon MR. Unipedal stance testing as an indicator of fall risk among older outpatients. *Arch Phys Med Rehabil.* 2000;81:587-591.

18. Bohannon RW. Single limb stance times: a descriptive meta-analysis of data from individuals at least 60 years of age. *Topics in Geriatr Rehab.* 2006;22:70-77.

19. American Physical Therapy Association. Guide to Physical Therapist Practice, 2nd ed. *Phys Ther.* 2001;81:9-746.

20. Longo UG, Loppini M, Denaro L, Maffulli N, Denaro V. Osteoporotic vertebral fractures: current concepts of conservative care. *Br Med Bull.* 2011; Nov 29. [Epub ahead of print]

21. Hodges PW, Richardson CA. Inefficient muscular stabilization of the lumbar spine associated with low back pain. A motor control evaluation of transversus abdominis. *Spine.* 1996;21:2640-2650.

22. Hodges PW, Richardson CA. Contraction of the abdominal muscles associated with movement of the lower limb. *Phys Ther.* 1997;77:132-142.

23. Hides JA, Jull GA, Richardson CA. Long-term effects of specific stabilizing exercises for first-episode low back pain. *Spine.* 2001;26:E243-E248.

24. Sinaki M, Mikkelsen BA. Postmenopausal spinal osteoporosis: flexion versus extension exercises. *Arch Phys Med Rehabil.* 1984;65:593-596.

25. Briggs AM, van Dieën JH, Wrigley TV, et al. Thoracic kyphosis affects spinal loads and trunk muscle force. *Phys Ther.* 2007;87:595-607.

26. Schultz AB, Andersson GBJ, Haderspeck K, Ortengren R, Nordin M, Bjork R. Analysis and measurement of lumbar trunk loads in tasks involving bends and twists. *J Biomech.* 1982;15:669-675.

27. Bennell KL, Matthews B, Greig A, et al. Effects of an exercise and manual therapy program on physical impairments, function and quality-of-life in people with osteoporotic vertebral fracture: a randomised, single-blind controlled pilot trial. *BMC Musculoskelet Disord.* 2010;11:36.

28. Ball JM, Cagle P, Johnson BE, Lucasey C, Lukert BP. Spinal extension exercises prevent natural progression of kyphosis. *Osteoporos Int.* 2009;20:481-489.

29. Katzman WB, Sellmeyer DE, Stewart AL, Wanek L, Hamel KA. Changes in flexed posture, musculoskeletal impairments, and physical performance after group exercise in community-dwelling older women. *Arch Phys Med Rehabil.* 2007;88:192-199.

30. Sinaki M, Itoi E, Wahner HW, et al. Stronger back muscles reduce the incidence of vertebral fractures: a prospective 10 year follow-up of postmenopausal women. *Bone.* 2002;30:836-841.

31. Nelson ME, Fiatarone MA, Morganti CM, Trice I, Greenberg RA, Evans WJ. Effects of high-intensity strength training on multiple risk factors for osteoporotic fractures. A randomized controlled trial. *JAMA.* 1994;272:1909-1914.

32. Howe TE, Shea B, Dawson LJ, et al. Exercise for preventing and treating osteoporosis in postmenopausal women. *Cochrane Database of Syst Rev.* 2011;Jul 6(7):CD000333.

33. Papaioannou A, Adachi JD, Winegard K, et al. Efficacy of home-based exercise for improving quality of life among elderly women with symptomatic osteoporosis-related vertebral fractures. *Osteoporos Int.* 2003;14:677-682.

34. Malmros B, Mortensen L, Jensen MB, Charles P. Positive effects of physiotherapy on chronic pain and performance in osteoporosis. *Osteoporos Int.* 1998;8:215-221.

Pressure Ulcer

Rose Hamm

A 39-year-old female was transferred from another hospital 4 days after an automobile accident resulting in an incomplete spinal cord injury (SCI) at C5-6 and a burst fracture at T5. She was transferred to the current hospital for neurosurgery to decompress and stabilize her spine. Upon the current admission, she was found to have a suspected deep tissue injury (SDTI) in the sacral area. After 2 days, it progressed to an unstageable pressure ulcer (PU). On the third day (1 week after her initial accident), the patient had spine surgery. On postoperative day 1 (POD 1), the physical therapist is asked to evaluate and treat the sacral pressure ulcer. The patient is married, lives with her husband and two children in a two-story home, and works part-time as a paralegal.

▶ Based on the patient's diagnosis, what do you anticipate may be the contributing factors to the pressure ulcer?
▶ What is the role of rehabilitation in optimizing healing potential?
▶ What are the most appropriate interventions?
▶ Identify referrals to other medical team members.

KEY DEFINITIONS

BURST FRACTURE: Comminuted fracture of the vertebral body that results in bone fragments that may scatter and damage surrounding tissue

INCOMPLETE SPINAL CORD INJURY: Injury that does not completely sever the spinal cord, resulting in partial sensory and/or motor function below the neurological level of injury, including some function of the lowest sacral segment

SUSPECTED DEEP TISSUE INJURY (SDTI): Localized area of discolored purple or maroon intact skin or blood-filled blister due to damage of underlying soft tissue from pressure and/or shear; may be preceded by tissue that is painful, firm, mushy, boggy, warmer, or cooler as compared to adjacent tissue[1]

UNSTAGEABLE PRESSURE ULCER: Full thickness tissue loss in which the base of the ulcer is covered by slough (yellow, tan, gray, green, or brown) and/or eschar (tan, brown, or black) in the wound bed[1]

Objectives

1. Perform a subjective and objective evaluation of a patient with a pressure ulcer.

2. Diagnose a pressure ulcer by depth of tissue involvement and accurately stage according to the National Pressure Ulcer Advisory Panel (NPUAP) Staging Classification.

3. Identify special equipment needed to facilitate wound healing.

4. Develop a strategy to eliminate contributing factors based on patient and wound evaluation.

5. Implement appropriate strategies to prevent other lesions from developing.

6. Select appropriate pressure redistribution surfaces for a patient with a pressure ulcer.

7. Develop a treatment plan to optimize wound healing including debridement method, dressing selection, and biophysical technologies.

8. Describe the focus of patient and family education for the individual with pressure ulcers.

9. Recommend appropriate care after discharge from the acute care setting.

Physical Therapy Considerations

PT considerations during management of the individual with a pressure ulcer:

▶ **General physical therapy plan of care/goals:** Prevent further tissue loss at wound site; optimize wound healing with debridement, moist wound healing, and biophysical modalities; educate patient, family, and/or caregivers to perform repositioning to help off-load wound location; prevent infection; optimize function without causing friction or shear to wound site; select appropriate pressure redistribution surface to enhance wound healing

▶ **Physical therapy interventions:** Patient, family, and/or caregiver education on contributing factors and strategies to eliminate those factors, especially repositioning and proper transfer techniques; debridement of necrotic tissue; appropriate dressing selection to maintain moisture balance, decrease bacterial load, and protect wound from external environment; apply biophysical technologies (*e.g.*, ultrasound, negative pressure, electrical stimulation) to enhance wound healing

▶ **Precautions during physical therapy:** Infection precautions, spine precautions, positioning for off-loading, moisture management (from wound and from incontinence), pain management

▶ **Complications interfering with physical therapy:** Protein energy malnutrition, adverse drug reactions (ADRs), immobility, decreased sensation, strength and range of motion deficits, aspiration precautions, comorbidities, poor blood glucose control

Understanding the Health Condition

In 2004, the Centers for Medicare and Medicaid Service (CMS) initiated "present on admission" standards for hospitals and long-term care facilities that resulted in increased awareness that all healthcare professionals in these facilities are responsible for prevention and treatment of pressure ulcers. The CMS standard states: "Based on the comprehensive assessment of an individual, the facility must ensure that an individual who enters the facility without pressure sores does not develop pressure sores unless the individual's clinical condition demonstrates that they were unavoidable."[2] As a result, full thickness pressure ulcers classified as stage III or IV (Table 22-1) became part of a list of "never-events," meaning that pressure ulcers should never occur on patients for whom they are reasonably preventable.[2] While CMS regulations have certainly improved education provided to healthcare professionals and preventive measures in all settings, the national prevalence of pressure ulcers in acute care facilities averages 14% to 17%[3] and the incidence in acute care facilities was reported as 7% in 2000.[4] The latter statistic is especially troubling because it indicates that 7% of individuals admitted to an acute care facility acquired pressure ulcers *during* that hospital stay, so preventive measures have not been 100% effective.

A PU is defined by the NPUAP as "a localized injury to the skin and/or underlying tissue usually over a bony prominence, as a result of pressure, or pressure in combination with shear and/or friction."[1] The contributing factors to the development of pressure ulcers include pressure, shear, friction, and moisture. Understanding how each of these forces affects tissue and causes necrosis is important in both prevention and treatment of pressure ulcers.

Pressure is the force per unit area exerted perpendicular to any surface of an object. A perpendicular force over (or under) a bony surface results in injury to the deep soft tissue directly adjacent to the bony prominence. However, this initial injury may not immediately surface to the more superficial skin layers and thus may not be observable upon skin assessment until days after the initial injury occurs. An example of this kind of pressure occurs over the ischial tuberosity of a person who

Table 22-1 INTERNATIONAL NPUAP-EPUAP PRESSURE ULCER CLASSIFICATION SYSTEM[10]

Category/stage I: nonblanchable erythema	Intact skin with nonblanchable redness of a localized area usually over a bony prominence. Darkly pigmented skin may not have visible blanching; its color may differ from the surrounding area. The area may be painful, firm, soft, warmer or cooler as compared to adjacent tissue. Category/stage I may be difficult to detect in individuals with dark skin tones. May indicate "at risk" persons.
Category/stage II: partial thickness skin loss	Partial thickness loss of dermis presenting as a shallow open ulcer with a red or pink wound bed, without slough. May also present as an intact or open/ruptured serum-filled blister. Presents as a shiny or dry shallow ulcer without slough or bruising.* This category/stage should not be used to describe skin tears, tape burns, perineal dermatitis, maceration, or excoriation. *Bruising indicates suspected deep tissue injury.
Category/stage III: full thickness skin loss	Full thickness tissue loss. Subcutaneous fat may be visible but bone, tendon, or muscle is not exposed. Slough may be present but does not obscure the depth of tissue loss. May include undermining and tunneling. Depth of a category/stage III pressure ulcer varies by anatomical location. The bridge of the nose, ear, occiput, and malleolus do not have subcutaneous tissue and category/stage III ulcers can be shallow. In contrast, areas of significant adiposity can develop extremely deep category/stage III pressure ulcers. Bone/tendon is not visible or directly palpable.
Category/stage IV: full thickness tissue loss	Full thickness tissue loss with exposed bone, tendon, or muscle. Slough or eschar may be present on some parts of the wound bed. Often include undermining and tunneling. Depth of a category/stage IV pressure ulcer varies by anatomical location. The bridge of the nose, ear, occiput, and malleolus do not have subcutaneous tissue and these ulcers can be shallow. Category/stage IV ulcers can extend into muscle and/or supporting structures (*e.g.*, fascia, tendon, or joint capsule), making osteomyelitis possible. Exposed bone/tendon is visible or directly palpable.
Unstageable: depth unknown	Full thickness tissue loss in which the base of the ulcer is covered by slough (yellow, tan, gray, green, or brown) and/or eschar (tan, brown, or black) in the wound bed. Until enough slough and/or eschar is removed to expose the base of the wound, the true depth, and therefore category/stage, cannot be determined. Stable (dry, adherent, intact without erythema or fluctuance) eschar on the heels serves as "the body's natural (biological) cover" and should not be removed.
Suspected deep tissue injury: depth unknown	Purple or maroon localized area of discolored intact skin or blood-filled blister due to damage of underlying soft tissue from pressure and/or shear. The area may be preceded by tissue that is painful, firm, mushy, boggy, warmer, or cooler as compared to adjacent tissue. Deep tissue injury may be difficult to detect in individuals with dark skin tones. Evolution may include a thin blister over a dark wound bed. The wound may further evolve and become covered by thin eschar. Evolution may be rapid exposing additional layers of tissue even with optimal treatment.

spends long periods of time in a wheelchair without a cushion or without other means of pressure relief and/or redistribution. The amount of time required for tissue necrosis to occur is dependent on both the time and the amount of pressure. For example, a pressure ulcer can result from a low amount of pressure for a long period of time or a high amount of pressure for a short period of time. The time of pressure required to cause tissue damage also depends on the patient's body composition and amount of soft tissue covering the bony prominences. Direct unrelieved pressures four to six times an individual's systolic blood pressure can cause tissue necrosis in less than 1 hour, whereas pressures less than systolic blood pressure may require 12 hours to produce tissue injury.[5]

Shear differs from pressure in that it is force per unit area exerted *parallel* to the surface of an object. Shear tends to occur between bony prominences and soft tissue during sliding activities (*e.g.*, when a patient slides down in bed, performs sliding transfers, or sits with slumping posture in a wheelchair). These shear forces distort capillaries beneath the epidermis, cause interstitial bleeding, and promote hypoxia to deeper tissue. Shear forces tend to create undermining and sinuses in addition to the wound directly over the bony prominence. As with pressure, there may be significant time between the initial tissue injury and observable changes in the skin.

Friction is resistance to motion in a parallel direction when two surfaces rub against each other. Friction causes serum-filled blisters or partial thickness abrasions (*e.g.*, a blister on the heel as it slides up and down on bed linens or in a new shoe). The clear fluid in the blister indicates that there has been superficial injury in the epidermis and/or dermis with an inflammatory response, but there has been no bleeding.

Moisture contributes to wound formation by decreasing the strength of the skin, making it more susceptible to abrasion, and opening portals for bacteria to enter the skin and deeper tissue. The moisture may be from urinary or fecal incontinence, perspiration, wound drainage, or lymphatic weeping.

In addition to the mechanical forces of pressure, shear, friction and moisture, there are intrinsic and extrinsic factors that increase an individual's risk for development of a pressure ulcer. These include protein malnutrition, low body mass index (BMI < 21 with involuntary weight loss[6]), age-related skin changes, hemodynamic instability that is exacerbated with changes of position in bed, dry and cracking skin, immobility, medications, motor and sensory neuropathy, contractures, and the need to wear orthoses or prosthetics.[7] Three specific conditions that place individuals with spinal cord injuries at high risk for PU development are immobility as a result of paralysis below the level of injury, associated sensory loss that prevents detection of increased pressure and tissue injury, and inadequate tissue blood flow as a result of impaired neural and metabolic regulatory mechanisms.[7]

Pressure ulcers are classified according to the depth of tissue injury using a staging system developed by the NPUAP and the European Pressure Ulcer Advisory Panel (EPUAP) that was last revised in 2007 (Table 22-1). Classifying the PU using the criteria, signs, and symptoms listed in the staging system can help the clinician identify the specific mechanism of tissue injury and thereby develop a more effective treatment plan. For example, if the PU presents as a fluid-filled blister, activities that cause friction of that particular area can be modified to eliminate the friction. If, however, the PU presents with deep undermining, positions and activities that produce shear should be identified and eliminated. When staging wounds using the NPUAP system, wounds are not staged in reverse. For example, a stage III PU that has fully re-epithelialized with changes in skin color is not defined as a stage I PU. Instead, it is described as a stage III PU in the remodeling phase of wound healing.

Optimizing pressure ulcer healing at any stage involves participation of the entire medical team (physicians, nurses, physical and occupational therapists, registered dieticians, social workers, and case management) in the care of the individual patient. Medical management of all disease processes is important for maintaining skin nutrition and for the systemic support of local wound healing, especially if the patient has diabetes mellitus. Blood glucose values less than 180 mg/dL are recommended for optimal wound healing.[8] Elevated blood glucose levels can be an indication of undetected infection, especially if the wound has undermining and sinuses that may be the site of hidden abscesses. Low BMI has also been associated with high risk for PU development, and protein malnutrition impedes healing because the substrates necessary for wound healing are not available.[7,9]

Physical Therapy Patient/Client Management

For any patient in the acute care setting who is at risk for or has a PU, multidisciplinary involvement is required to prevent and/or treat the patient successfully. CMS requires that on hospital admission, a complete skin assessment must be performed and that the physician document any wound that is present.[11] In addition, a risk assessment is recommended by the NPUAP to help determine the patient's overall risk for PU formation, to identify specific risk factors, and to help develop an individualized care plan for prevention or treatment.[1] The most frequently used tool for predicting PU risk is the **Braden Scale** that has been validated for adult patients with different skin colors in all settings.[12,13] Table 22-2 shows the Braden Scale with six individual risk factors (sensory perception, moisture, activity, mobility, nutrition, and friction and shear) that are assessed on a scale of 1 to 4 or 1 to 3. A total score for the six risk factors ranges from 6 to 23. The lower the total score, the higher the risk of PU development. Any hospitalized adult with a score < 16 is considered at risk for PU development, and older adults with a score < 18 may be considered at risk.[14] In a prospective study of 200 older adults admitted to a skilled nursing facility, the risk of PU development was effectively predicted by individuals' Braden Scale scores upon admission. Individuals scoring 15 and 16 had a 50% to 60% chance of developing a stage I pressure ulcer. Individuals scoring 12 to 14 were at moderate risk, with 65% to 90% chance of developing a stage I or II pressure ulcer. Those scoring < 12 were at the highest risk, with 90% to 100% risk of developing a stage II or deeper pressure ulcer.[15]

The role of the physical therapist extends from developing and teaching prevention strategies (consistent with NPUAP recommendations and based upon the therapist's knowledge of movement analysis) to aggressive and extensive treatment of the existing PU. Physical therapists' involvement in treatment of pressure ulcers varies among facilities depending on state practice acts (*e.g.*, sharp debridement), department competencies, and individual hospital culture (*i.e.*, whether wound management responsibilities are shared among physical therapists and certified

Table 22-2 BRADEN SCALE FOR PREDICTING PRESSURE ULCER RISK[16]

Sensory Perception Ability to respond meaningfully to pressure related discomfort	1. *Completely limited:* Unresponsive (does not moan, flinch, or grasp) to painful stimuli, due to diminished level of consciousness or sedation, Or Limited ability to feel pain over most of body surface.	2. *Very limited:* Responds only to painful stimuli Cannot communicate discomfort Except by moaning or restlessness Or Has a sensory impairment, which limits the ability to feel pain or discomfort over ½ of body.	3. *Slightly limited:* Responds to verbal commands but cannot always communicate discomfort or need to be turned Or Has some sensory impairment, which limits ability to feel pain or discomfort in 1 or 2 extremities.	4. *No impairment:* Responds to verbal command. Has no sensory deficit which would limit ability to feel pain or voice pain or discomfort.
Moisture Degree to which skin is exposed to moisture	1. *Constantly moist:* Perspiration, urine, etc. keep skin moist almost constantly. Dampness is detected every time patient is moved or turned.	2. *Moist:* Skin is often but not always moist. Linen must be changed at least once a shift.	3. *Occasionally moist:* Skin is occasionally moist, requiring an extra linen change approximately once a day.	4. *Rarely moist:* Skin is usually dry; linen requires changing only at routine intervals.
Activity Degree of physical activity	1. *Bedfast:* Confined to bed.	2. *Chairfast:* Ability to walk severely limited or nonexistent. Cannot bear own weight and/or must be assisted into chair or wheelchair.	3. *Walks occasionally:* Walks occasionally during day but for very short distances, with or without assistance. Spends majority of each shift in bed or chair.	3. *Walks frequently:* Walks outside the room at least twice a day and inside the room at least once every 2 hours during walking hours.
Mobility Ability to change and control body position	1. *Completely immobile:* Does not make even slight changes in body or extremity position without assistance.	2. *Very limited:* Makes occasional slight changes in body or extremity position but unable to make frequent or significant changes independently.	3. *Slightly limited:* Makes frequent though slight changes in body or extremity position independently.	4. *No limitations:* Makes major and frequent changes in position without assistance.

(Continued)

Table 22-2   BRADEN SCALE FOR PREDICTING PRESSURE ULCER RISK[16] (CONTINUED)

	1. Very poor:	2. Probably inadequate:	3. Adequate:	4. Excellent:
Nutrition Usual food intake pattern	Never eats a complete meal. Rarely eats > ⅓ of any food offered. Eats ≤ 2 servings of proteins (meat or dairy products) per day. Takes fluids poorly. Does not take a liquid dietary supplement, Or Is NPO and/or maintained on clear liquids or IV for > 5 days.	Rarely eats a complete meal and generally eats only about ½ of any food offered. Protein intake includes only 3 servings of meat or dairy products per day. Occasionally will take a dietary supplement, Or Receives less than optimum amount of liquid diet or tube feeding.	Eats > ½ of most meals. Eats a total of 4 servings of protein (meat, dairy products) each day. Occasionally will refuse a meal, but will usually take a supplement if offered, Or Is on tube feeding or TPN regimen, which probably meets most of nutritional needs.	Eats most of every meal. Never refuses a meal. Usually eats a total of 4 or more servings of meat and dairy products. Occasionally eats between meals. Does not require supplementation.
	1. Problem:	2. Potential problem:	3. No apparent problem:	
Friction and shear	Requires moderate to maximum assistance in moving. Complete lifting without sliding against sheets is impossible. Frequently slides down in bed or chair, requiring frequent repositioning with maximum assistance. Spasticity, contractures, or agitation leads to almost constant friction.	Moves feebly or requires minimum assistance. During a move, skin probably slides to some extent against sheets, chair, restraints, or other devices. Maintains relatively good position in chair or bed most of the time but occasionally slides down.	Moves in bed and in chair independently and has sufficient muscle strength to lift up completely during move. Maintains good position in bed or chair at all times.	
			TOTAL SCORE	

Abbreviations: IV, intravenous; NPO, *nil per os* (nothing by mouth).

nursing staff). The most important criterion is that the clinician treating the patient is specifically trained in evidence-based wound management. However, entry-level physical therapists are trained in basic wound care, including the use of specific modalities such as electrical stimulation and ultrasound to facilitate wound healing.

For the patient who is immobile or limited in activity, a physical therapy evaluation is appropriate to optimize patient function and to involve the patient in repositioning as much as possible. An individualized turning schedule should be visible in the patient's room so that all disciplines involved in the patient's care can be consistent with positioning the patient to avoid prolonged pressure on any one body part. Although the traditional positioning schedule has been to reposition or turn a patient every 2 hours, studies have shown that tissue damage may occur in less than 2 hours in some situations. Therefore, the NPUAP recommendation is to schedule repositioning based upon patient risk factors and the support surface being used.[10] Furthermore, the shear forces produced between the bony surfaces and adjacent soft tissue are higher than those at the surface and potentially cause deep tissue injury that can progress to deep sinuses and undermining.[12] In addition to repositioning, **NPUAP recommends that patients with increased risk of pressure ulcers** be placed on a higher specification foam mattress, an active support surface, or an alternating-pressure mattress or overlay. All positioning and turning should be carried out with techniques to eliminate or minimize shear and friction, especially at the sacrum, heels, and elbows (e.g., using a "lift and carry" technique when moving the patient up in bed rather than sliding).

For patients with acute spinal cord injuries with limited or lack of ability to participate in repositioning, additional precautions may be needed, especially before stabilization surgery. Any turning should be accomplished with the log roll technique (i.e., avoiding spinal rotation) with enough personnel to maintain a stable spine position during the movement, and the patient should be transitioned to a rotational bed as soon as possible.[17] In order to avoid shear on the sacrum, the bed should be kept as flat as possible at all times.[18] One study of factors that influenced the development of pressure ulcers during the acute phase after SCI found that immobilization for more than 6 hours was associated with ulcer formation.[19] After acute SCI, blood flow to the sacral skin after 2 hours of pressure loading was less than that for subjects with orthopaedic injuries or normal (uninjured) subjects, with a longer reperfusion time and a shorter time to develop reactive hyperemia.[20] Based on these studies, more frequent turning times may be indicated for patients with acute SCI.

Issues of malnutrition are referred to the dietician who may recommend protein supplementation based on the patient's prealbumin measurements. If needed, a speech therapist may be involved to assess safety with swallowing. Incontinence of bowel and bladder are managed by nursing with meticulous skin care for the perineal region.

Recommendations for patients who have existing pressure ulcers depend on the stage, location of the wound, and healing phase (inflammation, proliferation, or remodeling).[10] For individuals with stage I/II pressure ulcers or deep tissue injuries, repositioning, protection of the skin with silicone-backed foam dressings and/or moisture barriers, optimal nutrition, and patient/caregiver education are recommended to prevent progression of tissue injury.[1] Other risk factors that are identified at the time of initial assessment should also be addressed. Once tissue injury is observed, more frequent skin assessment is advised to detect any wound progression. In most cases, specialty beds (*e.g.*, air flow mattresses, fluidized air beds) are not necessary if the patient is able to independently reposition; however, avoidance of prolonged elevation of the head of the bed or sitting/lying in a slouched position is necessary to prevent further shear on the sacrum and coccyx. Sitting on the edge of the bed for eating is preferable to sitting up in the bed due to the decreased shear at the sacrum.

Stage III/IV ulcers require more intensive local care, in addition to more attention to repositioning in order to eliminate any position that places direct pressure on the involved area. For example, if the patient has a PU on the right greater trochanter, the turning schedule would only include supine and 30° sidelying on the left (30° sidelying is defined as lying with the sacrum supported by pillows or a foam wedge at a 30° angle with the bed). For the current patient with a sacral unstageable PU (which could be stage III/IV after debridement), the positioning schedule should include left and right 30° sidelying with pillows or a foam wedge, but no supine positioning. **Debridement, antimicrobial filler dressings to maintain proper moisture balance, and biophysical technologies** are recommended to facilitate healing, whether or not surgical closure is anticipated. Low-air-loss, air-fluidized, or alternating-pressure beds are recommended, with the choice being influenced by the patient's functional status and the extent, number, and location of pressure ulcers.[21] If the heels are involved, an overhead trapeze is beneficial for the patient to use during bed mobility in order to avoid friction and direct pressure. Placing pillows under the calves and using foot protectors are recommended so that the heels are "floating" to eliminate direct contact with the bed.[10]

Physical therapists who specialize in wound care may be involved in sharp/selective debridement, dressing selection, and application of biophysical technologies, depending on state practice act and facility policy. **Direct contact electrical stimulation**[10] and negative pressure wound therapy have been shown to facilitate wound healing for stage II, III, and IV pressure ulcers, and early studies have shown that non-contact, low-frequency ultrasound may help heal deep tissue injury.[22] The physical therapist works closely with the entire team to determine goals regarding management of the PU (*e.g.*, closure by secondary intention vs. surgical closure with a flap). Functional activities that form the basis of the physical therapist's plan of care may need to be modified to avoid direct pressure, shear, or friction on the affected area.

Examination, Evaluation, and Diagnosis

Patient evaluation begins with a thorough chart review to determine risk factors, comorbidities, and any other history that may have contributed to the wound formation and/or impeded wound healing. Medications that inhibit the wound healing cascade need to be identified. These include glucocorticoids, nonsteroidal anti-inflammatories, cancer chemotherapy agents, and immunosuppressive medications.

In some cases, working with the physician to alter the medications during the healing process may be helpful. Anticoagulants may cause the patient to bleed easily during treatment, in which case, ultrasonic, enzymatic, or autolytic debridement may be advised instead of mechanical or sharp debridement. Identification of pain medications that can be administered prior to treatment if needed can be gathered from subjective history, chart review, and discussion with the patient's nurse. Laboratory values that indicate the patient may have impaired wound healing include: prealbumin < 16 mg/dL; albumin < 3.5 g/dL with normal hydration; transferrin < 179 mg/dL; hemoglobin < 12 g/dL; hematocrit < 33%; serum cholesterol < 160 mg/dL; total lymphocyte count < 1800 mm^3; blood urea nitrogen/creatinine > 10:1; blood glucose level > 200 mg/dL.[7]

The therapist should also check the patient's chart for platelet value and International Normalized Ratio (INR): a low platelet count or high INR indicates the patient is at a higher risk for bleeding.

The chart review is followed by a subjective evaluation which can often be more informative about the wound etiology than the wound evaluation itself. Specific questions about any event that occurred at or before the wound was detected can help identify the precipitating cause. The physical therapist should evaluate the patient's recumbent and sitting positions, support surfaces, and functional status (*e.g.*, how the patient moves in bed, transfers, sits, and ambulates). This information further assists in determining the specific cause of the wound(s). A musculoskeletal evaluation (range of motion, strength, and bony abnormalities) of the involved body areas is indicated, especially if rigid foot protectors are being considered. The neurologic examination emphasizes assessment of sensation, reflexes, spasticity, and visual field deficits that may impair self-mobility.[7]

Pain can be assessed using a Visual Analog Scale, the Wong-Baker FACES pain rating scale (See Fig. 2-1) or the Critical-Care Pain Observation Tool. Determining the cause of the pain may give some indication to the cause of the wound. For example, if the patient has orthotic devices, casts, or tubes and complains of pain in that area, the device may be the cause of the pressure and resulting tissue damage.

Next, a complete wound assessment is performed. Table 22-3 includes the components of the wound evaluation.

The type of tissue in the wound is used to determine the depth of injury and make a staging diagnosis. Healing phase (inflammatory, proliferative, or remodeling) is

Table 22-3   WOUND ASSESSMENT
• Measurement of length, width, depth, and any undermining or sinuses that can be probed
• Tissue visualized within the wound, including eschar, slough, muscle, bone, tendon, fascia, granulation, and subcutaneous fat
• Presence of drainage, including type (serous, sanguineous, purulent, and combinations thereof) and amount (scant, minimal, moderate, heavy, copious)
• Condition of the periwound skin (*e.g.*, erythema, maceration, discoloration, excoriation)
• Status of the wound edges (*e.g.*, even or uneven, rolled, epithelializing) that may give an indication of the wound healing phase or lack of healing progression
• Presence of odor that may indicate presence of infection

also determined by tissue type. For example, if the wound is primarily devitalized tissue, the wound is still in the inflammatory phase of healing. If there is substantial granulation tissue, the wound is in the proliferative phase of healing. If the wound is epithelialized, the wound is in the remodeling phase of healing. Written documentation of the wound is confirmed with digital photographs that can be included in the written or electronic chart.

Plan of Care and Interventions

The most important component of treating a PU of any stage is pressure redistribution. During the acute phase of SCI, log-roll turning requires multiple staff members in order to maintain the patient's neutral spine throughout the task. Active support surfaces that change the pressure against a patient's skin regardless of whether the patient moves in the surface may be preferable to reduce the risk of spinal motion during the turning process. Examples include alternating pressure or lateral rotation mattresses. These are recommended as soon as possible after SCI, especially if stabilization surgery is delayed for any reason.[23] When safely possible, the family and/or caregivers are included in assisting with repositioning. All disciplines need to be consistent in the education of the patient and family in order for care to be most effective. Patients with unstable spine fractures may need to have local wound care delayed until after stabilization surgery in order to minimize the risk for further spinal cord damage; however, strategies for pressure relief are still recommended during this time.

Local wound care, dependent upon the extent of tissue injury and healing phase, is addressed in detail in the 2009 NPUAP recommendations.[10] Briefly, stage I and II wounds are usually successfully treated with conservative care (repositioning, covering with a protective dressing, and optimizing nutrition). Dressings without adhesives (e.g., silicone-backed foams) are recommended to avoid skin tears and periwound skin maceration. More frequent reassessments of the affected area with the risk assessment tool are recommended to assist in preventing ulcer progression.

Stage III and IV pressure ulcers require more aggressive pressure relief with more frequent turning or specialized beds (e.g., low-air loss mattresses or air-fluidized beds). Debridement of necrotic tissue is the first step of topical wound care. This process may be performed at the bedside with sharp debridement because the individual with a SCI usually does not experience pain (the individual with an incomplete SCI may be the exception). Pulsed lavage with suction is often used to soften and loosen necrotic tissue and to cleanse the wound of exudate and bacteria. Enzymatic debridement may help soften the eschar and facilitate the sharp debridement process; however, it is not sufficient alone for extensive tissue loss that occurs with a stage III or IV PU. The selection of the primary dressing (the dressing on or in the wound bed) is based on the presence of microbes within the wound and the amount and type of drainage present. Primary dressings for infected wounds include non-cytotoxic substances like ionic or nanocrystalline silver, cadexomer iodine, or manuka honey. The selection of the secondary dressing (the dressing that anchors or contains the primary dressing) is based on the activity level of the patient.

If the wound is staged as deep tissue injury, low-frequency non-contact ultrasound may help prevent the tissue from becoming necrotic eschar.[22] Once the wound is debrided of all necrotic tissue, negative pressure wound therapy (NPWT) is indicated if there is any depth to the wound. For the current patient (whose sacral ulcer was initially unstageable but after debridement was classified as stage IV because of tissue loss to the bone), NPWT was initiated in the acute care setting and continued after transfer to an acute rehabilitation facility. Electrical stimulation may also be included in the plan of care, since it has been proven to facilitate wound closure in all phases of healing.[24] The care plan is developed in collaboration with the physician, who determines if the wound will be allowed to heal by secondary intention (without surgery) or if a flap will be indicated. Again, biophysical technologies (those modalities that promote a biological, cellular change when applied to the wound) need to be deferred until after spinal stabilization has been performed and the patient can tolerate positioning for effective treatment.

Evidence-Based Clinical Recommendations

SORT: Strength of Recommendation Taxonomy

A: Consistent, good-quality patient-oriented evidence
B: Inconsistent or limited-quality patient-oriented evidence
C: Consensus, disease-oriented evidence, usual practice, expert opinion, or case series

1. The Braden Scale can be used for predicting the risk of pressure ulcers and has been validated for adults with different skin colors in all clinical settings. **Grade A**

2. Frequent repositioning, protein supplementation, and higher-specification foam mattresses or alternating pressure active support overlays are recommended preventative strategies for patients at risk for pressure ulcer formation as well as for treatment of existing pressure ulcers. **Grade A**

3. Removal of necrotic tissue and the use of wound dressings that maintain moisture balance, provide antimicrobial agents, and minimize friction and shear are recommended for stage II, III, and IV pressure ulcers. **Grade A**

4. Direct contact electrical stimulation is recommended to facilitate healing of stage II, III, and IV pressure ulcers. **Grade A**

COMPREHENSION QUESTIONS

22.1 A patient presents with a complaint of pain on her right heel. Upon examination, the physical therapist finds a clear fluid-filled blister about 2 cm in diameter. Based on NPUAP staging, the wound would be diagnosed as a:

   A. Suspected deep tissue injury
   B. Stage I
   C. Stage II
   D. Unstageable

22.2 The support surface recommended for a patient with a stage III pressure ulcer on the sacrum would be:

   A. Memory foam mattress
   B. Air-filled overlay
   C. Egg-crate overlay
   D. Low-air loss mattress

22.3 Sinuses and undermining are frequently seen with stage III and IV pressure ulcers on the coccyx. Which of the following functional tasks is *most* likely a contributing factor in a mobile patient?

   A. Sitting up in bed with the head raised 45° to 60°
   B. Performing sliding board transfers from bed to wheelchair
   C. Sitting in a wheelchair without a support cushion
   D. Rolling from side to side on a regular mattress

22.4 Which of the following medications is *most* likely to inhibit wound healing of a patient who has systemic lupus erythematosus?

   A. Anticoagulants
   B. Glucocorticoids
   C. Tylenol
   D. Antihypertensives

ANSWERS

22.1 **C.** The fluid-filled blister indicates an inflammatory response *between* the layers of the skin and is therefore only partial thickness. If the blister is blood-filled, indicating capillary damage in the subcutaneous tissue, it is termed suspected deep tissue injury (option A). A stage I pressure ulcer is *intact* skin that demonstrates nonblanchable redness (option B). An unstageable pressure ulcer is one with full thickness tissue loss with the wound evolution potentially including a thin blister over a *dark* wound bed, not the clear fluid-filled blister described (option D).

22.2 **D.** Beds with alternating pressures (*e.g.*, low-air loss mattress) are recommended for any patient who has a stage III or IV pressure ulcer. Options A, B, and C would not *consistently* reduce the pressure at the site of tissue injury.

22.3 **A.** Sitting up in the bed produces shear in the deep tissue adjacent to the sacrum and coccyx, thereby causing deep tissue damage that becomes sinuses and undermining. Sliding board transfers cause friction on the gluteal region (option B), and sitting in a wheelchair without a cushion is more likely to cause direct pressure on the ischial tuberosities (option C). Rolling from side to side on a regular mattress is an accepted method of repositioning for a mobile patient (option D).

22.4 **B.** Glucocorticoids inhibit wound healing because of their anti-inflammatory effects. The cells necessary for wound healing to progress through the inflammatory phase are not attracted to the injured tissue and healing cannot progress.

REFERENCES

1. National Pressure Ulcer Advisory Panel. Available at: http://www.npuap.org/pr2.htm. Accessed September 25, 2011.

2. Black JM, Edsberg LE, Baharestani MM, et al. Pressure ulcers: avoidable or unavoidable? Results of the National Pressure Ulcer Advisory Panel Consensus Conference. *Ostomy Wound Manage.* 2011;57:24-37.

3. Whittington KT, Briones R. National prevalence and incidence study: 6-year sequential acute care data. *Adv Skin Wound Care.* 2004;17:490-494.

4. Whittington K, Patrick M, Roberts JL. A national study of pressure ulcer prevalence and incidence in acute care hospitals. *J Wound Ostomy Continence Nurs.* 2000;27:209-215.

5. Salcido R, Lee A, Ahn C. Heel pressure ulcers: purple heel and deep tissue injury. *Adv Skin Wound Care.* 2011;24:374-380.

6. Posthauer ME. Nutritional assessment and healing. In: Sussman C, Bates-Jensen B, eds. *Wound Care: A Collaborative Practice Manual for Health Professionals.* 3rd ed. Baltimore, MD: Lippincott Williams & Wilkins; 2007:52-84.

7. Rappl LM, Sprigle SH, Lane RT. Prevention and treatment of pressure ulcers. In: McCulloch JM, Kloth LC, eds. *Wound Healing: Evidence-based Management.* 4th ed. Philadelphia, PA: FA Davis; 2010: 292-332.

8. Bloomgarden ZT. Intensive diabetes management. Available at: http://www.medscape.com/viewarticle/480753. Accessed January 22, 2012.

9. Patterson GK, Martindale. Nutrition and wound healing. In: McCulloch JM, Kloth LC, eds. *Wound Healing: Evidence-based Management.* 4th ed. Philadelphia, PA: FA Davis; 2010:44-50.

10. European Pressure Ulcer Advisory Panel and National Pressure Ulcer Advisory Panel. Prevention and treatment of pressure ulcers: quick reference guide. Washington DC: National Pressure Ulcer Advisory Panel; 2009. Available at: http://www.npuap.org/wp-content/uploads/2012/02/Final_Quick_Prevention_for_web_2010.pdf. Accessed May 25, 2012.

11. Welker K. How to code for present on admission. *Today's Hospitalist.* Posted 9/2008. Available at: http://www.todayshospitalist.com/index.php?b=articles_read&cnt=649. Accessed January 21, 2012.

12. Braden B, Bergstrom N. Clinical utility of the Braden Scale for predicting pressure sore risk. *Decubitus* 1989;2:44-46, 50-51.

13. Kring DL. Reliability and validity of the Braden Scale for predicting pressure ulcer risk. *J Wound Ostomy Continence Nurs.* 2007;34:399-406.

14. Bates-Jensen BM. Pressure ulcers: pathophysiology and prevention. In: Sussman C, Bates-Jensen B, eds. *Wound Care: A Collaborative Practice Manual for Health Professionals.* 3rd ed. Baltimore, MD: Lippincott Williams & Wilkins; 2007:336-373.

15. Bergstrom N, Braden B. A prospective study of pressure sore risk among institutionalized elderly. *J Am Geriatr Soc.* 1992;40:747-758.

16. Prevention Plus. Home of the Braden Scale. Available at: http://www.bradenscale.com/products. htm. Accessed January 21, 2012.

17. Denton M, McKinlay MA. Cervical cord injury and critical care. *Cont Edu Anaesth Crit Care Pain.* 2009;9:82-86.

18. Wuermser L, Ho CH, Chiodo AE, Priebe MM, Kirshblum SC, Scelza WM. Spinal cord injury medicine. 2. Acute care management of traumatic and non-traumatic injury. *Arch Phys Med Rehabil.* 2007;88:S55-S61.

19. Curry K, Casady L. The relationship between extended periods of immobility and decubitus ulcer formation in the acutely spinal-cord injured individual. *J Neurosci Nurs.*1992;24:185-189.

20. Sae-Sai W, Wipke-Tevis DD, Williams DA. The effect of clinically relevant pressure duration on sacral skin blood flow and temperature in patients after acute spinal cord injury. *Arch Phys Med Rehabil.* 2007;88:1673-1680.

21. Norton L, Couutts P, Sibbald RG. Beds: practical pressure management for surfaces/mattresses. *Adv Skin Wound Care.* 2011;24:324-332.

22. Honaker J, Forston M, Davis E, Wiesner M, Morgan J. Effect of noncontact low-frequency ultrasound treatment on suspected deep tissue injury healing. Poster presentation at NPUAP 2011 National Conference.

23. Rechtine GR, Conrad BP, Bearden BG, Horodyski MB. Biomechanical analysis of cervical and thoracolumbar spine motion in intact and partially and completely unstable cadaver spine models with kinetic bed therapy or traditional log roll. *J Trauma: Injury, Infection, Crit Care.* 2007;62: 383-388.

24. Gardner SE, Frantz RA, Schmidt FL. Effect of electrical stimulation on chronic wound healing: a meta-analysis. *Wound Repair Regen.* 1999;7:495-503.

Chronic Inflammatory Demyelinating Polyneuropathy

Doris Chong
Leslie B. Glickman
Paz Susan Cabanero-Johnson

CASE 23

A 55-year-old female with a past medical history of leukemia, hepatitis C, and liver cirrhosis went to the hospital with progressive low back pain, fatigue, extremity numbness, and generalized weakness. The initial diagnosis made by her primary care physician was sciatica and questionable cancer relapse. Further diagnostic tests during this hospital admission, which included a lumbar puncture and repeated nerve conduction studies, confirmed a diagnosis of chronic inflammatory demyelinating polyneuropathy (CIDP). The patient was admitted to the hospital for medical work-up and interventions. Her medical therapy included oral prednisone, plasmapheresis, and intravenous immunoglobulin (IVIg) treatment, lactulose, morphine, pantoprazole, enoxaparin, oxycodone, temazepam, and gabapentin. On hospital admission day 2, the physical therapist is asked to evaluate and treat the patient as well as provide discharge recommendations. The patient was working as an accountant prior to the onset of her symptoms. She lives in a single-story house with her husband, who is available to provide full-time care.

▶ Based on her health condition including past medical history and onset of present illness, what do you anticipate will be the contributors to activity limitations?
▶ What are the physical therapy examination priorities?
▶ What are the most appropriate physical therapy outcome measures?
▶ What are the most appropriate physical therapy interventions?
▶ What precautions should be taken during physical therapy examination and interventions?
▶ What are possible complications interfering with physical therapy?

KEY DEFINITIONS

INTRAVENOUS IMMUNOGLOBULIN (IVIg): Blood product extracted from plasma that contains immunoglobulin antibody G; it is administered intravenously and is commonly used to treat autoimmune diseases or acute infections

NERVE CONDUCTION STUDY: Electrical test commonly performed in both sensory and motor nerves that is used to determine the adequacy of the conduction of the nerve impulse

Objectives

1. Describe the medical diagnosis and differential diagnoses of chronic inflammatory demyelinating polyneuropathy (CIDP).
2. Describe common clinical presentations of CIDP.
3. Describe commonly used medical interventions for CIDP.
4. Explain adverse drug reactions (ADRs) of CIDP medical interventions that may affect physical therapy examination and/or interventions.
5. Describe the importance of combined medical and rehabilitation therapy and interdisciplinary collaboration in the management of CIDP.
6. List factors that may impact physical therapy prognosis for the patient with CIDP.
7. Design an appropriate plan of care for the patient with CIDP, taking comorbidities and variable medical course into consideration.

Physical Therapy Considerations

PT considerations during management of the individual with CIDP:

▶ **General physical therapy plan of care/goals:** Prevent or minimize loss of range of motion, strength, and aerobic functional capacity; minimize pain and fatigue; maximize functional activity tolerance and safety while minimizing secondary impairments; improve quality of life

▶ **Physical therapy interventions:** Patient and caregiver education regarding functional mobility, prognosis, and physical therapy plan of care; pain management; range of motion and strength training; functional mobility training; gradual activity tolerance training; sitting balance training; interdisciplinary collaboration

▶ **Precautions during physical therapy:** Monitor and respect pain by not overworking the patient; monitor overwork fatigue; monitor vital signs, especially after IVIg; monitor fall risk due to severe weakness

▶ **Complications interfering with physical therapy:** Pain; patient's response to medical therapy; patient's comorbidities; delayed onset of medical therapy due to difficulty with diagnosis; severe weakness and deconditioning

Understanding the Health Condition

CIDP is an uncommon autoimmune disorder of the peripheral nerves that leads to progressive weakness, sensory loss, and areflexia.[1] Distinguishing CIDP from other neurological conditions may be difficult due to its heterogeneity. The pathology and pathogenesis of CIDP is complex and not well understood. An unknown trigger releases substances that cross the blood-nerve barrier and damage the myelin sheath and axons of peripheral nerves through cytotoxicity of lymphokines.[2,3] Studies have found that CIDP might occur subsequent to influenza vaccination, tetanus toxoid immunization, or hepatocellular carcinoma.[4-6]

The reported prevalence of CIDP ranges from 1.24 to 7.7 per 100,000 across the world.[7-12] In the United States, the annual incidence is between 1.6 and 8.9 per 100,000.[13] CIDP affects individuals of all ages and both genders, but is most prevalent in people 40 to 60 years of age.[14] There are three typical clinical courses of CIDP: monophasic, relapsing, and progressive. Patients with a monophasic course have one single episode of deterioration followed by sustained improvement. A relapsing course has at least two separate deteriorations and at least one improvement between relapses. A progressive course shows unremitting gradual deterioration. The clinical course of CIDP is heterogeneous and therefore prognoses may vary. Sixty-one percent of patients with a relapsing or monophasic course demonstrated minimal non-disabling symptoms.[15] In contrast, only 8% of patients with a progressive course had minor symptoms.[15] To diagnose CIDP and categorize the condition into possible, probable, or definite categories, certain clinical, laboratory, and electrodiagnostic criteria are used.[16,17] The mandatory clinical presentations to meet the criteria for CIDP diagnosis include the following: (1) at least 2 months progressive onset of symptoms; (2) majority of motor dysfunction; (3) symmetrical weakness both proximally and distally; and (4) areflexia or hyporeflexia.[16,17] All of the above clinical presentations must be present for either a definite, probable, or possible CIDP diagnosis. However, laboratory and electrodiagnostic criteria for a definitive diagnosis of CIDP vary between experts and institutions in terms of level of sensitivity and specificity.[18] For laboratory criteria, a cerebrospinal fluid protein level of > 45 mg/dL is required to consider the diagnosis.[17] Nerve biopsy results that indicate predominant demyelination and/or inflammation is another laboratory criterion for CIDP diagnosis.[17] For electrodiagnostic criteria, it is generally accepted that the presence of three of the following abnormal four features is required for a definite CIDP diagnosis: (1) reduction in conduction velocity in two or more motor nerves; (2) abnormal conduction block/temporal dispersion in one or more motor nerves; (3) prolonged distal latency in two or more motor nerves; and (4) absent F-wave or prolonged minimum F-wave latencies in two or more motor nerves.[16,17] It is important to realize that no consensus on one single set of electrodiagnostic criteria for CIDP exists. At least 16 sets of electrodiagnostic criteria were identified in the literature and their sensitivity and specificity vary.[19] Selection of criteria set depends on goals of examination (research vs. clinical trials and diagnosis vs. treatment effect).[19]

Although there is a lack of consensus on laboratory and electrodiagnostic criteria for CIDP, successful treatment trial in the absence of clinical, laboratory, and electrodiagnostic features may also help confirm a diagnosis of demyelinating neuropathy.[16,20,21]

Although it is not within physical therapists' scope of practice to diagnose a patient medically, possessing this knowledge helps to facilitate medical referral if they suspect CIDP.

Since CIDP is an extremely heterogeneous condition, the exact clinical manifestation differs from person to person. The typical clinical presentation of CIDP encompasses chronic progressive symptoms developed over 2 months or more, with symmetrical weakness of both proximal and distal extremity muscles, motor and/or sensory involvement, absent or reduced deep tendon reflexes, with or without cranial nerve involvement, and may be progressive or relapsing in the disease course.[16,22] Clinical variants may be classified by involved structures such as cranial nerves or central nervous system[22-26] or by clinical presentations such as distal versus proximal and symmetrical versus asymmetrical.[27,28] Another suggested classification is by functional symptoms such as pure motor, pure sensory, or ataxic pattern.[29-32]

Differential diagnosis of CIDP may include polyneuropathy associated with monoclonal gammopathy of undetermined significance (MGUS), polyneuropathy organomegaly endocrinopathy M protein and skin changes (POEMS), and Charcot-Marie-Tooth disease (CMT). The age of onset, clinical course, electrophysiological presentation, and response to medical therapy of these diagnoses are different from CIDP.[33-35] Knowledge of atypical symptoms, clinical variants, differential diagnoses, and their different responses to medical management assists physical therapists in differentiating the condition from others, and in formulating a more accurate rehabilitation prognosis and plan of care.

The most commonly used first-line medical therapy for CIDP includes prednisone, plasmapheresis, and IVIg. A Cochrane systematic review showed similar short-term efficacy among these three agents.[36] Thus, the first choice of medical therapy might depend on the individual's medical history and concurrent medical status, cost, ADRs, and administration factors.

Prednisone is a popular primary and cost-effective medical intervention.[29] Literature suggests the initial dose of 1.0 to 1.5 mg/kg/day or 60 to 100 mg/day.[14,17,29,37,38] Patients with CIDP showed improved strength and disability scores as early as 2 weeks after the initiation of prednisone.[39] Treatment continues until strength returns to normal or the condition reaches a plateau, which is usually between 3 and 6 months.[17]

Plasmapheresis and IVIg are also common first-line intervention for CIDP, which may be prescribed simultaneously with prednisone.[40,41] IVIg therapy has demonstrated a high response rate and long-term efficacy.[40] However, IVIg is more expensive compared to prednisone. It is generally administered at a dosage of 2.0 g/kg given over 2 to 5 days.[14,17,29,37,38] Plasmapheresis is less commonly used due to its invasive nature, the need for special equipment, and high cost.[41,42] There is no specific guideline on the frequency and schedule of treatment; the general practice is to perform five plasma exchanges over 7 to 10 days.[29,42] Although plasmapheresis provides fast improvement in patients with CIDP, the effects of this medical therapy are temporary—usually lasting for only 4 to 8 weeks.[17]

Alternative therapies are considered when patients do not respond readily to traditional intervention or when their condition has relapsed.[29,43] Regardless of the choice of medical therapies, initiating medical intervention as early as possible until improvement reaches a plateau is a common recommendation.[38]

As with clinical presentations and course of condition, prognosis of CIDP is heterogeneous. Patients with CIDP often present with decreased functional balance, diminished quality of life, and increased fatigue.[44] In general, patients with a sub-acute onset, symmetrical symptoms, and distal nerve abnormalities in nerve conduction studies have better outcomes compared to those with a chronic onset, asymmetrical presentation, and demyelination in the proximal nerve segments.[9,45]

Physical Therapy Patient/Client Management

Since CIDP is heterogeneous and the search for an accurate diagnosis may be extensive, it is not uncommon for physical therapists in acute care settings to manage patients with questionable demyelinating neuropathies before a definitive diagnosis is confirmed. It is important for physical therapists not to educate the patient on medical diagnosis and prognosis, but to facilitate early communication with physicians if the clinical presentation is suggestive of CIDP or differential diagnoses. In acute care settings, the treatment team for patients with suggested or confirmed CIDP generally consists of neurologists, physiatrists, or specialists on electrodiagnostic studies, nurses, psychologists, social workers, case managers, respiratory therapists, and rehabilitation specialists. Physical therapists play an important role by communicating the patient's neurologic function and functional mobility status with the multidisciplinary team in a timely and objective manner. Neurologists use this information to assist with diagnosis, assess the patient's response to medical therapies, and determine if modification or alternative therapy is necessary. Should the patient show no response to medical therapies, differential diagnosis may need to be considered.

The primary role of the physical therapist in acute care settings for patients with CIDP is to assess functional mobility and to prepare for the next level of care. The specific roles of the physical therapist are to examine and treat musculoskeletal, neurological, cardiopulmonary, and integumentary systems. In particular, interventions include: maintaining and/or improving range of motion, strength, pain, activity tolerance, and functional mobility; preventing or minimizing complications associated with immobility; implementing a mobility program based on the patient's functional status; educating the nursing team on safe and early mobility; educating the patient and family regarding pain, positioning, and mobility; monitoring ADRs from medical therapies such as IVIg and plasmapheresis; and, monitoring the patient's response to medical therapies to facilitate a better overall plan of care. Successful management of the patient with CIDP depends upon both medical and rehabilitative interventions as medical therapies are essential to reverse the inflammatory process, which allows the patient to optimally benefit from rehabilitation.

Examination, Evaluation, and Diagnosis

Prior to seeing the patient, it is beneficial for the physical therapist to review the history of the present illness and current clinical presentation. The information may assist the physical therapist in differentiating the condition from other possible diagnoses, and in formulating a more accurate rehabilitation prognosis and plan of care.

In addition, knowing the chief clinical presentation assists prioritization of examination procedures since the patient has impairments in multiple systems.

The physical therapist needs to acquire information from the patient's medical chart on lab values, medications, electrodiagnostic test results, and any exercise or mobility restrictions. Since this patient has a history of leukemia and liver disease, the physical therapist should check the patient's hemoglobin, hematocrit, platelet count, and liver function tests. The physical therapist should also review the medication list and anticipate possible ADRs and their potential disruption on patient management.

Prednisone, which is used to reduce and potentially reverse the inflammatory process caused by CIDP, has several significant ADRs. The most relevant ADRs for a patient in the inpatient setting include emotional lability, weight gain, osteoporosis, steroid myopathy, increased blood pressure, increased risk of infections, glaucoma, cataracts, Cushingoid appearance, and skin thinning.[29] The physical therapist should keep in mind the ADRs of prednisone and exercise precautions during activities. The physical therapist should be prepared for a patient's emotions to vacillate between euphoria and tearfulness—even within the same therapy session. In this case, the therapist can help reassure the patient and her husband that this emotional lability is a common ADR of prednisone.

Intravenous immunoglobulin has proven effectiveness in the treatment of CIDP. The reported ADRs of IVIg include chills, nausea, myalgias, rash, headaches, anaphylaxis, renal failure, and thromboembolic events.[29,38] It is common for nursing staff to monitor the patient's vital signs at frequent intervals (e.g., every 5 minutes) during initial IVIg administration. Generally, the physical therapist is not recommended to work with the patient undergoing IVIg and should therefore schedule therapy sessions around the IVIg administration schedule.

Plasmapheresis is less commonly used due to its invasive nature, the need for special equipment, and high cost.[41,42] The physical therapist should monitor vital signs closely for possible acute responses such as lightheadedness, fatigue, anemia, paresthesias, hypotension, nausea, vomiting, and cardiac arrhythmia.[29,41] The identification of these adverse reactions ensures patient safety during physical therapy management.

In addition to the primary medical therapies for CIDP, this patient is also taking lactulose for liver cirrhosis, pantoprazole (Protonix) for gastroesophageal reflux, enoxaparin (Lovenox) for preventative anticoagulation due to decreased mobility, temazepam (Restoril) for sleeplessness and anxiety, and morphine, oxycodone, and gabapentin for pain. Since pain is a major complaint for this patient, adequate pain control optimizes the patient's participation in physical therapy. The physical therapist should work closely with nursing staff on pain premedication and with other rehabilitation therapists on spacing of therapy sessions.

The physical therapist begins the physical examination by performing a systems review. Since CIDP may affect multiple systems, it is important to screen the cardiopulmonary, integumentary, musculoskeletal, and neuromuscular systems and use the findings to guide and prioritize detailed examination. For the cardiopulmonary system, the physical therapist should assess vital signs in different patient positions, if possible. For the integumentary system, special attention should be given to skin condition as patients with CIDP often have a rapid decrease in mobility. Together with impaired sensation, patients are at risk for developing skin breakdown. In addition, prednisone delays wound healing and increases the risk of skin breakdown. The musculoskeletal system screen provides information about the patient's gross range of motion (ROM) and strength. The neuromuscular system screen provides information on the patient's cognition and gross sensorimotor function such as coordination and balance.

Common impairment examination for patients with CIDP includes assessing pain, ROM, strength, sensation, coordination, and deep tendon reflexes. Since the patient in this case is alert and cognitively intact, the Numeric Pain Rating Scale (NPRS) is an appropriate test for pain examination. The NPRS is an ordinal scale where 0 = no pain and 10 = worst possible pain. It is also a responsive scale for patients with low back pain.[46] In acute care settings, ROM and strength are usually examined initially through observation of functional mobility to determine which joint(s) need to be further examined. Detailed examination can be performed by goniometry and manual muscle testing; however, the patient's position may need to be modified due to limited mobility. Sensory impairment is common in patients with CIDP. Examination procedures on light touch, temperature, proprioception, kinesthesia, vibration, and two-point discrimination should be included in the physical therapy examination. The tests are usually performed from distal to proximal regions of the extremities. In acute care settings, due to time constraints, attention is usually given to light touch and proprioception initially. It is important to realize that patients with CIDP often present with an array of sensory impairments; additional sensory examination procedures may need to be included as the patient progresses.

Coordination may be affected in patients with CIDP secondary to impaired strength and sensation. Alternatively, coordination problems may result from ataxic variants of CIDP.[30-32] Performing the finger-nose-finger and rapid alternating movements tests provides preliminary information on the patient's coordination and how impaired coordination may impact functional mobility. Areflexia is a key clinical presentation and diagnostic criterion for CIDP. Assessing deep tendon reflexes using a reflex hammer at major tendons (i.e., biceps, triceps, quadriceps, and Achilles) must therefore be included in the physical therapy examination. If deep tendon reflexes are intact, differential diagnoses may need to be considered.

Physical therapy activity examination includes assessing the patient's general functional mobility, gait, and balance (as applicable). There are no disease-specific standardized activity outcome measures that are validated in patients with CIDP; therefore, generic standardized outcome measures are often employed. For general functional mobility, the **Functional Independence Measure (FIM)** has been shown to be reliable across different types of settings, patients, and raters.[47] If the patient has sufficient ability to perform gait and dynamic balance activities, tests on these categories should be included. Since functional abilities vary widely in patients with CIDP, the choice of tests depends largely on the mobility status of the patient. In addition, time and equipment are common considerations in the acute care setting when selecting standardized outcome measures. The Berg Balance Scale,[48,49] Timed Up and Go,[50] and gait speed[51] are examples of standardized outcome measures on balance and gait that are validated and appropriate for patients in acute care settings with a variety of diagnoses. Nonetheless, the physical therapist should select tests that possess good psychometric properties.

Plan of Care and Interventions

Because patients with CIDP usually present with an array of different clinical presentations, it is important to prioritize physical therapy interventions to maximize functional recovery and to prepare the patient for the next level of care. For this patient, the priorities include decreasing low back pain to facilitate participation in functional mobility, improving sitting upright tolerance to increase endurance and to prevent secondary complications, and improving overall functional mobility. Since the patient's response to medical interventions has yet to be determined, the physical therapist must be cautious when educating the patient on functional prognosis. The physical therapist should vigilantly monitor changes in the patient's function and initiate changes in the treatment plan and revise the prognosis as appropriate.

To manage low back pain, a combination of medications and physical therapy interventions may be employed. The cause of pain may be related to overstretch of the demyelinated nerves and weak muscles, and pain may be the result of immobility. Gentle ROM exercises within physiological limits and pain tolerance, together with early mobility, may help to decrease pain in this patient. Collaborating with nursing staff on premedication prior to physical therapy sessions may enhance the patient's participation. It has not been reported if heat or electrical stimulation is effective for pain management in patients with CIDP. However, if patients present with sensory impairments, applying heat or electrical stimulation may not be appropriate. As with other patient populations, testing the patient's sensation prior to applying these modalities is necessary. In addition, communicating with the neurologists is helpful to identify if a trial of these interventions would be appropriate.

Improving sitting tolerance is another common physical therapy goal for patients in the acute care setting, especially for patients whose disposition is to an inpatient rehabilitation setting because these facilities often require patients to be able to tolerate at least 3 hours of rehabilitation therapies. To achieve this goal, multidisciplinary collaboration between physical therapy, occupational therapy, and nursing is the essence for success. All disciplines should recognize and appreciate the importance of increasing the patient's time out of bed in order to encourage and assist the patient to improve sitting tolerance. In addition to increasing the time of sitting, it is well-known that early mobility is key to prevent secondary complications such as pneumonia, deep vein thrombosis, and skin breakdown.[52] The benefits of increasing sitting tolerance and early mobility are important first steps to the patient's functional recovery.

Fatigue is another common complaint in patients with CIDP.[44] It is therefore important to monitor the patient's response to rehabilitation therapies to avoid over-fatigue. Increased pain and decreased functional status are **common signs of overwork**. In this case, the therapist should educate the patient, her husband, and other interdisciplinary team members on signs of overwork and should respect the patient's symptoms by stopping or modifying the intensity of interventions, if necessary. A common practice is to alternate interventions between functional mobility and gentle ROM and/or strengthening exercises, at least in the acute stage of the condition. In addition, strengthening with functional mobility is preferred over strengthening alone. In the chronic stage of CIDP, patients seem to be able to tolerate **high-intensity exercise** with positive outcomes on fatigue and quality of life.[53] Researchers showed that a 12-week high-intensity (70%-90% of age-predicted heart rate maximum) bicycle exercise program yielded significant improvement in cardiovascular fitness, muscle strength, quality of life, and a 20% reduction of fatigue in patients with CIDP and Guillain-Barré syndrome. However, the results may not apply to acute care patients and therefore close monitoring of pain and fatigue in the acute stage is necessary.

Interdisciplinary collaboration is an important aspect of the overall physical therapy plan of care in this patient.[54] In addition to collaborating with team members on early mobility and pain medication schedule, the physical therapist plays an important role in alerting the team on observed positive or negative effects of medical therapy, since there is a positive relationship between response to medical therapy and functional status. While functional and motor improvements are strong signs of positive response to medical therapy, neurologic changes and functional decline may indicate ADRs and should be communicated to the team promptly. In addition, frequent and detailed communication may help to decrease the patient's frustrations and increase motivation toward recovery.

Evidence-Based Clinical Recommendations

SORT: Strength of Recommendation Taxonomy

A: Consistent, good-quality patient-oriented evidence
B: Inconsistent or limited-quality patient-oriented evidence
C: Consensus, disease-oriented evidence, usual practice, expert opinion, or case series

1. In patients with CIDP, physical therapists can use the functional independence measure (FIM) to establish baseline functional mobility status and to measure changes. **Grade C**

2. Close monitoring of fatigue and signs and symptoms of overwork minimizes adverse effects of rehabilitation therapy and promotes gradual functional improvement. **Grade C**

3. A high-intensity exercise program in the *chronic* stage of CIDP decreases fatigue and improves physical fitness and quality of life. **Grade B**

4. Interdisciplinary collaboration and communication on medication schedule, early mobility, and functional status improve the overall plan of care through dynamic medical and rehabilitation therapy adjustments. **Grade C**

COMPREHENSION QUESTIONS

23.1 A physical therapist has been providing ROM and strengthening exercises and functional mobility training to a patient with CIDP in the acute care setting. On day 3 of physical therapy, the patient complains of increased pain and soreness in her lower extremities. Which of the following is the *most* appropriate course of action?

A. Test the patient's lower extremities' sensation and apply heat if sensation is intact.

B. Examine the patient's functional mobility and note changes and stop strengthening exercise.

C. Report the patient's symptoms to the neurologist and ask for changes in drug therapy.

D. Allow the patient to rest for the day, reassess the next day, and note changes.

23.2 A patient in the hospital with CIDP reported to the physical therapist that she was dizzy and felt heart palpitations. The patient had just received a medical intervention. Which medical intervention is *most* likely responsible for this adverse drug reaction?

A. Prednisone

B. IVIg

C. Plasmapheresis

D. Gabapentin

23.3 Which of the following exercises is *most* appropriate for a patient in the hospital with CIDP who has quadriceps weakness and is able to ambulate with minimal assistance with a walker?

A. Knee extension exercise in supine with 2-lb weights, 10 repetitions, 2 to 3 sets per day

B. Walk up and down a flight of stairs with assistance, 1 to 2 times per day

C. Recumbent bicycle for 30 minutes at 70% of age-predicted heart rate maximum

D. Sit to stand with walker for support, 5 repetitions, 2 to 3 sets per day

ANSWERS

23.1 **B.** A complaint of increased pain and soreness in a major body area may indicate overwork fatigue. Another key sign of overwork is functional decline. Therefore, examining the patient's functional status and comparing results to the *previous* day can give the therapist an idea if therapy was too intense. Reassessing the patient's functional status after a day of rest does not provide the therapist a clear idea if therapy is too intense (option D). The usual practice is to stop strengthening exercise and focus on gentle ROM exercises and functional mobility. Communicating with neurologists about changes in the patient's symptoms is an appropriate course of action; however, it is beyond physical therapists' scope of practice to determine medication appropriateness (option C).

23.2 **C.** It is very common for patients to experience acute hypotension and cardiac arrhythmia during or immediately post-plasmapheresis due to the mechanism of the therapy. Usual practice is for rehabilitation therapists to work with patients *prior* to plasmapheresis since patients are unlikely to be able to tolerate upright postures or exercise after plasmapheresis. Therapists should monitor heart rate and blood pressure when working with patients undergoing a course of plasmapheresis.

23.3 **D.** Strengthening with functional mobility is recommended over strengthening exercises alone (options A and C). This patient requires minimal assistance for ambulation, so it is likely unsafe to use stair negotiation as a strengthening exercise (option B). Stair training may also be too vigorous and lead to overwork fatigue. Therefore, the best option is to use sit-to-stand transfers as a method to strengthen the quadriceps; this is a functional and appropriate task for the patient's functional status.

REFERENCES

1. Hughes RA, Bouche P, Cornblath DF, et al. European Federation of Neurological Societies/ Peripheral Nerve Society guideline on management of chronic inflammatory demyelinating polyradiculoneuropathy: report of a joint task force of the European Federation of Neurological Societies and the Peripheral Nerve Society. *Eur J Neurol.* 2006;13:326-332.

2. Kieseier BC, Dalakas MC, Hartung HP. Immune mechanisms in chronic inflammatory demyelinating neuropathy. *Neurology.* 2002;59(Suppl 6):S7-S12.

3. Rezania K, Gundogdu B, Soliven B. Pathogenesis of chronic inflammatory demyelinating polyradiculoneuropathy. *Front Biosci.* 2004;9:939-945.

4. Brostoff JM, Beitverda Y, Birns J. Post-influenza vaccine chronic inflammatory demyelinating polyneuropathy. *Age Ageing.* 2008;37:229-230.

5. Pritchard J, Mukherjee R, Hughes RA. Risk of relapse of Guillain-Barre syndrome or chronic inflammatory demyelinating polyradiculoneuropathy following immunisation. *J Neurol Neurosurg Psychiatry.* 2002;73:348-349.

6. Arguedas MR, McGuire BM. Hepatocellular carcinoma presenting with chronic inflammatory demyelinating polyradiculoneuropathy. *Dig Dis Sci.* 2000;45:2369-2373.

7. McLeod JG, Pollard JD, Macaskill P, Mohamed A, Spring P, Khurana V. Prevalence of chronic inflammatory demyelinating polyneuropathy in New South Wales, Australia. *Ann Neurol.* 1999;46:910-913.

8. Lunn MP, Manju H, Choudhary PP, Hughes RA, Thomas PK. Chronic inflammatory demyelinating polyradiculoneuropathy: a prevalence study in south east England. *J Neurol Neurosurg Psychiatry*. 1999;66:677-680.

9. Mygland A, Monstad P. Chronic polyneuropathies in Vest-Agder, Norway. *Eur J Neurol*. 2001;8: 157-165.

10. Chio A, Cocito D, Bottacchi E, et al. Idiopathic chronic inflammatory demyelinating polyneuropathy: an epidemiological study in Italy. *J Neurol Neurosurg Psychiatry*. 2007;78:1349-1353.

11. Lijima M, Koike H, Hattori N, et al. Prevalence and incidence rates of chronic inflammatory demyelinating polyneuropathy in the Japanese population. *J Neurol Neurosurg Psychiatry*. 2008;79:1040-1043.

12. Rajabally YA, Simpson BS, Beri S, Bankart J, Gosalakkal JA. Epidemiologic variability of chronic inflammatory demyelinating polyneuropathy with different diagnostic criteria: study of a UK population. *Muscle Nerve*. 2009;39:432-438.

13. Laughlin RS, Dyck PJ, Melton LJ, Leibson C, Ransom J, Dyck PJ. Incidence and prevalence of CIDP and the association of diabetes mellitus. *Neurology*. 2009;73:39-45.

14. Kissel JT. The treatment of chronic inflammatory demyelinating polyradiculoneuropathy. *Semin Neurol*. 2003;23:169-180.

15. Mygland A, Monstad P, Vedeler C. Onset and course of chronic inflammatory demyelinating polyneuropathy. *Muscle Nerve*. 2005;31:589-593.

16. Lewis RA. Chronic inflammatory demyelinating polyneuropathy. *Neurol Clin*. 2007;25:71-87.

17. Saperstein DS. Chronic acquired demyelinating polyneuropathies. *Semin Neurol*. 2008;28:168-184.

18. Magda P, Latov N, Brannagan TH III, Weimer LH, Chin RL, Sander HW. Comparison of electrodiagnostic abnormalities and criteria in a cohort of patients with chronic inflammatory demyelinating polyneuropathy. *Arch Neurol*. 2003;60:1755-1759.

19. Bromberg MB. Review of the evolution of electrodiagnostic criteria for chronic inflammatory demyelinating polyradiculoneuropathy. *Muscle Nerve*. 2011;43:780-794.

20. Latov N. Diagnosis of CIDP. *Neurology*. 2002;59(Suppl 6):S2-S6.

21. Rotta FT, Sussman AT, Bradley WG, Ram Avyar D, Sharma KR, Shebert RT. The spectrum of chronic inflammatory demyelinating polyneuropathy. *J Neurol Sci*. 2000;173:129-139.

22. Misra UK, Kalita J, Yadav RK. A comparison of clinically atypical with typical chronic inflammatory demyelinating polyradiculoneuropathy. *Eur Neurol*. 2007;58:100-105.

23. Alwan AA, Mejico LJ. Ophthalmoplegia, proptosis, and lid retraction caused by cranial nerve hypertrophy in chronic inflammatory demyelinating polyradiculoneuropathy. *J Neuroophthalmol*. 2007;27:99-103.

24. Hemmi S, Kutoku Y, Inoue K, Murakami T, Sunada Y. Tongue fasciculations in chronic inflammatory demyelinating polyradiculoneuropathy. *Muscle Nerve*. 2008;38:1341-1343.

25. Kokubun N, Hirata K. Neurophysiological evaluation of trigeminal and facial nerves in patients with chronic inflammatory demyelinating polyneuropathy. *Muscle Nerve*. 2007;35:203-207.

26. Pineda AAM, Ogata K, Osoegawa M, et al. A distinct subgroup of chronic inflammatory demyelinating polyneuropathy with CNS demyelination and a favorable response to immunotherapy. *J Neurol Sci*. 2007;255:1-6.

27. Katz JS, Saperstein S, Gronseth G, Amato AA, Barohn RJ. Distal acquired demyelinating symmetrical neuropathy. *Neurology*. 2000;54:615-620.

28. Lewis RA, Summer AJ, Brown MJ, Asbury AK. Multifocal demyelinating neuropathy with persistent conduction block. *Neurology*. 1982;32:958-964.

29. Gorson KC, Ropper AH. Chronic inflammatory demyelinating polyradiculoneuropathy (CIDP): a review of clinical syndromes and treatment approaches in clinical practice. *J Clin Neuromuscul Dis*. 2003;4:174-189.

30. Yato M, Ohkoshi N, Sato A, Shoji S, Kusunoki S. Ataxic form of chronic inflammatory demyelinating polyradiculoneuropathy (CIDP). *Eur J Neurol*. 2000;7:227-230.

31. Ohkoshi N, Harada K, Nagata H, et al. Ataxic form of chronic inflammatory demyelinating polyradiculoneuropathy: clinical features and pathological study of the sural nerves. *Eur Neurol*. 2001;45:241-248.

32. Mazzucco S, Ferrari S, Mezzina C, Tomelleri G, Bertolasi L, Rizzuto N. Hyperpyrexia-triggered relapses in an unusual case of ataxic chronic inflammatory demyelinating polyradiculoneuropathy. *J Neurol Sci*. 2006;27:176-179.

33. Notermans NC, Franssen H, Eurelings M, Van der Graaf Y, Wokke JH. Diagnostic criteria for demyelinating polyneuropathy associated with monoclonal gammopathy. *Muscle Nerve*. 2000;23:73-79.

34. Dispenzieri A. POEMS syndrome. *Hematology Am Soc Hematol Educ Program*. 2005:360-367.

35. Pareyson D. Differential diagnosis of Charcot-Marie-Tooth disease and related neuropathies. *J Neurol Sci*. 2004;25:72-82.

36. van Schaik IN, Winer JB, De Hann R, Vermeulen M. Intravenous immunoglobulin for chronic inflammatory demyelinating polyradiculoneuropathy (Review). *Cochrane Database Syst Rev*. 2002;2:CD001797.

37. Said G. Chronic inflammatory demyelinating polyneuropathy. *Neuromuscul Disord*. 2006;16:293-303.

38. Toothaker TB, Brannagan TH. Chronic inflammatory demyelinating polyneuropathies: current treatment strategies. *Curr Neurol Neurosci Rep*. 2007;7:63-70.

39. Hughes R, Benas S, Willison H, et al. Randomized controlled trial of intravenous immunoglobulin versus oral prednisolone in chronic inflammatory demyelinating polyradiculoneuropathy. *Ann Neurol*. 2001;50:195-201.

40. Hughes R. The role of IVIg in autoimmune neuropathies: the latest evidence. *J Neurol*. 2008;225(Suppl 3):7-11.

41. Hahn AG, Bolton CF, Pillay N, et al. Plasma-exchange therapy in chronic inflammatory demyelinating polyneuropathy: a double-blind, sham-controlled, cross-over study. *Brain*. 1996;119:1055-1066.

42. Mehndiratta MM, Singh AC. Plasmapheresis for chronic inflammatory demyelinating polyradiculoneuropathy. *Curr Allergy Asthma Rep*. 2007;7:274-279.

43. Kuitwaard K, van Doorn PA. Newer therapeutic options for chronic inflammatory demyelinating polyradiculoneuropathy. *Drugs*. 2009;69:987-1001.

44. Westblad ME, Forsberg A, Press R. Disability and health status in patients with chronic inflammatory demyelinating polyneuropathy. *Disabil Rehabil*. 2008;24:1-6.

45. Kuwabara S, Misawa S, Mori M, Tamura N, Kubota M, Hattori T. Long term prognosis of chronic inflammatory demyelinating polyneuropathy: a five year follow up of 38 cases. *J Neurol Neurosurg Psychiatry*. 2006;77:66-70.

46. Childs JD, Piva SR, Fritz JM. Responsiveness of the numeric pain rating scale in patients with low back pain. *Spine (Phila Pa 1976)*. 2005;30:1331-1334.

47. Ottenbacher KJ, Hsu Y, Granger CV, Fiedler RC. The reliability of the functional independence measure: a quantitative review. *Arch Phys Med Rehabil*. 1996;77:1226-1232.

48. Berg KO, Wood-Dauphinee SL, Williams JI, Maki B. Measuring balance in the elderly: validation of an instrument. *Can J Public Health*. 1992;83(Suppl 2):S7-S11.

49. Graham D, Newton RA. Relationship between balance abilities and mobility aids in elderly patients at discharge from an acute care setting. *Physiother Res Int*. 1999;4:293-301.

50. Podsiadlo D, Richardson S. The timed "Up & Go": a test of basic functional mobility for frail elderly persons. *J Am Geriatr Soc*. 1991;39:142-148.

51. Salbach NM, Mayo NE, Higgins J, Ahmed S, Finch LE, Richards CL. Responsiveness and predictability of gait speed and other disability measures in acute stroke. *Arch Phys Med Rehabil*. 2001;82:1204-1212.

52. Morris PE. Moving our critically ill patients: mobility barriers and benefits. *Crit Care Clin.* 2007;23:1-20.

53. Garssen MP, Bussman JB, Schmitz PI, et al. Physical training and fatigue, fitness, and quality of life in Guillain-Barré syndrome and CIDP. *Neurology.* 2004;63:2393-2395.

54. Chong DY, Glickman LB, Cabanero-Johnson PS. Chronic inflammatory demyelinating polyradiculoneuropathy from a physical therapist's perspective: a case report. *J Acute Care Phys Ther.* 2010;1:4-13.

Peripheral Neuropathy in HIV/AIDS

Judith R. Gale

CASE 24

duration is important

A 52-year-old male was admitted to the hospital 4 days ago with a 1-week history of sharp abdominal pain, fever, nausea, and vomiting. Computed tomography (CT) scan revealed acute pancreatitis. He was placed on intravenous (IV) antibiotics, opiate analgesics, and total parenteral nutrition (TPN). He has been NPO since admission. His relevant medical history includes acquired immune deficiency syndrome (AIDS) diagnosed 13 years ago and associated wasting syndrome and peripheral neuropathy. His CD4 count is 54 and viral load is undetectable. Current medications include fentanyl, imipenem/cilastatin, testosterone transdermal, atazanavir, abacavir, and lamivudine. The patient works as a lawyer and lives with his partner of 11 years. The physical therapist is asked to see the patient today for strengthening, endurance, and gait activities. He is expected to be hospitalized for another 3 to 4 days, and then will be discharged home.

▶ What functional limitations may you expect based on his health history?
▶ What are the examination priorities?
▶ What are the most appropriate physical therapy interventions?
▶ What precautions should be taken during physical therapy examination and interventions?
▶ What potential complications may limit the effectiveness of your interventions?

KEY DEFINITIONS

CD4 COUNT: Number of T cells expressing CD4 that are circulating in the blood, described as number of cells/μL blood; CD4 cells are sometimes called T-helper cells and are critical in initiating the coordinated immune response to foreign organisms; normal value is ~500 to 1500 cells/μL

NPO: Abbreviation for Latin phrase *nil per os*, meaning "nothing through the mouth"; individuals with instructions to be NPO are not allowed to eat or drink for various medical reasons

TOTAL PARENTERAL NUTRITION (TPN): Supplying all of a person's nutritional needs intravenously, thereby bypassing the gastrointestinal tract; nutritional source when individuals cannot eat or drink

VIRAL LOAD: Amount of human immunodeficiency virus (HIV) circulating in the blood, described by number of copies of HIV/mL blood; values range from undetectable (meaning none was found) to > 50,000/mL

WASTING SYNDROME: Unintentional loss of lean body mass, often associated with AIDS

Objectives

1. Understand the implications of the CD4 count and viral load in the health of a person infected with HIV.

2. Describe the signs and symptoms of HIV-related peripheral neuropathy.

3. Identify the causes and sequelae of wasting syndrome.

4. Discuss the benefits of aerobic and resistance exercise in the management of HIV-related wasting, weakness, and deconditioning.

Physical Therapy Considerations

PT considerations during management of the individual with HIV/AIDS with HIV wasting syndrome and peripheral neuropathy:

▶ **General physical therapy plan of care/goals:** Maximize function by increasing general strength; increase endurance to allow independent performance of activities of daily living (ADLs); decrease pain and dysesthesia associated with peripheral neuropathy; independent ambulation with or without assistive device

▶ **Physical therapy interventions:** Patient education regarding loss of strength and endurance with bedrest; general strengthening and endurance exercise; gait training on flat surfaces and stairs; joint mobilization, soft tissue mobilization, stretching, and microcurrent to the feet

CD4 vs. viral load

▶ **Precautions during physical therapy:** Standard precautions; monitor vital signs before and during exercise

▶ **Complications interfering with physical therapy:** Nausea/vomiting; peripheral neuropathy

Understanding the Health Condition

There are nearly 1.2 million people in the United States living with HIV infection. More than 490,000 are living with Acquired Immune Deficiency Syndrome (AIDS), the chronic, progressive, and potentially life-threatening disease caused by HIV. There are about 50,000 new HIV infections each year.[1,2] Thus, it seems quite likely that physical therapists will come in contact with patients with this illness at some time during their careers. While the term "HIV" is used for the virus and the infection itself and "AIDS" is used for later stages of HIV infection, the virus and the disease are frequently referred together as HIV/AIDS. To successfully treat those with HIV/AIDS, healthcare providers should be knowledgeable about the typical response to medical management and physical therapy interventions, laboratory values used to monitor disease progression, stages of HIV infection and AIDS, pharmacologic interventions and anticipated adverse drug reactions (ADRs), and common comorbidities.

Lab values important in monitoring HIV/AIDS include CD4 count and viral load. The CD4 count indicates how well the immune system is working (*i.e.*, how many CD4 cells are still circulating) and the viral load shows how successful the medications are in treating the infection (*i.e.*, how many infectious HIV particles have been destroyed). Individuals with low CD4 counts (< 350 cells/μL) are more susceptible to opportunistic infections because they have fewer CD4 cells to combat infection. Those with high viral loads (> 10,000 copies/mL) have the potential to become sicker as the virus destroys more of the CD4 cells.[3] Antiretroviral drug treatment is recommended for those with CD4 counts < 500 cells/μL.[4] Many individuals who are HIV seropositive (*i.e.*, have circulating antibodies against HIV) have CD4 counts of > 500 cells/μL, an undetectable viral load, and can be relatively "healthy" for many years. HIV/AIDS is commonly classified by three stages. Stage 1 is when the individual is HIV seropositive, has a CD4 count ≥ 500 cells/μL, and no AIDS-defining conditions (Table 24-1). Stage 2 is when the individual has a CD4 count 200 to 499 cells/μL, may have recurrent illnesses, but does not have an AIDS-defining condition. Individuals in stage 2 respond normally to treatment for their recurrent illnesses. Stage 3 is when the individual's CD4 count drops below 200 cells/μL or the person has been diagnosed with one or more AIDS-defining conditions.[5,6]

Because newer medications and protocols have dramatically slowed the progression of HIV/AIDS, individuals are living longer and beginning to have many comorbidities and chronic health problems. In addition to the chronic problems that affect the general aging population, people with HIV/AIDS get many illnesses that those with healthy, intact immune systems do not. Their recovery can be slower and less complete. Diseases and conditions that commonly affect those with HIV/AIDS include hepatitis B, hepatitis C, tuberculosis, wasting syndrome, pancreatitis, peripheral neuropathy, and hyperlipidemia.[4]

Table 24-1 AIDS-DEFINING ILLNESSES OR OPPORTUNISTIC INFECTIONS[7]
Candidiasis of bronchi, trachea, lungs, esophagus
Cervical cancer, invasive
Coccidioidomycosis, disseminated or extrapulmonary
Cryptococcosis, extrapulmonary
Cryptosporidiosis, chronic intestinal for > 1 month
Cytomegalovirus disease (other than liver, spleen, or lymph nodes) Cytomegalovirus disease, retinitis
Encephalopathy (HIV-related)
Herpes simplex: chronic ulcers for > 1 month or bronchitis, pneumonitis, or esophagitis
Histoplasmosis, disseminated or extrapulmonary
Isosporiasis, chronic intestinal for > 1 month
Kaposi's sarcoma
Lymphoma, Burkitt's, immunoblastic, or primary brain
Mycobacterium avium complex
Mycobacterium, other species, disseminated or extrapulmonary
Mycobacterium tuberculosis, any site
Pneumocystis jiroveci pneumonia (*Pneumocystis carinii*)
Pneumonia, recurrent
Progressive multifocal leukoencephalopathy
Salmonella septicemia, recurrent
Toxoplasmosis of the brain
Wasting syndrome due to HIV

Acute pancreatitis is fairly common in patients with HIV/AIDS. It is found to occur as many as 800 times more frequently in this population than in the general population.[8,9] It is more common in females and is often associated with opportunistic infections such as cytomegalovirus or some of the medications used to treat HIV/AIDS. Declining CD4 counts, indicating increased immunosuppression, are also associated with acute pancreatitis.[9-11] Patients hospitalized with acute pancreatitis typically complain of sharp abdominal pain that may be associated with eating, nausea, and vomiting. Food and liquids are completely restricted (*i.e.*, NPO) to significantly limit the secretion of pancreatic enzymes to allow the inflammation of the pancreas to resolve. Patients are then placed on TPN. They may require intravenous opiates for pain relief.[9] Decreased mobility because of pain, nausea, and vomiting often leads to generalized weakness and deconditioning.

HIV-associated wasting syndrome is a common complication of HIV/AIDS and is defined as an involuntary weight loss of greater than 10% of initial weight in the past year or 5% during the past 6 months, often accompanied by diarrhea or weakness and fever. It is characterized by a preferential loss of lean body mass due to inadequate nutrition (due to altered taste secondary to medications, anorexia, nausea/vomiting, diarrhea, gastrointestinal infections, oral lesions), malabsorption, and altered metabolism or hormonal deficiencies. These complications and contributing factors are more common in individuals with AIDS than in the earlier stages of HIV infection. Wasting can lead to complications such as generalized weakness, decreased function, depressed immune function, and significantly increased morbidity and mortality.[12,13] Wasting is treated by administration of hormones, anabolic steroids, and nutritional supplements, and by controlling viral load and immune competence.[12]

Distal symmetric peripheral neuropathy is a non-life-threatening health problem typically associated with AIDS, although it can occur at any stage of HIV infection. It is the most common neurological problem found in individuals with HIV/AIDS.[14,15] The exact cause is unknown, but it appears to be associated with the virus itself, ADRs of the antiretroviral medications, low CD4 count, and high viral load. Other risk factors include aging, nutritional factors, cytomegalovirus infection, and weight loss.[7,14,16] Although it is not considered a medically serious condition, it can be debilitating and have a profound impact on quality of life. Individuals can present with various symptoms in the feet and sometimes in the hands. Signs and symptoms include dysesthesia, painful numbness, burning, tingling, decreased sensation, intrinsic muscle atrophy, and areflexia at the ankles. The discomfort can become so severe that just the touch of bed sheets can be intolerable. Signs and symptoms of neuropathy lead to gait deviations, loss of function, and decreased independence. Current medical management includes the use of over-the-counter (OTC) and prescription analgesics, anti-seizure medications, and antidepressants. In a study of 450 individuals on self-management for HIV-related peripheral neuropathy, complementary therapies (reflexology and meditation) were rated higher in effectiveness than activities (taking a hot bath, elevating the feet, rubbing the feet), exercise (walking), medications (OTC and prescribed), supplements (vitamin B, calcium, magnesium), and substance use (alcohol, street drugs).[17] Evidence supporting the use of topical capsaicin to decrease symptoms of peripheral neuropathy has been inconsistent, although in some cases it appears to work well.[18-20] While there is no cure for HIV/AIDS, there are several different classes of medications that significantly inhibit the progression of the disease. These include nucleoside and nucleotide reverse transcriptase inhibitors, non-nucleoside reverse transcriptase inhibitors, protease inhibitors, entry inhibitors, fusion inhibitors, and integrase inhibitors. Each class of drugs works at a different part of the HIV life cycle. All these medications have adverse effects, most commonly fatigue, diarrhea, nausea and vomiting, anorexia, and abdominal cramping.[13] Since the introduction of highly active antiretroviral therapy (HAART) in 1996, which *combines* several classes of drugs into the therapeutic regimen, survival rates for people with HIV/AIDS have dramatically increased. Life expectancy following diagnosis was 6.8 years in 1993, 10.5 years in 1996, and increased to 30 to 50 years in 2008.[21,22]

In October 2011, the United States Department of Health and Human Services released the most recent **antiretroviral treatment guidelines**[23] recommending when pharmacological treatment for HIV/AIDS should be initiated (Table 24-2).

Table 24-2   GUIDELINES FOR INITIATION OF ANTIRETROVIRAL TREATMENT FOR HIV[23]
History of an AIDS-defining illness
CD4 count < 350
Pregnant women to prevent vertical transmission
Diagnosis of HIV-associated nephropathy, regardless of the CD4 cell count
People coinfected with hepatitis B virus (HBV) and HIV, regardless of the CD4 cell count, when HBV treatment is recommended
Patients with CD4 counts between 350 and 500
There is no consensus regarding initiation of antiretroviral treatment in patients with CD4 counts >500; about 50% of the expert panel recommended it while the other 50% viewed it as optional

Physical Therapy Patient/Client Management

The patient hospitalized with complications of HIV/AIDS typically requires physical therapy to maximize independence and to return to prior level of function. Frequently, some degree of physical endurance and strength compromise is apparent. This patient has been acutely ill for almost 2 weeks when the physical therapist evaluates him. In addition to the nausea, vomiting, and pain related to the acute pancreatitis, he also has signs and symptoms related to wasting syndrome and peripheral neuropathy. The wasting will be exacerbated by the recent history of gastrointestinal disturbance, NPO status, and prolonged bedrest. The peripheral neuropathy can lead to further deterioration of the patient's functional status due to altered sensation in the feet and consequent balance impairment. Physical therapy intervention should be initiated as soon as the patient's constitutional symptoms and pain are controlled.

Examination, Evaluation, and Diagnosis

The chart review informs the physical therapist of the patient's social and medical history, current medications, lab values, vital signs, and any restrictions in activities. With this patient, the therapist should be aware of potential ADRs of the two new medications he has started during this hospitalization: fentanyl and imipenem/cilastatin. The ADRs include dizziness, drowsiness, respiratory depression, and seizure. Lab values of interest with this patient are his very low CD4 count and undetectable viral load. Clinically, these reflect that even though the virus itself is not replicating rapidly, the patient is quite susceptible to illness or infection because his immune function is not robust. Thus, the physical therapist should be especially vigilant about following standard precautions. Red blood cell values (hematocrit and hemoglobin) are also important to review since anemia is a frequent problem in this patient population, and low values predict the ability to participate in the physical examination and interventions.

Given the acuteness of the patient's pain and the degree of deconditioning, an efficient yet thorough examination is advised. However, examination of this patient should not require many special tests and measures. The subjective history likely corroborates what was found during the chart review, and allows the therapist to assess the patient's level of consciousness, appropriateness, and willingness to participate in physical therapy interventions. The general physical therapy examination should begin with measuring vital signs, including heart rate, respiratory rate, and blood pressure. This can be followed by assessment of bed mobility, generalized strength, and transfers. Because of the patient's documented peripheral neuropathy and recent immobility, examination of the signs and symptoms of peripheral neuropathy should be prioritized. This involves testing sensation, lower extremity reflexes, strength, range of motion (ROM) in the lower extremities and balance. While sensation of the lower legs is sometimes assessed using light touch with a cotton ball, most individuals with peripheral neuropathy do not tolerate this on their feet. Dysesthesia, an unpleasant sensation to light touch, is common and thus, these individuals respond better to a firm rather than a light touch. Semmes Weinstein monofilament sensation assessments are better tolerated. Sensation is typically decreased in a symmetrical stocking pattern, although it may be limited to just the feet. Reflexes are usually intact at the knees and absent at the ankles. The toe extensors and Achilles tendons are likely to be very tight, limiting ROM, and perhaps pulling the toes into a hammer toe-like position. Delayed muscle recruitment at the ankle has been documented, leading to decreased ability to recover from lateral lean.[24] Therefore, both static and dynamic balance assessments should be performed prior to beginning gait activities. These might include standing with eyes open, eyes closed, single leg stance, and adding perturbations. A formal test that incorporates these activities, such as the **Tinetti Performance Oriented Mobility Assessment (POMA)**[25] or Berg Balance Test,[26] might be appropriate to assess risk of falling. While the POMA is a reliable and valid clinical test of balance and gait in older adults, it has also been used in individuals with peripheral neuropathy.[27] If the patient presents with endurance sufficient to tolerate 10 to 15 minutes of activity, the POMA is an easily administered test in the acute care setting, requiring only a hard armless chair, a short walkway, and a stopwatch. The POMA is scored using a three-point ordinal scale ranging from 0 to 2, with "0" indicating the highest level of impairment and "2" indicating no impairment. A perfect score (*i.e.*, lack of impairment) on the balance component is 16 and a perfect score on the gait component is 12, for a total POMA test score of 28. Individuals scoring 19 to 24 out of 28 have a "moderate" risk of falling, and those scoring < 19 have a "high" risk of falling.[28] Finally, since the patient works and ambulates independently in the community, his ability to negotiate stairs should be observed. Vital signs should be reassessed following these activities and any signs of distress or exercise intolerance noted during performance.

Applying the International Classification of Functioning, Disability and Health Model (ICF) to this case, there are obvious body structure and function limitations based on his current illness and prior history of wasting syndrome and peripheral neuropathy. These impairments are likely limiting his activities and participation because of fatigue, weakness, generalized deconditioning, and gait disturbances.[6] Physical therapy diagnoses for this patient include decreased strength, primarily in the lower extremities, decreased endurance related to prolonged bedrest and wasting syndrome, HIV-related peripheral neuropathy, and impaired balance.

Plan of Care and Interventions

Because this patient will be discharged home in a few days, emphasis should be on maximizing independent functioning. It has been shown that strengthening and balance exercises significantly decrease risk of falls in individuals with diabetic peripheral neuropathy.[24,29] Since HIV-related and diabetic peripheral neuropathies present very similarly, these exercises would likely benefit those with HIV-related neuropathy. Table 24-3 presents a sample daily exercise program for individuals with peripheral neuropathy.

Resistance and moderate intensity aerobic exercise have been shown to be safe and beneficial for those with HIV/AIDS. Exercise does not decrease CD4 count nor does it increase viral load, so it does not further compromise the patient's immune system. There is also no association between exercise and development of illnesses. In addition, resistance exercise increases lean body mass and improves strength in those infected with HIV.[13,30] Exercise helps decrease depression and anxiety in this patient population.[30] Moderate intensity aerobic exercise has been shown to

Table 24-3 STRENGTHENING AND BALANCE EXERCISES FOR INDIVIDUALS WITH PERIPHERAL NEUROPATHY[24,29]

Exercise	Description and Progression
Single leg stance	Progress from holding onto a firm counter support with 2, 1, or no hands. Stand as long as possible on one leg, to the point of fatigue or loss of balance. Repeat with opposite leg.
Toe raises/heel raises	Progress to no hands and from bilateral to single leg. Begin with 1 set of 10 repetitions and increase by 1 set every 5 exercise sessions.
Wall slides	Stand with back against wall and feet ~12-20 inches from wall. Bend hips and knees to ~45° knee flexion—pretend to "sit in a chair." Progression: gradually increase the hold time for "sitting in the chair."
Figure 8	Walk in a figure 8 while holding therapist's or partner's hand. Progress to independent walking in figure 8 pattern.
Tandem walking	Walk "heel-to-toe" with hand to the side on a firm counter support. Perform 4 sets of at least 10 steps. Progress to tandem walking with no hands.
Ball toss on gymnastic ball	Sit on gymnastic ball and throw small ball back and forth with therapist or partner. The ball is tossed directly to the patient at first. Progressively challenge balance by tossing ball in directions that require patient to increase amount of weight shift necessary to catch the ball.
Ankle inversion/eversion	Stand on one leg and hold on to firm support with one or both hands. Shift weight medially and laterally (causing ankle inversion and eversion), to the point of fatigue or loss of balance. Progress to weight shift without support of hands.
Walking on exercise mat or other uneven surface	Begin with arms out to sides for balance. Progress to arms folded across chest.

significantly increase maximal oxygen consumption (VO_2 max) and time to fatigue in individuals with HIV/AIDS participating in an aerobic and a resistance exercise training program.[31,32] Exercises included treadmill training at 50% to 70% of age-predicted heart rate maximum and resistance exercises using free weights, pneumatic, and plated exercise equipment.[31] Although this might be beyond this patient's current capabilities, he could benefit from a combined aerobic and resistance exercise program once his current illness has resolved. Hopefully he will be able to begin a lower intensity program prior to discharge. The physical therapist could help the patient initiate resistance exercises by prescribing a light resistance home exercise program using resistance bands or tubing (*e.g.*, yellow Theraband).

Peripheral neuropathy can respond directly to physical therapy intervention. In a case study involving two individuals with HIV-related peripheral neuropathy, a combination of **microcurrent, joint and soft tissue mobilization, and stretching** decreased the symptoms of HIV-related peripheral neuropathy.[33] Joint mobilizations of the feet, toes, and ankles are an appropriate intervention since many patients with neuropathy present with decreased passive accessory and passive physiological movements in the feet and ankles[34] in addition to numbness/tingling or dysesthesia. Individuals received grades III and IV anterior-posterior mobilizations to the small joints of the feet and toes, as well as to the talocrural joint.[33] Dysesthesia and/or paresthesia can respond to soft tissue mobilization, typically tolerated best with a firm grasp on the feet. Deep tissue massage utilizing a firm grip was performed on the feet to decrease sensitivity to touch, improve soft tissue pliability, and promote circulation. This intervention resulted in decreased use of pain medications, improved quality of gait, and independent functioning.[33] Stretching of the toe extensors and Achilles tendons may also allow a more normal foot-to-floor contact during the stance phase of gait.

Evidence-Based Clinical Recommendations

SORT: Strength of Recommendation Taxonomy

A: Consistent, good-quality patient-oriented evidence

B: Inconsistent or limited-quality patient-oriented evidence

C: Consensus, disease-oriented evidence, usual practice, expert opinion, or case series

1. Antiretroviral drug therapy should be initiated when CD4 count is < 350 and/or the individual has a history of an AIDS-defining illness. **Grade A**

2. The Tinetti Performance Oriented Mobility Assessment (POMA) can be used to predict the risk of falls in adults with peripheral neuropathy. **Grade C**

3. Both resistance exercise and moderate intensity aerobic exercise are safe and beneficial for individuals with HIV/AIDS. **Grade A**

4. Microcurrent, joint mobilization, and soft tissue mobilization applied to the feet of individuals with peripheral neuropathy decreases use of opiate analgesics, improves quality of gait, and promotes independent functioning. **Grade B**

COMPREHENSION QUESTIONS

24.1 A patient with long-standing HIV/AIDS and acute pancreatitis becomes dizzy, lightheaded, and short of breath while the physical therapist is performing a balance assessment. The medication *most* likely to cause this is:

A. Abacavir

B. Fentanyl

C. Lamivudine

D. Atazanavir

24.2 A patient diagnosed with AIDS has a CD4 count of 112 and a viral load of 15,000. This means that:

A. The patient's immune system is strong and the medications are controlling the virus well.

B. The patient's immune system is weakened, but the medications are controlling the virus well.

C. The patient's immune system is strong, but the medications are not controlling the virus adequately.

D. The patient's immune system is weakened and the medications are not controlling the virus adequately.

24.3 Individuals with wasting syndrome:

A. Should avoid drugs such as anabolic steroids that promote muscle growth.

B. Can improve endurance by exercising at 50% of age-predicted heart rate maximum.

C. Cannot gain lean muscle by using nutritional supplements.

D. Should not be concerned because this is not a serious complication of HIV/AIDS.

ANSWERS

24.1 **B.** Fentanyl is an opiate analgesic. The ADRs include dizziness, drowsiness, lightheadedness, and respiratory depression. The medications used to treat HIV infection typically cause gastrointestinal upset (options A, C, D).

24.2 **D.** Normal CD4 count ranges from about 500 to 1500 cells/µL. The CD4 count reflects the health of the immune system. A cell count of 112 indicates that an inadequate number of CD4 cells are available to fight off infections and illness. Viral load reflects how well the medications are controlling the virus. Ideally, the viral load is undetectable. When it is above 10,000 copies/mL, it indicates that the medications are not as effective as they should be.

24.3 **B.** Wasting syndrome is a serious complication of HIV infection (option D). It can lead to increased morbidity and mortality in addition to decreasing functional status and quality of life. Aerobic exercise at 50% to 70% of age-predicted heart rate maximum has been shown to increase VO_2 max and time to fatigue in patients with HIV wasting syndrome. Other treatments for wasting syndrome include use of anabolic steroids (option A), hormones, and nutritional supplements (option C).

REFERENCES

1. Centers for Disease Control and Prevention: HIV in the United States. Available at: http://www.cdc.gov/hiv/resources/factsheets/us.htm. Accessed January 11, 2012.

2. AVERTing HIV and AIDS. Available at: http://www.avert.org/usa-statistics.htm. Accessed January 11, 2012.

3. Hopkin TB. *Lab Notes: Guide to Lab and Diagnostic Tests*. Philadelphia, PA: FA Davis Company; 2005.

4. National Institutes of Health: AIDSinfo; HIV and its treatment. Available at: http://aidsinfo.nih.gov/education-materials/fact-sheets. Accessed January 12, 2012.

5. 2012 Case Definitions: Nationally Notifiable Conditions Infectious and Non-Infectious Case. Atlanta, GA; Centers for Disease Control and Prevention; 2012. Available at: wwwn.cdc.gov/nndss/document/2012_Case%20Definitions.pdf. Accessed January 12, 2012.

6. US Department of Health and Human Services, Health Resources and Services Administration, HIV/AIDS Bureau. Guide for HIV/AIDS Clinical Care. HIV classification: CDC and WHO staging systems. Rockville, MD. 2011. Available at: www.newarkema.org/pdf/reports/CM_Jan2011.pdf. Accessed January 12, 2012.

7. Centers for Disease Control and Prevention. MMWR - Recommendations and Reports. Available at: http://www.cdc.gov/mmwr/preview/mmwrhtml/00018871.htm. Accessed January 2, 2013.

8. Bush ZM, Kosmiski LA. Acute pancreatitis in HIV-infected patients: are etiologies changing since the introduction of protease inhibitor therapy? *Pancreas*. 2003;27:e1-e5.

9. Trindade AJ, Huysman AM, Huprikar SS, Kim MK. A case study and review of pancreatitis in the AIDS population. *Dig Dis Sci*. 2008;53:2616-2620.

10. Riedel DJ, Gebo KA, Moore RD, Lucas GM. A ten-tear analysis of the incidence and risk factors for acute pancreatitis requiring hospitalization in an urban HIV clinical cohort. *AIDS. Patient Care STDS*. 2008;22:113-121.

11. Leurquin-Sterk G, Schepers K, Delhaye M, Goldman S, Verset L, Matos C. Diffuse pancreatic lesion mimicking autoimmune pancreatitis in HIV-infected patient: successful treatment by antiretroviral therapy. *J Pancreas*. 2011;12:477-481.

12. Polsky B, Kotler D, Steinhart C. Treatment guidelines for HIV-associated wasting. *HIV Clin Trials*. 2004;5:50-61.

13. Dudgeon WD, Phillips KD, Carson JA, Brewer RB, Durstine JL, Hand GA. Counteracting muscle wasting in HIV-infected individuals. *HIV Med*. 2006;7:299-310.

14. Dorsey SG, Morton PG. HIV peripheral neuropathy: pathophysiology and clinical implications. *AACN Clinical Issues*. 2006;17:30-36.

15. Gonzalez-Duarte A, Cikurel K, Simpson DM. Managing HIV peripheral neuropathy. *Curr HIV/AIDS Rep*. 2007;4:114-118.

16. Evans SR, Ellis RJ, Chen H, et al. Peripheral neuropathy in HIV: prevalence and risk factors. *AIDS*. 2011;25:919-928.

17. Nicholas PK, Kemppainen JK, Canaval GE, et al. Symptom management and self-care for peripheral neuropathy in HIV/AIDS. *AIDS Care*. 2007;19:179-189.

18. Paice JA, Ferrans CE, Lashley FR, Shott S, Vizgirda V, Pitrak D. Topical capsaicin in the management of HIV-associated peripheral neuropathy. *J Pain Symptom Manag.* 2000;19:45-52.

19. Gonzalez-Duarte A, Cikurél K, Simpson D. Managing HIV peripheral neuropathy. *Curr HIV/AIDS Rep.* 2007;4:114-118.

20. Tesfaye S, Selvarajah D. Recent advances in the pharmacological management of painful diabetic neuropathy. *Br J Diabetes Vasc Dis.* 2009;9:283-287.

21. Harrison KM, Song R, Zhang X. Life expectancy after HIV diagnosis based on national HIV surveillance data from 25 states, United States. *J Acquir Immune Defic Syndr.* 2010;53:124-130.

22. Antiretroviral Therapy Cohort Collaboration. Life expectancy of individuals on combination antiretroviral therapy in high-income countries: a collaborative analysis of 14 cohort studies. *Lancet.* 2008;372:293-299.

23. US Department of Health and Human Services. Panel on Antiretroviral Guidelines for Adults and Adolescents. Guidelines for the use of antiretroviral agents in HIV-1-infected adults and adolescents. 2011;34. Available at: http://www.aidsinfo.nih.gov/ContentFiles/AdultandAdolescentGL.pdf. Accessed January 11, 2012.

24. Richardson JK, Sandman D, Vela S. A focused exercise regimen improves clinical measures of balance in patients with peripheral neuropathy. *Arch Phys Med Rehabil.* 2001;82:205-209.

25. Tinetti ME. Performance oriented assessment of mobility problems in elderly patients. *J Am Geriatr Soc.* 1986;34:119-126.

26. Berg K, Wood-Dauphinée SL, Williams JI, Gayton D. Measuring balance in the elderly: preliminary development of an instrument. *Physiother Canada.* 1989;41:304-308.

27. Volkert V, Hassan A, Hassan MA, et al. Effectiveness of monochromatic infrared photo energy and physical therapy for peripheral neuropathy: changes in sensation, pain, and balance—a preliminary, multi-center study. *Phys Occup Ther Geriatr.* 2005;24:1-17.

28. Shumway-Cook A, Wollacott MH. *Motor Control: Theory and Practical Applications.* 2nd ed. Baltimore, MD: Lippincott Williams & Wilkins; 2001.

29. Kruse RL, LeMaster JW, Madsen RW. Fall and balance outcomes after an intervention to promote leg strength, balance, and walking in people with diabetic peripheral neuropathy: "feet first" randomized controlled trial. *Phys Ther.* 2010;90:1568-1579.

30. Dudgeon WD, Phillips KD, Bopp CM, Hand GA. Physiological and psychological effects of exercise interventions in HIV disease. *AIDS Patient Care STDS.* 2004;18:81-98.

31. Hand GA, Phillips KD, Dudgeon WD, Lyerly GW, Durstine JL, Burgess SE. Moderate intensity exercise training reverses functional aerobic impairment in HIV-infected individuals. *AIDS Care.* 2008;20:1066-1074.

32. O'Brien K, Tynan AM, Nixon S, Glazier RH. Effects of progressive resistive exercise in adults living with HIV/AIDS: systematic review and meta-analysis of randomized trials. *AIDS Care.* 2008;20:631-653.

33. Gale J. Physiotherapy intervention in two people with HIV or AIDS-related peripheral neuropathy. *Physiother Res Int.* 2003;8:200-209.

34. Williams DS III, Brunt D, Tanenberg RJ. Diabetic neuropathy is related to joint stiffness during late stance phase. *J Appl Biomech.* 2007;23:251-260.

Terminal Illness: Hospice Physical Therapy

Karen Mueller

A 91-year-old ectomorphic male with a 25-year history of Parkinson's disease (PD) was transported by ambulance to the emergency department with complaints of confusion and weakness. The patient lives with his 70-year-old daughter who reported finding her father confused, disoriented, and unable to get out of bed that morning. She denied any change in his medication schedule, but was concerned that her father might have become dehydrated from being outside in the heat the previous day. Approximately 3 years ago, the patient had been active in the community and was independent in activities of daily living (ADLs) and mobility. Over the past 2 years, the patient's cognitive and physical status declined significantly. He needed to use a walker for ambulation and he also lost 20 lb. The patient had been receiving outpatient physical therapy intervention until 3 months ago when he developed a severe urinary tract infection requiring a 3-day hospitalization. According to the patient's daughter, his energy level declined considerably. At this point, the patient moved into his daughter's home, and appointed her as his power of attorney. Over the last month, the patient's ambulation declined to the point of short household distances with minimal assist. He also experienced two choking episodes during meals in the past week. Home health physical therapy had just been initiated to address functional decline. The patient has several comorbidities including: hypertension, hyperlipidemia, osteoporosis, and a cardiac pacemaker placement 3 years ago due to bradycardia. His home medications included alendronate, Aricept, carbidopa/levidopa, Celebrex, citalopram, Cozaar, Namenda, aspirin, and calcium. The patient was admitted to the hospital for further testing and follow-up. Chest x-ray revealed increased basilar opacities and vascular congestion with small left effusion, consistent with pneumonia. A computed tomography (CT) scan of the head was unchanged from 3 years prior, and normal except for atrophy and chronic small vessel ischemic change. Over a 2-week inpatient hospital stay, the patient experienced multisystem failure. He continued to demonstrate moderate confusion and orientation deficits and was agitated at times. On several occasions, he reported seeing "strange objects" in his room. Wheezing and upper respiratory expiratory noises were pronounced after meals; diagnosis of aspiration pneumonia was confirmed and swallowing precautions were initiated. The option of placing a percutaneous endoscopic gastrostomy tube into the jejunum (J-PEG) was considered, but the patient and his daughter decided against this measure. He continued to exhibit decreased appetite, resulting in a 7-lb weight loss. Inpatient physical therapy assessment noted impairments of rigidity, akinesia/bradykinesia, and loss of trunk, pelvic girdle, and lower extremity extension that contributed to loss of functional mobility. Ten physical therapy interventions were provided over 30-minute sessions. The emphasis was on optimizing range of motion of trunk and extremities, strengthening, and activities to promote functional mobility. The patient made minimal progress due to general malaise, weakness, and severe rigidity. At times, he appeared restless and in pain. His bed mobility varied from maximal to moderate assist and he required maximal assistance for standing pivot transfers. He could stand for 5 to 10 seconds with maximal assistance, but was unable to ambulate. He required maximal assistance in all ADLs including feeding. The patient was initially expected to return to his daughter's home once his condition stabilized. However, given the patient's complete dependence in ADLs, this was no longer considered a feasible option. The patient's physician suggested a referral for placement in a hospice residential home. The daughter agreed, stating that her father had an advanced directive that stated that he wanted no aggressive treatment once he became dependent in mobility.

▶ As the physical therapist treating this patient in the acute hospital, on what basis might you support the recommendation of a hospice evaluation for this patient?
▶ What is the role of the physical therapist in the hospice setting?
▶ Which outcome measures are recommended for physical therapy assessment in the hospice setting?
▶ Given the patient's impairments, which interventions might be appropriate in terms of comfort, mobility, and pain management?
▶ How would you prioritize this patient's impairments and functional limitations for effective intervention?

KEY DEFINITIONS

ADVANCED DIRECTIVE: Legal document that details options for the provision of health care when a person is incapacitated. Specific elements include a Healthcare Power of Attorney (written authorization given by an individual for another person to act on his/her behalf with respect to healthcare decisions) and a Living Will (includes preferences with respect to use of life-sustaining treatment and other interventions). It may also include a Do Not Resuscitate (DNR) order and a Mental Health Power of Attorney.

END-OF-LIFE CARE: Interdisciplinary approach to promotion of comfort, dignity, and quality of life for persons with terminal conditions

HOSPICE CARE: Focuses on patient comfort and quality of life rather than curing disease; generally appropriate for someone with terminal illness and life expectancy of 6 months or less

PALLIATIVE CARE: Aims to enhance quality of life of individuals who are faced with a serious, chronic illness; focuses on increasing comfort through prevention and treatment of distressing symptoms; patients receiving palliative care may still be involved in curative measures such as chemotherapy and radiation treatment

POWER OF ATTORNEY: Written authorization given by an individual for another person to act on his/her behalf with regards to any legal matters

Objectives

1. Describe the typical progression of Parkinson's disease and which symptoms are indications for referral to hospice.
2. Describe the Medicare hospice benefit provided for physical therapy services.
3. List the service providers considered part of the core interdisciplinary team (IDT) in Medicare-certified hospice facilities.
4. Describe strategies that might be useful for a physical therapist that is interested in providing services to the population of individuals receiving hospice care.
5. Define education provided by the physical therapist that might be helpful for the IDT and nursing staff at a hospice residence.
6. List the requirements for initiation of Medicare hospice services.
7. Describe reliable and valid assessment tools that would be appropriate for an individual receiving hospice care.

Physical Therapy Considerations

PT considerations during management of the older adult with end-stage Parkinson's disease during the transition to hospice care:

▶ **General physical therapy plan of care/goals:** Minimize loss of range of motion (ROM), strength, and aerobic functional capacity; decrease pain; promote decreased rigidity to optimize functional movement patterns, improve quality of life

▶ **Physical therapy interventions:** Patient and family education regarding positioning for comfort and skin protection; modified mobility training to optimize functional movement patterns; energy conservation techniques; breathing and relaxation exercises to reduce pain and congestion; edema reduction strategies

▶ **Precautions during physical therapy:** Slow transition to upright to reduce the risk of orthostatic hypotension; graded activity to prevent cardiovascular distress

▶ **Complications interfering with physical therapy:** Severe pain, agitation, terminal restlessness, transition to active death

Understanding the Health Condition

PD is generally recognized as a chronic, progressive, neurologic disorder involving cardinal motor signs of bradykinesia, resting tremor, and postural instability. An objective measure of PD-related motor impairments can be identified either along a five-stage continuum (from Stage 1 with unilateral signs, to Stage 5 involving full incapacitation) described by Hoehn and Yahr in 1967,[1] or by the Unified Parkinson's Disease Rating Scale which was first published in 1987.[2]

While there is substantial evidence supporting the value of physical therapy intervention in optimizing physical functioning, strength, balance, gait speed, and health-related quality of life for patients with PD in the early and middle stages (Hoehn and Yahr Stages 1-3),[3-6] such evidence is minimal for those with end-stage disease.

As the trajectory of PD continues into the later stages, physical function deteriorates to the point of full incapacitation, whereby the person is bedridden or in a wheelchair unless assisted (Hoehn and Yahr Stage 5). The later stages of the disease are further complicated by progressive dementia and in some cases, the onset of psychotic symptoms such as hallucinations. Although the exact pathogenesis of this late stage dementia is unclear, emerging evidence attributes this to Lewy body infiltration into the cerebral cortex, brainstem nuclei, and basal forebrain cholinergic system.[7] Furthermore, it has been postulated that the signs and symptoms of Parkinson's disease with dementia (PDD) and dementia with Lewy bodies (DLB) may overlap.[8] Therefore, in the absence of reliable and valid objective measures that enable accurate differential diagnoses of these conditions, clinicians must rely on clinical observation and existing methods of intervention. For example, visual hallucinations are often present in patients with DLB, but not in those with PDD.[8]

In addition to the development of progressive dementia, patients with PD face a host of systemic complications in the end stages. Autonomic system failure (implicated by Lewy body infiltration into the hypothalamus, pre-ganglionic parasympathetic projection neurons of the Vagus nerve, and post-ganglionic sympathetic projection neurons of the spinal cord)[9] leads to cardiovascular complications including orthostatic hypotension, respiratory sinus arrhythmia, and decreased heart rate variability. In the case of the current patient, cardiovascular impairments necessitated the placement of cardiac pacemaker for severe bradycardia. Lewy body infiltration has also been implicated in PD-related autonomic dysfunction of the submandibular gland (which, along with a forward head posture, contributes to drooling) and the lower esophagus and larynx (which contributes to dysphagia and speech deficits). These autonomic deficits combined with respiratory muscle deficits result in both obstructive and restrictive dysfunction,[10,11] placing patients with PD at high risk for choking and aspiration pneumonia. Accordingly, respiratory dysfunction is one of the leading causes of death in persons with end-stage PD.[12]

Gastrointestinal system function becomes severely impaired in end-stage PD, threatening the ability to maintain optimal oral nutrition. Impairments include constipation, olfactory decline, early satiety, decreased gastric transit time, and nausea. In one systematic review of 1134 patients with PD, up to 24% were identified as being malnourished, and up to 60% were identified as at risk for malnutrition.[13] Nausea and vomiting may also be adverse drug reactions (ADRs) of dopamine replacement therapy. Higher intakes of these medications have been associated with a lower body mass index.[13]

The presence of pain in PD is poorly understood, but recent evidence suggests that the prevalence of pain is as high as 83%.[14] Five different types of pain have been described in patients with PD: musculoskeletal pain (due to rigidity, rheumatological disease, or skeletal deformity), radicular-neuropathic pain (due to a root lesion, or focal or peripheral neuropathy), dystonic pain (related to effects of anti-Parkinson's medication), central neuropathic pain (related to effects of anti-Parkinson's medication) and akathisia (unpleasant perception of restlessness—an ADR of anti-Parkinson's medication).[15] Despite the apparently high prevalence of pain among patients with PD, this symptom is often unrecognized, possibly because many patients are unable to vocalize their discomfort. Consequently, up to 40% of patients with PD do not receive appropriate analgesic medications, further increasing their level of debility.[15]

Despite the severity of total system decline in PD, patients with end-stage disease do not receive palliative and hospice care as often as those with other neurodegenerative diseases such as amyotrophic lateral sclerosis (ALS) and multiple sclerosis.[16,17] To address possible reasons for this disparity, a recent study compared the experiences of 50 caregivers of persons with end-stage ALS to 52 caregivers of persons with end-stage PD.[17] The authors intentionally selected ALS, a terminal disease with a well-established need for hospice intervention in order to highlight the unmet hospice and palliative care needs of patients with PD. Caregivers were surveyed about their loved ones' symptoms, distress levels, and psychosocial experiences in the last month of life. In addition, the study explored caregivers' perceptions of their loved ones' use of healthcare services and their treatment preferences. The results revealed striking similarities in the experiences of patients with ALS and PD. Specifically, both groups rated their level of suffering as 4 out of 6 (1 = none and 6 = severe). Pain was rated as moderately severe or greater (a rating of ≥ 4) in 42% of patients with PD and 52% of patients with ALS. However 27% of patients with PD received no pain medication in the last month compared to only 19% of those with ALS. Patients with PD demonstrated more severe confusion than those with ALS, but there was no difference between groups with respect to the prevalence and severity of depression and anxiety. While dyspnea and respiratory distress were significantly higher in the patients with ALS, both groups rated difficulty eating as the most common and severe physical symptom of their diseases. Although 56% of patients with PD received hospice care as did 64% of those with ALS, the average length of hospice services was significantly shorter for the patients with PD (3 weeks) compared to those with ALS (8 weeks). Finally, only 25% of the patients with PD died at home in contrast to over 50% of those with ALS. The authors concluded with the following statement: "Patients with PD experienced suffering comparable to that of patients with ALS, with more frequent and severe confusion, yet patients with PD receive fewer weeks of hospice benefit prior to death. Prospective research would serve this population . . . to improve quality of care at the end of life."[18]

The disparities described in this study are particularly relevant given the growing prevalence of PD compared to ALS (1 million individuals compared to 30,000, respectively).[19,20] Thus, patients with PD are likely at risk for continued underutilization of hospice services at a time when increasing numbers of individuals will need them. In order to best meet the healthcare needs of current and future patients with PD, barriers to hospice access must be identified and addressed. Two recent studies have provided valuable insights into the nature and impact of such barriers. Hasson et al.[21] explored caregiver perceptions of palliative and hospice care needs of 15 patients with PD. The study revealed that many caregivers were unaware of the appropriateness of hospice intervention in the end stages of PD, and that communication with medical providers was inadequate to promote understanding of such benefits. Furthermore, the unpredictable nature of end-stage PD, with its potential for rapid onset of potentially fatal complications (e.g., aspiration pneumonia), made it difficult to determine the optimal timeframe for the initiation of palliative and hospice care. Further evidence suggests that confusion about the hospice and palliative care needs of patients with end-stage PD also occurs among healthcare providers. A study of allied health professionals' views on palliative care needs for patients with PD suggested that the value of their services as a comfort measure is often overlooked. Furthermore, many providers are not cognizant of the multisystem issues facing patients with end-stage PD, which limits the patients' access to hospice and palliative care services.[22]

The National Hospice and Palliative Care Organization (NHPCO) released an annual report to track patterns of hospice utilization in the United States over the past several years.[23] According to the 2010 report, 83% of the 1.56 million patients receiving end-of-life related services in 2009 were covered under the Medicare hospice benefit.[23] The Medicare hospice benefit began in 1982. Appropriate initiation of hospice services has proven to be a cost-effective approach to end-of-life care. A study from Duke University reported that the use of hospice services reduced Medicare expenditures by an average of $2309 during the last year of life—a time period when 25% of all Medicare expenditures occur.[24]

For the past several years, NHPCO has reported an ongoing decline in the number of patients receiving hospice services for cancer. Although this diagnosis is still the most common for individuals receiving these services, it has decreased from 50% to 41% in the past decade. The second most common diagnosis (13.1% in 2009) is a condition known as, "debility, unspecified" (ICD-9 CM 799.3), which pertains to progressive system failure ultimately leading to adult failure to thrive. Patients who qualify for the Medicare hospice benefit under the debility unspecified diagnosis typically demonstrate general system failure from a host of comorbidities related to chronic degenerative disease or trauma. In the absence of a recognized diagnostic category specifically related to PD, the debility unspecified diagnosis provides a guideline that enables these patients to qualify for the Medicare hospice benefit. Accordingly, patients with end-stage PD must first demonstrate one or more of the following in the previous 12 months[25]: muscle wasting (cachexia), failure to maintain nutritional needs (inanition) as evidenced by a 10% decline in body weight, recurrent fever, septicemia, aspiration pneumonia, or recurrent urinary tract infection. In addition to these criteria, Medicare requires that a physician provide certification of patient life expectancy of 6 months or less. Furthermore, in order to accept the Medicare hospice benefit, patients must certify that they are no longer seeking curative measures for their condition. In the case of a patient with PD accessing hospice through the debility unspecified diagnosis, this would involve withholding life-prolonging treatment measures unless used solely for comfort.[23] At the current time, the role of anti-Parkinson's medication in the context of *comfort* is unclear. As a result of this lack of consensus, when the patient in this case study was admitted to hospice, his anti-Parkinson's medications were initially discontinued until it was evident that their withdrawal increased his pain, rigidity, and cognitive symptoms. Accordingly, an increasing number of hospice physicians now recommend the continued use of anti-Parkinson's medication as a *comfort* measure, insuring their coverage under the Medicare hospice benefit.

Patients who elect the Medicare hospice benefit services (under Part A) are provided two initial 90-day periods, followed by unlimited 60-day periods as long as documentation shows the *continued need and appropriateness* for services. This caveat leads to a feature of hospice care that is not widely recognized—the possibility of discharge from hospice care due to improving health status beyond hospice admission criteria. Patients may also revoke their hospice benefit at any time (*e.g.*, to resume curative measures). In fact, the 2010 NHPCO report stated that 243,000 patients were discharged from services in 2009 (exact numbers of patients who either improved or sought curative measures were not provided).[23] Once patients elect the Medicare hospice benefit, depending on their desires along with available resources in their community, they may receive services in their home (68.6% of all patients in 2010), in a hospice residential facility (21.2% in 2009) or in a nursing home (18.9% in 2010).[23]

Physical Therapy Patient/Client Management

Medicare-certified hospice facilities require the involvement of several distinct health professionals who comprise the core IDT. The core IDT includes physicians, nurses, social workers, and chaplains. Coverage for core services, medications, and durable medical equipment is provided to Medicare-certified hospices through a specified, daily, or *per diem* rate for each patient. In 2010, this *per diem* rate was $163.00. Physical therapists are not a required "core service" on the hospice IDT. This means that Medicare does not require physical therapy services to be provided to all patients. Instead, physical therapists are among a group of healthcare professionals (along with occupational therapists and speech-language pathologists) whose services must be made available on a consultative or "as needed" basis. This level of involvement is supported by a Medicare policy change (section 418.92 "conditions of participation") that occurred in 2008. This policy change was revised to include the following statement: "Physical therapy, occupational therapy and speech-language pathology must be available, and when provided, consistent with accepted standards of practice, and furnished by personnel who meet the qualifications specified in part 484 of this chapter (individuals who are licensed in their relevant disciplines)."[26]

Although the Medicare policy change suggests that physical therapy is an important component of the IDT, individual hospice programs must develop their own guidelines for inclusion. Most importantly, physical therapists must be educated about the value of therapy services in end-of-life care in order to address the full societal spectrum of patient/client need. Physical therapists must work toward the elimination of educational, institutional, and policy barriers that prevent patients from timely, coordinated, and efficient entry into the hospice system. Furthermore, physical therapists must advocate for the inclusion of their services through the development of outcomes research, education and policy initiatives within their practice settings as well as within their community, societal, and professional realms of influence.

In 2008, the American Physical Therapy Association (APTA) approved the formation of a Hospice and Palliative Care special interest group (HPC-SIG) within the Oncology section. Since its inception, the HPC-SIG has provided education to the APTA membership about the role of physical therapists in the hospice setting, and has developed alliances with NHPCO and other related agencies to promote these efforts. In 2011, the APTA House of Delegates (the policy-making body of the organization) unanimously approved a motion entitled "The Role of Physical Therapy in Hospice and Palliative Care" (APTA House of Delegates RC 17-11).[27] Approval of this motion resulted in the formation of a 17-member group that is currently developing an action plan to promote education, research, and clinical practice related to physical therapy intervention in end-of-life care.

Physical therapists who provide services in the hospice setting do so under a variety of billing arrangements. These include direct contract arrangements or through employment in hospitals, home health agencies, or nursing homes. Payment for physical therapy services is administered as part of the daily *per diem* for each patient that includes covered core services (*i.e.*, medications, equipment and nursing, medical and social work services). Physical therapists must demonstrate the value of their services in relation to the benefits of the core services. Many physical therapists (including this author) are successfully demonstrating their role as a valued member of the hospice IDT.

All patient interventions in the hospice setting are administered in the context of a coordinated interdisciplinary plan of care. The Medicare Conditions of Participation (which provides guidelines for reimbursement of care under the hospice benefit)[26] mandates that each patient in a Medicare-certified hospice receives an interdisciplinary plan of care at the time of admission and the team must update this plan at least every 2 weeks. Thus, most hospices hold weekly IDT meetings that facilitate the coordination of care for both new and existing patients. The reports of each core discipline provide a comprehensive picture of the status of each patient and his/her support system. The patient and family members may also request the option to attend the IDT. The IDT model of hospice care prevents many of the communication pitfalls that can impede quality of care and create patient dissatisfaction. By the thoughtful coordination of every aspect of care, patients and their families can have every element of their quality of life addressed at a time when it is most needed. Because physical therapists are not considered a core member of the IDT, they may not feel that their presence at the weekly meetings is appropriate or necessary. However, it has been the experience of this author that a consistent presence at weekly IDT meetings is invaluable for educating team members about the value of physical therapy services. In addition, physical therapists can identify patients who could benefit from physical therapy examination and interventions.

Examination, Evaluation, and Diagnosis

Regardless of the patient's position in the continuum of care (*i.e.*, acute inpatient hospitalization, rehabilitation, or palliative/hospice care), the role of the physical therapist remains the same. In the context of the World Health Organization's International Classification of Functioning, Disability and Health (ICF),[28] this role pertains to the assessment and treatment of body systems and structures that coordinate and execute goal-directed movement.

In the hospice setting, functional measures related to endurance, gait speed, and balance can provide useful information on which to base targeted interventions. For example, measures such as the **Timed Up and Go test (TUG)** and the 10-m walk test provide important information about gait speed, which has recently been identified as the "sixth vital sign."[29] Recent studies have correlated declining gait speed with functional decline,[30] increased fall risk,[31] and higher mortality rates.[32] In these studies, gait speeds of 0.6 m/s or less were identified as the threshold of risk for adverse events. At this speed, individuals are limited to household ambulation (usually with an assistive device such as a walker). In the hospice setting, patients often demonstrate significantly decreased walking speeds due to a variety of musculoskeletal, neurological, or physiological causes. In patients with end-stage PD, rigidity, bradykinesia, and loss of postural stability all contribute to decreased walking speed. The TUG involves instructing the patient to come to standing from a chair with arms, walk 3 m, turn around, walk back to the chair, and sit down. Age-referenced normative values have been established for adults over the age of 59 years. In frail older adults, scores of over 30 seconds are predictive of the need for an assistive device and dependence in ADLs.[33] Ongoing studies are utilizing the

TUG in a population of patients in hospice and palliative care settings; these results may provide data regarding the trajectory of declining gait speed in this population. Furthermore, these data may assist in defining the TUG's potential use in defining appropriate interventions as well as their timing.

The ability to move from sitting to standing is a critical prerequisite for walking. The loss of sit-to-stand ability may result from lower extremity weakness and balance deficits, both of which contribute to increased fall risk.[34] The **Five Times Sit to Stand Test (FTSST)** involves having the person come to stand five times as quickly as possible with his arms across his chest. Age-referenced test norms have been developed for the FTSST, with increased fall risk in those taking: more than 11.4 seconds for persons between the ages of 60 to 69 years, more than 12.6 seconds (ages 70-79 years), and more than 14.8 seconds (ages 80-89 years).[35] A 2011 study of 7421 community-dwelling women (mean age 80 years) also found a relationship between a score of over 15 seconds on the FTSST and cognitive impairment.[36]

There are several assessments typically used in hospice and palliative care settings that are used to prognosticate the likelihood of death.[37,38] The **Palliative Performance Scale (PPS)** is a reliable and valid assessment tool that assesses five domains on an 11-point scale.[38] Patient performance is measured in 10% decrements which range from 100% (healthy) to 0% (death). The five domains and their end-range descriptors include: (1) ambulation (from "full" to "bed bound"); (2) evidence of disease (from "no disease" to "extensive disease"); (3) self-care (from "full" to "total care"); (4) oral intake (from "normal" to "mouth care only"); and, (5) level of consciousness (from "full" to "drowsy or coma"). Based on the mean score for each of these five factors, estimated median survival is anywhere from 1 day to 145 days. The PPS has established survival norms for patients with cancer and for those with all diagnoses admitted to either an inpatient palliative care or acute hospice unit. Depending on the specific identifiers for extent of disease, the patient in this case might have scored anywhere from 40 (estimated median survival time of 18 days in a hospice setting) to 60 (estimated median survival of 29 days). Recent studies are providing additional information on the contributions of specific symptoms to the PPS score.[38,39] For example, a recent study correlated lower PPS scores with higher levels of dyspnea.[39] Although the PPS is used widely as a hospice admission tool to quantify the elements of the "debility unspecified" diagnosis, there are no studies that specifically follow the trajectory of patients with PD. Such studies would be helpful to identify specific benchmarks for the multisystem impairments of end-stage PD.

Downing et al.[37] proposed a three-level progressive framework that can be used to target physical therapy assessment and intervention in the hospice setting. This framework is known as function, safety, and comfort (FSC). Patients in the "function" and "safety" domains of this framework might undergo physical therapy examinations targeted to assessing strength, endurance, mobility, and balance. Patients in the "comfort" domain may undergo examinations related to physiological responses such as heart rate, respiratory rate, pain scale ratings, circumferential limb measures (for patients with edema), and oxygen saturation. These latter measures provide a useful means to assess the effectiveness of comfort-based interventions.

Assessment of quality of life is an important feature of physical therapy assessment, and many tools exist for this purpose. Some of these measures are disease-specific such as the Stroke Impact Scale.[40] At the end of life, there are also several measures that can be found on websites such as the City of Hope Pain & Palliative Care Resource Center[41] and the Toolkit of Instruments to Measure End of Life Care (TIME).[42] These assessments include those targeted to the patient, caregivers, and the healthcare team.

The patient described in this case study was admitted to hospice and a physical therapy initial consult was provided 2 days later. Prior to this consult, the hospice physical therapist contacted the patient's home health and acute care physical therapists for the patient's status at discharge and strategies to optimize the transfer of care. The hospice physical therapy assessment included functional measures of bed mobility, sitting balance, and transfers. Body structure/function assessment included ROM respiratory rate, cough effectiveness, and orientation.

Plan of Care and Interventions

Limited research examining the impact of **physical therapy in the hospice setting** suggests that patients benefit from interventions related to improving function,[43] respiratory status,[44] fatigue,[45] stress reduction,[46] and patient/family education.[47] Although these studies are based on clinical observation of a small number of subjects, they provide a valuable starting point for the continued exploration of optimal interventions and outcomes.

In a study by Mueller and Decker[48], 164 consecutive hospice admissions were screened in weekly interdisciplinary team meetings during a 1-year period. Of the 164 subjects, 47 were referred for physical therapy. Only 12 of the 47 subjects who received a physical therapy referral survived long enough to complete both pre- and post-physical therapy intervention assessments. The Patient Specific Functional Scale (PSFS)[49-51] was used to identify and quantify patient-desired outcomes for therapy interventions. Subjects identified five problem areas. The most frequently identified problem areas were decreased mobility and pain. The remaining three areas were edema, dyspnea, and anxiety. Each of the seven subjects with mobility concerns made a clinically significant change in at least one of their targeted outcomes on the PSFS. The functional goals of these subjects included bed mobility, transfers, standing, and walking. For the five subjects who reported pain as their major problem, physical therapy intervention produced a statistically significant reduction. The study identified nine unique patient interventions. The two most commonly delivered were mobility training (92%) and family education (83%). These were followed by non-pharmacological interventions for pain control (38%) including transcutaneous electrical nerve stimulation (TENS), massage, stretching, splinting, and guided relaxation. Findings from this study highlight the facts that patients in a hospice setting continue to have goals related to the improvement or maintenance of function and physical therapy interventions can include effective non-pharmacological approaches to pain management. This study found that patients in hospice could achieve improvements through education in energy conservation, appropriate introduction of assistive devices, and family education. Many patients in hospice have specific functional goals that may require short-term physical therapy intervention. For example, one of the patients in the study requested physical therapy intervention so that he would be able to walk to his dining room for Thanksgiving dinner. After accomplishing this goal, the patient declined further physical therapy services and died shortly after. This example underscores the idea that the needs of patients in hospice are better served by slightly different approaches to physical therapy intervention.

Briggs has termed these approaches as "rehabilitation in reverse" and "rehabilitation light."[52] Rehabilitation in reverse is the idea of directing interventions toward the increasing need for safe and effective mobility assistance in the face of physical decline. For example, a patient with ALS and his family will need ongoing modifications to optimize function and independence, which might first involve the use of a cane for optimizing mobility. As the disease progresses, the patient would require a walker, and finally a power wheelchair. Thus, a primary role of the physical therapist is to integrate ongoing patient assessment with knowledge of the disease in order to assist the patient and family in adjusting to these changes. In the case of the patient presented here, rehabilitation in reverse would entail identifying safe and effective strategies and assistive devices for bed mobility, transfers to a wheelchair, and appropriate positioning. This patient required a hospital bed to assist rolling and coming to sitting. In addition, an air mattress was recommended to maintain skin integrity. An adjustment of bed height facilitated ease of transfers. The use of a sliding board facilitated transfers between level surfaces. In addition, both the hospice staff and the patient's daughter were instructed in methods to safely assist the patient, and the option of a mechanical sling lift was considered for future use. The patient required the use of a reclining wheelchair with elevating leg rests. Trunk supports were added to assist with midline positioning.

Rehabilitation light is essentially a concept of adjusting the frequency, intensity, and duration of treatment sessions to optimize the patient's level of participation and skill development. While daily physical therapy intervention is a prominent feature of conventional rehabilitation programs, patients receiving hospice services are more likely to receive sessions on a *weekly* basis. In many cases, a physical therapy consult may be completed in one or two visits, with subsequent interventions being carried out by the patient and family. Physical therapy involvement may also be episodic, based on changes in the patient's status and needs. Many patients with end-stage disease cannot tolerate more than a few minutes of continuous activity before tiring. Thus, the physical therapist must monitor signs of fatigue, offer frequent rest periods, and modify activities within the patient's tolerance. Furthermore, the physical therapist can help the patient prolong his activity tolerance through instruction in energy conservation techniques. For example, patients with end-stage respiratory disease become increasingly short of breath during functional activities. The perception of air hunger provokes anxiety, leading to a cycle of ineffective breathing strategies and further emotional distress. In such cases, the physical therapist can provide instruction in slow pursed-lips breathing as well as breathing exercises to promote relaxation. These techniques can be taught to the patient's caregivers as well.

A critical element of pharmacological management in hospice is pain control. In order to reduce pain, agitation, and anxiety, the current patient was prescribed 30 mg MS Contin every 12 hours for baseline pain control. Morphine sulfate liquid and Ativan were delivered sublingually as needed for breakthrough pain. Due to the highly constipating effect of opioids, the patient was also placed on a bowel management protocol (involving the use of stool softeners). The patient's anti-Parkinson's medications (carbidopa and levodopa) were initially discontinued (as was his Aricept and Namenda) upon his admission to hospice. Subsequently, a significant increase in rigidity was noted, along with more frequent periods of confusion and disorientation. After 1 month, the patient's daughter requested that these medications be resumed. Recognizing the importance of these medications as a comfort measure, the hospice team physician agreed.

Comfort care is a central element of physical therapy provided in the hospice setting. Interventions such as ROM gentle mobilization, lymphedema management, and the use of modalities can be valuable additions to pharmacological measures. In the case of the patient presented here, an emphasis of treatment was to optimize chest mobility to promote segmental breathing patterns. Exercises to promote trunk extension and rotation were utilized to maintain muscle length and reduce tension. The value of these interventions as a comfort measure was noted by the observation that the patient slept more soundly on the days these were provided. Physical therapy intervention also included gentle massage and compression wrapping the patient's legs to reduce edema. The hospice staff was encouraged to transfer the patient to his wheelchair for meals. The patient enjoyed sitting on the front porch of the hospice residence with his friends and family members, and it was noted that he was less agitated after spending time in this manner.

For the patient in this case, physical therapy interventions were targeted toward preserving function for sitting in a wheelchair, optimizing transfers, and bed mobility. Staff and family education was provided on active assisted ROM, bed exercises focusing on trunk rotation, assisting the patient from supine to sit, sliding board transfers, and optimal positioning in his recliner wheelchair for assisted feeding. Comfort-based treatment included ROM of extremities and trunk (particularly of the thoracic rib cage to facilitate chest expansion), and assisted coughing. The patient was seen once per week for 1 month, with follow-up care provided by the patient's family and hospice staff. These interventions enabled the patient to be up in a wheelchair twice per day for 2 hours during which time he had meals, visited with friends, and sat on the porch of the hospice home with his daughter. The patient's pain and constipation were well managed. However, despite his swallowing limitations, his daughter requested that he be allowed to eat and drink as desired. The patient continued to decline, refusing food and fluids in the last week. His congestion increased markedly in the last 3 days; however, his pain was effectively managed and he died peacefully.

Evidence-Based Clinical Recommendations

SORT: Strength of Recommendation Taxonomy

A: Consistent, good-quality patient-oriented evidence

B: Inconsistent or limited-quality patient-oriented evidence

C: Consensus, disease-oriented evidence, usual practice, expert opinion, or case series

1. The Timed Up and Go test (TUG) can be used to determine whether an older individual's gait speed is 0.6 m/s or less, a threshold value for adverse events such as functional decline, increased fall risk, and higher mortality rates. **Grade A**

2. An older adult's time to complete the Five Times Sit to Stand Test (FTSST) can be calculated to determine increased fall risk. **Grade B**

3. For individuals in inpatient palliative care or acute hospice units, performance on the five domains within the Palliative Performance Scale (PPS) can be used to estimate median survival (from 1 day to 145 days). **Grade A**

4. Physical therapy provided to patients in the hospice setting decreases stress and improves function, respiratory status, and fatigue. **Grade B**

COMPREHENSION QUESTIONS

25.1 An individual with Hoehn and Yahr Stage 4 Parkinson's disease is being considered for hospice admission. Which of the following would confirm the appropriateness of a hospice referral?

A. The individual must meet one or more of the criteria for "debility unspecified."

B. The individual can no longer benefit from medications for PD.

C. The individual's physician must certify a probable life expectancy of 6 months or less.

D. A and C.

25.2 Elements of physical therapy intervention in a hospice setting include:

A. Non-pharmacological approaches to pain management

B. Interventions directed toward comfort

C. Interventions for optimizing function

D. All of the above

25.3 The Medicare hospice conditions of participation for hospice reimbursement state that physical therapy services:

A. Are solely up to the discretion of the hospice medical director

B. Must be made available and provided by licensed providers

C. Must be made available and may be provided by non-licensed providers

D. Must be offered to every patient admitted to hospice

ANSWERS

25.1 **D.** Option B is the least desirable answer because of the growing recognition that medications for PD can help maintain optimal motor function, swallowing, speech, and cognitive function. The use of these medications may also help to minimize pain and discomfort, which are central goals of hospice intervention.

25.2 **D.** All of these answers represent evidence-based benefits of physical therapy intervention in the hospice setting. Some patients may even be capable of increasing strength and function while in a hospice setting. Based on the patient's level of disease, interventions may also be targeted to optimize safety and function in the midst of declining health.

25.3 **B.** Physical therapy services must be made available and provided by licensed personnel. Option A is not correct because any member of the hospice IDT can refer a patient for a physical therapy consult. The patient can also request a referral. Not every hospice patient will be appropriate for a physical therapy consult because some are admitted in the active stages of death (option D).

REFERENCES

1. Hoehn MM, Yahr MD. Parkinsonism: onset, progression and mortality. *Neurology*. 1967;17: 427-442.

2. Fahn S, Elton RL, Committee UD. Unified Parkinson's disease rating scale. In: Fahn S, Marsden CD, Calne D, Goldstein M, eds. *Recent Developments in Parkinson's Disease*. Florham Park, NJ. Macmillan Healthcare Information; 1987;153-163.

3. Pellecchia MT, Grasso A, Biancardi LG, Squillante M, Bonavita V, Barone P. Physical therapy in Parkinson's disease: an open long-term rehabilitation trial. *J Neurol*. 2004;251:595-598.

4. Nieuwboer A, De Weerdt W, Dom R, Bogaerts K. Prediction of outcome of physical therapy in advanced Parkinson's disease. *Clin Rehabil*. 2002;16:886-893.

5. Schenkman M, Ellis T, Christiansen C, et al. Profile of functional limitations and task performance among people with early- and middle-stage Parkinson disease. *Phys Ther*. 2011;91:1339-1354.

6. Goodwin VA, Richards SH, Taylor RS, Taylor AH, Campbell JL. The effectiveness of exercise interventions for people with Parkinson's disease: a systemic review and meta-analysis. *Mov Disord*. 2008;23:631-640.

7. Metzler-Baddeley C. A review of cognitive impairments in dementia with Lewy bodies relative to Alzheimer's disease and Parkinson's disease with dementia. *Cortex*. 2007;43:583-600.

8. Henchcliffe C, Dodel R, Beal MF. Biomarkers of Parkinson's disease and dementia with Lewy bodies. *Prog Neurobiol*. 2011;95:601-613.

9. Jain S. Multi-organ autonomic dysfunction in Parkinson disease. *Parkinsonism Relat Disord*. 2011;17:77-83.

10. Yamada H, Murahashi M, Takahashi H, et al. Respiratory function impairment in patients with Parkinson's disease: a consideration on the possible pathogenetic relation to autonomic dysfunction. *Rinsho Shinkeigaku*. 2000;40:125-130.

11. De Pandis MF, Starace A, Stefanelli F, et al. Modification of respiratory function parameters in patients with severe Parkinson's disease. *Neurol Sci*. 2002 Sept;23(Suppl 2):569-570.

12. Ebihara S, Saito J, Kanda A, et al. Impaired efficacy of cough in patients with Parkinson disease. *Chest*. 2003;124:1009-1015.

13. Sheard JM, Ash S, Silburn PA, Kerr GK. Prevalence of malnutrition in Parkinson's disease: a systemic review. *Nutr Rev.* 2011;69:520-532.

14. Boivie J. Pain in Parkinson's disease (PD). *Pain.* 2009;141:2-3.

15. Beiske AG, Loge JH, Ronningen A, Svensson E. Pain in Parkinson's disease: prevalence and characteristics. *Pain.* 2009;141:173-177.

16. Goy ER, Carter J, Ganzini L. Neurologic disease at the end of life: caregiver descriptions of Parkinson disease and amyotrophic lateral sclerosis. *J Palliat Med.* 2008;11:548-554.

17. Campbell CW, Jones EJ, Merrills J. Palliative and end-of-life care in advanced Parkinson's disease and multiple sclerosis. *Clin Med.* 2010;10:290-292.

18. Alliance for Aging Research. Prevalence and incidence of neurological disease. In: *Chronic Disease and Medical Innovation in an Aging Nation: The Silver Book.* Available at: http://www.silverbook.org/browse.php?id=49. Accessed January 4, 2012.

19. Snell K, Pennington S, Lee M, Walker R. The place of death in Parkinson's disease. *Age Ageing.* 2009;38:617-619.

20. ALS Association. Who gets ALS? Available at: http://www.alsa.org/about-als/who-gets-als.html. Accessed January 4, 2012.

21. Hasson F, Kernohan WG, McLaughlin M, et al. An exploration into the palliative and end-of-life experiences of carers of people with Parkinson's disease. *Palliat Med.* 2010;24:731-736.

22. Waldron M, Kernohan WG, Hasson F, Foster S, Cochrane B, Payne C. Allied health professional's views on palliative care for people with advanced Parkinson's disease. *Int J Ther Rehab.* 2011;18:48-58.

23. National Hospice and Palliative Care Organization. NHPCO Facts and Figures: Hospice Care in America: 2010 edition. Available at: http://www.nhpco.org/files/public/Statistics_Research/Hospice_Facts_Figures_Oct-2010.pdf. Accessed January 4, 2012.

24. Taylor DH, Ostermann J, Van Houtven CH, Tulsky JA, Steinhauser K. What length of hospice use maximizes reduction in medical expenditures near death in the US Medicare program? *Social Sci Med.* 2007;65:1466-1478.

25. Briggs R, Mueller K. Hospice and end of life. In: Guccione AA, Wong RA, Avers D, eds. *Geriatric Physical Therapy.* 3rd ed. St. Louis: Elsevier; 2011.

26. Centers for Medicare and Medicaid Services. Medicare conditions of participation, section 418.92. 2008. Available at: http://edocket.access.gpo.gov/cfr_2008/octqtr/pdf/42cfr418.98.pdf. Accessed January 4, 2012.

27. American Physical Therapy Association. House passes position and plan on PT role in hospice and palliative care. *PT in Motion.* June 17, 2011. Available at: http://www.apta.org/PTinMotion/NewsNow/2011/6/17/HospicePalliative/. Accessed January 15, 2012.

28. World Health Organization. Towards a common language for functioning, disability and health: ICF: The international classification of functioning, disability and health; 2002. Available at: www.who.int/classifications/icf/training/icfbeginnersguide.pdf. Accessed May 28, 2012.

29. Fritz S, Lusardi M. White paper: "walking speed: the sixth vital sign". *J Geriatr Phys Ther.* 2009;32:46-49.

30. Brach JS, VanSwearingen JM, Newman AB, Kriska AM. Identifying early decline of physical function in community-dwelling older women: performance-based and self-report measures. *Phys Ther.* 2002;82:320-328.

31. Maki BE. Gait changes in older adults: predictors of falls or indicators of fear. *J Am Geriatr Soc.* 1997;45:313-320.

32. Hardy SE, Perera S, Roumani YF, Chandler JM, Studenski SA. Improvement in usual gait speed predicts better survival in older adults. *J Am Geriatr Soc.* 2007;55:1727-1734.

33. Bohannon RW. Reference values for the timed up and go test: a descriptive meta-analysis. *J Geriatr Phys Ther.* 2006;29:64-68.

34. Whitney SL, Wrisley DM, Marchetti GF, Gee MA, Redfern MS, Furman JM. Clinical measurement of sit-to-stand performance in people with balance disorders: validity of data for the Five-Times-Sit-to-Stand Test. *Phys Ther.* 2005;85:1034-1045.

35. Bohannon RW. Reference values for the five-repetition sit-to-stand test: a descriptive meta-analysis of data from elders. *Percept Mot Skills* 2006;103:215-222.

36. Annweiler C, Schott AM, Abellan van Kan G, et al. The Five-Times-Sit-to-Stand test, a marker of global cognitive functioning among community-dwelling older women. *J Nutr Health Aging.* 2011;15:271-276.

37. Downing GM, Lynd PJ, Gallaher R, Hoens A. Challenges in understanding functional decline, prognosis and transitions in advanced illness. *Topics in Geriatric Rehabilitation.* 2011;27:18-28.

38. Anderson F, Downing GM, Hill J, Casorso L, Lerch. Palliative performance scale (PPS): a new tool. *J Palliat Care.* 1996;12:5-11.

39. Olajide O, Hanson L, Usher BM, Qaqish BF, Schwartz R, Bernard S. Validation of the palliative performance scale in the acute tertiary care hospital setting. *J Palliat Med.* 2007;10:111-117.

40. Duncan PW, Bode RK, Min Lai S, Perera S. Rasch analysis of a new stroke-specific outcome scale: the Stroke Impact Scale. *Arch Phys Med Rehabil.* 2003;84:950-963.

41. City of Hope Pain & Palliative Care Resource Center. Available at: http://prc.coh.org/res_inst.asp. Accessed January 13, 2012.

42. TIME: Toolkit of Instruments to Measure End of Life Care. Available at: http://www.chcr.brown.edu/pcoc/toolkit.htm. Accessed January 13, 2012.

43. Mackey KM, Sparling JW. Experiences with older women with cancer receiving hospice care: significance for physical therapy. *Phys Ther.* 2000;80:459-469.

44. Syrett E, Taylor J. Non-pharmacological management of breathlessness: a collaborative nurse-physiotherapist approach. *Int J Palliat Nurs.* 2003;9:150-156.

45. Donnelly CM, Lowe-Strong A, Rankin JP, Campbell A, Allen JM, Gracey JH. Physiotherapy management of cancer-related fatigue: a survey of UK current practice. *Supportive Care Cancer.* 2010;18:817-825.

46. Marcant D, Rapin CH. Role of physiotherapist in palliative care. *J Pain Symptom Manage.* 1993;8:68-71.

47. Toot J. Physical therapy and hospice: concept and practice. *Phys Ther.* 1984;64:665-671.

48. Mueller K, Decker I. Impact of physical therapy intervention on patient-centered outcomes in a community hospice. *Topics in Geriatric Rehabilitation.* 2011;27:2-9.

49. Physical Therapy Resources: The Patient Specific Functional Scale. Government of Western Australia. *Transport Accident Commission.* Available at: http://www.tac.vic.gov.au/upload/Patient-specific.pdf. Accessed September 6, 2010.

50. Chatman AB, Hyams SP, Neel JM, et al. The patient-specific functional scale: measurement properties in patients with knee dysfunction. *Phys Ther.* 1997;77:820-829.

51. Stratford P, Gill C, Westaway M, Binkley J. Assessing disability and change on individual patients: a report of a patient specific measure. *Physiother Can.* 1995;47:258-262.

52. Briggs R. Clinical decision making for physical therapists in patient-centered end-of-life care. *Topics in Geriatric Rehabilitation.* 2011;27:10-17.

Burn Injury— Pediatric Case

David John Lorello

A 6-year-old male is admitted to the burn intensive care unit (ICU) after sustaining 40% total body surface area (TBSA) burns to bilateral lower extremities, buttocks, genitals, lower abdomen, and lower back. The patient was playing around a campfire with his older siblings when he tried jumping over the campfire and he caught his pants on fire. In a panic, the patient began to run away. The patient's family was eventually able to catch the child and put the fire out. Upon arrival at the hospital, it was determined that the patient developed compartment syndrome in both legs and was emergently taken to the operating room (OR), where escharotomies were performed on both lower extremities. The patient returned from the OR intubated and sedated. The physical therapist will evaluate the patient less than 12 hours post-admission. The patient will be returning to the OR in the afternoon for surgical excision of the burns as well as possible grafting. After this surgery, the patient will be extubated.

▶ What are the examination priorities?
▶ Based on his health condition, what do you anticipate will be contributors to activity limitations?
▶ What are the most appropriate physical therapy interventions?
▶ What are possible complications interfering with physical therapy?

KEY DEFINITIONS

AUTOGRAFT: Skin that is taken from an unburned area of the patient and transplanted to cover an injured area of the same patient

ESCHAROTOMY: Incision through burn eschar (rigid barrier of dead tissue) used to relieve the pressure inside a limb, digit, or the trunk to restore circulation to potentially viable tissue

FASCIOTOMY: Incision made through the fascia to relieve the pressure inside a limb, or within the trunk

GRANULATION TISSUE: Vascularized tissue comprised of fibroblasts and inflammatory cells that forms in healing wounds; appears as red, moist tissue

Objectives

1. Describe the classification of burn injuries.
2. Understand burn wound physiology, including systems affected and the phases of wound healing.
3. Understand the major impairments associated with a severe burn.
4. Describe the appropriate plan of care for each phase of wound healing.

Physical Therapy Considerations

PT considerations during management of the child with a severe burn injury:

▶ **General physical therapy plan of care/goals:** Prevent loss of range of motion (ROM) or contracture; achieve pre-injury level of strength and cardiovascular endurance; maximize functional independence with mobility and gait

▶ **Physical therapy interventions:** ROM and stretching; tendon gliding; splinting and positioning; aerobic and resistance exercise; mobility training; gait training; family education regarding exercise and mobility

▶ **Precautions during physical therapy:** Monitor vital signs; post-surgical limitations

▶ **Complications interfering with physical therapy:** Compartment syndrome; exposed tendons; heterotopic ossification

Understanding the Health Condition

Advancement in the medical management of large burns including surgical techniques, wound care and dressings, and artificial skin has made a previously non-survivable injury one that is routinely survivable. However, burn injuries leave physical impairments that can take years to rehabilitate. It is the job of the physical therapist to help prevent these impairments and to help these survivors regain the function that they have lost. The physical therapist must have a strong knowledge

Table 26-1   STATISTICS FOR BURN INJURIES IN CHILDREN IN THE UNITED STATES[1]
~88,000 children ≤ 14 years of age were treated at hospital emergency rooms for burn-related injuries.
~62,000 burn injuries were thermal and ~26,000 were scald.
Majority of children ≤ 4 years of age who are hospitalized for burn-related injuries suffer from scald burns (65%) or contact burns (20%).
Most scald burns to small children are caused by hot foods or liquids spilled in the kitchen.
More than 1/3 of children ages 6-14 years reportedly have played with fire at least once. Boys are two times as likely to play with fire.

of the anatomy of the skin, wound healing, and wound care to accomplish this task. Table 26-1 shows the incidence of burn injuries in the United States in children.[1]

As the largest organ of the body, the skin protects the body from infection and injury, prevents the loss of body fluid, regulates body temperature, receives external stimuli, serves as an indicator of internal events (*e.g.*, erythema seen in the skin as result of infection), and helps to determine one's identity. Burn injuries can cause a loss to some or all of these functions.

The skin consists of the epidermis, dermis, and the subcutaneous tissue beneath which are structures such as fascia, muscles, tendons, ligaments, nerves, bone, and organs (Fig. 26-1). A thorough knowledge of these skin layers is necessary to classify the depth of a burn injury and to predict what functions will be lost depending on

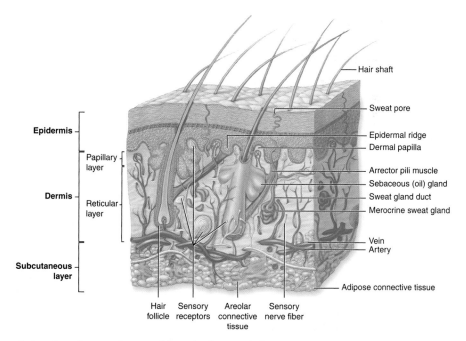

Figure 26-1. Schematic diagram of three skin layers with their associated appendages, vasculature, and major sensory receptors. (Reproduced with permission from Mescher AL. *Junqueira's Basic Histology: Text and Atlas.* 12th ed. Available at: http://www.accessmedicine.com. Copyright © The McGraw-Hill Companies, Inc. All rights reserved.)

the depth and extent of the injury. The most superficial layer, the epidermis, has a thickness that varies from 0.05 to 1.5 mm. This avascular layer receives its necessary cellular nutrients from the vascular plexus within the deeper dermis.[2-4] There are five layers within the epidermis: stratum corneum, stratum lucidum (found only in the palms of the hand and soles of the feet), stratum granulosum, stratum spinosum, and stratum basale.[2-4] The deepest layer of the epidermis is the stratum basale that contains the keratinocytes that produce the protective protein keratin. Other important cells within the epidermis are melanocytes (produce the pigment melanin), Merkel cells (mechanoreceptors that provide information on light touch), and Langerhans cells (dendritic cells that regulate immune responses in the skin).[2-5]

Important structures within the epidermis include hair follicles (lined with epithelium that are continuous with the epidermis), sebaceous glands (contained within the hair follicle and produce sebum that lubricates the skin and hair), and sudoriferous glands (secrete sweat to assist the body in dissipating heat and cooling the body).[2-4] The basement membrane is connective tissue between the epidermis and dermis. This membrane acts as scaffolding where ridges in the epidermis fit within projections in the dermis. This series of ridges—known as rete pegs—anchors the dermis to the epidermis, preventing shearing forces between the layers.[2-4]

Beneath the epidermis is the thicker dermis. It can range in thickness from 2 to 4 mm. It is a highly vascularized layer, providing nutrition to both the dermis and epidermis. The dermis consists of two distinct layers. The papillary dermis is the top layer and it conforms to the epidermis. The deeper, thicker layer is the reticular dermis that contains collagen bundles that provide the skin with its extensibility.[2-4] Structures within the dermis include smooth muscle that causes hair follicles to elevate (i.e., goose bumps), blood vessels (provide nutrition and help in thermoregulation), lymphatic vessels, and nerves (afferent fibers that supply sensory information on temperature, pain, touch, itch, and pressure).[2-4] Beneath the dermis is a subcutaneous layer consisting of adipose tissue and connective tissue that provides energy, cushioning, and insulation to deeper structures.[2-4]

Burn injuries are classified based on the mechanism, depth, and the size of the injury. The six primary mechanisms of injury include scald, flame, contact, chemical, electrical, and radiation. Knowing the mechanism of injury can help give a physical therapist clues as to how severe an injury may be. Mechanisms that generate higher temperatures will cause greater injury. For example, skin exposed to water at 158°F for 1 second can cause a deep partial thickness burn. Hot grease can typically be greater than 350°F.[4] Because oil can remain at higher temperatures for longer periods of time than water, soups or broths can cause deeper burns than hot water.

The traditional method of classifying burn depth was as first, second, and third degree burns. These classifications have been replaced with the more descriptive clinical terms superficial (1st degree), superficial partial thickness and deep partial thickness (2nd degree), and full thickness (3rd degree).[6] Superficial burns involve only the epidermis. The skin appears red with no blistering. Healing takes 3 to 7 days as the outer epidermal cells peel away. An example of this type of burn would be a painful sunburn.[6-8] Superficial partial thickness burns involve the entire epidermis as well as the papillary (top) layer of the dermis. Superficial partial thickness burns are red, moist, and weepy (Fig. 26-2). Blisters may be present. The wound blanches easily.

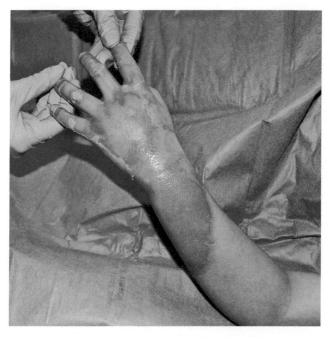

Figure 26-2. Superficial partial thickness burn on dorsum of hand and forearm.

These are extremely painful burns because nerve endings in the dermis are exposed or damaged. Since the deeper structures of the dermis are intact, superficial partial thickness wounds typically heal within 7 to 21 days with minimal scarring.[6-8] A deep partial thickness burn involves not only the epidermis and papillary layer of the dermis, but also the reticular layer of the dermis (Fig. 26-3). Deep partial thickness burns can appear mottled white, pink, or deep red. Blisters are large, and the burn can still be very painful since many nociceptors remain intact. Because some hair follicles and sebaceous glands remain undamaged, the wound may be able to re-epithelialize. If the burn is large or likely to take longer than 21 days to heal, a surgeon may consider skin grafting to achieve faster wound closure. Deep partial thickness burns are at risk for hypertrophic scarring and contracture. With poor nutrition or infection, these burns are at risk of converting to full thickness injuries.[6-8] Full thickness burns involve the epidermis, the entire dermis, and the subcutaneous tissue (Fig. 26-4). They can appear white, yellow, brown, charred, and/or leathery. Because all of the blood vessels have thrombosed and nociceptors and other skin receptors have been destroyed by the burn injury, the wound is dry and there is little to no pain. Since the hair follicles are destroyed, any remaining hair pull out easily. If the wound is very small, it may be allowed to heal on its own by epithelial ingrowth, but most often these wounds require surgical debridement and skin grafting. Full thickness wounds are also at risk for hypertrophic scarring and contracture.[6-8]

In addition to the depth of a burn, the percentage of TBSA of a burn must be calculated. Only areas of partial thickness and full thickness injury are included in

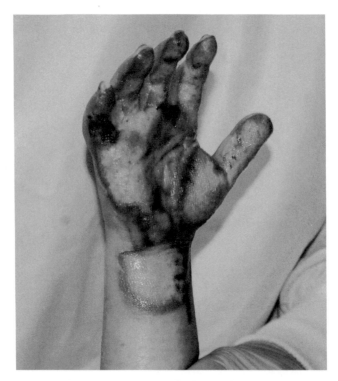

Figure 26-3. Deep partial thickness burn on palm of child's hand. Burn can appear mottled white, pink, and deep red.

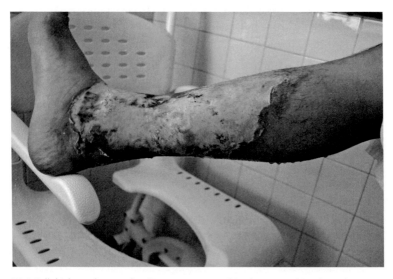

Figure 26-4. Full thickness burn on leg. Burn can appear white, brown, and/or charred.

the TBSA calculation. Methods of calculating TBSA include the Rule of Nines and the Lund-Browder classification.[3] The Rule of Nines, in which each part of the body represents 9% or a multiple of 9% of the body surface, is the simplest and most common way to calculate TBSA. However, this method is not accurate when calculating TBSA of a child or infant. The **Lund-Browder classification system** accounts for the fact that a child's head represents a larger area and the lower limbs a smaller area than in an adult. It is a more accurate system of calculating TBSA with infants and children.[9]

Major burns encompassing more than 25% TBSA result in systemic responses by the body.[9] One of the first systems affected by a major burn is the cardiovascular system. Almost immediately, there is a massive increase in capillary permeability, resulting in edema. Plasma fluid is lost at the site of injury through evaporation. This state of hypovolemia, also known as shock, causes decreased cardiac output and blood pressure, increased heart rate, decreased urine output and can eventually lead to renal failure.[8,10] Pulmonary failure is one of the leading causes of death for the burn patient. Inhalation injuries can cause increased airway resistance, pulmonary arterial hypertension, and reduced pulmonary compliance. Burns to the torso can cause edema, leading to decreased chest expansion and impaired ventilation.[8,10] The gastrointestinal system responds with gastric dilation and paralytic ileus can occur in response to shock. Burn patients also have an increased incidence of ulcers.[11] In response to the burn injury, the body enters a hypermetabolic state to provide the energy required to initiate wound healing. Energy stores are mobilized from fat and muscle. The increased muscle catabolism can lead to muscle wasting.[8,10] Due to the metabolic demands of the burn injury and the prolonged bedrest that can accompany these injuries, patients can develop a loss of bone mineral density. This places patients at an increased risk for fractures.[12] Scoliotic changes in pediatric patients with asymmetrical burns to the trunk can also develop.[13] Another leading cause of burn morbidity and mortality is infection. In addition to the loss of skin that is the body's primary immunological defense, large TBSA burns can cause immunosuppression. This predisposes the patient to sepsis and multi-organ failure.[8,10]

Wound healing can be divided into three phases: inflammatory, proliferative, and remodeling/maturation.[3] The inflammatory phase begins at the time of injury and can last 2 to 5 days. There is an immediate vascular response: vasoconstriction to stop bleeding, shortly followed by vasodilation to bring nutrients to the surrounding tissues.[3,14,15] There is also a cellular response in which neutrophils and macrophages begin to rid the wound of bacteria and foreign debris. The wound is characterized by redness, edema, warmth, pain, and decreased range of motion (ROM).[3,14] The proliferative phase begins around the third to fifth day after injury and can last up to 3 weeks. It is characterized by angiogenesis (formation of new blood vessels), granulation tissue formation (fibroblasts enter the wound and produce extracellular matrix of collagen and elastin, appearing as moist, red tissue within the wound bed), wound contraction (myofibroblasts pull wound margins together), and epithelialization (keratinocytes at wound margins and within hair follicles migrate across the wound).[3,14,15] The end of epithelialization marks the beginning of the remodeling/maturation phase. This final phase can last from 6 months to 3 years. During this time, collagen becomes more parallel in formation and creates stronger bonds.

New collagen is being created in the wound while older collagen is being removed (collagen turnover). Collagen synthesis should be equal to collagen degradation during this phase—leaving a flat, pliable scar. If collagen synthesis is greater than collagen degradation, hypertrophic scarring can occur.[3,14]

All phases of wound healing require oxygen. Burns develop necrotic tissue on the wound surface that impedes oxygen delivery, supports bacteria, encourages infection, and prolongs healing. More superficial burns can heal using a variety of different wound dressings that simply provide a clean and moist environment. Full thickness burns typically require surgical eschar removal. When it is determined that a burn wound will take longer than 21 days to heal, surgical intervention is required. Burns that take longer than 21 days to heal are at an increased risk for hypertrophic scarring and contracture. Removal of eschar through tangential excision allows a surgeon to preserve underlying tissue.[7,16] In tangential excision, the surgeon debrides thin layers of burned tissue until healthy, viable tissue is reached.[7,16] Once the burned tissue has been removed, the wound needs to be covered by new skin. There are two types of skin grafts: split-thickness (containing the epidermis and a thin portion of the dermis) and full-thickness (containing the epidermis and the entire dermis).[3,7,16] Sometimes the excised wound bed is not healthy enough to accept the patient's own skin. With larger TBSA burns, the patient may not have enough unburned skin to cover the large surface area of injury. In these instances, temporary grafts are used. Cadaver skin (known as allograft or homograft) or porcine skin (xenograft) may be used until a donor site (area of unburned skin) is available or when the wound is healthy enough to graft with the patient's own skin (autograft).[3,7,16] Other methods of wound closure include skin substitutes and biosynthetic wound dressing such as cultured epithelial autografts (CEAs), Biobrane, and Integra. Patients who have large TBSA burns and limited donor sites available for harvesting may benefit from CEAs. For this procedure, a biopsy of the patient's healthy skin is taken. This biopsy is sent to a laboratory where epidermal cells from the biopsy are grown into skin sheets. After 3 weeks, the cells are ready for placement over the patient's clean burn injury site. The CEAs are less durable than autografts because there is no dermis present.[7,16] Biobrane is a wound dressing with a two-layer membrane: an inner layer of nylon mesh that allows fibrovascular ingrowth and an outer layer of silastic (silicone and plastic) that serves as a barrier.[7] Fluid and exudate may collect beneath the membrane and the dressing needs to be removed daily. Integra is another type of bilayer membrane wound dressing that is used with full thickness wounds and on areas with exposed tendons. The top layer is silicone, which acts as a neoepidermis to control moisture loss. The bottom layer is a dermal replacement made of bovine collagen that serves as a matrix for fibroblasts. After 2 to 3 weeks, the silicone layer can be removed and a thin autograft can be placed over the wound.[7,17]

Physical Therapy Patient/Client Management

The physical therapist is a member of a large team that manages the patient with severe burn injuries. The burn team consists of the patient and his family, general surgeons and plastic surgeons, physician extenders (e.g., physician assistants and nurse practitioners), nurses, dieticians, clinical pharmacologists, respiratory therapists, child life specialists, occupational therapists, speech-language pathologists, psychologists, case managers, social workers, and researchers. Each member of the burn team is critical to the functional recovery of the burn survivor. This model of care assists each discipline in reaching goals and ensuring the patient achieves the best functional outcome.

In the management of a patient with severe burns, physical therapy is often initiated within 24 hours of admission to the ICU and occurs concurrently with all phases of wound healing. Management includes preventing loss of ROM, strength and cardiovascular training, as well as mobility and gait training. Phase of wound healing and surgical management often dictate treatment and development of goals.

Examination, Evaluation, and Diagnosis

Prior to seeing the patient for the first time, it is important for the physical therapist to do a thorough chart review. It is important to know the mechanism of injury, TBSA, location and depth of the burns, and whether there was concomitant trauma. This helps the physical therapist have an idea of what to expect before entering the patient's room. The physical therapist should learn if there were any surgical procedures performed since admission to the ICU, whether there is significant past medical history, pre-injury level of mobility, and social history including family dynamics and school environment. It is important to speak with the patient's nurse before entering the room. Nurses are invaluable sources of information. Sometimes not all of the information makes it into the chart and pertinent things can be learned about the patient and his family. It is also important to learn from the nurse what medical devices are currently being used. Typically, patients in the ICU have peripheral intravenous lines, nasoenteral feeding tubes, cardiac monitors, and urinary catheters.

Of utmost importance, the physical therapist must learn the patient's current medication regimen for decreasing pain and how well the patient's pain is being controlled. Typically, the patient in the burn ICU has medications for background pain, breakthrough pain, and procedural pain. Common medications prescribed include: opioid analgesics (morphine, oxycodone, fentanyl, hydromorphone, methadone), benzodiazepines (midazolam, lorazepam), and anesthetic agents (ketamine, propofol) that can be used for procedural sedation.[18,19] Controlling the patient's pain throughout his ICU stay is important not only for the relationship between the therapist and the patient, but also for the nurse-patient, nurse-therapist, family-patient, and family-therapist relationships as well. Occasionally, it takes time to achieve the correct analgesia. The nurse may indicate that the patient is in too much pain to be evaluated by the therapist. If the physical therapist knows that the patient is going to surgery later in the day, this is an excellent opportunity to take advantage of the patient being under anesthesia to assess passive ROM (PROM). Once all this information has been gathered, the physical therapist can begin the evaluation.

It is important to first assess whether the patient is alert and able to follow any commands. If the patient is sedated, it is important to monitor the patient's vital signs during the evaluation. It is common for patients to have tachycardia as a result of the injury, but the therapist needs to pay attention to whether or not any of the assessment causes inappropriate increases in heart rate or blood pressure.

The physical therapist should seek every opportunity to be involved with either the dressing change or to be present in the operating room to be able to view the wounds. ROM may be limited by wound dressings, so it is important to assess ROM with the dressings removed. Assessments of active range of motion (AROM) should be performed with an alert patient, even if he is on a ventilator. In addition, some bed mobility can be assessed with a ventilated patient if a respiratory therapist and nurse are present. If the patient is sedated and unable to follow commands, then PROM can be assessed. If resistance is encountered during the examination, then pain may not be adequately controlled. The examination may have to wait until better pain control can be achieved, possibly during a dressing change or before surgery. Goniometric measurements of ROM should be prioritized for joints affected by the burn, but should also be taken for unaffected joints. Since the medical plan is for this patient to be extubated after the next surgical procedure, strength, mobility, and gait will need to be assessed at a later time. During the first 48 hours after ICU admission, the patient also receives fluid resuscitation to prevent burn shock. Mobility and gait are often delayed until the patient has been fully resuscitated.

Goals are based upon a number of factors including the phase of wound healing, extent and depth of burn, patient's current health status, age, and physical and mental condition. Goals change frequently based on surgical procedures due to postoperative mobility restrictions and the changes in the patient's status. The foremost goal is to prevent loss of ROM, especially for joints directly affected by the burn. Other goals include returning to pre-injury level of strength, cardiovascular endurance, mobility, gait, and independence with activities if daily living (ADLs). For small children and infants, a common goal is to demonstrate age-appropriate gross and fine motor developmental milestones.

Plan of Care and Interventions

Initially the patient is in the inflammatory phase of wound healing. He is also receiving fluid resuscitation. Edema may be prevalent for the first few days. Since he may not be able to mobilize out of bed until he is more medically stable, edema control is one of the major goals. **Active ROM and positioning of the burned extremities** *above* the level of the heart help decrease edema. Positioning is important not only to decrease edema, but also to prevent contracture. In burn care, it is not uncommon to hear the phrase: "The position of comfort is the position of deformity." Whenever a patient is unable to move his joints, it is important to keep the tissues elongated to prevent soft tissue contractures. Table 26-2 describes proper positioning for affected areas of the body as well as the effects of improper positioning. This patient (with burns to bilateral lower extremities, abdomen, and back) should be positioned with knees in extension, hips in neutral rotation and neutral extension, and ankles in neutral dorsiflexion. Because elevation of his head is important while he is being ventilated, placing the bed in reverse Trendelenburg (i.e., feet below head) allows

Table 26-2   POSITIONING AREAS AFFECTED BY BURNS

Splinted Area	Desired Position	Effects of Improper Positioning
Neck/head (anterior aspect)	• Neutral • Slight extension • Head of bed elevated 30°-45°	• Side-bending contractures • Rotation contractures • Flexion contractures • Facial muscle contractures
Axilla	• Abduction to 90° • Forearm supinated (palm facing up) • Horizontal adduction to 20° (to keep shoulder in the scapular plane)	• Decreased shoulder ROM • Impaired functional ability • Decreased ability to perform overhead movements • Impingement syndrome • Rotator cuff injury/tear
Elbow	• Elbow in full extension • Forearm supinated • Elbow elevated above the level of shoulder	• Inability to fully flex and/or extend elbow • Impaired hand-to-mouth movements • Impaired functional ability/ADLs
Hand	• Wrist: 15°-40° extension • MCPs: 70°-90° flexion • IPs fully extended • Thumb positioned to preserve 1st web space • Hand elevated above level of the elbow and the heart	• Decreased fine motor coordination • Impaired functional ability/ADLs • Impaired gross motor movements
Trunk	• Midline	• Scoliosis • Perceived leg length discrepancy • Impaired full trunk ROM • Impaired rib/chest expansion • Respiratory impairment
Hip	• Abduction 15°-20° • Neutral (or increased) extension • Neutral rotation	• Impaired gait • Decreased erect posture • Low back pain • Perceived leg length discrepancy • Sciatica-type symptoms
Knee	• Full extension	• Impaired gait • Perceived leg length discrepancy
Foot/ankle	• Neutral dorsiflexion	• Plantar flexion contracture • Equinovarus deformity

Abbreviations: IPs, interphalangeal joints; MCPs, metacarpophalangeal joints.

safe elevation of the head of the bed while avoiding hip flexion (to decrease the risk of hip flexion contractures). However, since edema control is critical in the first few days post-burn, elevating his legs to decrease edema is a greater concern than positioning the hips in neutral extension. Once the anterior hips have been autografted, reverse Trendelenburg position is optimal for hip positioning.

In addition to the physiologic sequelae associated with burn injuries (tightening skin, loss of muscle mass, decreased aerobic capacity), the bedrest resulting from a significant burn injury has deleterious effects including decreased muscle mass and decreased aerobic capacity.[20,21] Patients with burn injuries have a difficult time mobilizing because of their injuries. Keeping them in bed only exacerbates the problem. Once the patient is medically stable, mobility and gait should be started as soon as possible. Since pain can be the principal limiting factor, the patient may require extra time to figure out how to move. Burns to the lower extremities are *not* a contraindication to mobility and gait. Prior to standing, lower extremities should be wrapped using compression/elastic dressings to prevent venous pooling and orthostatic hypotension that often occurs upon standing. Once he can tolerate standing and taking steps, gait should be progressed throughout hospitalization. For patients who have been intubated for long periods of time or are too medically fragile to begin mobility and gait, a tilt table can be utilized to begin upright positioning and promote upright tolerance. Burns to the plantar surface of the foot can be extremely painful to ambulate on, but patients should still be out of bed and gait should be encouraged. Off-the-shelf cast shoes that are padded with foam can be used to protect the bottom of the foot during weightbearing activity.

It is important that the patient not only mobilizes during therapy, but also during scheduled times out of bed throughout the day. It is important to work with the burn team to have each patient on a regular schedule. An example would be to have this patient up for all meals and out of bed for all visitors. The more a patient moves, the easier it will be to move. To inhibit the progressive decrease in muscle mass and aerobic capacity seen with these patients, our facility (Arizona Burn Center) initiates therapeutic exercise early in the ICU stay. Baker et al.[22] assessed the physical and psychological rehabilitation outcomes for 83 young adults (18-28 years of age) who were burned as children. Subjects had minimum of 30% TBSA burns at least 2 years prior to the assessments. Physical outcome measures included strength, mobility, and performance of ADLs. Psychological outcomes included behavioral problems and incidence of psychiatric illness. The area most impaired was wrist flexor strength, which limited ADL performance. Higher TBSA burns also correlated with overall lower mean strength. Subjects with higher TBSA burns (> 50%) also demonstrated decreased pinch and grip strength. The authors concluded that rehabilitation professionals should include programs that develop overall muscle strength in severely burned children.[22]

Exercise programs for pediatric burn patients have demonstrated increased strength,[23-25] increased lean body mass,[24-26] increased pulmonary function,[27] and decreased number of required surgical interventions up to two years after discharge from the inpatient setting.[28] These exercise programs were conducted within outpatient programs 6 months post-discharge; however, all authors stressed the importance of exercise for pediatric burn patients. This is why our facility incorporates therapeutic exercise early in patients' rehabilitation. For young children that may not be able to follow a regimented exercise program, play should be incorporated into rehabilitation. In addition to helping increase strength and mobility, play helps develop social learning skills and coping behaviors.[29] Many hospitals have child life specialists with expertise in assisting children and families deal with challenging life events. They can assist in providing play activities for children that help carry over to achievement of rehabilitation goals (*e.g.*, using the burned extremity to pick up toys, ambulating to the play room).

In the care of the burn patient, there are instances when movement is contraindicated. The physical therapist should be familiar with every post-surgical protocol.

For temporary grafts such as an allograft or xenograft, ROM and mobility are typically encouraged on the first post-operative day (POD 1). However, once a patient has received an autograft, protocols may dictate immobilization of the extremity or body part that was grafted until POD 5. Five days is usually how long it takes for the new autograft to become vascularized and for enough collagen to form between the graft and the wound bed to prevent shear.[14] Integra, a bilayer matrix wound dressing, may take 10 days to adhere, so the surgeon may require immobilization during that entire time. Cultured epithelial autografts are extremely fragile, so mobilization of the grafted area may not be possible until POD 14. During this time, the grafted joint is splinted to maintain maximum tissue elongation. The physical therapist should become adept with the casting and splinting skills necessary to properly position a joint. There are a number of excellent resources for splints that the therapist can use.[30-34] While the grafted joint is immobilized, it is important to continue exercise for non-grafted and uninvolved areas. Patients who have only upper extremity involvement may still be able to mobilize out of bed; the physical therapist should teach the patient how to move without using the grafted upper extremity.

Once it has been determined that the autograft is adhered, it is important to begin movement of the autografted area as soon as possible. The wound is now in the maturation phase of healing and begins to contract. The **contractile nature of scar tissue**—whether it is injured tissue that heals on its own or it is an autograft—requires an opposing force to maintain tissue length either through movement or splinting.[35] Movement may be difficult because the areas where donor skin was harvested are extremely painful. Indeed, most patients report the pain associated with the donor site is more painful than the original burn injury.

There are a few complications of the burn injury that the physical therapist should be aware of when treating the burn patient. The first is exposed tendons. The physical therapist must know each surgeon's protocols for mobilizing joints with exposed tendons. Some facilities do not allow *any* ROM to ensure that the tendon remains intact. Other facilities may allow gentle tendon gliding to prevent adhesions to the tendons provided that the tendon is kept moist with dressings throughout the entire movement session. The second complication is compartment syndrome developing in patients with circumferential limb burns. The combination of edema and the inelastic burn eschar surrounding the limb can cause increased pressure *inside* the limb. This causes a decrease in blood flow to muscles and nerves, resulting in tissue necrosis. Patients that have compartment syndrome need emergent surgery to relieve the pressure by either an escharotomy or a fasciotomy. Alert patients that report numbness or tingling at the distal limb should be immediately brought to the attention of the burn team. For sedated patients, the physical therapist should palpate the distal limb for pulses as well as temperature. Distal limbs that feel cold to the touch and/or pulses that cannot be palpated should be brought to the attention of the burn team. Another complication that can occur in patients with burn injuries is heterotopic ossification (HO). HO is the development of mature lamellar bone in soft tissue.[36] For burn patients, it typically occurs around the joints affected by the burn.[36,37] It most commonly affects the elbow, shoulder, hip, and knee.[36] It has been hypothesized that the frequent immobilization of joints along with forcible ROM during therapy may trigger HO.[37] Signs and symptoms of HO include sudden loss of ROM at a joint, swelling, and erythema. Patients often complain of pain at the affected joint. Since a patient may be sedated and unable to verbally express pain and erythema is difficult to see because of the injured skin, the physical therapist is often the first person to suspect HO because of the sudden loss in ROM. At an early stage, HO may not be visible with imaging. A sudden loss of ROM without another explanation (e.g., wound contracture) should be brought to the attention of the burn team and HO should be suspected. Aggressive ROM and stretching of the affected joint with possible HO is contraindicated. If the patient is alert, he can perform AROM in a pain-free range. If the patient is sedated, then gentle PROM can be performed up to the point of resistance in the affected joint.

Eventually, the patient's burn wounds will be covered. This can be a hectic time as discharge planning is the primary goal of the burn team. The transition from the hospital to an inpatient rehabilitation setting, a skilled nursing facility, a subacute facility, or to home with outpatient therapy can be an extremely stressful time for the patient and his family. There is often a delay in restarting physical therapy during this transition, so it is not uncommon for a patient to lose some ROM and function. The physical therapist can be instrumental in making the transition as easy as possible, by laying the foundation throughout the patient's inpatient stay. Providing continuous education to the patient and his family, having the patient out of bed and mobilizing regularly, teaching family members to provide regular exercise and play activities for the patient, and educating the patient and family about all positioning devices and splints help make this transition easier. The physical therapist should provide a home exercise program that can be utilized to help provide a bridge during the transition. Last, it is important that the acute care physical therapist provide contact information for the therapist that will be treating the patient after discharge.

Evidence-Based Clinical Recommendations

SORT: Strength of Recommendation Taxonomy

A: Consistent, good-quality, patient-oriented evidence
B: Inconsistent or limited-quality, patient-oriented evidence
C: Consensus, disease-oriented evidence, usual practice, expert opinion, or case series

1. In children with burn injuries, the Lund-Browder classification system is more accurate than the Rule of Nines for calculating the percentage of total body surface area (TBSA). **Grade A**

2. Active ROM and positioning of burned extremities above the level of the heart decrease edema. **Grade B**

3. Exercise training 6 months post-burn enhances strength and lean muscle mass, improves pulmonary function, and leads to fewer surgical releases of burn scar contractures in severely burned children. **Grade B**

4. Active and passive ROM, positioning, and splinting prevent decreases in ROM associated with burn injury. **Grade C**

COMPREHENSION QUESTIONS

26.1 The clinical signs of a superficial partial thickness burn are
 A. White, charred, leathery, and dry wound that is insensate
 B. Moist, red, weepy wound that is extremely painful
 C. Mottled white, pink, or deep red and moist wound that is painful
 D. Red, painful, no blisters present

26.2 You are evaluating an adult patient who sustained a combination of deep partial thickness and full thickness flame burns to the face, proximal half of the anterior trunk, circumferentially around the right upper extremity, and on the anterior left upper extremity. Using the Rule of Nines, what is the patient's TBSA?
 A. 25% TBSA
 B. 27% TBSA
 C. 36.5% TBSA
 D. 40% TBSA

26.3 The *most* appropriate plan of care for the patient who is POD 5 for an autograft to the right knee would be:
 A. AROM exercises for all extremities, dangling at the edge of bed, transfer training, and gait training
 B. Right knee splinted into extension, AROM bed exercises for the left lower extremity, and bilateral upper extremities
 C. Bedrest
 D. Bedrest with AROM of all extremities, except for the right lower extremity

ANSWERS

26.1 **B.** Superficial partial thickness burns involve the entire epidermis as well as the (top) papillary layer of the dermis. The appearance is red, moist, and weepy. Blisters may be present. The wound blanches easily. Superficial burns involve only the epidermis; the skin is red and has no blisters (option D). Deep partial thickness burns appear mottled white, pink, or deep red and are also painful (option C). Full thickness burns involve the epidermis, entire dermis, and the subcutaneous tissue; they are white, yellow, brown, charred, and/or leathery. This is little to no pain because of the destruction of all the nociceptors (option A).

26.2 **B.** To calculate TBSA on an adult using the Rule of Nines, the face would be 4.5%, the proximal half of the anterior trunk would be 9%, the circumferential right upper extremity would be 9%, and the anterior left upper extremity would be 4.5%. Thus, the total TBSA is 27%.

26.3 **A.** By POD 5, the graft has become vascularized enough that collagen has formed between the graft and the wound bed to prevent shear. The patient may begin AROM of the grafted joint, and should begin to mobilize out of bed. Keeping the right knee splinted increases the risk of loss of ROM around this joint (option B). Gait training may be introduced at this time to help combat the inherent risks associated with bedrest. Bedrest should not be encouraged (options C and D) because it is associated with loss of muscle mass, development of pressure ulcers, and increased risk of deep vein thrombosis and pneumonia.[38,39]

REFERENCES

1. Fire Safety and Burn Injury Statistics (2011). Available at: http://www.childrenshospital.org/az/Site903/mainpageS903P0.html. Accessed January 15, 2011.

2. Falkel JE. Anatomy and physiology of the skin. In: Richard RL, Staley MJ, eds. *Burn Care and Rehabilitation: Principles and Practice*. Philadelphia, PA: FA Davis; 1993:10-28.

3. Myers BA. *Wound Management: Principles and Practice*. New Jersey: Prentice Hall; 2004.

4. Pham TN, Gibran NS, Heimbach DM. Evaluation of the burn wound. In: Herndon DN, ed. *Total Burn Care*. Philadelphia, PA: Elsevier Saunders; 2007:119-126.

5. Kaplan DH, Jenison MC, Saeland S, Shlomchik WD, Sclomchik MJ. Epidermal langerhans cell-deficient mice develop enhanced contact hypersensitivity. *Immunity*. 2005;23:611-620.

6. Bessey PQ. Wound Care. In: Herndon DN, ed. *Total Burn Care*. Philadelphia, PA: Elsevier Saunders; 2007:127-135.

7. Muller M, Gahankari D, Herndon DN. Operative wound management. In: Herndon DN, ed. *Total Burn Care*. Philadelphia, PA: Elsevier Saunders; 2007:177-195.

8. Johnson C. Pathologic manifestations of burn injury. In: Richard RL, Staley MJ, eds. *Burn Care and Rehabilitation: Principles and Practice*. Philadelphia, PA: FA Davis; 1993:29-48.

9. Hartford CE, Kealy P. Care of outpatient burns. In Herndon DN. *Total Burn Care*. Philadelphia, PA: Elsevier Saunders; 2007:67-80.

10. Cakir B, Yegen BC. Systemic responses to burn injury. *Turk J Med Sci*. 2004;34:215-226.

11. Wolf SE. Critical care in the severely burned: organ support and management of complications. In Herndon DN, ed. *Total Burn Care*. Philadelphia, PA: Elsevier Saunders; 2007:454-476.

12. Mayes T, Gottschlich M, Scanlon J, Warden GD. Four-year review of burns as an etiologic factor in the development of long bone fractures in pediatric patients. *J Burn Care Rehabil*. 2003;24:279-284.

13. Dutcher K, Johnson C. Neuromuscular and musculoskeletal complications. In: Richard RL, Staley MJ, eds. *Burn Care and Rehabilitation: Principles and Practice*. Philadelphia, PA: FA Davis; 1993:576-602.

14. Greenhalgh DG, Staley MJ. Burn wound healing. In: Richard RL, Staley MJ, eds. *Burn Care and Rehabilitation: Principles and Practice*. Philadelphia, PA: FA Davis; 1993:70-102.

15. Sussman C, Bates-Jensen BM. Wound healing physiology and chronic wound healing. In: Sussman C, Bates-Jensen BM, eds. *Wound Care: A Collaborative Practice Manual for Physical Therapists and Nurses*. Gaithersburg, MD: Aspen Publishers; 2001.

16. Miller SF, Staley MJ, Richard RL. Surgical Management of the Burn Patient. In: Richard RL, Staley MJ, eds. *Burn Care and Rehabilitation: Principles and Practice*. Philadelphia, PA: FA Davis; 1993:177-197.

17. Integra Bilayer Matrix Wound Dressing. Available at: http://ww.integra-ls.com/products/?product=122. Accessed November 3, 2008.

18. Meyer WJ, Patterson DR, Jaco M, Woodson L, Thomas C. Management of pain and other discomforts of burn patients. In Herndon DN, ed. *Total Burn Care*. Philadelphia, PA: Elsevier Saunders; 2007:797-818.

19. Richardson P, Mustard L. The management of pain in the burns unit. *Burns.* 2009;35:921-936.

20. Bloomfield SA. Changes in musculoskeletal structure and function with prolonged bed rest. *Med Sci Sports Exerc.* 1997;29:197-206.

21. Convertino VA, Bloomfield SA, Greenleaf JE. An overview of the issues: physiological effects of bed rest and restricted physical activity. *Med Sci Sports Exerc.* 1997;29:187-190.

22. Baker CP, Russell WJ, Meyer W III, Blakeney P. Physical and psychologic rehabilitation outcomes for young adults burned as children. *Arch Phys Med Rehabil.* 2007;88(12 Suppl 2):S57-S64.

23. Cucuzzo NA, Ferrando A, Herndon DN. The effects of exercise programming vs traditional outpatient therapy in the rehabilitation of severely burned children. *J Burn Care Rehabil.* 2001;22: 214-220.

24. Suman OE, Thomas SJ, Wilkins JP, Mlcak RP, Herndon DN. Effect of exogenous growth hormone and exercise on lean mass and muscle function in children with burns. *J Appl Physiol.* 2003;94: 2273-2281.

25. Suman OE, Spies RJ, Celis MM, Mlcak RP, Herndon DN. Effects of a 12-wk resistance exercise program on skeletal muscle strength in children with burn injuries. *J Appl Physiol.* 2001;91: 1168-1175.

26. Al-Mousawi AM, Williams FN, Mlcak RP, Jeschke MG, Herndon DN, Suman OE. Effects of exercise training on resting energy expenditure and lean mass during pediatric burn rehabilitation. *J Burn Care Res.* 2010;31:400-408.

27. Suman OE, Mlcak RP, Herndon DN. Effect of exercise training on pulmonary function in children with thermal injury. *J Burn Care Rehabil.* 2002;23:288-293.

28. Celis MM, Suman OE, Huang TT, Yen P, Herndon DN. Effect of a supervised exercise and physiotherapy program on surgical interventions in children with thermal injury. *J Burn Care Rehabil.* 2003;24:57-61.

29. Mahaney NB. Restoration of play in a severely burned three-year-old child. *J Burn Care Rehabil.* 1990;11:57-63.

30. Coppard BM, Lohman H. *Introduction to Splinting: A Clinical Reasoning and Problem-Solving Approach.* 3rd ed. St. Louis, MO: Mosby Elsevier; 2008.

31. Jacobs M, Austin A. *Splinting the Hand and the Upper Extremity: Principles and Process.* Baltimore, MD: Lippincott Williams & Wilkins; 2003.

32. Goga-Eppenstine P, Hill JP, Philip PA, Philip M, Seifert TM, Yasukawa AM. *Casting Protocols for the Upper and Lower Extremities.* Gaithersburg, MD: Aspen Publishers; 1999.

33. Ricks NR, Meagher DP Jr. The benefits of plaster casting for lower-extremity burns after grafting in children. *J Burn Care Rehabil.* 1992;13:465-468.

34. Daugherty MB, Car-Collins JA. Splinting techniques for the burn patient. In: Richard RL, Staley MJ, eds. *Burn Care and Rehabilitation: Principles and Practice.* Philadelphia, PA: FA Davis; 1993:242-323.

35. Richard RL, Staley MJ. Evaluation and treatment planning. In: Richard RL, Staley MJ, eds. *Burn Care and Rehabilitation: Principles and Practice.* Philadelphia, PA: FA Davis; 1993:201-220.

36. Chen HC, Yang JY, Chuang SS, Huang CY, Yang SY. Heterotopic ossification in burns: our experience and literature reviews. *Burns.* 2009;35:857-862.

37. Vanden Bossche L, Vanderstraeten G. Heterotopic ossification: a review. *J Rehabil Med.* 2005;37: 129-136.

38. Schweinberger MH, Roukis TS. Effectiveness of instituting a specific bed protocol in reducing complications associated with bed rest. *J Foot Ankle Surg.* 2010;49:340-347.

39. Dittmer DK, Teasell R. Complications of immobilization and bed rest. Part 1: musculoskeletal and cardiovascular complications. *Can Fam Physician.* 1993;39:1428-1437.

Burn Injury to Dorsal Hand— Adult Case

David John Lorello

A 42-year-old male is admitted to the burn unit after sustaining a 2% total body surface area (TBSA) propane flash/flame burn to the dorsum of his right hand while he was attempting to light a gas grill (Fig. 27-1). The patient's burns were determined to be deep partial thickness burns. The patient is medically stable and is in a non-intensive care unit room. His hand is currently dressed in silver sulfadiazine, gauze, and burn netting. The physical therapist has received orders to evaluate the patient 18 hours post-admission to the hospital.

▶ What examination signs may be associated with this diagnosis?
▶ What are possible complications interfering with physical therapy?
▶ Describe a physical therapy plan of care based on each stage of the health condition.

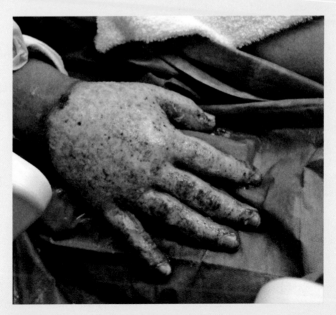

Figure 27-1. Deep partial thickness dorsal hand burn.

KEY DEFINITIONS

BOUTONNIERE DEFORMITY: Rupture of the central tendinous slip of the extensor hood resulting in hyperextension of the MCP, flexion of the PIP, and extension of the DIP

HYPERTROPHIC SCARRING: Scar that rises above the height of the original area of injury

SYNDACTYLY: Loss of the dorsal web space through contraction

Objectives

1. Understand complications associated with burns to the dorsum of the hand.
2. Develop a plan of care for each phase of wound healing.
3. Identify the risks for hypertrophic scarring and interventions designed to minimize its occurrence.

Physical Therapy Considerations

PT considerations during management of the individual with dorsal hand burns:

▶ **General physical therapy plan of care/goals:** Prevent loss of range of motion (ROM)/contracture; achieve pre-injury level of strength; maximize functional independence with activities of daily living (ADLs)

▶ **Physical therapy interventions:** ROM exercises, stretching, tendon gliding, splinting and positioning, resistance exercise, ADL training, patient education regarding exercise and splint-wearing schedule

▶ **Precautions during physical therapy:** No ROM to PIP joints, if the integrity of the extensor tendons is unknown; postsurgical limitations

▶ **Complications interfering with physical therapy:** Compartment syndrome, exposed tendons, hypertrophic scarring

Understanding the Health Condition

In the adult, the hand comprises < 5% of total skin surface area. Even with such a small surface area, there is inherent potential for permanent functional deficits and abnormal scarring after a burn injury. For this reason, the American Burn Association referral criteria for who should be transferred to a verified burn center includes burns to the hand.[1] For the clinician treating patients with burns, it is helpful to consider the hand as an "organ" of the body with thin, highly mobile skin on the dorsal surface and thicker, sensory-enriched skin on the palmar surface, and a delicately balanced musculotendinous system.[2] Damage to any of these areas from a burn can have deleterious effects for the patient. For detailed descriptions of skin anatomy, burn wound physiology, and the phases of wound healing, please refer to Case 26.

A successful outcome is dependent upon a team effort to ensure timely healing. Superficial partial thickness burns typically heal in less than 21 days if the wound remains infection-free. Deep partial thickness burns can take longer to heal, so the surgeon may elect to surgically excise the burn eschar and apply a graft to heal the wound quickly. Full thickness burns need to be excised and skin grafted. The goal is to heal the burn wound in *less than* 21 days. Burn wounds that take longer than 21 days to heal are at a higher risk for hypertrophic scarring.[3] In addition to length of time to heal, there are other factors that increase a patient's risk for abnormal scarring. Infection, young age, darker pigmented skin, burn location (sternum, upper back, and shoulder), and areas of tension (shoulder and upper back) are all risk factors for hypertrophic scars.[3]

To decrease the likelihood of hypertrophic scarring associated with lengthy healing, the hand is one of the areas that is autografted as soon as possible. The surgeon typically uses a split-thickness skin graft, and if enough unburned skin is available (*e.g.*, a small TBSA burn), the surgeon uses a sheet graft. A sheet graft is an autograft that is not altered in any way after it is harvested. If there is not enough skin available, the harvested skin is meshed with a mechanical meshing instrument. When available, it is always best to use a sheet graft because sheet grafts have a better cosmetic appearance and are less likely to develop contracture.[4,5]

Physical Therapy Patient/Client Management

Physical therapy examination is often initiated within 24 hours of admission to the hospital. Treatments begin immediately thereafter, and a plan of care is formulated for every phase of wound healing. Management includes preventing loss of ROM, strengthening, and maximizing independence with ADLs. Treatments can include therapeutic exercise, splinting, and functional activities. Therapy goals and interventions are influenced and frequently modified by surgical management and the phases of wound healing.

Examination, Evaluation, and Diagnosis

The physical therapist must begin with a thorough chart review. It is important to know the mechanism of injury, TBSA, the location of injuries, and the depth of the burns. Whether there was concomitant trauma is also important to know. Did the patient fall during the injury? If so, does the patient have pain anywhere besides the burned area? Often a patient does not realize that he has sustained other injuries because the burn injury is so painful. Did the patient hit his head? These are all questions that must be answered through the chart review or from interviewing the patient, if this is possible. The physical therapist should learn if any surgical procedures such as surgical debridement, escharotomies, or fasciotomies have been performed. Learning of an *impending* surgery gives immediate clues that the burn is deep enough that it will not heal on its own. The physical therapist should ascertain whether there is significant past medical history, especially the presence of any health conditions that may slow the healing process (*e.g.*, diabetes mellitus, peripheral vascular disease). Finally, any information regarding the patient's social history including family dynamics and work environment should be gathered.

The physical therapist should speak to the patient's nurse prior to the evaluation to learn when the patient will have his next wound dressing change. Ideally, the physical therapist should initially evaluate the patient with all wound dressings removed. This allows visualization of the wounds and more accurate goniometric measurements. The physical therapist must also learn the patient's pain regimen. Burn patients have medications for background pain, breakthrough pain, and procedural pain. The physical therapist should learn from the nurse if the patient's pain has been well-controlled and if he is tolerating the current medications. For burn patients, it is the standard of care that medications are prescribed and provided for background pain and for procedural pain (*e.g.*, dressing changes, therapy). If the patient is in too much pain with only the background pain medications administered, it may be more appropriate to hold the initial physical therapy evaluation until procedural medications can be administered.

The first step in the examination is to assess whether the patient is alert and able to follow commands. If the patient's dressing change does not correspond with the time of the evaluation, the physical therapist can get a thorough history from the patient regarding the mechanism of injury, past medical history, hand dominance, and his family and social support network. Evaluating active ROM (AROM) for joints unaffected by the burn injury can be done at this time, as well as a cursory assessment of the patient's mobility and ability to perform ADLs. If the injured hand is completely covered by dressings, the therapist should ask the patient questions regarding intactness of sensation in the hand. The therapist should specifically ask if he feels any numbness or tingling because these can be symptoms of compartment syndrome and must be brought to the attention of the medical team immediately. If the patient has been admitted to the hospital promptly after injury, he is in the inflammatory phase of wound healing and edema will be present. The patient's affected hand should be elevated above the level of the heart and he should be educated regarding edema prevention and requisite elevated positioning (see Table 26-2). The physical therapist will need to return to complete the evaluation when the dressings are removed.

There are two critical reasons why the burned hand *must* ultimately be evaluated without the wound dressings on. First, accurate ROM cannot be measured with the dressings in place. Second, the dorsal skin is very thin and the extensor tendons lay just beneath. Pressure exerted from the dressings and from the edema can cause damage to these delicate structures, resulting in permanent injury such as a boutonniere deformity. The therapist should assess ROM (active and passive) during the patient's dressing change. Measurements of ROM should be taken for joints affected by the burn and for those unaffected as well. If the integrity of the extensor tendons at the proximal interphalangeal (PIP) joints cannot be determined, **ROM of the PIP joints** must not be performed. Tendon ischemia can occur as a result of pressure between the inelastic eschar and the head of the proximal phalanx during PIP flexion.[2,6] With dressings removed, sensation of the hand should also be assessed. Initial physical therapy goals will be based upon a number of factors including the phase of wound healing, extent and depth of burn, patient's current health status, age, and physical and mental condition. Goals change frequently based on surgical procedures and post-surgical movement restrictions. The foremost goal is to prevent loss of ROM. Other goals include maintaining the patient's pre-injury level of aerobic capacity, strength, and independence with ADLs.

Plan of Care and Interventions

In the initial inflammatory phase (2-5 days from time of injury), edema control is one of the primary goals. In addition to the possibility of compartment syndrome, the resulting pressure from edema beneath the dorsal skin of the hand can cause hyperextension of the metacarpophalangeal joints (MCPs). Prolonged hyperextension of the MCPs can lead to flexion of the PIPs. This presents like a boutonniere deformity, but without the true injury to the central slip of the extensor hood at the PIP joint. This deformity is referred to as a pseudo-boutonniere deformity.[7] The physical therapist can utilize positioning and AROM during this phase to decrease edema. The affected hand should be positioned above the level of the heart. Pillows or foam wedges are helpful to achieve elevation. Active flexion of the MCPs and active abduction and adduction of the fingers should be initiated during this phase. The muscle pump action provided from these motions helps reduce edema.[2,6,8] Patients with deep partial thickness burns and full thickness burns should not perform active or passive flexion of the PIP joints until the integrity of the extensor tendons is known. Composite flexion exercises such as making a fist should be avoided. However, the patient may actively flex the distal interphalangeal (DIP) joint while the PIP joint remains blocked into extension; gutter splints placed on the volar side of the PIP joints allow the patient to move the MCP joints and DIP joints while maintaining PIP extension. After the first 36 hours post-burn, patients that cannot tolerate performing AROM because of pain or difficulty moving through full range due to inelastic burn eschar may be candidates for splinting. The splint of preference for the dorsal hand burn is known as the "anti-deformity splint," "resting hand splint," or "burn hand splint."[2,6-8] The goal of the splint is to provide flexion of the MCPs to prevent the hyperextended position that these joints naturally adopt due to the dorsal hand burn injury and subsequent edema. The patient should be placed in the "intrinsic plus" position in the splint: flexion of the MCP joints and extension of the interphalangeal joints. There is not a true consensus regarding the exact position of the hand and wrist joints in the intrinsic plus position. Our facility (Arizona Burn Center) aims to place the wrist at 15° to 40° of extension, 70° to 90° of MCP flexion, and full extension of the interphalangeal joints. The thumb should be placed somewhere between radial or palmar abduction, depending on where in the first web space the burn is located. Care must be taken, however, when splinting during the inflammatory phase. If the patient's hand cannot be placed into position because of edema, the joints must not be forced into optimal positioning. The result could be ischemia to the underlying structures, which can lead to permanent injury.

From about the third or fifth day post-burn until approximately three weeks post-burn, the patient is in the proliferative phase of wound healing. During this time, eschar is being removed from the burn either surgically or during the dressing changes. The physical therapist should continue treating the patient during dressing changes in order to visualize the tissue. If the surgeon determines that the extensor tendons are intact and if edema is controlled, then the patient can begin AROM of the PIP joints. Every effort should be made for the patient to perform all ROM actively. If the patient cannot tolerate ROM because the pain is not well controlled, the physical therapist can take advantage of seeing the patient in the operating room to perform passive ROM (PROM) when the patient is unconscious or provide therapy interventions during procedural sedation. It is not uncommon for procedural sedation to be ordered and performed solely for the purpose of ROM in the acute setting. Procedural sedation, sometimes referred to as conscious sedation, is when analgesics and sedatives are administered to the patient by the medical team to minimize the patient's pain and awareness and preserve spontaneous respiration during a therapeutic intervention.[9] Common medications administered include ketamine (anesthetic with analgesic properties), midazolam (sedative with amnestic effects), and fentanyl (opiate analgesic).[9] Midazolam and fentanyl are usually used in combination to achieve both sedation and analgesia.[9] Aggressive PROM and stretching should be avoided during the proliferative phase because some burn clinicians and researchers have theorized that damage to granulation tissue during stretching prolongs inflammation and may lead to hypertrophic scarring.[3,10-12] Visualization of the burn injury allows inspection of whether there are exposed tendons. Our facility allows for gentle tendon gliding of exposed tendons to prevent adhesions along their length as long as the tendons are kept moist with dressings during the gliding. In tendon gliding, the patient contracts the agonist muscle to glide the tendon in one direction, and then contracts the antagonist muscle to glide the tendon in the opposite direction. Movements are never taken to end range during tendon gliding. At all other times, the joint with an exposed tendon is kept splinted.

In addition to guiding ROM exercises during dressing changes, the physical therapist should also see the patient to progress exercise and to practice functional activities with the involved hand. During periods of rest, the patient's hand should be placed in the intrinsic plus position in the resting hand splint. Once it has been determined that the patient's wound is healthy and has an adequate blood supply, it is ready for a skin graft. For dorsal hand burns, the surgeon often uses a sheet graft. Immediately prior to the surgery, the physical therapist should be present to perform PROM to the hand, as this is the last opportunity for the hand to be mobilized until the graft has adhered. The physical therapist should also be involved with determining the optimal positioning of the wound bed for graft application to allow full functional ROM postoperatively. The graft is often attached with sutures and an occlusive petroleum gauze dressing is placed on the hand to keep the graft moist. In our burn center, the physical therapist is present in the operating room to wrap the fingers and the hand with cohesive bandages immediately after surgery. Cohesive bandages (*e.g.*, Coban or Co-Flex) inhibit edema and fluid collection underneath the graft. After application of the cohesive bandages, a new burn hand splint must be fabricated to maintain tissue length during graft healing and to accommodate changes in the size of the hand because of decreases in edema and in the amount of wound dressings applied. During the five days while the patient's hand is kept immobile to allow the sheet graft to adhere, other non-grafted joints should be exercised so the patient maintains strength and endurance. The physical therapist must ensure that the patient keeps his grafted hand elevated during all activities.

On the second postoperative day (POD 2), the dressings are removed so that the graft can be visually inspected. Any areas of fluid that have collected beneath the graft are evacuated because fluid acts as a barrier that prevents adherence between the graft and the wound bed. New dressings are then applied to the hand and the splint is put back on.

If it is determined that the graft is well-vascularized and adhered on POD 5, active exercises with the grafted hand can be resumed. The splint is typically removed and ROM can begin. ROM should begin with the dressings removed to prevent any shearing caused by the cohesive bandages. The patient is placed in less restrictive dressings to continue to keep the graft moist while allowing greater movement. The splint schedule can be modified so that the patient only has to wear the splint at night. Exercise can be initiated and should encompass ROM for individual joints as well as composite flexion exercises. The patient should progressively work up to performing exercises 5 times per day. Once the patient's pain is adequately controlled and he has the ability to either perform the dressing changes independently, or it has been established that he has support at home with dressing changes, discharge planning will commence. The patient should have a home exercise program (HEP) in place, as well as a splint-wearing schedule. Prior to discharge, outpatient therapy should be arranged by the case manager or the social worker.

After hospital discharge, the patient's burn is usually in the maturation phase of healing. This phase lasts an average of 1.5 years but can be as long as 3 years. At this time, the patient is most often seen in the outpatient setting for exercise, ROM, splinting, and scar management. The primary goals in this phase are for the patient to have full AROM and normal strength of the hand, independent performance of ADLs, and the presence of a flat pliable scar. Common hand deformities during the maturation phase include boutonniere deformity (Fig. 27-2), swan-neck deformity (hyperextension of the PIP with MCP and DIP flexion; Fig. 27-3) and syndactyly (Fig. 27-4). These deformities often occur when therapy is not initiated soon enough, therapy is not performed frequently enough, or if patients are non-compliant with the physical therapy plan of care.[2,3,6,8]

Hypertrophic scarring can limit ROM and cause joint contractures and extreme pain. The prevalence of hypertrophic scarring in burn survivors is between 32% and 72%.[13] Risk factors include young age, longer time to heal (> 21 days), darker pigmented skin, burn wound infection, and area of the body burned (neck and upper extremity).[13-16] Various modalities may influence, prevent, or decrease hypertrophic scarring after a burn. These include pressure therapy, scar massage, and silicone gel. Pressure therapy provided by the use of **pressure garments** and custom inserts is often used for the prevention and/or minimization of burn scars. It has been postulated that pressure therapy limits collagen synthesis and promotes the realignment of collagen already present in the scar by restricting the supply of blood, oxygen,

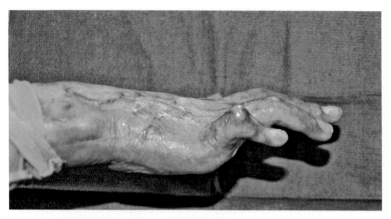

Figure 27-2. Boutonniere deformity of the right fifth finger.

and nutrients to the scar tissue.[17] Engrav et al.[18] evaluated the effectiveness of pressure garment therapy over a 12-year period and found that scars were significantly softer, thinner, and had improved clinical appearance, but this effect was only observed with scarring that was moderate to severe. These authors recommended that custom pressure garments be used for: deep partial thickness burns that have healed spontaneously over weeks, burns in children and young adults, burns in individuals with darker pigmented skin, and in instances where vascular support or protection is needed. Our facility usually initiates pressure therapy once the graft is fully adhered and no open areas remain. An off-the-shelf interim glove is used. In addition to providing pressure on the graft, the interim glove helps prevent edema

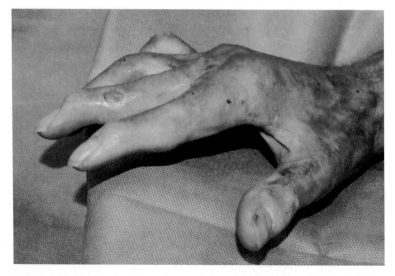

Figure 27-3. Swan-neck deformities (hyperextension of the PIP with MCP and DIP flexion) of the right second and third digits.

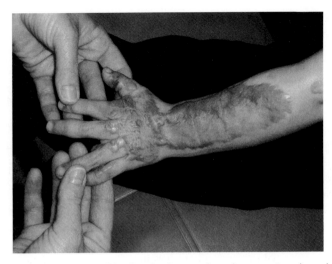

Figure 27-4. Syndactyly, or the loss of the dorsal web space through contraction, shown between the left third and fourth digits.

in the hand. After 2 weeks, the patient is measured for custom pressure garments. Patients are advised to wear the garments 23 hours per day and remove them only for bathing and scar massage. It is important that the patient uses sunscreen underneath the pressure garments because newly grafted skin sunburns easily and becomes permanently discolored due to sun exposure. Massage has also been advocated in the treatment of hypertrophic scarring. Massage has been thought to encourage collagen remodeling, decrease itching, desensitize the scar, and provide moisture and pliability through the use of moisturizers.[3,19-21] Studies in patients with burn injuries have shown that scar massage decreases itching and pain and improves anxiety and depression.[19-21] **Silicone gel** is another modality frequently used in the treatment of hypertrophic scars. The exact mechanism of action is unknown, although it has been postulated that silicone works by increasing scar hydration, increasing pressure on the scar, and increasing the temperature of the scar.[10-12] A randomized, double-blinded, placebo-controlled trial by Momeni et al.[22] studied the efficacy of silicone gel sheeting applied to hypertrophic burn scars. Participants were selected 2 to 4 months after injury, and had a hypertrophic scar measuring at least 5 × 5 cm. For each participant, the scar was divided in half. Half the scar received silicone gel sheeting, and the other half received a placebo (non-silicone) sheeting. Sheeting was held in place using tape. Wearing time of either sheeting started at 4 hours per day and was increased by 4 hours each week until wearing time was 24 hours per day. Outcome measures included pigmentation, vascularity, pliability, pain, and itching. Participants were seen at 1 month and at 4 months after enrollment in the study. At 4 months, the portion of the scar that received silicone gel sheeting had significantly improved from baseline scores in all areas except pain. In contrast, the portion of the scar that had received the non-silicone sheeting had slightly lower scores from baseline scores, but these scores were not significant. Li-Tsang et al.[23] investigated the effect that silicone gel sheeting had on hypertrophic scars. This prospective randomized clinical trial divided participants with a previous burn (time since burn not provided) that resulted in hypertrophic scarring into two groups. The silicone group wore silicone gel sheeting over the hypertrophic scar 24 hours per day. The control group received a 15-minute lanolin massage to the hypertrophic scars two times per day. At 6 months, the silicone group had significantly decreased scar thickness and improved scar pliability compared to the control group. The silicone group also reported improvements in scar pigmentation and scar pain; however, these latter results were not statistically significant. Our facility recommends use of silicone gel sheeting on hypertrophic scars for 12 hours per day. If the patient has been issued pressure garments, the silicone gel sheeting is worn beneath the garments. If the patient does not have garments, the silicone gel sheeting is held in place using tape or cohesive bandages.

Finally, education is paramount during this phase of healing. The physical therapist must design and prescribe a home exercise program that builds upon what has been learned during therapy sessions. In addition to exercise, the patient needs continued instruction and education regarding use of splints, pressure garments, and silicone, if those modalities are utilized. It is important for the physical therapist to begin education and instruction early in rehabilitation and to reinforce it throughout the entire plan of care. Rehabilitation of the patient with burn injuries is a dynamic process in which the parameters of the plan of care are dependent on the phase of wound healing and the presentation of the patient.

Evidence-Based Clinical Recommendations

SORT: Strength of Recommendation Taxonomy

A: Consistent, good-quality, patient-oriented evidence
B: Inconsistent or limited-quality, patient-oriented evidence
C: Consensus, disease oriented evidence, usual practice, expert opinion, or case series

1. In dorsal hand burns, active and passive ROM of the PIP joints should be avoided unless the integrity of the extensor tendon is known. **Grade C**

2. Pressure garments worn 23 hours per day in the maturation phase of wound healing minimize hypertrophic scarring. **Grade B**

3. Silicone gel sheets worn 24 hours per day increase pliability and decrease thickness, pigmentation, pain, vascularity, and itching of hypertrophic scars. **Grade B**

COMPREHENSION QUESTIONS

27.1 Which of the following increases the risk of hypertrophic scarring?
    A. Aggressive stretching
    B. Deeper burns
    C. Infection
    D. All of the above

27.2 A finger deformity that presents as hyperextension of the PIP with flexion of the MCP and DIP is known as:

   A. Boutonniere deformity

   B. Mallet finger

   C. Swan-neck deformity

   D. Syndactyly

27.3 The most appropriate plan of care for the patient who has a hand burn that is in the proliferative phase of wound healing would be:

   A. Tendon gliding exercises, strengthening exercises, night splinting, functional activities

   B. Positioning the hand at the level of the heart, AROM exercises to promote muscle pump action to decrease edema

   C. Strengthening exercises, stretching, functional activities, scar massage, fitting for pressure garments

   D. No exercises during this phase of wound healing

ANSWERS

27.1 **D.** Age, darker pigmentation, infection, tension, location of burn, and burn wounds that take longer than 21 days to heal are all factors that increase the risk of hypertrophic scarring.

27.2 **C.** Swan-neck deformity is hyperextension of the PIP joint and flexion of both the MCP and DIP joints. Boutonniere deformity is PIP flexion and DIP hyperextension (option A). Mallet finger is an abnormal flexion resting position of the DIP (option B). Syndactyly is loss of the dorsal web space through contraction (option D).

27.3 **A.** Tendon gliding exercises, strengthening exercises, night splinting, and functional activities are all appropriate during the proliferative phase of healing. Option B is most appropriate for the inflammatory phase; option C is most appropriate for the maturation phase. Option D is not appropriate because without interventions, contractures are likely.

REFERENCES

1. Guidelines for the operation of burn centers (2006). Available at: http://ameriburn.org/Chapter14.pdf?PHPSESSID=6306abbb623fb6829f248897646f8792. Accessed July 28, 2011.

2. Howell JW. Management of the acutely burned hand for the nonspecialized clinician. *Phys Ther.* 1989;69:1077-1090.

3. Richard RL, Staley MJ. Scar management. In: Richard RL, Staley MJ, eds. *Burn Care and Rehabilitation: Principles and Practice.* Philadelphia, PA: FA Davis; 1993:380-418.

4. Greenhalgh DG, Staley MJ. Burn wound healing. In: Richard RL, Staley MJ, eds. *Burn Care and Rehabilitation: Principles and Practice.* Philadelphia, PA: FA Davis; 1993:70-102.

5. Greenhalgh DG. Wound healing. In: Herndon DN, ed. *Total Burn Care*. Philadelphia, PA: Elsevier Saunders; 2007:578-595.

6. Moore ML, Dewey WS, Richard RL. Rehabilitation of the burned hand. *Hand Clin.* 2009;25:529-541.

7. Simpson RL, Gartner MC. Management of burns in the upper extremity. In: Hunter JM, Macklin EJ, Callahan AD, eds. *Rehabilitation of the Hand and Upper Extremity*. St. Louis, MO: Mosby; 2002:1475-1491.

8. Grigsby deLinde L, Knothe B. Therapist's management of the burned hand. In: Hunter JM, Macklin EJ, Callahan AD, eds. *Rehabilitation of the Hand and Upper Extremity*. St. Louis, MO: Mosby; 2002:1492-1526.

9. Brown TB, Lovato LM, Parker D. Procedural sedation in the acute care setting. *Am Fam Physician.* 2005;71:85-90.

10. Slemp AE, Kirschner RE. Keloids and scars: a review of keloids and scars, their pathogenesis, risk factors, and management. *Curr Opin Pediatr.* 2006;18:396-402.

11. Wolfram D, Tzankov A, Pülzl P, Piza-Katzer H. Hypertrophic scars and keloids—a review of their pathophysiology, risk factors, and therapeutic management. *Dermatol Surg.* 2009;35:171-181.

12. Bloemen MC, van der Veer WM, Ulrich MM, van Zuijlen PP, Niessen FB, Middelkoop E. Prevention and curative management of hypertrophic scar formation. *Burns.* 2009;35:463-475.

13. Lawrence JW, Mason ST, Schomer K, Klein MB. Epidemiology and impact of scarring after burn injury: a systematic review of the literature. *J Burn Care Res.* 2012;33:136-146.

14. Gangemi EN, Gregori D, Berchialla P, et al. Epidemiology and risk factors for pathologic scarring after burn wounds. *Arch Facial Plast Surg.* 2008;10:93-102.

15. Deitch EA, Wheelahan TM, Rose MP, Clothier J, Cotter J. Hypertrophic burn scars: analysis of variables. *J Trauma.* 1983;23:895-898.

16. Baker RH, Townley WA, McKeon S, Linge C, Vijh V. Retrospective study of the association between hypertrophic burn scarring and bacterial colonization. *J Burn Care Res.* 2007;28:152-156.

17. Macintyre L, Baird M. Pressure garments for use in the treatment of hypertrophic scars—a review of the problems associated with their use. *Burns.* 2006;3:10-15.

18. Engrav LH, Heimbach DM, Rivara FP, et al. 12-Year within-wound study of the effectiveness of custom pressure garment therapy. *Burns.* 2010;36:975-983.

19. Field T, Peck M, Scd, Hernandez-Reif M, Krugman S, Burman I, Ozment-Schenck L. Postburn itching, pain, and psychological symptoms are reduced with massage therapy. *J Burn Care Rehabil.* 2000;21:189-193.

20. Patino O, Novick C, Merlo A, Benaim F. Massage in hypertrophic scars. *J Burn Care Rehabil.* 1999;20:268-271.

21. Field T, Peck M, Krugman S, et al. Burn injuries benefit from massage therapy. *J Burn Care Rehabil.* 1998;19:241-244.

22. Momeni M, Hafezi F, Rahbar H, Karimi H. Effects of silicone gel on burn scars. *Burns.* 2009;35:70-74.

23. Li-Tsang CW, Lau JC, Choi J, Chan CC, Jianan L. A prospective randomized clinical trial to investigate the effect of silicone gel sheeting (Cica-Care) on post-traumatic hypertrophic scar among the Chinese population. *Burns.* 2006;32:678-683.

Juvenile Dermatomyositis

Kristi Whitney-Mahoney
Jo-Anne Marcuz

CASE 28

A previously well, 8-year-old boy presented to the emergency room with a 2.5-month history of worsening skin rash, fatigue, progressive muscle weakness and recent 2-day history of choking on food and drinks. He has had increasing difficulty negotiating stairs and reported several recent falls. A rheumatic disease was suspected and he was admitted to the hospital for further work-up. Investigations revealed diffuse, symmetrical muscle weakness (most prominent in the proximal muscle groups), a waddling gait, and a positive Gower's sign. Heliotrope rash and Gottron's papules (on hands, elbows, and knees) were present. On nailfold capillaroscopy, capillary dilation and dropout was observed. Video fluoroscopic feeding assessment confirmed clinical dysphagia and parenteral nutrition was initiated. Laboratory investigations revealed elevated serum muscle enzymes and acute phase reactants. Magnetic resonance imaging (MRI), electromyography (EMG), nerve conduction studies (NCS), and muscle biopsy were consistent with myositis. The diagnosis of juvenile dermatomyositis (JDM) was made. On the second day after hospital admission, a physical therapy consult for evaluation and treatment was requested.

▶ What examination signs may be associated with this diagnosis?
▶ What are the most appropriate examination tests?
▶ What are the examination priorities?
▶ What are the most appropriate physical therapy outcome measures for muscle strength and endurance?
▶ Describe a physical therapy plan of care based on each stage of the disease.
▶ Identify referrals to other medical team members.

KEY DEFINITIONS

DYSPHAGIA: Difficulty (or inability) to swallow

GOWER'S SIGN: Physical sign indicating proximal lower limb weakness; describes when a patient flexes his trunk, places his hands on his knees and moves them up his legs in order to extend the trunk

GOTTRON'S PAPULES: Erythematous, maculopapular rash most commonly found on extensor surfaces of the hands (especially proximal interphalangeal joints), as well as elbows, knees and less often, medial malleoli; erythematous rash without papules in this distribution is known as Gottron's sign

HELIOTROPE RASH: Violet-colored rash of (primarily) the upper eyelids

NAILFOLD CAPILLAROSCOPY: Non-invasive test in which skin capillaries at the base of the fingernail (nailfold) are examined under a microscope to evaluate vascular abnormalities; test assists in diagnosis, classification, and prediction of clinical outcome in connective tissue disorders

VIDEOFLUOROSCOPY FEEDING STUDY: Also known as dysphagia barium swallow; test to determine oral and pharyngeal swallowing difficulties that uses videotaping, barium, and x-ray while a patient swallows varying consistencies of food and liquids

Objectives

1. Identify the signs and symptoms of JDM.
2. Identify valid and reliable outcome tools to measure muscle strength and endurance in this population.
3. Recognize the complications of JDM.
4. Understand the medical treatments for JDM and their relevance to physical therapy management.
5. Design an appropriate physical therapy program for a child with JDM in the hospital.

Physical Therapy Considerations

PT considerations during management of the child with newly diagnosed juvenile dermatomyositis:

► **General physical therapy plan of care/goals:** Prevent/minimize loss of range of motion (ROM), strength, and aerobic functional capacity; maximize physical function and safety; minimize secondary impairments; optimize health-related quality of life

► **Physical therapy interventions:** Patient/family education regarding JDM and the risk of: muscle contracture development, further deterioration of muscle strength and potential falls; caregiver training for bed positioning, ROM, stretching, and safe assisted lift/transfer techniques; exercises to optimize muscle strength in a graded fashion with a focus on return to independent, daily functional activities and ultimately, school, play, and sports; facilitate home exercise program and/ or referral to community rehabilitation providers, if appropriate upon discharge; monitor progress with valid and objective outcome measures

▶ **Precautions during physical therapy:** Physical supervision to enhance safety and prevent falls; monitor ability to manage airway; monitor positioning of medical lines

▶ **Complications during physical therapy:** Vertebral compression fractures, pain, behavior/mood changes

Understanding the Health Condition

JDM is the most common of the childhood inflammatory myopathies.[1,2] It is thought that the inflammation in JDM primarily affects the blood vessels supplying the muscle, skin, and to varying degrees, the internal organs. The exact etiology is unknown. Both genetic and infectious agents are thought to be important.[3] JDM has a worldwide distribution and an estimated annual incidence of two to three cases per 1 million children in the Western population.[4-6] It can occur at any time in childhood with an average age at onset of 7 years.[4,7] It seems to be more common in girls than boys (ratio of 2-3:1).[7]

Classic JDM is characterized by symmetrical proximal muscle weakness, raised serum concentration levels of several muscle enzymes (*e.g.*, creatine kinase, lactate dehydrogenase, aldolase, alanine aminotransferase, aspartate aminotransferase), and pathognomonic Gottron's and heliotrope skin rashes. A variety of other photosensitive rashes (*e.g.*, malar, V sign, and shawl sign) and non-specific rashes can also be seen.[8] In addition to elevated muscle enzyme levels, non-specific indicators of inflammation (*e.g.*, erythrocyte sedimentation rate, C-reactive protein) can be elevated and help differentiate JDM from non-inflammatory conditions. Constitutional symptoms such as fever, anorexia, weight loss, and general malaise can also occur at presentation. Parents often report that their child has become irritable and note difficulties with gross motor function or regression of motor milestones.[3] For example, a child may ask to be carried frequently and become unable to climb stairs independently. Significant periungal erythema, cuticular overgrowth and marked nailfold capillary changes (vessel dilation, dropout, tortuosity) are noted in most children with JDM.[3,9] Internal organ involvement, such as heart, lungs, and gastrointestinal tract are not infrequent and can be important features of illness.[10] A non-deforming, transient arthritis can occur.[3,4] Dysphagia secondary to weakness of oropharyngeal, laryngeal, and esophageal musculature is common[4,8,11] and recognition of this problem is important in the prevention of aspiration and respiratory complications. Videofluoroscopic swallowing study is the preferred diagnostic test.[12-14] Signs and symptoms of JDM are generally insidious and often predate the diagnosis by 3 to 6 months.[3]

The 1975 diagnostic criteria established by Bohan and Peter[15] for JDM are widely applied in the diagnosis of JDM. The five criteria include: symmetrical proximal muscle weakness, presence of at least one characteristic rash (Gottron's, heliotrope), increased serum muscle enzyme levels (*e.g.*, creatine kinase, aldolase), myopathic changes on electromyography, and pathological changes on muscle biopsy. Presence of four of the five criteria is designated as definite JDM; presence of three criteria is designated as probably JDM, and presence of only two criteria is designated as possible JDM. However, the sensitivity and specificity of these criteria have not been validated. A probable diagnosis of JDM requires the presence of a pathognomonic rash (Gottron's or heliotrope) and two of the five other criteria. A definitive diagnosis of JDM requires a rash with at least three of the other criteria.[15,16] With the emergence of non-invasive diagnostic tools such as MRI, invasive testing such as muscle biopsy, and even electromyography and nerve conduction studies, are performed less frequently. These latter tests are often reserved for uncertain cases. MRI is a sensitive test for determining the presence of muscle inflammation, although it is not specific to the diagnosis of myositis or myopathy. In a prevalence sample of 102 patients with childhood myositis, only 76% had an abnormal MRI.[11] Despite this, many rheumatologists endorse MRI as an important diagnostic test that should be included in any revised diagnostic criteria for JDM.[17]

Many of the clinical features of JDM are seen in other conditions that must be considered in the differential diagnosis. Weakness alone could be attributed to muscular dystrophies or myopathies related to metabolic, endocrine, or even drug-induced causes. Rash associated with JDM can be confused with psoriasis, eczema, and allergic reactions. These skin conditions should be considered in the absence of overt muscle weakness. Infections, both viral and bacterial, can also mimic JDM. Other rheumatic diseases such as systemic lupus erythematosus, juvenile idiopathic arthritis and scleroderma, must be excluded as well as other inflammatory conditions (*e.g.*, inflammatory bowel disease).[18,19]

Complications of JDM include dystrophic calcification, also referred to as calcinosis. This can occur in up to 30% of patients.[20,21] The most common sites affected are pressure points such as the elbows, knees, digits, and buttocks.[21] Calcinosis is typically a late manifestation of JDM occurring 1 to 3 years after the onset of illness, but it has been described both at initial presentation and as long as 20 years later.[21,22] Calcinosis can result in skin ulcerations, pain, and contracture. Calcinosis is associated with delayed diagnosis and long duration of disease, chronic disease course, and inadequate glucocorticoid therapy.[8] Cutaneous ulcerations affect less than 10% of patients with JDM and may predict a more severe illness characterized by persistent weakness, widespread calcinosis, and poor response to therapy.[22,23] Serious gastrointestinal complications such as ulceration, hemorrhage, or perforation can occur secondary to vasculopathy of the intestines.[22]

Previously, the prognosis for JDM was poor with mortality reported in one third of patients and significant physical impairments in another third.[24] Treatment with glucocorticoids revolutionized the treatment and dramatically improved prognosis for children with JDM.[3] It is generally accepted that glucocorticoid therapy is a required pharmacological intervention. However, the dosing regimen and route of administration vary among physicians. Most protocols implement dosing in the range of 2 mg/kg of glucocorticoids (most commonly prednisone) with a tapering protocol of about 10% per month over 9 to 12 months.[25] The concomitant use of disease-modifying agents, such as methotrexate, has allowed for a reduction in the total amount and duration of prednisone therapy.[26] Other frequently used steroid-sparing agents include cyclosporine,[27] azathioprine,[28] mycophenolate mofetil (MMF),[29] and hydroxychloroquine[30] and more recently, biologic agents such as infliximab[31] or rituximab.[32] In instances of inadequate drug response, the addition of monthly intravenous immunoglobulin infusions can be beneficial.[33] In more severe or resistant cases of JDM, stronger immune suppression with agents such as cyclophosphamide may be required.[34]

Prolonged, high-dose glucocorticoid therapy can lead to multiple adverse drug reactions (ADRs) and complications. The development of significant osteopenia and osteoporosis frequently leads to vertebral compression fractures. Vertebral compression fractures can lead to significant pain and subsequently further limit physical function and progression of the physical therapy program. Treatment with bisphosphonate agents and calcitonin may improve pain associated with compression fractures and thus facilitate physical function and physical therapy progression. **Calcium and vitamin D supplementation is routinely prescribed and weightbearing activities** are promoted in an attempt to prevent some of the deleterious bone effects of glucocorticoids.[35] Growth delay, cataracts, weight gain, avascular necrosis, and hypertension are other glucocorticoid-related ADRs.[25]

Earlier diagnosis and better treatments have led to a significant decline in mortality and improvements in functional outcomes.[20] However, for many patients, the disease course of JDM is chronic and requires long-term pharmacological treatment. It has been reported that up to 35% of children were still receiving medications for disease treatment after a median of 7 years of follow-up.[20,25]

Physical Therapy Patient/Client Management

Management of the child with JDM requires a multidisciplinary team approach. The team for a newly diagnosed child with JDM just admitted to the hospital may include a pediatric rheumatologist, physical therapist, occupational therapist, social worker, dietitian, and nurse. The physical therapist works with the patient, family, and team to provide an objective assessment of the patient's specific functional abilities and impairments (e.g., muscle strength, flexibility, endurance). The overall goal is to determine potential safety risks, monitor change in status over time, and develop an appropriate physical therapy regimen that promotes optimal physical function and quality of life. Patient and family education is an important aspect of physical therapy. Physical therapy treatments may include stretching, strengthening, aerobic training, safe transfer training, and ongoing education to the patient, family/caregivers, and possibly educators or administrators at the patient's school. Liaising with other team members to address issues pertaining to nutrition, coping, and discharge planning is required. To prepare for hospital discharge, the physical therapist must evaluate the patient's ability to safely return to home and school as well as make necessary recommendations and referrals for community support. This could range from a home program to be carried out with the assistance of parents/caregivers to a referral for specialized inpatient rehabilitation.

Examination, Evaluation, and Diagnosis

Prior to seeing the patient, the physical therapist needs to obtain information regarding the patient's current status and relevance to the physical therapy plan. This includes vital signs, current medications, timing of analgesic medications (if appropriate), and test results (e.g., MRI). There may be other team members (e.g., neurologists, infectious disease specialists) within the hospital that are still carrying out tests to rule out differential diagnoses. Patients connected to peripheral or central lines may be somewhat limited in their ability to participate in therapeutic activities. Timing therapy around times of day when the patient may have peripheral lines capped or locked may facilitate participation in physical therapy. Muscle pain may be a feature of acute JDM, so planning physical therapy sessions around analgesic medication administration may be necessary.

History taking is an important first step in forming a rapport with the patient and his family and in clarifying the patient's gross motor abilities and developmental progression *prior* to the onset of symptoms. This helps the therapist develop motivating activities and guide short- and long-term goal setting.

The assessment for a patient with JDM is comprehensive, including strength, ROM, flexibility, gait, safety, and functional mobility. The primary objectives of physical therapy assessment are to determine mobility-related safety risks and to document the degree of physical impairments, in particular muscle strength. Manual muscle testing (MMT) using a 5- or 10-point scale, is the most commonly implemented strength assessment method.[36] Table 28-1 illustrates the 5-point and 10-point muscle grading systems.[37] The MMT is employed as a major endpoint in most JDM-related studies and is important in the longitudinal follow-up of this population.[38-40] The MMT has demonstrated good reliability and sensitivity to change in children (over the age of 5 years) with JDM with moderate to severe muscle weakness.[41] Expert consensus established that the strength testing of a core subset of eight muscle groups (MMT8) is valid, performs as well as the strength assessment of 24 muscle groups, and is more time-efficient and less tiring for patients.[38] The MMT8 is a frequently reported outcome in clinical trials and practice with this population. The muscles tested in the MMT8 include neck flexors, deltoids, biceps, wrist extensors, gluteus maximus, gluteus medius, quadriceps, and ankle dorsiflexors. Each muscle is graded on the 1- to 10-point scale and a summary score of 0 to 70 (unilateral testing) or 0 to 140 (bilateral testing) is calculated. A standard script of commands for completing manual muscle testing in children is available on the National Institute of Environmental Health Sciences—The International Myositis Assessment and Clinical Studies Group (IMACS) Web site.[41] This script ensures consistency among examiners and provides helpful guidelines for therapists unfamiliar with testing children.

Table 28-1   MANUAL MUSCLE TESTING WITH 5-POINT AND 10-POINT SCORING

Muscle Function	0-10 Point Scale	0-5 Point Scale	Grade
No Movement			
No palpable muscle contraction	0	0	Zero
Palpable contraction but no visible movement	T	1	Trace
Test Movement in the Horizontal Plane			
Moves through partial range, gravity eliminated	1	2–	Poor –
Moves through full range, gravity eliminated	2	2	Poor
Test Movement—Anti-Gravity Position			
Moves through partial range	3	2+	Poor +
Test Position—Anti-Gravity Position			
Gradual release from test position	4	3–	Fair –
Holds test position, no resistance	5	3	Fair
Holds test position against slight resistance	6	3+	Fair +
Holds test position against slight to moderate resistance	7	4–	Good –
Holds test position against moderate resistance	8	4	Good
Holds test position against moderate to strong resistance	9	4+	Good +
Holds test position against strong resistance	10	5	Normal

Reproduced with permission from Kendall FP, McCreary EK, Provance PG. Muscles: Testing and Function. Baltimore, MD: Williams & Wilkins; 1993.

Strength can also be assessed using various quantitative measures that may be more objective and sensitive to change than MMT; however, they are not always clinically practical.[42] For isometric strength testing, the modified sphygmomanometer and hand-held dynamometer[43] can be used. For isokinetic strength testing, examples include the Cybex and Biodex machines.[44] The modified sphygmomanometer consists of a modified blood pressure cuff and manometer. It is a portable and inexpensive tool that can easily be utilized in the clinical setting. It has been shown to be sensitive and reproducible and potentially adaptable in all 24 different muscle groups.[45]

Range of motion and flexibility should be thoroughly assessed. Limitations are most commonly seen in the hip and shoulder girdle, biceps, forearm flexors, and gastrocnemius and soleus muscles. Standard goniometry can be utilized to assess joint ROM. Special tests, such as the Thomas test (for hip flexor tightness), prone knee bend (for knee flexor tightness), passive straight leg raise (for hamstring tightness) and others are objective methods of documenting and tracking muscle flexibility.[46]

The **Childhood Myositis Assessment Scale** (CMAS) is a 14-item observational, performance-based instrument that was developed to evaluate proximal muscle strength, physical function, and endurance in patients across a wide age range (2 years to adult) that have idiopathic inflammatory myopathies (IIM).[42,47] It has been shown to possess excellent intra- and inter-rater reliability and good validity and responsiveness.[42,47] Normative data are available for nine CMAS maneuvers in healthy children, 4 to 9 years of age.[48] The CMAS is widely used internationally in the quantitative assessment of muscle function in children with inflammatory myositis, including JDM. Testing is easy and practical (generally takes 15-20 minutes to complete) to employ in daily clinical practice. Detailed descriptions of each maneuver and a video of the test being conducted are available online.[41]

The Childhood Health Assessment Questionnaire (CHAQ) is another physical function measure initially adapted from the adult Health Assessment Questionnaire.[49] The CHAQ is commonly employed in the evaluation of children with arthritis, but has also been validated in the JDM population.[50] The CHAQ is a parent- or self-report measure that consists of a discomfort index that assesses pain and a disability index. The disability index consists of 30 items in 8 domains of physical function. A summary score is calculated ranging from 0 to 3, with 0 indicating no reported disability.[49] The International Myositis Assessment and Clinical Studies Group endorses the use of at least one measure of physical function as part of a core set of disease activity measures.[41]

The physical therapist must look at several safety considerations that take into account the patient's age and both cognitive and physical developmental levels. Issues may arise with safety on stairs, transfers (especially sit to stand and floor to sit/stand), ambulating on uneven ground and/or ambulating with distractions. A child with JDM may present so significantly weakened that he has lost protective reflexes. A small stumble or nudge in a crowd could send him falling without the ability to protect himself, which could lead to a possible head injury. Due to the proximal and symmetrical weakness characteristic of JDM, the appropriateness of a walker or rollator must also be assessed. If the patient is significantly weak in his upper extremities, a walker may not necessarily be a practical option. In such instances, a wheelchair or scooter may be required to facilitate safe and efficient mobility. Use of this equipment is generally temporary and rarely required in the long term. A patient who is profoundly weak requires head and neck support during transfers as well as special considerations for positioning and a pressure-relief surface to avoid development of pressure ulcers.

Plan of Care and Interventions

Physical therapy intervention should address the impairments found on assessment. Therapeutic exercises are developed to address the muscular tightness and weakness that results from the inflammatory process. Muscle weakness in JDM relates to the pathological inflammation. Muscle biopsies demonstrate muscle fiber degeneration,

SECTION II: THIRTY-ONE CASE SCENARIOS

necrosis and inflammatory infiltration. Atrophied fibers and some abnormal architecture have also been noted.[51] In addition to specific muscle weakness, generalized deconditioning and reduced exercise capacity are also observed.

It is well accepted that it is safe to initiate **moderate intensity strengthening and endurance exercises** with children who have active JDM without risk of exacerbating or flaring their inflammation.[52] The strengthening and stretching exercises should be done to the patient's tolerance. There may be discomfort, but no pain should be elicited with the exercises thereby not aggravating active inflammation within the muscle. A combination of eccentric and concentric exercises has been shown to be the most effective training program for all ages.[53,54] Most often, family/caregivers must be taught to carry out and/or assist the child with stretching and strengthening exercises. The program should be developed with the patient's developmental stage in consideration. Distraction is often a very important tool when trying to complete stretches with a child of any age. For example, watching a favorite movie or singing and talking can be effective distraction techniques for younger children. Table 28-2 provides an example of an appropriate exercise program for an

Table 28-2	SAMPLE INPATIENT EXERCISE PROGRAM FOR A CHILD WITH JDM
Exercise	Instructions
Prone knee bends	In prone, patient brings heel to his buttock and therapist/parent helps hold in position of stretch.
Hamstring stretch	In supine, patient's hip is flexed to 90° and knee is straightened to point of stretch.
Heel cord stretch	Patient stands in front of wall in lunge position or stands on edge of step with heels hanging over edge to point of stretch.
Active assisted shoulder flexion	In supine or sitting with arms straight at sides, patient flexes arm up and above head as far as able. Therapist or parent assists movement as needed, then helps support arm above head while stabilizing scapula to allow for stretch.
Active assisted shoulder abduction	In supine or sitting, patient is assisted as needed with abducting shoulder as far as able. Therapist or parent helps support arm at end range to allow for stretch.
Elbow extension stretch	With patient in supine, therapist or parent helps patient achieve end range elbow extension and hold this position.
Prayer position stretch	Sitting patient pushes palms together into a prayer-like position and elevates elbows laterally while trying to keep fingers fully extended.
Bridging	In hooklying, patient pushes through feet and raises buttocks off bed as far as possible. If patient is able, hold for 3-5 seconds before returning to start position.
Knee extension in sitting	Sitting with/without support, patient extends knee to straightest position possible. If patient is able, hold for 3-5 seconds before returning to start position.
Sit-to-stands	Sitting on plinth or hospital bed raised to height that enables patient to stand independently. Patient stands then sits. Try to do "slow motion" sits, if patient able.

inpatient with acute moderate to severe JDM, like the current patient. The exercises address impairments commonly found in patients with JDM. Each stretch should be held for a minimum of 30 seconds and repeated 3 to 5 times per session, as tolerated. Ideally, the patient should perform the exercise program twice per day. The exercise program must be progressed when improvement is observed in order to continually challenge the patient.

If medically stable, the patient can participate in daily gym sessions, where he is engaged through play to work on further general conditioning. Activities may include taking shots on a basketball net, playing catch with a football or volleyball, playing soccer in either standing with close supervision or sitting, throwing bean bags at targets, and navigating through obstacle courses. If the patient is safe and able, he can work on squatting activities such as picking up items and passing back to the physical therapist (*e.g.*, bean bags or balls). Timing activities can often motivate children to complete tasks and beat their personal bests. Active video games have also been increasingly used to promote upper and lower extremity strengthening and conditioning.

Hydrotherapy has been used in the treatment of many musculoskeletal disorders. With safety modifications, hydrotherapy has been endorsed as enjoyable by adults and children with arthritis.[51,55] In addition, hydrotherapy for rheumatic diseases has been reported as the treatment of choice by parents and children in preference to land-based therapy alone.[55] If the patient has a peripheral line and can be unattached from the line, he can participate in a hydrotherapy session with care to wrap the site to maintain dryness of the dressing/site. Therapy in a warm pool addresses the same goals as land-based therapy (*i.e.*, addressing impairments found on examination, especially muscle weakness and tightness), but hydrotherapy has several inherent benefits. Buoyancy alleviates the painful effect of gravity on muscles and joints. Hydrostatic pressure improves circulation. The warmth of the water eases muscle pain and spasm. Therapy pools typically operate in the range of 33.5°C to 35.5°C, which allows for lengthy immersion durations and exercise activities without chilling or overheating.[56] Properties of water such as turbulence and drag can be utilized to grade the difficulty of exercises in all planes and ranges of movement. Walking can be done safely without the fear of falling and injury. The combination of improved circulation, muscle relaxation, decreased weightbearing, and pain relief improves the ability for soft tissues to stretch and buoyancy can facilitate a greater ROM. Hypertension, which may occur as a result of glucocorticoid therapy, would be a relative contraindication for prolonged submersion in heated pools if the hypertension were not medically controlled.

Heat (*e.g.*, hot packs, heating pads) and ice can be used per the patient's preference for easing pain in muscles and joints. Though these modalities do not produce a significant change in temperature approximately 1 to 2 cm below the skin, many patients find relief with superficial thermal agents.[57] Anecdotally, children frequently favor heat over cold.

If the patient has had a long history of symptoms resulting in decreased mobility and participation prior to diagnosis, he may be at risk of decreased bone mineral density (BMD). In combination with the initiation of systemic glucocorticoids, it is important to educate the patient and his family/caregivers on activity precautions to reduce the risk of fractures. For example, upon hospital discharge he should not participate in contact sports or climb on jungle gyms. Such precautions need to be followed until glucocorticoid therapy is ceased and follow-up assessment of bone health (*e.g.*, BMD test) is completed. Weightbearing activities to encourage positive bone stress should be encouraged. Education supporting the recommended vitamin D and calcium supplementation is important. The team dietitian can determine the specific supplementation needs. Vitamin D supplementation is of particular importance given that natural vitamin D production (originating from sun exposure) is reduced because patients need to avoid sun exposure due to the photosensitive nature of the rashes of JDM. It has been suggested that disease activity in general may be exacerbated with ultraviolet radiation exposure. Therefore, it is often recommended that individuals with JDM use sunscreen throughout the year. For patients with vertebral compression fractures, education regarding the avoidance of twisting and diagonal movements while encouraging appropriate posture and exercise is important. In some cases, back supports are used as temporary measures to provide pain relief.

Discharge planning should include strategies to ensure safety as well as a follow-up plan for the ongoing monitoring of physical functional status and activity progression. Referral to a community rehabilitation hospital, home therapy, or outpatient therapy is likely required. In choosing discharge disposition recommendations, the physical therapist should consider assessment of home and school safety and equipment needs. Short-term use of equipment such as raised toilet seats or a wheelchair may be required until strength and endurance improve. The age and size of the patient are also important considerations. A 5-year-old that is unable to safely climb stairs or rise from the floor can usually be easily managed by parents/caregivers as compared to a 15-year-old with the same impairments. For the current patient case, an 8-year-old that has difficulty rising from the floor will likely need close supervision on the stairs at home, assistance with bathing and accommodations at school to ensure safety. Specific recommendations for return to school and sport may include modifications. For example, alteration to physical education classes and recess participation, additional travel time between classes, and use of an elevator are common modifications for children with moderate to severe JDM. A long-term link to physical therapy services is also essential to ensure monitoring of physical status and progression of an appropriate exercise program with graded return to sport/activity.

Evidence-Based Clinical Recommendations

SORT: Strength of Recommendation Taxonomy

A: Consistent, good-quality patient-oriented evidence

B: Inconsistent or limited-quality patient-oriented evidence

C: Consensus, disease-oriented evidence, usual practice, expert opinion or case series

1. Calcium and vitamin D supplementation in combination with weightbearing activity (while avoiding body contact/impact sports) minimize the deleterious effects of glucocorticoid therapy and chronic disease. **Grade B**

2. The Childhood Myositis Assessment Scale is a reliable, valid tool to assess proximal muscle strength, physical function, and endurance that is sensitive to change in children with juvenile dermatomyositis. **Grade A**

3. A moderate intensity strengthening and aerobic endurance program for children with JDM is likely to be beneficial without exacerbating the disease process. **Grade B**

4. A hydrotherapy exercise program is beneficial for children with JDM. **Grade C**

COMPREHENSION QUESTIONS

28.1 Muscle weakness in JDM is
   A. Predominantly symmetrical and proximal
   B. Results from capillary inflammation
   C. Associated with elevated serum muscle enzyme levels
   D. All of the above

28.2 The adverse effects of glucocorticoids include:
   A. Calcinosis
   B. Vertebral compression fractures
   C. Hypotension
   D. All of the above

28.3 Which of the following statements is true regarding strengthening exercises prescribed to children with JDM?
   A. Strengthening exercises are contraindicated in acute JDM.
   B. Strengthening exercises are safe to perform only after normalization of muscle enzymes.
   C. Strengthening exercises result in exacerbation of chronic myositis.
   D. Strengthening exercises can be safely performed in children with JDM.

ANSWERS

28.1 **D.** Complement activation and deposition causes lysis of capillaries and perivascular inflammation. This is thought to lead to reduced capillary density and compensatory dilation of the remaining capillaries, as well as muscle ischemia, muscle fiber degeneration (which leads to increased serum concentration of muscle enzymes), and perifasicular atrophy.[2] Although the muscle weakness in JDM is frequently widespread, it is more prominent in the proximal and core or postural muscles.

28.2 **B.** Adverse skeletal effects of oral glucocorticoids can manifest rapidly and are related to daily dose.[58] Vertebral compression fractures are seen clinically in JDM with associated symptoms and deleterious effects on physical function. Physical therapy strategies are directed toward symptom control and preventative education.

28.3 **D.** It was previously believed that resistance training in the context of active myositis would lead to exacerbation of the pathological inflammatory process (options A and C). However, improvements in strength, muscle function, and aerobic endurance have been achieved in JDM patients with exercise training *without* evidence of disease exacerbation.[52,59]

REFERENCES

1. Mendez EP, Lipton R, Ramsey-Goldman R, Roettcher P, Bowyer S, Dyer A, Pachman LM. US incidence of juvenile dermatomyositis, 1995-1998: results from the National Institute of Arthritis and Musculoskeletal and Skin Diseases Registry. *Arthritis Rheum.* 2003;49:300-305.

2. Dalakas MC, Hohlfeld R. Polymyositis and dermatomyositis. *Lancet.* 2003;362:971-982.

3. Petty RE, Laxer RM, Petty RE, Lindsley CB. *Textbook of Pediatric Rheumatology.* 6th ed., Philadelphia, PA; Saunders Elsevier; 2011:375-413.

4. Ramanan AV, Feldman BM. Clinical features and outcomes of juvenile dermatomyositis and other childhood onset myositis syndromes. *Rheum Dis Clin N Am.* 2002;28:833-857.

5. Symmons DP, Sills JA, Davis SM. The incidence of juvenile dermatomyositis: results from a nationwide study. *Brit J Rheumatol.* 1995;34:732-736.

6. Oddis CV, Conte CG, Steen VD, Medsger TA Jr. Incidence of polymyositis-dermatomyositis: a 20-year study of hospital diagnosed cases in Allegheny County, PA 1963-1982. *J Rheumatol.* 1990;17:1329-1334.

7. Pachman LM, Lipton R, Ramsey-Goldman R, et al. History of infection before the onset of juvenile dermatomyositis: results from the National Institute of Arthritis and Musculoskeletal and Skin Diseases Research Registry. *Arthritis Rheum.* 2005;53:166-172.

8. Pachman LM, Hayford JR, Chung A, et al. Juvenile dermatomyositis at diagnosis: clinical characteristics of 79 children. *J Rheumatol.* 1998;25:1198-1204.

9. Feldman BM, Rider LG, Dugan L, Miller FW, Schneider R. Nailfold capillaries as indicators of disease activity in juvenile idiopathic inflammatory myopathies. *Arthritis Rheumatism.* 1999; 42(Suppl 9):S181.

10. Huber AM, Juvenile dermatomyositis: advances in pathogenesis, evaluation and treatment. *Pediatr Drugs.* 2009;11:361-374.

11. McCann LJ, Juggins AD, Maillard SM, et al. The Juvenile Dermatomyositis National Registry and Repository (UK and Ireland)—clinical characteristics of children recruited within the first 5 year. *Rheumatology.* 2006;45:1255-1260.

12. McCann LJ, Garay SM, Ryan MM, Harris R, Pilkington CA. Oropharyngeal dysphagia in juvenile dermatomyositis (JDM): an evaluation of videofluoroscopy swallow study (VFSS) changes in relation to clinical symptoms and objective muscle scores. *Rheumatology.* 2007;46:1363-1366.

13. Arvedson J, Rogers B, Buck G, Smart P, Msall M. Silent aspiration prominent in children with dysphagia. *Intl J Pediatr Otorhinolarngology.* 1994;28:173-181.

14. Zerilli KS, Sefans VA, DiPietro MA. Protocol for the use of videofluoroscopy in pediatric swallowing dysfunction. *Am J Occupational Ther.* 1990;44:441-446.

15. Bohan A, Peter JB. Polymositis and dermatomyositis (first of two parts). *N Engl J Med.* 1975;292:344-347.

16. Bohan A, Peter JB. Polymyositis and dermatomyositis (second of two parts). *N Engl J Med.* 1975;292:403-407.

17. Brown VE, Pilkington CA, Feldman BM, Davidson JE, Network for Juvenile Dermatomyositis PRES. An international consensus survey of the diagnostic criteria for juvenile dermatomyositis (JDM). *Rheumatology.* 2006;45:1255-1260.

18. Nirmalananthan N, Holton JL, Hanna MG. Is it really myositis? A consideration of the differential diagnosis. *Curr Opin Rheumatol.* 2004;16:684-691.

19. Compeyrot-Lacasssagne S, Feldman BM. Inflammatory myopathies in children. *Pediatr Clin N Am.* 2005;52:493-520.

20. Huber AM, Lang B, LeBlanc CM, et al. Medium- and long-term functional outcomes in a multi-centre cohort of children with juvenile dermatomyositis. *Arthritis Rheum.* 2000;43:541-549.

21. Rider LG. Calcinosis in JDM: Pathogenesis and current therapies. *Pediatr Rheumatol Online J.* 2003;1:119-123.

22. Feldman BM, Rider LG, Reed AM, Pachman LM. Juvenile dermatomyositis and other idiopathic inflammatory myopathies of childhood. *Lancet.* 2008;372:2201-2212.

23. Bowyer SL, Blane CE, Sullivan DB, Cassidy JT. Childhood dermatomyositis: factors predicting functional outcome and development of dystrophic calcification. *J Pediatr.* 1983;103:882-888.

24. Bitnum S, Daeschner CW Jr, Travis LB, Dodge WF, Hopps HC. Dermatomyositis. *J Pediatr.* 1964;64:101-131.

25. Ramanan AV, Campbell-Webster N, Ota S, et al. The effectiveness of treating juvenile dermatomyositis with methotrexate and aggressively tapered corticosteroids. *Arthritis Rheum.* 2005;52:3570-3578.

26. Stringe E, Bohnsack J, Bowyer S, et al. Treatment approaches to juvenile dermatomyositis (JDM) across North America: the childhood arthritis and rheumatology research alliance (CARRA) JDM treatment survey. *J Rheumatol.* 2010;27:1953-1961.

27. Reiff A, Rawlings DJ, Shaham B, et al. Preliminary evidence for cyclosporin A as an alternative in the treatment of recalcitrant juvenile rheumatoid arthritis and juvenile dermatomyositis. *J Rheumatology.* 1997;24:2436-2443.

28. Bunch TW. Prednisone and azathioprine for polymyositis: long-term followup. *Arthritis Rheum.* 1981;24:45-48.

29. Edge JC, Outland JD, Dempsey JR, Callen JP. Mycophenolate mofetil as an effective corticosteroid-sparing therapy for recalcitrant dermatomyositis. *Arch Dermatol.* 2006;142:65-69.

30. Pelle MT, Callen JP. Adverse cutaneous reactions to hydroxychloroquine are more common in patients with dermatomyositis than in patients with cutaneous lupus erythematosus. *Arch Dermatol.* 2002;138:1231-1233.

31. Riley P, McCann LJ, Maillard SM, Woo P, Murray KJ, Piklington CA. Effectiveness of infliximab in the treatment of refractory juvenile dermatomyositis with calcinosis. *Rheumatology.* 2008;47(6):877-880.

32. Cooper MA, Willingham DI, Brown ED, French AR, Shih FF, White AJ. Rituximab for the treatment of juvenile dermatomyositis: a report of four pediatric patients. *Arthritis Rheum.* 2007;56:3107-3111.

33. Lang BA, Laxer RM, Murphy G, Silverman ED, Roifman CM. Treatment of dermatomyositis with intravenous gammaglobulin. *Am J Med.* 1991;91:169-172.

34. Riley P, Maillard SM, Wedderburn LR, Woo P, Murray KJ, Pilkington CA. Intravenous cyclophosphamide pulse therapy in juvenile dermatomyositis. A review of efficacy and safety. *Rheumatology.* 2004;43:491-496.

35. Alsufayani KA, Ortiz-Alvarez O, Cabral DA, et al. Bone mineral density in children and adolescents with systemic lupus erythematosus, juvenile dermatomyositis, and systemic vasculitis: relationship to disease duration, cumulative corticosteroid dose, calcium intake, and exercise. *J Rheumatol.* 2005;32:729-733.

36. Huber AM, Rennebohm RM, Maillard SM. Assessing muscle strength, endurance and function. In: Rider LG, Pachman LM, Miller FW, Bollar H, eds. *Myositis and You: A Guide to Juvenile Dermatomyositis for Patients, Families and Healthcare Providers.* Washington, DC: The Myositis Association; 2007:139-152.

37. Kendall FP, McCreary EK, Provance PG. *Muscles: Testing and Function.* Baltimore, MD: Williams & Wilkins; 1993.

38. Rider LG, Koziol D, Giannini EH, et al. Validation of manual muscle testing and a subset of eight muscles for adult and juvenile idiopathic inflammatory myopathies. *Arthritis Care Res.* 2010;62: 465-472.

39. Miller FW, Rider LG, Chung YL, et al. Proposed preliminary core set measures for disease outcome assessment in adult and juvenile idiopathic inflammatory myopathies. *Rheumatology.* 2001;40: 1262-1273.

40. Oddis CV, Rider LG, Reed AM, et al. International consensus guidelines for trials of therapies in the idiopathic inflammatory myopathies. *Arthritis Rheum.* 2005;52:2607-2615.

41. National Institute of Environmental Health Sciences—National Institutes of Health. The International Myositis Assessment and Clinical Studies Group (IMACS). Disease Activity Core Set Measures. Available at: http://www.niehs.nih.gov/research/resources/collab/imacs/diseaseactivity. cfm. Accessed October 12, 2011.

42. Lovell DJ, Lindsley CB, Rennebohm RM, et al. Development of validated disease activity and damage indices for the juvenile idiopathic inflammatory myopathies. II. The childhood myositis assessment scale (CMAS): A quantitative tool for the evaluation of muscle function. *Arthritis Rheum.* 1999;42:2213-2219.

43. Stoll T, Bruhlmann P, Stucki G, Seifert B, Michel BA. Muscle strength assessment in polymyositis and dermatomyositis: evaluation of the reliability and clinical use of a new, quantitative, easily applicable method. *J Rheumatol.* 1995;22:473-477.

44. Rider LG. Assessment of disease activity and its sequelae in children and adults with myositis. *Curr Opin Rheumatol.* 1996;8:495-506.

45. Helewa A, Goldsmith AH, Smythe JA. The modified sphygmomanometer—an instrument to measure muscle strength: a validation study. *J Chronic Dis.* 1981;34:353-361.

46. Magee DJ. *Orthopedic Physical Assessment.* 5th ed. Saunders; 2008.

47. Huber AM, Feldman BM, Rennebohm RM, et al. Validation and clinical significance of the Childhood Myositis Assessment Scale for assessment of muscle function in the juvenile idiopathic inflammatory myopathies. *Arthritis Rheum.* 2004;50:1595-1603.

48. Rennebohm RM, Jones K, Huber AM, et al. Normal scores for nine maneuvers of the Childhood Myositis Assessment Scale. *Arthritis Rheum.* 2004;51:365-370.

49. Singh G, Athreya BH, Fries JF, Goldsmith DP. Measurement of health status in children with juvenile rheumatoid arthritis. *Arthritis Rheum.* 1994;37:1761-1769.

50. Feldman BM, Ayling-Campos A, Luy L, Stevens D, Silverman ED, Laxer RM. Measuring disability in juvenile dermatomyositis: validity of the childhood health assessment questionnaire. *J Rheumatol.* 1995;22:326-331.

51. Takken T, Van Der Net J, Kuis W, Helders PJ. Aquatic fitness training for children with juvenile idiopathic arthritis. *Rheumatology.* 2003;42:1408-1414.

52. Maillard SM, Jones R, Owens CM, et al. Quantitative assessments of the effects of a single exercise session on muscles in juvenile dermatomyositis. *Arthritis Rheum.* 2005;53:558-564.

53. Brindle TJ, Nyland J, Ford K, Coppola A, Shapiro R. Electromyographic comparison of standard and modified closed-chain isometric knee extension exercises. *J Strength Cond Res.* 2002;16: 129-134.

54. Proske U, Morgan DL. Muscle damage from eccentric exercise: mechanism, mechanical signs, adaptation and clinical applications. *J Physiology.* 2001;537:333-345.

55. Scott JM. Hydrotherapy or land-based exercises: a patient satisfaction survey. *Ann Rheum Dis.* 2000;59:748-749.

56. Becker BE. Aquatic therapy: scientific foundations and clinical rehabilitation applications. *PMR.* 2009;1:859-872.

57. Low J, Reed A. *Electrotherapy Explained: Principles and Practice.* 3rd ed. Philadelphia, PA: Elsevier; 2000.

58. van Staa TP, Leufkens HG, Abenheim L, Zhang B, Cooper C. Oral corticosteroids and fracture risk: relationship to daily and cumulative doses. *Rheumatology.* 2000;39:1383-1389.

59. Omorio C, Prado DM, Gualano B, et al. Responsiveness to exercise training in juvenile dermatomyositis: a twin case study. *BMC Musculoskelet Disord.* 2010;11:270.

Osteogenesis Imperfecta

Amanda Stoltz

CASE 29

An 8-year-old female diagnosed with osteogenesis imperfecta (OI) type IV returns to the hospital today for a scheduled admission of spica cast removal. Six weeks ago, she underwent bilateral femoral intramedullary rodding with multiple right corrective femoral osteotomies, and hip spica cast application due to significant progressive anterior bowing of her femurs. The child has typical features of OI with loose joints and short stature. She has had more than 25 fractures over her lifespan, including multiple fractures of bilateral humeri, right ulna, bilateral femurs, and the left tibia. She has mild scoliosis, her right leg is shorter than her left by 2 cm, and she has mild to moderate anterior bowing of her tibias. She wears bilateral lower leg orthoses (left hinged ankle foot orthosis and right UCBL orthosis) for planovalgus feet. The patient has been on bisphosphonate medication since she was 3 years old. This was discontinued 7 months prior to surgery per her metabolic and orthopaedic physicians' recommendations. Prior to surgery, the patient complained of mild bilateral thigh and knee pain, primarily with walking and standing. She had full hip and knee extension and hip and knee flexion to at least 120°. She lacks 20° of elbow extension bilaterally and has mild radial deformities of her wrists. The patient has a rear-wheeled walker and a lightweight manual wheelchair. Over the past 2 years, she has used the walker "off and on" as needed to heal from various fractures and for minimizing lower extremity pain. In the 2 months prior to surgery, she used the walker in the school classroom and in the community. At home, she did not use an assistive device for ambulation; she either walked or knee-walked, depending on pain severity. In general, she uses her wheelchair during healing of fractures and she is independent with propulsion. Prior to surgery, she was also independent with all transfers. The patient has one step to enter her home and she was able to negotiate the step with one handrail and one arm-hold assist. Since surgery, she has been non-weightbearing on bilateral lower extremities and has been using a reclining wheelchair with elevating leg rests for dependent mobility. Her parents have been lifting her for all transfers. Today, the physical therapist is asked to evaluate and treat the patient for initiation of lower extremity weightbearing. She is allowed to bear weight as tolerated, though she must initially use knee immobilizers if weightbearing on land. The radiographs from today show stable healing of bilateral femurs. The patient is seen at bedside with her spica cast already removed and with her mother in the room. She has pressure sores from the cast on her left calcaneus and bilateral anterior knees. The nurse has administered pain medication in anticipation of physical therapy. Although the patient is tearful and states she is scared to start standing, the patient's and mother's short-term goals for this admission are to complete standing transfers with a walker and to sit comfortably in her personal wheelchair. Her long-term goal is to return to community distance ambulation with her rear-wheeled walker. It is anticipated that she will have 5 days of inpatient rehabilitation, with physical therapy twice per day.

▶ Based on the patient's diagnosis and prior health condition, what do you anticipate will be contributing factors to activity limitations?
▶ What are the examination priorities?
▶ What precautions should be taken during physical therapy?
▶ What are the most appropriate physical therapy interventions?
▶ Identify psychological factors apparent in this case.

KEY DEFINITIONS

ANKLE FOOT ORTHOSIS (AFO): Custom or off-the-shelf brace worn on the lower leg and foot to increase stability, maintain correct joint positions, and/or correct foot-drop

BISPHOSPHONATES: Drug class that helps prevent loss of bone mass by inhibiting osteoclast activity, which in turn decreases bone resorption; used off-label in individuals with OI

INTRAMEDULLARY ROD: Also known as an intramedullary (IM) nail; long rod made of steel or titanium that is surgically placed into the medullary canal of long bone in order to add stability to the bone (Fig. 29-1)

OSTEOTOMY: Surgical cutting of the bone usually performed to realign a bone deformity

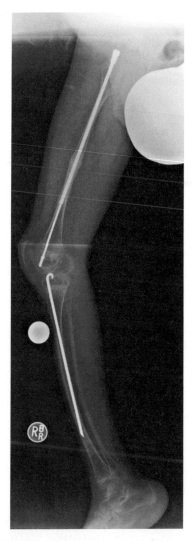

Figure 29-1. Intramedullary rods in right femur and tibia of a child.

SPICA CAST: Cast that extends from the chest down to one or both legs; usually the hips are positioned in wide abduction and the cast has a peri-care cutout to allow for toileting

UCBL: Rigid foot orthotic with a molded heel cup that is placed inside a shoe to stabilize a flexible flat-foot deformity; named after the University California Berkeley Laboratory where it was developed

Objectives

1. Describe typical characteristics of individuals diagnosed with osteogenesis imperfecta (OI) and potential complications associated with OI.

2. Describe the goals and limitations of intramedullary rodding surgery for a child with OI.

3. Understand potential benefits and limitations of bisphosphonates in the medical treatment of OI.

4. Design appropriate short-term goals and interventions for a child with OI status/post rodding surgery.

5. Describe the benefits of aquatic therapy as an intervention for post-rodding surgery.

Physical Therapy Considerations

PT considerations during management of the child diagnosed with OI, status/post intramedullary rodding surgery:

▶ **General physical therapy plan of care/goals:** Improve lower extremity strength, range of motion (ROM) and endurance; increase mobility; maximize safe, functional independence while minimizing risk for fracture; improve tolerance to sitting upright with optimal alignment

▶ **Physical therapy interventions:** Transfer training, active ROM, gentle strengthening, home exercise program, initiate weightbearing through aquatic therapy with a progression to weightbearing on land

▶ **Precautions during physical therapy:** High risk of fracture, pain, weakness, and deconditioning; maintain close proximity to patient to decrease risk of fall or injury; close monitoring of skin, especially with knee immobilizers and AFOs, which may increase progression of pressure ulcers; no passive twisting, rotating, or forceful ROM to the extremities or trunk

▶ **Complications interfering with physical therapy:** Pressure ulcers, especially while using knee immobilizers and AFO; pain; patient and parent anxiety of fracturing; bowing of upper extremities may complicate use of a walker and upper extremity weightbearing for mobility

Understanding the Health Condition

The majority of cases of OI are caused by an autosomal dominant genetic disorder that affects type 1 collagen production. Type 1 collagen is the most abundant collagen type in the body, comprising the major connective tissue substance in bones, ligaments, tendons, skin, dentin, cornea, and lung. The disease has varying degrees of manifestation, depending on the specific gene mutation. In the United States, the prevalence of OI is estimated to be one in 20,000 to 50,000 infants, although the prevalence may actually be higher due to frequent underdiagnosis or misdiagnosis.[1] OI was originally classified into four types; however, there are now at least seven to eight different types delineated.[1,2] The eight types (type I-VIII) are based on clinical and radiographic presentation and inheritance pattern. All individuals with OI have fragile bones that fracture easily, joint laxity, and weak muscles. Most have resulting bone deformities. The rate of bone healing is normal although it may be affected by the amount of bowing in long bones[3] and possibly also by bisphosphonate use. Individuals with OI may also have hearing loss, poor dentition, blue sclera, easy bruising, excessive sweating, short stature, scoliosis, and fatigue. The disorder does not affect intelligence. Initial diagnosis of OI can be made clinically, but definitive diagnosis is confirmed by specific genetic testing. Individuals with mild to moderate forms of OI have a normal life expectancy. Moderate to severe types of OI (type III and IV) have a higher mortality rate related to respiratory compromise, cardiovascular failure (from severe kyphoscoliosis), neurologic causes (such as brainstem compression) and cranial trauma.[2] Type II OI is considered fatal in the neonatal period. Many different providers are typically involved in the care of the child with OI, including: a primary care physician, orthopaedic surgeon, endocrinologist, metabolic geneticist, physical therapist, occupational therapist, and case manager.

Bisphosphonates are a class of drugs (taken orally or intravenously) that have been used to treat children with OI since the early 1990s. Bisphosphonates increase bone density by inhibiting osteoclast activity. In individuals with OI, bisphosphonates have been shown to increase bone density in the spine, femoral neck, hip, and tibia.[4,5] A systematic review of eight studies evaluating the effect of bisphosphonates in children with OI found that bisphosphonates increased bone density and many (but not all) studies demonstrated a reduction in fracture rate[5]; however, taking bisphosphonates neither eliminated fracture risk nor obviated the need for rodding surgery in this population.[1,6-8] Because bisphosphonates have been found to potentially delay surgical osteotomy healing (but not fracture healing),[1] children taking these drugs may be instructed to discontinue use prior to a scheduled orthopaedic surgery. Children are usually able to resume bisphosphonate use 3 to 6 months after surgery. Bone density changes that may occur during this bisphosphonate-free interim have not been thoroughly studied. Therefore, there are no specific recommendations for altering a child's activity level during this time. Additional unknowns surrounding bisphosphonate use in this population include dosing, efficacy of oral versus intravenous routes of administration, which specific medication is optimal, how long a patient should be treated, and long-term effects.[2,5,7] While the use of bisphosphonates has been approved by the Food and Drug Administration for other diagnoses, it continues to be used "off-label" in individuals diagnosed with OI. Recent recommendations suggest that the use of bisphosphonates in the OI population should be driven by clinical severity, not based discretely on bone density measurements.[7] It has been recommended that bisphosphonates be used in conjunction with orthopaedic surgery and physical therapy, and not as a replacement for these interventions.[6]

The standard surgical method to treat bowing deformities in children with OI is placement of intramedullary rods into the long bones.[1,9] This surgery is indicated in a child who is attempting to stand, or in the child who has had multiple fracture sites of the long bones. **Intramedullary rodding surgery** reduces fracture recurrence at a given site and improves alignment and stability of the bone to allow for weightbearing.[1,3,9,10] The goal of rodding surgery is to improve a child's function, comfort, gross motor development, and ability to stand and walk.[1] When the rod is placed, osteotomies with wedge cuts may additionally be performed to correct the alignment of the bone. The steel or titanium rods are placed in the intramedullary cortex of the bone. Therefore, the bone must be large enough in diameter to accommodate the rod. Differing styles of rods may be used depending on many factors including the purpose for the surgery and the child's age.[10,11] The extremity is then typically immobilized in a cast for 6 to 8 weeks to allow sufficient healing. At times, rods may need to be revised or replaced.

The child in this case study has type IV OI. Individuals with OI type IV are moderately affected (severity between type I and III) and life expectancy is typically unchanged. Short stature and bowing of the long bones is common and few to multiple fractures are experienced over the lifespan. Typically, most fractures occur before puberty. A diagnosis of OI may not be made until the child is mobile because fractures often do not occur until the child starts ambulating. The prognosis for type IV OI is good for some form of upright ambulation. Issues that need to be considered in this population are (1) preventing the cycle of fracture and immobility; (2) timing of rodding surgery, monitoring scoliosis; (3) developing compensations for short stature and fatigue (e.g., lowering work surfaces, keeping frequently used items at a lower level and using assistive devices/wheeled mobility for community ambulation in order to keep up with peers); (4) choosing appropriate and meaningful age-appropriate exercise; and (5) making decisions about the use of bisphosphonates. Because of the complex nature of impairments and treatments, families need emotional support to help care for the needs of their child with OI.[10,12]

Adaptive equipment and bracing may need to be utilized to promote safe functional mobility. Socialization may be increasingly difficult because the child cannot physically keep up with her peers and she is unable to participate in high impact activities. The additional anxiety of fracturing and heightened guarding may further prevent the child from being fully integrated with her peers.[8] While there are typical characteristics for each type of OI, treatment should focus on the specific needs of the individual and should be guided by patient presentation, not by diagnosed OI type.

Physical Therapy Patient/Client Management

Postoperative physical therapy management for the child who has had a spica cast removed after intramedullary rodding should focus on gentle active ROM within the child's pain tolerance and non-aggressive isometric and open kinetic chain strengthening exercises. The physical therapist should frequently communicate with the child's orthopaedic physician and nursing staff regarding the child's progress to maintain consistent expectations of the child's abilities and limitations and to monitor any pain complaints. Pain could be an indicator of overly stressed bones, muscle weakness, or generalized discomfort with weightbearing. Gaining trust from the child is important because it is likely that she is moving in a guarded manner related to fear of pain and apprehension of fracturing. Rapport, trust, and confidence are facilitated if consistent therapist(s) treat the child. Including the child in treatment planning and goal setting for each session can motivate and allow her to gain a sense of shared control over the session and participation expectations. For example, if the therapist would like the child to walk with the walker in the pool during a treatment session, the therapist could ask how many lengths of the pool does the child think she can walk? Making the treatment session a game with mutually set goals not only increases participation, but also enjoyment. Creating a tracking grid for exercises completed outside of treatment sessions can be an additional motivator and visual aid to help the child feel a sense of accomplishment.

Examination, Evaluation, and Diagnosis

Prior to seeing the patient, the physical therapist needs to know the child's postsurgical weightbearing restrictions and any mobility precautions. The therapist should obtain information from the chart regarding past surgical and fracture history. Prior to mobilizing the child in any way, the therapist should also gather information from the child and parents regarding the patient's and parents' preferred method of post-operative lift transfers, current equipment, orthotics and braces the child uses or will be using, inpatient physical therapy goals, and the child's pain level. Additional interview questions should include prior level of function with transfers and mobility (during non-postoperative times), previous extracurricular gross motor activities, and interventions and goals during any previous outpatient physical therapy.

Pain should be reassessed throughout the physical examination and during interventions. The examination and interventions should be closely timed with administration of pain medication to minimize pain as much as possible. The child's pain level should be assessed using either a visual analog scale or the Wong-Baker FACES Pain Rating scale. The **Wong-Baker FACES Pain Rating scale** is a visual scale of six faces in a series of differing levels of "happiness" (see Figure 2.2). The faces correspond to numbers 0 through 10, with written descriptors of "no hurt" (0), to "hurts worst" (10). The clinician shows the face scale to the child with simple instructions to choose the face that best depicts or describes how she is feeling. The Wong-Baker Faces Pain Rating scale has been found to be reliable and valid in children from age 3 to 18 years of age.[13]

During the examination, the therapist evaluates the child's active assisted hip and knee flexion and extension with gentle hands-on guidance for support of the limb. The therapist also assesses the child's strength by asking the child to move her leg against gravity if possible, supporting the limb as needed. In general, applying resistance to test muscle strength should be withheld to decrease the risk of fracture. The child's general tolerance to activity should be noted. To facilitate trust and avoid injury, the parent should initially transfer the child until the child is comfortable with the therapist. The therapist should move slowly and gently and discuss the plan for mobilizing the child *before* actually assisting the child with mobilization. Mutual goals for the rehabilitation admission should be agreed upon with the parent and child.

Plan of Care and Interventions

Physical therapy interventions should focus on impairments and activity limitations noted in the evaluation with the overall goal of promoting safe functional independence. If possible, initiating physical therapy in a pool is optimal. **Aquatic therapy** is ideal because the buoyancy of the water decreases the amount of force on the limbs and allows the child to move in a safe environment.[10,12] Being unweighted in the water allows the child to move more freely than she would be able to on land. The child is able to master skills in a less challenging and less fearful environment, and can then progress these skills on land. The water also provides resistance along the entire length of the bone, allowing the child to strengthen muscles while also being protected from fracturing.[10] The therapist should consider supported weightbearing in the pool with the use of a walker. Although the child's postsurgical precautions are weightbearing as tolerated, she has an increased risk for fractures not only due to her fragile bones, but also due to muscle wasting and weakness from being immobilized for the past 6 weeks. The walker can provide her the necessary added stability and support in the pool. The child can begin walking in the water at chest level, and gradually transition to more shallow water as she tolerates progressively more weightbearing and her strength improves. The therapist can progress her from a walker to using a less stable surface such as a kick board or other floatation device. The pool is also an ideal environment for the therapist to provide strengthening, ROM, and endurance activities.

Therapy should be transitioned to land with isometric and open kinetic chain exercises. Supported by the therapist, the child can begin standing on land (with knee immobilizers and bilateral lower leg orthoses on) while using a walker. As the child gains strength and balance, the time spent standing is progressed. The knee immobilizers are used to help stabilize the bones and provide added support until she is able to stand comfortably and confidently without them. There are no specific guidelines for the use of knee immobilizers after intramedullary rodding surgery; they are used at the discretion of the orthopaedic surgeon and the physical therapist. After spica cast removal, knee immobilizers may be used for only one therapy session or up to 2 days, depending on how quickly the child progresses. However, the patient may be discharged from the hospital still using them, if it is deemed necessary. The child's AFO and UCBL for lower leg and foot support should also be used. The therapist should maintain close proximity to the child with hands-on support for safety, especially as the child participates in a new or more challenging standing activity. Breaking down activities such as a stand pivot transfer with a walker into component parts may help the child be more successful. Allow rest breaks between repetitions as needed to avoid overstraining the musculoskeletal system. The therapist needs to use conservative clinical judgment to determine whether and when the child is physically capable to progress beyond the child's comfort in her own skill level. This clinical judgment can be influenced by the patient's and parents' anxiety of a new fracture, and the child's pain complaints related to muscle fatigue. It is important to validate both child's and parents' concerns while still encouraging functional independence with mobility and activities of daily living. As the child gains hip and knee flexion ROM, she can begin sitting in her own manual wheelchair and propelling short distances to promote endurance. Discharge planning should include a thorough home exercise program and discussion regarding how she will enter the home. The child needs to practice stepping up and down a step with parental assistance prior to discharge, or be transported up the step in her wheelchair. The child also needs to continue physical therapy on an outpatient basis until her preoperative status is met or surpassed.

Evidence-Based Clinical Recommendations

SORT: Strength of Recommendation Taxonomy

A: Consistent, good-quality patient-oriented evidence
B: Inconsistent or limited-quality patient-oriented evidence
C: Consensus, disease-oriented evidence, usual practice, expert opinion, or case series

1. Bisphosphonates decrease fracture rate in children with osteogenesis imperfecta. **Grade B**

2. Femoral intramedullary rodding surgery decreases fracture recurrence in the long bones and minimizes progression of bowing deformity in children with OI. **Grade A**

3. The Wong-Baker FACES Pain Rating scale is a reliable and valid tool to assess pain in children between the ages of 3 and 18 years old with a variety of health conditions. **Grade A**

4. Aquatic therapy is an optimal modality for strengthening weak muscles, while protecting fragile bones in children with OI. **Grade C**

COMPREHENSION QUESTIONS

29.1   It is common practice to use a gait belt when working with an individual in an acute care setting who is at risk for falls. Which of the following statements describes the *most* appropriate situation for a physical therapist to use a gait belt when working with a child with OI?

A.   It is only needed when the child is performing activities that challenge her balance.

B.   The therapist should always use a gait belt no matter what the situation is.

C.   The therapist should not use a gait belt when working with children with moderate to severe OI.

D.   It is only needed when the child is standing or walking without an assistive device.

29.2   A physical therapist has discharged a patient with OI from an inpatient rehabilitation facility. Which of the following is *not* an appropriate exercise to strengthen quadriceps for a home exercise program?

A.   Long-arc quads

B.   Single leg squats

C.   Straight leg raises

D.   Quad sets in standing

29.3   At discharge from the acute care setting, the child in this case study is able to perform a stand pivot transfer (without any knee immobilizers) using a walker with stand-by assistance. She is also able to gingerly and slowly take six steps using the walker. The mother and the child would like her to return to school as soon as possible. Discharge instructions for return to school should include:

A.   The child should not return to school until she can safely ambulate community distances without an assistive device.

B.   The child should return to school using both her wheelchair and walker as needed in the classroom.

C.   The child should return to school once she can walk with only handhold assistance from an adult.

D.   Children with OI are too fragile to be in school; they should be homeschooled.

ANSWERS

29.1   **C.** Children with OI typically have a short trunk and fragile ribs. The gait belt will most likely reside on the child's ribs, applying pressure that could potentially cause a rib fracture. It is generally a safer practice for the therapist to instead place his/her hands gently on the child's pelvis for safety during mobility training.

29.2 **B.** Individuals with OI should not be put in positions of compromising balance or potential rotation of the extremity due to risk of falling and fracturing.

29.3 **B.** The child should return to school primarily using her manual wheelchair. She may need to start with half days until she can tolerate a full day. She should have an adult with her in the restroom until she is able to transfer safely on and off a toilet. She will most likely be ready to ambulate in the classroom with a walker when she is consistently walking household distances at home with a stable and efficient gait. She should initially walk in the classroom with as few distractions and few classmates surrounding her as possible. It is recommended that a school physical therapist be involved with her school-based needs to make more specific recommendations regarding safety within the school environment.

REFERENCES

1. Esposito P, Plotkin H. Surgical treatment of osteogenesis imperfecta: current concepts. *Curr Opin Pediatr.* 2008;20:52-57.

2. Starr SR, Roberts TT, Fischer PR. Osteogenesis imperfecta: primary care. *Pediatr Rev.* 2010;31:e54-e64.

3. Staheli L. *Pediatric Orthopaedic Secrets.* Philadelphia, PA: Hanley and Belfus Inc; 1998.

4. Bishop N, Harrison R, Ahmed F, et al. A randomized, controlled dose-ranging study of risedronate in children with moderate and severe osteogenesis imperfecta. *J Bone Miner Res.* 2010;25:32-40.

5. Castillo H, Samson-Fang L; American Academy for Cerebral Palsy and Developmental Medicine Treatment Outcomes Committee Review Panel. Effects of bisphosphonates in children with osteogenesis imperfecta: an AACPDM systematic review. *Dev Med Child Neurol.* 2009;51:17-29.

6. Rauch F, Glorieux FH. Treatment of children with osteogenesis imperfecta. *Curr Osteoporos Res.* 2006;4:159-164.

7. Falk MJ, Heeger S, Lynch KA, et al. Intravenous bisphosphonate therapy in children with osteogenesis imperfecta. *Pediatrics.* 2003;111:573-578.

8. Astrom E, Jorulf H, Soderhall S. Intravenous pamidronate treatment of infants with severe osteogenesis imperfecta. *Arch Dis Child.* 2007;92:332-338.

9. Luhmann SJ, Sheridan JJ, Capelli AM, Schoenecker PL. Management of lower-extremity deformities in osteogenesis imperfecta with extensible intramedullary rod technique: a 20-year experience. *J Pediatr Orthop.* 1998;18:88-94.

10. Campbell SK, Vander Linden DW, Palisano RJ. *Physical Therapy for Children.* 2nd ed. Philadelphia, PA: W.B. Saunders Company; 1994.

11. Hartman J. *Osteogenesis Imperfecta: A Guide for Nurses.* Gaithersburg, MD: Osteogenesis Imperfecta Foundation; 2005.

12. Osteogenesis Imperfecta Foundation. Available at: www.oif.org. Accessed October 7, 2011.

13. Keck JF, Gerkensmeyer JE, Joyce BA, Schade JG. Reliability and validity of the Faces and Word Descriptor Scales to measure procedural pain. *J Pediatr Nurs.* 1996;11:368-374.

Pediatric Spinal Cord Injury

Larisa Reed Hoffman

CASE 30

A 5-year-old boy was admitted to the regional trauma center through the emergency department (ED) following a motor vehicle accident 4 days ago. He was a restrained passenger in the front seat during a highway collision. His injuries are consistent with a cervical flexion injury. He was immediately placed on full spine precautions. Results from cervical spine radiographs and computed tomography (CT) scan reveal no overt vertebral abnormality. A T2-weighted magnetic resonance imaging (MRI) scan shows widespread edema in the interspinous ligaments and paraspinal muscles from C4 to T1. In the ED, his American Spinal Injury Association Impairment Scale (AIS) classification was C4, AIS B. He was immediately started on methylprednisolone and immobilized with a hard cervical collar. Three days ago, he was transferred to the pediatric intensive care unit (PICU). He was fitted for and currently immobilized in a rigid cervicothoracic brace (Guilford brace). In the PICU, his AIS classification was found to be C6, AIS C (Fig. 30-1). The following spinal precautions have been advised from the spinal orthopaedist: the patient can be out of bed, but the Guilford brace must be worn at all times. The patient's mother and younger sister were also involved in the accident. His mother sustained multiple musculoskeletal injuries including pelvic fracture and abdominal lacerations. She was also admitted to the same hospital. His sister had only minor injuries and was discharged home with their father. The physical therapist has been asked to examine the child and design a plan of care. He is expected to be discharged to a pediatric inpatient rehabilitation center in a week and a half.

► What are the examination priorities?
► Based on his health condition, what do you anticipate may be the contributors to activity limitations?
► What is his rehabilitation prognosis?
► What are the most appropriate physical therapy interventions?
► What precautions should be taken during physical therapy examination and/or interventions?
► Identify the psychological (or psychosocial) factors apparent in this case.

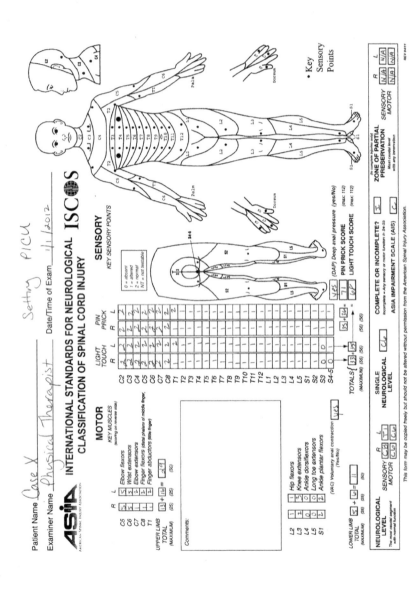

Figure 30-1. American Spinal Injury Association Neurological Classification of Spinal Cord Injury form for the case patient. (Reproduced with permission from American Spinal Injury Association: *International Standards for Neurological Classification of Spinal Cord Injury*, revised 2011; Atlanta, GA. Reprinted 2011.)

Muscle Function Grading

0 = total paralysis

1 = palpable or visible contraction

2 = active movement, full range of motion (ROM) with gravity eliminated

3 = active movement, full ROM against gravity

4 = active movement, full ROM against gravity and moderate resistance in a muscle specific position.

5 = (normal) active movement, full ROM against gravity and full resistance in a muscle specific position expected from an otherwise unimpaired peson.

5* = (normal) active movement, full ROM against gravity and sufficient resistance to be considered normal if identified inhibiting factors (i.e. pain, disuse) were not present.

NT = not testable (i.e. due to immobilization, severe pain such that the patient cannot be graded, amputation of limb, or contracture of >50% of the range of motion).

ASIA Impairment (AIS) Scale

☐ **A = Complete.** No sensory or motor function is preserved in the sacral segments S4-S5.

☐ **B = Sensory Incomplete.** Sensory but not motor function is preserved below the neurological level and includes the sacral segments S4-S5 (light touch, pin prick at S4-S5: or deep anal pressure (DAP)), AND no motor function is preserved more than three levels below the motor level on either side of the body.

☑ **C = Motor Incomplete.** Motor function is preserved below the neurological level**, and more than half of key muscle functions below the single neurological level of injury (NLI) have a muscle grade less than 3 (Grades 0-2).

☐ **D = Motor Incomplete.** Motor function is preserved below the neurological level**, and at least half (half or more) of key muscle functions below the NLI have a muscle grade ≥ 3.

☐ **E = Normal.** If sensation and motor function as tested with the ISNSCSI are graded as normal in all segments, and the patient had prior deficits, then the AIS grade is E. Someone without an initial SCI does not receive an AIS grade.

**For an individual to receive a grade of C or D, i.e. motor incomplete status, they must have either (1) voluntary anal sphincter contraction or (2) sacral sensory sparing with sparing of motor function more than three levels below the motor level for that side of the body. The Standards at this time allows even non-key muscle function more than 3 levels below the motor level to be used in determining motor incomplete status (AIS B versus C).

NOTE: When assessing the extent of motor sparing below the level for distinguishing between AIS B and C, the *motor level* on each side is used, whereas to differentiate between AIS C and D (based on proportion of key muscle functions with strength grade 3 or greater) the *single neurological level* is used.

Steps in Classification

The following order is recommended in determining the classification of individuals with SCI.

1. Determine sensory levels for right and left sides.

2. Determine motor levels for right and left sides.
   Note: in regions where there is no myotome to test, the motor level is presumed to be the same as the sensory level, if testable motor function above that level is also normal.

3. Determine the single neurological level.
   This is the lowest segment where motor and sensory function is normal on both sides, and is the most cephalad of the sensory and motor levels determined in steps 1 and 2.

4. Determine whether the injury is Complete or Incomplete. (i.e. absence or presence of sacral sparing)
   If voluntary anal contraction = No AND all S4-S5 sensory scores = 0 AND deep anal pressure = No, then injury is COMPLETE. Otherwise, injury is incomplete

5. Determine ASIA Impairment Scale (AIS) Grade:
   If YES, AIS=A and can record ZPP (lowest dermatome or myotome on each side with some preservation)

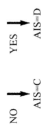

Is injury Complete?

NO → Is injury motor Incomplete? → If NO, AIS=B

YES → (Yes=voluntary anal contraction OR motor function more than three levels below the motor level on a given side, if the patient has sensory incomplete classification)

Are at least half of the key muscles below the single neurological level graded 3 or better?

NO → AIS=C

YES → AIS=D

If sensation and motor function is normal in all segments, AIS=E
Note : AIS E is used in follow-up testing when an individual with a documented SCI has recovered normal function. If at initial testing no deficits are found, the individual is neurologically intact, the ASIA Impairment Scale does not apply).

Figure 30-1. (*Continued*)

KEY DEFINITIONS

AMERICAN SPINAL INJURY ASSOCIATION (ASIA) CLASSIFICATION OF SPINAL CORD INJURY: Classification system used to determine an individual's neurological level of injury, create a prognosis, and predict outcomes for individuals with spinal cord injury

GUILFORD BRACE: Rigid cervicothoracic orthosis with anterior and posterior chest plates and a chin and occipital piece that are connected by shoulder straps; designed to limit flexion and extension from C3 to T2

SCIWORA: Acronym for Spinal Cord Injury without Radiologic Abnormality; disorder in which myelopathy occurs in the absence of a spinal abnormality

SECONDARY INJURY: Swelling, ischemia, excitotoxicity, and inflammatory response that occurs following neurologic injury

Objectives

1. Describe the anticipated prognosis in terms of participation restrictions, activity limitations, and impaired body functions and structures based on the patient's health condition (SCIWORA) and implications of the recent changes in his AIS classification.

2. Provide a rationale for measures obtained in a systems review for this individual.

3. Identify measures that should be performed to determine the individual's participation restrictions, activity limitations, and impaired body functions and structures.

4. Describe programs to improve tolerance to upright postures and differentiate between those that could be implemented by another health care provider (e.g., nurse) and those that could be safely implemented by family members.

5. Describe a flexibility program that would promote this individual's performance of activities.

6. Select activities for task-oriented training and provide a rationale for each activity that incorporates the decision to focus on compensatory strategies used by individuals with more severe injuries (AIS A and B) compared to those strategies used by individuals with more incomplete injuries (AIS C and D).

Physical Therapy Considerations

PT considerations during management of the child status/post spinal stabilization due to spinal cord injury:

▶ **General physical therapy plan of care/goals:** Improve functional mobility including bed mobility and transfers; improve tolerance and balance in upright postures (sitting or standing); improve locomotion (wheelchair mobility or walking)

▶ **Physical therapy interventions:** Positioning program to promote tolerance to upright postures (including use of garments and manual assistance); flexibility program to promote activities and reduce participation restrictions; task-oriented training focused on teaching compensatory strategies or the typical movement pattern (depending on prognosis for recovery of function); family education regarding guidelines for care and expectations for the rehabilitation process

▶ **Precautions during physical therapy:** Monitor blood pressure to avoid orthostatic hypotension and autonomic dysreflexia; swelling and redness in the leg potentially indicative of deep vein thrombosis; mobility restrictions due to spinal instability; positioning and skin shear to maintain skin integrity

▶ **Complications interfering with physical therapy:** Pain, spasticity, heterotopic ossification, bowel and bladder management

Understanding the Health Condition

A spinal cord injury (SCI) is particularly devastating to a child and his family, and while this is not a common health condition, the ramifications are global in nature. Further, there are unique concerns for SCI in children that include the influence of growth, development, and transitional phases into adulthood that require additional attention.[1] There are 1455 new traumatic spinal cord injuries in children each year in the United States.[2] The leading cause of pediatric SCI is motor vehicle accidents (56% of cases), followed by falls (14%), firearms (9%), and sports injuries (7%).[2] For children under 12 years of age, paraplegia (from thoracic injuries) is most common; for individuals over 12 years, tetraplegia (from cervical injuries) is more common.[3]

A traumatic SCI, defined as a compromise of neural structures from trauma, occurs as a result of one of four injury mechanisms: impact with compression, contusion, distraction, or laceration/translation injury.[4] Imaging (*e.g.*, spinal radiographs) is frequently used to identify spinal fractures. Following plain radiographs, computed tomography (CT) scans are used to further examine structural abnormalities.[5] There is some evidence that CT may have better sensitivity to identify spinal fractures than plain radiographs.[6]

Early spinal stabilization occurs through external immobilization (*i.e.*, by an orthotic) or surgical stabilization (internal fixation).[7] Traction for spinal realignment is not typically done in the pediatric population due to the thin cranial structures in children.[8] Some vertebral injuries (such as odontoid injuries) are successfully managed with closed reduction and immobilization with a halo vest, although surgical stabilization may be indicated if external immobilization fails.[8] Spinal surgery is often indicated to realign spinal structures and stabilize the spine.[7]

Medical intervention is directed at reducing the impact of secondary injury. While the direct trauma leads to local cellular death of neurons and glia, secondary injury can be just as damaging.[4] Secondary damage, which includes swelling, ischemia, excitotoxicity, and the inflammatory response, can continue for up to 4 weeks after the initial injury.[4] The inflammatory response that includes infiltration of immune cells necessary to clear cellular debris also increases pressure (via edema) on the damaged neural elements. Ischemia results from damage to local blood vessels, which reduces perfusion of the spinal cord. Excitotoxicity is related to excessive release of glutamate (primary excitatory neurotransmitter). When released into the extracellular space, glutamate causes an influx of calcium ions and subsequent apoptosis (cell death).[4] Apoptosis and excitotoxicity result in further release of free radicals that induces even more cell death. Several drugs are used to reduce the secondary damage to the neural elements following an SCI.[7] Neuroprotective therapies include methylprednisolone (potent anti-inflammatory glucocorticoid), neuroganglioside GM-1, gacyclidine (NMDA glutamate receptor antagonist), tirilazad (free radical scavenger), and naloxone.[7]

Spinal cord injury without radiographic abnormality (SCIWORA) is a disorder in which myelopathy occurs in the *absence* of spinal abnormality.[5,9] The actual frequency of occurrence is unknown, but it occurs most often in the pediatric population.[10] In children, the immature musculoskeletal system can withstand greater stresses than the neural tissues, resulting in SCIWORA injury.[10] SCIWORA can be visualized on MRI and subsequently classified into five categories for prognostic purposes.[10] The two categories with the worst prognosis are complete disruption of spinal cord due to severe distraction injury or severe flexion and major spinal cord hemorrhage. The remaining three categories (minor cord hemorrhage, edema only, or no findings on MRI) have much better prognosis for functional recovery.[10]

At the time of the injury, spinal precautions are initiated in the field and are maintained until the spine has been "cleared" by either the trauma medical team or the spine medical team. Common full spinal precautions include spinal immobilization with a cervical collar or thoracolumbosacral orthosis (TLSO), maintaining a neutral spine (no rotation) when moving the patient (through log rolling), limiting movement of the proximal extremities (no more than 90° of passive shoulder flexion or abduction and no active or passive hip flexion). Partial spinal precautions usually indicate external spinal immobilization through a cervical collar or TLSO, but allow the patient unrestricted movement at peripheral joints.

The severity of injury is determined based on the AIS.[11] The AIS is a measure that examines the integrity of the sensorimotor system following a spinal neurological insult. The motor component includes 10 *key* muscles used to represent different motor neurological levels. The representative muscles include the biceps brachii, extensor carpi radialis longus, triceps, flexor digitorum profundus, abductor digiti minimi, iliopsoas, quadriceps, tibialis anterior, extensor hallucis longus, and the gastrocnemius-soleus complex. The sensory section of the exam includes examining different dermatome levels and comparing the sensation (of a pin prick or cotton wisp) to an area of intact sensation (usually on the cheek).

An individual is classified as having a complete (AIS A) or incomplete (AIS B, C, D, or E) SCI based on the integrity of the final sacral segment (S4-S5). In general, individuals classified as having an AIS A SCI have limited sensory and motor function below the neurological level of injury and absence of sensorimotor function at the final sacral segment. Individuals classified as an AIS B (Sensory Incomplete) have sensory, but not motor preservation below the neurological level, including the final sacral segment. Individuals classified as an AIS C (Motor Incomplete) have motor function preserved below the neurological level, but at more than half of the key muscles have a manual muscle grade of *less than* 3/5. Individuals classified as an AIS D (Motor Incomplete) have motor function preserved below the neurological level, and at least half of the key muscles have manual muscle grade of *at least* 3/5.

Recovery of function is based on severity (AIS classification), neurologic level (AIS level of injury), and chronicity of injury. Children classified as having incomplete spinal cord injuries tend to demonstrate greater gains during rehabilitation than children classified with complete spinal cord injuries.[12] Not only do they make greater gains, but they tend to have fewer activity limitations. In adults with SCI, 50% of individuals classified as an AIS B are considered community ambulators compared to only 3% of individuals classified as an AIS A.[13] This is further elucidated with more incomplete injuries: 75% of individuals classified as an AIS C are community ambulators and 95% of individuals classified as AIS D are community ambulators.[13] Most studies define community ambulation as ability to walk using orthotics and assistive devices. The level of injury also influences the functional outcome. Children with an injury level at C6 tend to have greater recovery of function than children with an injury at C5, despite having similar functional status at admission.[12] The ability to *minimally* activate the wrist extensors, latissimus dorsi, and pectoralis major (muscles innervated by the C6 spinal segment) dramatically improves the ability to grasp objects (including an assistive device), transition from supine to sitting, and transfer to a level surface. Individuals with greater voluntary control over muscles innervated at C6 have greater independence with transfers from bed to wheelchair, toilet to wheelchair, and car to wheelchair.[14] Chronicity also impacts prognosis. Most motor recovery occurs in the first 6 months after the injury,[13] although physical therapy related improvements are seen in the chronic phase of recovery. While the prognostic value of the AIS is useful, special consideration must be taken when performing and interpreting the AIS classification in children. Children under the age of 4 years may have difficulty comprehending the instructions to complete the exam.[15] Further, low precision of outcomes has been found in children less than 15 years of age, with the sensory examination being most difficult for kids under 5 years.[15]

An acute SCI can cause dysfunction in multiple organ systems including cardiovascular, musculoskeletal, neuromuscular, and integumentary systems. The physical therapist must understand anticipated body system changes prior to performing examination and treatment, and also to properly educate the child and family. Acute cardiovascular impairments that must be addressed include hypotension, autonomic dysreflexia, and thromboembolic complications. Acutely, hypotension is a symptom of neurogenic shock resulting from denervation of the sympathetic nervous system (in individuals with SCI above T4).[16,17] Orthostatic hypotension results from the combination of arteriolar dilation with absent muscular venous pumps due to paralysis and lack of sympathetic nervous response.[16,17] Autonomic dysreflexia, in which there is an immediate sympathetic response to an irritant, is also caused by disruption of the autonomic nervous system.[7] Autonomic dysreflexia includes elevation of blood pressure coinciding with bradycardia. Other symptoms include a pounding headache, sweating, and flushing *above* the level of injury. The most common irritant provoking autonomic dysreflexia is the urinary system. Removal of the irritant usually resolves the autonomic response.[7] Adults with SCI have an increased risk of thromboembolic complications because of the lack of muscle pumps and the potential for venous pooling[7]; however, the risk has been found to be lower in children.[18] Symptoms of a deep vein thrombosis (DVT) include swelling and redness in the associated leg, although a DVT can be asymptomatic.

Musculoskeletal changes that accompany SCI include heterotopic ossification (HO)[19] and osteoporosis.[20] Heterotopic ossification is bone formation at ectopic sites and it occurs following traumatic neurologic injury such as SCI or traumatic brain injury.[19] In children and adults with a SCI, the most common joint affected is the hip, followed by the elbow, knee, and shoulder.[18] In children, HO is most common 14 months post-injury.[18] In the chronic phase of SCI, osteoporosis occurs due to the loss of weightbearing activities and the lack of muscle pull on bony structures.[20] This puts individuals with SCI at greater risk for fractures during typical daily activities.

Changes in the neuromuscular system include neuropathic pain[7,21] and spasticity.[18,22] Neuropathic pain is a pathological response related to trauma to the nervous system; it can occur at or below the level of the injury. Allodynia is a type of neuropathic pain in which there is a hypersensitivity to touch.[7] Spasticity is a result of an upper motor neuron deficit, and is therefore more likely in individuals with higher level injuries. More than half of individuals with spasticity have cervical level lesions, and 70% of individuals with spasticity have hypertonia in their lower extremities.[22] Interestingly, 40% of individuals with spasticity report that it promotes the performance of their daily activities, whereas only 20% report that it interferes with their daily activities (the remainder reported no effect).[22] Individuals with SCI also have an increased risk of acquiring decubitus ulcers because of the multiple risk factors associated with their injury.[7] Factors such as immobility, moisture, shear forces, and friction all increase risk of decubiti.[23]

Physical Therapy Patient/Client Management

Successful intervention and discharge planning for the child with SCI depends on a multidisciplinary team. The members of the trauma team vary based on institution, but the essential members include medicine (trauma, neurosurgery, and/or physiatry), nursing (pediatric trauma nursing or intensive care nursing), rehabilitation specialists (physical therapy, occupational therapy, speech language pathology, and recreational therapy), mental health services (pediatric psychiatry or rehabilitation psychology), and case management (social work or advanced practice nursing). The medical team and nursing ensure that the child is medically stable. Rehabilitation specialists primarily consider the child's activity limitations and impaired body functions and structures. Mental health specialists provide support for the child and his family as they identify new roles and challenges for each member of the family. Case managers facilitate the discharge planning process, identify resources, and ensure that the transition to the next level of care is successful for the unique needs of the family. Other members specific to the *pediatric* team also include a child life specialist and special educator. A child life specialist educates the family regarding expectations during the hospital stay and provides support and comfort to the child during the hospital stay. A special educator identifies areas of educational support to ensure a successful transition back to school. Members of the team work together to ensure a successful transition from the acute care hospital to the rehabilitation hospital.

Examination, Evaluation, and Diagnosis

The mean length of stay in an acute care hospital for a child with a SCI is 14 days.[2] This relatively short stay demonstrates the need for the physical therapist to conduct a thorough, yet efficient clinical examination and evaluation and design a plan of care for the child and his family. Prior to examining the child, the physical therapist should perform a thorough review of the medical record. This should include information relating to the injury itself including the date, mechanism, severity, and level of injury. This information frames the examination process and influences the prognosis for recovery. If the AIS has not been documented, the therapist should collect this information during the examination. Any spinal stabilization procedures should be noted, as well as spinal precautions. The therapist should also note other injuries that may have occurred at the time of the SCI. Closed head injuries, musculoskeletal injuries, and abdominal injuries are common.

Prior to assisting the patient to sitting at the edge of the bed, a brief systems review is necessary. For the cardiovascular system, heart rate and blood pressure must first be measured in the supine position to screen for bradycardia and hypotension,[24,25] as well as to monitor changes during movement. These initial measurements also serve as baseline measures to screen for autonomic dysreflexia. Normal values for systolic blood pressure in children *without* SCI can be estimated using the formula: systolic blood pressure = 90 + (2 times the child's age in years).[18] Published values for expected systolic and diastolic blood pressure in non-disabled children based on age and height are published and updated by the National Heart and Lung Institute of the Department of Health and Human Services.[26] The therapist should screen for HO (especially in the hip), although it is unlikely to present so soon following injury.[19] Symptoms of HO include fever, joint swelling, and unexplained loss of joint range of motion. The neuromuscular system should be screened for potentially undiagnosed traumatic brain injury, especially for individuals with cervical injury.[2] Neurogenic pain is not common in the acute phase, but in some individuals it is present within hours of the injury.[21] The integumentary system should be examined for skin integrity, especially under the occiput, elbows, sacrum, and heels.[27] Skin breakdown is possible from prolonged immobilization on the backboard, pressure garments, splints, or any surface that limits tissue profusion.[27]

After performing the systems review in the supine position, the physical therapist focuses the examination on the patient's functional mobility. Setting up the environment prior to assisting the child to sitting upright ensures greater success. Application of lower limb compression devices (such as elasticized wraps) and an abdominal binder reduce the risk of orthostatic hypotension. Positioning a reclining wheelchair with elevating leg rests near the bed provides an opportunity to transfer out of bed, contingent upon a successful transition to sitting. Following positioning the child in sitting, signs of orthostatic hypotension should be assessed.[7] The time tolerated, as well as the angle supported in an upright position should be documented.

Provided that an AIS has been completed, appropriate impairment level measures are selected based on the child's activity limitations that will be the focus for the intervention. Individuals with more severe SCI are able to perform many activities using compensatory strategies, while individuals with more incomplete injuries (as in this patient case) have a better prognosis of recovery of the typical movement pattern. If the therapist understands the kinematics and muscle activation patterns used by skilled individuals with chronic SCI, the efficiency of the examination improves. Table 30-1 shows typical and compensatory movement patterns, muscle activation, and force production required to perform several transfers and wheelchair propulsion.

Long sitting is an important position for an individual with a cervical injury because it provides a large base of support (compared to short sitting) and enables many self-care activities such as dressing. Impaired body functions that can restrict long sitting include orthostatic hypotension, hamstring flexibility, and sitting balance. Acutely, tolerance to sitting is usually limited by orthostatic hypotension, which, in adults, is defined as a drop in systolic blood pressure by 20 mm Hg or a drop in diastolic blood pressure by 10 mm Hg.[28] Hamstring length of 100° to 110° (measured through hip flexion with an extended knee) is required for long sitting. In an individual with a complete cervical injury, static sitting balance is maintained through reactive balance responses in the head and upper extremities, whereas in this case the individual likely has some (albeit weak) abdominal musculature to assist in the balance responses.

Scooting is a useful precursor to transferring to a wheelchair. Impaired body functions that can restrict the ability to scoot include impaired force production in the pectoralis major (innervated primarily at C6) and latissimus dorsi (innervated primarily at C6) or triceps muscles (innervated primarily at C7)[29]; flexibility in the shoulders (flexion, extension, and external rotation), elbow (extension) and hamstrings; and long sitting balance. If the individual has voluntary control of the triceps, then using a strategy of extending the shoulder and elbow during the movement pattern is frequently used.[29] However, if voluntary activation of the triceps is absent, then a compensatory strategy using more proximal musculature is required (Table 30-1). With the elbows locked in hyperextension, the latissimus dorsi can depress the shoulder and thereby unweight the body. Then, the pectoralis major can adduct the shoulder and bring the trunk toward the arm. In the case of this patient, his triceps are weak, although voluntary control is present (Fig. 30-1). This suggests that initial transfer training will likely require elbow hyperextension. However, during the rehabilitation process, the triceps may recover sufficiently to assist in unweighting the hips. Dynamic, anticipatory sitting balance in long sitting is also required to accomplish scooting. The use of speed and momentum of the head and upper trunk in the *opposite* direction of the hips can improve the ease of performing this task.

Transfer skills include transfer to surfaces of the same height (bed to wheelchair), slightly differing heights (wheelchair to toilet), and significantly different heights and larger distances (car transfers).[14] Impaired body functions related to the activity of transfers include force production of the pectoralis major, latissimus dorsi, deltoid (innervated primarily at C5), wrist extensors (innervated primarily at C6), triceps,

Table 30-1 BODY FUNCTION AND STRUCTURE REQUIREMENTS TO PERFORM TYPICAL AND COMPENSATORY MOVEMENT PATTERNS BY INDIVIDUALS WITH SPINAL CORD INJURY

Activity	Kinematics of Movement Pattern		Coordinated Muscle Activation Required	Muscle Force Production Required	Flexibility Required
Supine to sitting	Typical pattern	In supine, upper extremities push and reach. Trunk rotates and flexes to achieve sitting.		Triceps (C7) = 5/5 Abdominals (T1-T9) = 5/5	Shoulder: extension and external rotation Elbow: hyperextension Hip flexion with knee extension
	Compensatory pattern	In supine, the head is lifted and the arms and head rotate to transition to sidelying. The unweighted elbow is passively extended with shoulder external rotation. Child rolls onto the extended elbow and hand. The other arm is now unweighted and elbow is extended. From a reclined long sitting position, the child weight shifts and walks arms closer to pelvis and ends in long sitting propped on extended arms.		Pectoralis major (C6) = 5/5 Deltoid (C5) = 5/5 Serratus anterior (C5) = 5/5 Extensor carpi radialis (C6) = 5/5	

(Continued)

Activity	Kinematics of Movement Pattern		Coordinated Muscle Activation Required	Muscle Force Production Required	Flexibility Required
Scooting	Typical	In a sitting position with hands on the supporting surface, the elbows extend while the shoulders are depressed, thereby unweighting the pelvis. Shoulder adducts which brings the trunk toward the arm.	Deltoid followed by triceps, latissimus dorsi and pectoralis major	Triceps (C7) = 5/5	Shoulder: extension and external rotation Elbow: extension Hip flexion with knee extension
	Compensatory	In a sitting position with hands on the supporting surface, shoulders are externally rotated to lock the elbows in hyperextension, the shoulders are depressed and thereby unweight the pelvis. Shoulder adducts, which brings trunk toward the arm. Head and upper trunk move in *opposite* direction of hips.	Deltoid followed by latissimus dorsi and pectoralis major	Pectoralis major (C6) = 5/5 Deltoid (C5) = 5/5 Latissimus dorsi (C6) = 5/5	

Transfer to surface of same height	Typical	Lead arm is on new surface. Shoulders and elbows extend to unweight pelvis. Head and upper trunk rotate away from surface while pelvis rotates toward surface.	Pre-lift phase: Latissimus dorsi and deltoid (primarily in trailing arm). Lift phase: deltoid, pectoralis major, and triceps[31]	Pectoralis major (C6) = 5/5 Latissimus dorsi (C6) = 5/5 Deltoid (C5) = 5/5 Extensors carpi radialis (C6) = 5/5 Triceps (C7) = 5/5 Flexor carpi (C7) = 5/5 Flexor digitorum (C7) = 5/5	Shoulder: extension and external rotation Elbow: extension Wrist: extension
	Compensatory	Lead arm is on new surface. Shoulders are externally rotated to lock elbows into hyperextension. Head and upper trunk shift forward to unweight pelvis. Head and upper trunk rotate away from surface while pelvis rotates toward surface.	Pre-lift phase: latissimus dorsi and deltoid Lift phase: deltoid, pectoralis major, and extensor carpi radialis longus/brevis	Pectoralis major (C6) = 5/5 Latissimus dorsi (C6) = 5/5 Deltoid (C5) = 5/5 Extensors carpi radialis (C6) = 5/5	
Wheelchair propulsion	Typical	Push phase: hands grasp rims of the wheelchair and shoulders flex while elbows flex and then extend. Recovery phase: release rims and shoulders and elbows extend to reposition hands on the rims.	Push phase: anterior deltoid, pectoralis major, serratus anterior, and biceps Recovery phase: Middle/posterior deltoid, triceps	Deltoid (C5) = 5/5 Pectoralis major (C6) = 5/5 Serratus anterior (C5) = 5/5 Biceps (C5) = 5/5 Triceps (C7) = 5/5 Extensor carpi radialis (C6) = 3/5 Flexor digitorum (C7) = 3/5	Shoulder: flexion and extension Elbow: extension Wrist: extension Fingers: flexion
	Compensatory	Push phase: palmar surface/web space is touching knobs of the wheelchair with wrist extended. Shoulder flexes. Recovery phase: release the rims and the shoulder extends to reposition the hands on the rim.	Push phase: anterior deltoid, pectoralis major, serratus anterior, and biceps Recovery phase: middle/posterior deltoid, and extensor carpi radialis longus/brevis.	Deltoid (C5) = 5/5, Pectoralis major (C6) = 5/5 Serratus anterior (C5) = 5/5 Biceps (C5) = 5/5 Extensor carpi radialis (C6) = 3/5	

wrist flexors (innervated primarily at C7), and finger flexors (innervated primarily at C7),[30] flexibility in the shoulders (flexion, extension, and external rotation), elbow (extension), and short sitting balance. For the individual who has voluntary activation of the triceps, the typical activation pattern is deltoid first, followed by pectoralis major, and triceps.[31] Those individuals *without* voluntary activation of the triceps must rely on elbow hyperextension and reverse activation of proximal muscles including latissimus dorsi, deltoid, pectoralis major, and wrist extensors. Because wrist flexors and finger flexors are innervated at the same level as the triceps (primarily at C7), if the triceps activation is absent, it is likely these are absent as well. The current patient has voluntary control of the triceps, but they are very weak. Given that his injury was so recent, it is likely that greater recovery of triceps strength will occur over the next year. At 1 year post-injury, 90% of paretic muscles initially rated with manual muscle testing (MMT) as 1 or 2 recover to at least antigravity strength (MMT = 3).[13] Therefore, this individual has good prognosis for recovery of triceps muscle function, and the typical muscle activation pattern should be considered for this activity.

Depending on the prognosis for locomotion, the physical therapist should assess either the child's ability to propel a wheelchair or walk short distances. Wheelchair propulsion can be accomplished with or without voluntary control over the elbow extensors and finger flexors (both muscle groups primarily innervated at C7). However, without the voluntary control of these muscles, the activity is slow and energy-consuming.[32,33] Impaired body functions related to wheelchair propulsion include impaired force production of the biceps (primarily innervated at C5), pectoralis major (primarily innervated at C6), anterior deltoid (primarily innervated at C5), and trapezius (primarily innervated by cranial nerve XI),[32] and flexibility of the shoulder (extension) and elbow (extension). Wheelchair propulsion is characterized by two phases: a pull/push phase and a recovery phase.[32] In the pull/push phase, the shoulders are moving from extension to flexion—pulling and then pushing the rims of the chair. Muscles used in the pull/push phase are the biceps, pectoralis major, anterior deltoid, and trapezius. In the recovery phase, the shoulders move from shoulder flexion to extension. Muscles used in the recovery phase include the trapezius, deltoid, and triceps.[32]

Most families of a child with SCI will ask about the prognosis for walking. In adults with SCI, walking prognosis (household distances) is dependent on strength of the quadriceps and gastrocnemius-soleus muscles, cutaneous sensory function (light touch at L3 and S1), and age (less than 65 years).[34] While this can be used to guide clinical decision making in children, it is likely that children have a greater prognosis for recovery of walking ability for two important reasons. First, children have greater neuroplasticity, and therefore greater potential for recovery with appropriate interventions. Second, the small size of the child compared to the adult makes the management of large orthotic devices (reciprocating gait orthoses, hip-knee-ankle-foot orthoses, and knee-ankle-foot orthoses) more manageable for both the individual and the family. While these compensatory mechanisms provide opportunities for the very severely impaired child to regain walking, there is exciting new evidence that there is much recovery potential with interventions that focus on **locomotor training**.[35-38]

Finally, prior to discharge from the acute setting, an outcome measure that assesses participation restrictions and activity limitations should be performed to facilitate communication to the physical therapist at the next level of care and to document change. Two measures that have been used to document change during rehabilitation of children with SCI are the Wee Functional Independence Measure (WeeFIM)[12] and the **Pediatric Evaluation of Disability Inventory (PEDI)**.[39] For the WeeFIM, there are documented outcomes of children with complete and incomplete SCI from inpatient rehabilitation centers, which enables comparison.[12] The limitation of the WeeFIM is that it measures capability and not *typical* performance. The PEDI is a measure of both activity limitation and participation restriction; thus, it captures both capability and typical performance. It has been shown to be responsive to change in an inpatient rehabilitation setting.[39]

Plan of Care and Interventions

The four main goals during the acute care phase of the rehabilitation process include tolerance to upright postures, creating a flexibility program to promote future independence with activities, creating early strategies for new movement patterns, and education regarding care for the individual with SCI.

The most important goal for the child with SCI during the acute care phase is to improve tolerance to upright positioning, usually as it relates to sitting. Mobilizing to the edge of the bed should begin as soon as there are no medical or spinal contraindications.[7] There is evidence from adults with SCI that individuals with orthostatic hypotension related to SCI can improve their tolerance to standing with a standing program.[40] Using this rationale, it is a reasonable assumption that practicing sitting in upright positions reduces orthostatic hypotension. To avoid prolonged weightbearing on the sacrum, the reclined sitting position should not be used.[41]

A flexibility program is important for the child with SCI because many of the new movement patterns that will eventually become routine have specific flexibility requirements. The flexibility program should begin as soon as there are no medical/orthopaedic contraindications. Activities such as transferring to a wheelchair and transitioning from supine to sitting require shoulder extension (at least 90°) and elbow extension (0°). Evidence suggests that loss of shoulder range of motion is associated with pain during the rehabilitation process.[42] Hamstring length becomes especially important for the long sitting position. Straight leg raise (an estimate of hamstring length) should be increased to 110° of hip flexion with the knee extended. Sufficient knee flexion is also necessary to transition from the floor to the wheelchair. To perform this transfer, the individual needs at least 130° of knee flexion.

While it is important to maintain and in some cases increase range of motion at specific joints, it is equally important to allow shortening at other joints to gain function. Shortened paraspinal muscles promote a sitting posture and may improve balance. Shortened finger flexors allow an individual who does not have voluntary activation of the finger flexors to grasp objects using a functional tenodesis grip. Tenodesis is the grasping of objects through active wrist extension combined with the passive insufficiency of shorted finger flexors. In this patient case, the child has voluntary activation of finger flexors. Although they are weak, they are likely to recover significantly within the first year. A thoughtful reflection on the prognosis of the individual should be performed prior to initiating a splinting program to promote finger flexor shortening.

Task-oriented training of activity limitations identified in the examination should begin in the acute phase. Activities such as long sitting balance, weight shifting, scooting, wheelchair transfers, and wheelchair mobility are common activity limitations for individuals with more severe injuries. Individuals with more severe spinal cord injuries perform these activities differently from non-disabled individuals, and it is important to understand the kinematics and muscle activation patterns of compensatory patterns used by individuals with SCI (Table 30-1). Adaptive equipment should be used to increase independence in the early learning process. Equipment such as loops, transfer boards, and wheelchairs are essential. Individuals with less severe injuries may progress to activities such as transitioning from sitting to standing or walking. It is unlikely that the child will become fully independent with these activities in the acute phase, but intervention in this phase serves as a basis for those interventions in the next inpatient rehabilitation setting and eventual outpatient therapy setting.

Education regarding the rehabilitation process and the importance of early involvement of the family is an important role for the physical therapist in this setting. It is also important for the physical therapist to begin discussions about the signs of organ system dysfunction and guidelines for prevention of dysfunction. For example, individuals with SCI have an increased risk for decubitus ulcers. To reduce this risk, individuals must perform weight shift maneuvers every 20 to 30 minutes.[43] The maturity of the individual must be considered in determining who will be ultimately responsible for scheduling the weight shift maneuver. The 5-year-old child in this case is unlikely to be independent in following a schedule for unweighting. Thus, the physical therapist must educate the parents about the need, frequency, and technique of a weight shift. To further reduce risk, avoiding shearing forces to weightbearing surfaces[41] and repositioning every 2 hours is vital.[43] The importance of positioning on the immature musculoskeletal system must also be considered. Children with spinal cord injuries have an increased risk of scoliosis[44] and hip dysplasia.[45] The younger the child at the time of injury, the greater the risk of scoliosis and hip instability.[44,45]

Evidence-Based Clinical Recommendations

SORT: Strength of Recommendation Taxonomy

A: Consistent, good-quality patient-oriented evidence
B: Inconsistent or limited-quality patient-oriented evidence
C: Consensus, disease-oriented evidence, usual practice, expert opinion, or case series

1. The American Spinal Injury Association (ASIA) classification guidelines of spinal cord injury predict overall recovery, zone of injury recovery, and ambulation potential. **Grade B**

2. The Pediatric Evaluation of Disability Inventory (PEDI) detects changes in mobility and self-care in children with SCI. **Grade B**

3. Locomotor training improves walking ability in both acute and chronic cases of individuals with pediatric incomplete SCI. **Grade C**

COMPREHENSION QUESTIONS

30.1 Given the AIS classification C and sensorimotor scores in Fig. 30-1, what is the *most* likely prognosis for this individual's locomotor potential?

   A. Limited to power wheelchair mobility

   B. Currently limited to power wheelchair mobility, but ultimately relying on manual wheelchair mobility

   C. Currently limited to manual wheelchair mobility, but ultimately walking household distances

   D. Currently limited to walking household distances, but ultimately walking community distances

30.2 Physiological monitoring for the individual with an AIS C, C6 SCI should include monitoring heart rate and blood pressure during all activities to identify:

   A. Tachycardia

   B. Hypotensive response

   C. Hypertensive response

   D. Either a hypotensive or hypertensive response

30.3 The flexibility program that *best* promotes independence for the individual with an acute AIS A, C6 SCI would include stretching of the:

   A. Iliopsoas, flexor digitorum, and glenohumeral joint (into shoulder extension)

   B. Hamstrings, gastrocnemius-soleus muscle group, and glenohumeral joint (into shoulder extension)

   C. Hamstrings, flexor digitorum, and paraspinals

   D. Iliopsoas, gastrocnemius-soleus muscle group, and paraspinals

ANSWERS

30.1 **C.** This individual will be limited to manual wheelchair mobility, but ultimately he can likely regain walking household distances. He has strong innervations at C5 and C6, which suggests strong deltoid, pectoralis, serratus anterior, biceps, and wrist extensor muscles—all of which will enable him to propel a manual wheelchair. He has good potential to eventually walk at least short distances. He has voluntary control of his quadriceps and gastrocnemius-soleus muscle group (albeit weak), sensory function at the final sacral segment, and he is young.

30.2 **D.** This individual is at risk for both hypotension and hypertension. Hypotension is likely and is related to denervation of the sympathetic nervous system and lack of muscular venous pumps. He is also at risk for autonomic dysreflexia which manifests as a hypertensive response with bradycardia.

30.3 **B.** This individual needs flexibility in his hamstrings (to enable a long sitting position), gastrocnemius-soleus muscle group (to position in his wheelchair), and glenohumeral joint (to enable him to transition from supine to sitting independently). He would benefit from *shortened* paraspinals to support his sitting balance (options C and D) and shortened finger flexors to support his tenodesis (option A).

REFERENCES

1. Vogel LC, Hickey KJ, Klaas SJ, Anderson CJ. Unique issues in pediatric spinal cord injury. *Orthop Nurs.* 2004;23:300-308.

2. Vitale MG, Goss JM, Matsumoto H, Roye DP Jr. Epidemiology of pediatric spinal cord injury in the United States: years 1997 and 2000. *J Pediatr Orthop.* 2006;26:745-749.

3. Lee JH, Sung IY, Kang JY, Park SR. Characteristics of pediatric-onset spinal cord injury. *Pediatr Int.* 2009;51:254-257.

4. Oyinbo CA. Secondary injury mechanisms in traumatic spinal cord injury: a nugget of this multiply cascade. *Acta Neurobiol Exp (Wars).* 2011;71:281-299.

5. Vialle LR, Vialle E. Pediatric spine injuries. *Injury.* 2005;36(Suppl 2):B104-B112.

6. Berne JD, Velmahos GC, El-Tawil Q, et al. Value of complete cervical helical computed tomographic scanning in identifying cervical spine injury in the unevaluable blunt trauma patient with multiple injuries: a prospective study. *J Trauma.* 1999;47:896-903.

7. Consortium for Spinal Cord Medicine. Early acute management in adults with spinal cord injury: a clinical practice guideline for health-care providers. *J Spinal Cord Med.* 2008;31:403-479.

8. Anon. Management of pediatric cervical spine and spinal cord injuries. *Neurosurgery.* 2002; 50(3 Suppl):S85-S99.

9. Brown RL, Brunn MA, Garcia VF. Cervical spine injuries in children: a review of 103 patients treated consecutively at a level 1 pediatric trauma center. *J Pediatr Surg.* 2001;36:1107-1114.

10. Pang D. Spinal cord injury without radiographic abnormality in children, 2 decades later. *Neurosurgery.* 2004;55:1325-1343.

11. Maynard FM Jr, Bracken MB, Creasey G, et al. International Standards for Neurological and Functional Classification of Spinal Cord Injury. American Spinal Injury Association. *Spinal Cord.* 1997;35:266-274.

12. Garcia RA, Gaebler-Spira D, Sisung C, Heinemann AW. Functional improvement after pediatric spinal cord injury. *Am J Phys Med Rehabil.* 2002;81:458-463.

13. Consortium for Spinal Cord Medicine. Outcomes following traumatic spinal cord injury: clinical practice guidelines for health-care professionals. *J Spinal Cord Med.* 2000;23:289-316.

14. Mizukami M, Kawai N, Iwasaki Y, et al. Relationship between functional levels and movement in tetraplegic patients. A retrospective study. *Paraplegia.* 1995;33:189-194.

15. Mulcahey MJ, Gaughan J, Betz RR, Johansen KJ. The International Standards for Neurological Classification of Spinal Cord Injury: reliability of data when applied to children and youths. *Spinal Cord.* 2007;45:452-459.

16. Claydon VE, Krassioukov AV. Orthostatic hypotension and autonomic pathways after spinal cord injury. *J Neurotrauma.* 2006;23:1713-1725.

17. Gondim FA, Lopes AC Jr, Oliveira GR, et al. Cardiovascular control after spinal cord injury. *Curr Vasc Pharmacol.* 2004;2:71-79.

18. Greenberg JS, Ruutiainen AT, Kim H. Rehabilitation of pediatric spinal cord injury: from acute medical care to rehabilitation and beyond. *J Pediatr Rehabil Med.* 2009;2:13-27.

19. Betz RR. Unique management needs of pediatric spinal cord injury patients: orthopedic problems in the child with spinal cord injury. *J Spinal Cord Med.* 1997;20:14-16.

20. Giangregorio L, McCartney N. Bone loss and muscle atrophy in spinal cord injury: epidemiology, fracture prediction, and rehabilitation strategies. *J Spinal Cord Med.* 2006;29:489-500.

21. Siddall PJ, Taylor DA, McClelland JM, Rutkowski SB, Cousins MJ. Pain report and the relationship of pain to physical factors in the first 6 months following spinal cord injury. *Pain.* 1999;81:187-197.

22. Sköld C, Levi R, Seiger A. Spasticity after traumatic spinal cord injury: nature, severity, and location. *Arch Phys Med Rehabil.* 1999;80:1548-1557.

23. Krouskop TA, Noble PC, Garber SL, Spencer WA. The effectiveness of preventive management in reducing the occurrence of pressure sores. *J Rehabil R D.* 1983;20:74-83.

24. Abd AG, Braun NM. Management of life-threatening bradycardia in spinal cord injury. *Chest.* 1989;95:701-2.

25. Lehmann KG, Lane JG, Piepmeier JM, Batsford WP. Cardiovascular abnormalities accompanying acute spinal cord injury in humans: incidence, time course and severity. *J Am Col. Cardiol.* 1987;10:46-52.

26. Blood Pressure Tables for Children and Adolescents, NHLBI. Available at: http://www.nhlbi.nih.gov/guidelines/hypertension/child_tbl.htm. Accessed January 3, 2012.

27. Kosiak M. Prevention and rehabilitation of pressure ulcers. *Decubitus.* 1991;4:62-66.

28. Medow MS, Stewart JM, Sanyal S, Mumtaz A, Sica D, Frishman WH. Pathophysiology, diagnosis, and treatment of orthostatic hypotension and vasovagal syncope. *Cardiol Rev.* 2008;16:4-20.

29. van Drongelen S, van der Woude LH, Janssen TW, Angenot EL, Chadwick EK, Veeger DH. Glenohumeral contact forces and muscle forces evaluated in wheelchair-related activities of daily living in able-bodied subjects versus subjects with paraplegia and tetraplegia. *Arch Phys Med Rehabil.* 2005;86:1434-1440.

30. Beninato M, O'Kane KS, Sullivan PE. Relationship between motor FIM and muscle strength in lower cervical-level spinal cord injuries. *Spinal Cord.* 2004;42:533-540.

31. Gagnon D, Koontz AM, Brindle E, Boninger ML, Cooper RA. Does upper-limb muscular demand differ between preferred and nonpreferred sitting pivot transfer directions in individuals with a spinal cord injury? *J Rehabil Res Dev.* 2009;46:1099-1108.

32. Schantz P, Björkman P, Sandberg M, Andersson E. Movement and muscle activity pattern in wheelchair ambulation by persons with para- and tetraplegia. *Scand J Rehabil Med.* 1999;31:67-76.

33. Mulroy SJ, Farrokhi S, Newsam CJ, Perry J. Effects of spinal cord injury level on the activity of shoulder muscles during wheelchair propulsion: an electromyographic study. *Arch Phys Med Rehabil.* 2004;85:925-934.

34. van Middendorp JJ, Hosman AJF, Donders AR, et al. A clinical prediction rule for ambulation outcomes after traumatic spinal cord injury: a longitudinal cohort study. *Lancet.* 2011;377:1004-1010.

35. Prosser LA. Locomotor training within an inpatient rehabilitation program after pediatric incomplete spinal cord injury. *Phys Ther.* 2007;87:1224-1232.

36. Behrman AL, Harkema SJ. Physical rehabilitation as an agent for recovery after spinal cord injury. *Phys Med Rehabil Clin N Am.* 2007;18:183-202.

37. Fox EJ, Tester NJ, Phadke CP, et al. Ongoing walking recovery 2 years after locomotor training in a child with severe incomplete spinal cord injury. *Phys Ther.* 2010;90:793-802.

38. Behrman AL, Nair PM, Bowden MG, et al. Locomotor training restores walking in a nonambulatory child with chronic, severe, incomplete cervical spinal cord injury. *Phys Ther.* 2008;88:580-590.

39. Choksi A, Townsend EL, Dumas HM, Haley SM. Functional recovery in children and adolescents with spinal cord injury. *Pediatr Phys Ther*. 2010;22:214-221.

40. Harkema SJ, Ferreira CK, van den Brand RJ, Krassioukov AV. Improvements in orthostatic instability with stand locomotor training in individuals with spinal cord injury. *J Neurotrauma*. 2008;25:1467-1475.

41. Goetz LL, Brown GS, Priebe MM. Interface pressure characteristics of alternating air cell mattresses in persons with spinal cord injury. *J Spinal Cord Med*. 2002;25:167-173.

42. Waring WP, Maynard FM. Shoulder pain in acute traumatic quadriplegia. *Paraplegia*. 1991;29:37-42.

43. Consortium for Spinal Cord Medicine Clinical Practice Guidelines. Pressure ulcer prevention and treatment following spinal cord injury: a clinical practice guideline for health-care professionals. *J Spinal Cord Med*. 2001;24(Suppl 1):S40-S101.

44. Dearolf WW III, Betz RR, Vogel LC, Levin J, Clancy M, Steel HH. Scoliosis in pediatric spinal cord-injured patients. *J Pediatr Orthop*. 1990;10:214-218.

45. Rink P, Miller F. Hip instability in spinal cord injury patients. *J Pediatr Orthop*. 1990;10:583-587.

Child with Near-Drowning Episode

Mary Swiggum
Brooke B. Pettyjohn

CASE 31

A 2-year-old child was found face down in his family's backyard pool. The family lives in Florida and the estimated pool temperature at the time of the near-drowning incident was 85°F. The parents estimate that their son was in the water for 6 to 8 minutes before being pulled out. His father began CPR immediately and Emergency Medical Services (EMS) was called. When EMS arrived, CPR was continued, but intubation was unsuccessful. The patient's heart stopped three separate times before he was eventually stabilized in the emergency department. His body temperature in the emergency room was 94°F. He was unresponsive to painful and verbal stimuli and was reliant on mechanical ventilation. His pupils were fixed and dilated at 4 mm. On admission, he had a PGCS score of 3. Two days later, he had an NSE level of 38. Both parents were emphatic that their child be "saved." The patient is currently in the pediatric intensive care unit (PICU) 10 days after the near-drowning episode. His PGCS score is now 11. His eyes open spontaneously and he is beginning to focus on people. He is groaning and beginning to respond to tactile input by pulling the touched body part away. He is still intubated but the plan is to begin weaning him over the next few days.

▶ What are the possible neurologic consequences and secondary musculoskeletal impairments associated with an anoxic incident in a child?

▶ What is the role of the acute care physical therapist in preventing secondary impairments and preparing the child and family for transfer to a rehabilitation unit?

▶ What are possible medical and psychosocial complications interfering with physical therapy?

▶ What precautions should be taken during physical therapy interventions?

▶ What are function and participation expectations for a typical 2-year-old?

KEY DEFINITIONS

ANOXIA: Complete lack of oxygen in blood; after 4 minutes, brain cells may begin to die; after > 5 minutes, permanent brain injury can occur

DECORTICATE POSTURING: Abnormal posture usually indicative of midbrain dysfunction in which the body is stiff with flexed arms and extended legs

DROWNING: Death from asphyxia within 24 hours of submersion

HYPOXIA/HYPOXEMIA: Often used interchangeably; hypoxia is insufficient oxygenation of tissues; hypoxemia is insufficient oxygenation of arterial blood

MAGNETIC RESONANCE IMAGING (MRI): Diagnostic tool based on signals emitted by protons when placed in a magnetic field; may be utilized several days after injury to evaluate hypoxic-ischemic damage secondary to a near-drowning episode

NEAR-DROWNING: Submersion episode of sufficient severity to warrant medical attention

NEURON SPECIFIC ENOLASE (NSE): Enzymatic marker of ischemic brain damage; increased levels in cerebrospinal fluid (CSF) taken within 72 hours after severe neurologic incident have accepted predictive value for subsequent outcome; normal NSE concentrations in CSF reported as (mean ± SD) 17.3 ± 4.6 ng/mL[1,2]

OPISTHOTONOS: Extreme form of hyperextension of the body in which the head and heels are arched backward

PEDIATRIC GLASGOW COMA SCALE (PGCS): Modification of Glasgow Coma Scale designed for utilization with children; test scores of eye, verbal, and motor responses are summed and range from 3 (deep coma or death) to 15 (awake and aware); total score of < 8 indicates significant risk of mortality[3]

SUBMERSION INJURY: Submersion resulting in hospital admission or death

VISUALLY EVOKED RESPONSE (VER): Diagnostic measure that records electrical impulses generated by a visual stimulus; performed to detect abnormalities in visual pathways

Objectives

1. Describe the body's physiologic response to near-drowning and the implications for physical therapy management of the near-drowning victim.
2. Identify reliable and valid tools to assess motor and functional skills in a child following a near-drowning episode.
3. Identify reliable, valid, and developmentally appropriate tools to assess pain in a child following a near-drowning episode.
4. Identify neurodiagnostic tests that would typically be performed in a child following a near-drowning episode.
5. Identify medications that may be administered to address abnormal muscle tone and seizure activity and any adverse drug reactions (ADRs) that would affect physical therapy evaluation and/or interventions.

Physical Therapy Considerations

PT considerations during management of the near-drowning childhood survivor with development of significant anoxic brain injury:

▶ **General physical therapy plan of care/goals:** Prevention of secondary impairments (*e.g.*, joint contracture, muscle atrophy, skin breakdown); improve or maintain ventilation and oxygenation; encourage purposeful developmentally appropriate movement patterns; improve cognitive level using multimodal stimuli; address functional, gross and fine motor, and visuomotor skills such as attention, arousal, and medical stability

▶ **Physical therapy interventions:** Family/caregiver education regarding current condition and activities to enhance performance such as functional range of motion (ROM) activities, positioning to prevent asymmetries, contractures, and skin breakdown; developmentally appropriate movement re-education and cognitive-behavioral stimulation; prolonged stretching; splinting, as warranted

▶ **Precautions during physical therapy:** Monitor vital signs; monitor responses to stimulation; utilize caution around equipment, especially ventilator

▶ **Complications interfering with physical therapy:** Decreased level of consciousness, ADRs

Understanding the Health Condition

Nearly 2000 children die annually in the United Sates as a result of drowning.[2,4,5] Near-drowning is a significant cause of morbidity and is defined as an episode in which someone survives a period of underwater submersion.[5] Morbidities associated with near-drowning include dysfunction of the cardiorespiratory, neuromuscular, musculoskeletal, neurobehavioral, renal, and gastrointestinal systems. The ultimate mechanism of injury is hypoxemia and ischemia-induced organ damage.[5,6]

During a near-drowning episode, the victim typically undergoes a period of panic, struggling, and automatic swimming movements. Apnea occurs and continues until the $Paco_2$ and Pao_2 levels reach a threshold at which involuntary breathing occurs and water is aspirated.[7-9] Some individuals aspirate a small amount of fluid during the initial apneic phase, which results in laryngospasm. In most, the laryngospasm eventually relaxes and further aspiration occurs. For approximately 10% of drowning victims, laryngospasm does not resolve and they drown without aspirating fluid.[10] However, if these victims are resuscitated, they may eventually aspirate gastric contents. The volume of fluid aspirated influences the risk of pneumonia. Inadequate oxygenation of the tissues, whether or not fluid is aspirated, eventually leads to neuronal injury, circulatory collapse, myocardial damage, dysfunction of multiple organ systems, and further ischemic brain injury.

The most devastating outcome of a near-drowning episode is hypoxic-ischemic brain injury or anoxic brain injury. In general, neurons die when there is a lack of oxygen for periods of 5 to 10 minutes. Certain areas of the brain are particularly sensitive to a lack of oxygen. These include the subcortical regions such as the basal ganglia, hippocampus, and limbic structures.[9] When oxygen shortage is severe and/or prolonged, increasing numbers and types of neurons are affected and the resulting sequelae are more severe.[11] The temperature of the water at the time of near-drowning can affect the extent of neurologic damage, with better outcomes reported when near-drowning occurs in cold water.[12] Additional factors that affect morbidity include duration of submersion, initial neurologic evaluation, time to first breath, and initial blood pH.[13]

The acute medical management of a child following a near-drowning episode involves efforts to support ventilation and prevent further neurologic injury. Mechanical ventilation is instituted. Extra-corporeal membrane oxygenation (ECMO) may also be instituted. ECMO is a respiratory system intervention in which blood is oxygenated mechanically outside of the body to allow the lungs to rest after an injury. Ventilation is frequently used in conjunction with pharmacologic paralysis of the musculoskeletal system. This may place the child at increased risk for contractures, muscle weakness, and atrophy during the acute phase.[14] Cardiac function is continuously electrically monitored. A urinary catheter is placed and fluid output monitored hourly to monitor renal function.[15] A nasogastric tube is placed as soon as possible and stomach contents are removed to reduce the risk of vomiting and aspiration. Metabolic acidosis occurs in 70% of near-drowning victims and is treated with sodium bicarbonate if the pH is below 7.[16] Radiographs may be performed to rule out musculoskeletal injury and to assess pulmonary status. Serial neurologic observations using the Pediatric Glasgow Coma Scale may occur.[16] Additional neurodiagnostic tests performed in the acute care environment may include CT scan, MRI, NSE test, VER, and brainstem auditory evoked response.[2,17,18] These tests are done to monitor the evolution of the neurologic injury and to assist in more accurate prognosis.

Determining prognosis for children who experience a near-drowning episode is complex, partly due to the nature of the disorder and partly because children are developing and growing. In a retrospective chart review of 44 children who had experienced near-drowning episodes, the authors found that children who were awake and had spontaneous, purposeful movements, and normal brainstem function 24 hours after near-drowning had satisfactory recovery. In contrast, children without spontaneous, purposeful movements and abnormal brain stem function 24 hours after near-drowning suffered severe neurologic deficits or death.[17] Another study looked at results of the **brainstem auditory evoked response (BAER)** as an indicator of future recovery.[19] This diagnostic test uses electrical impulses to determine abnormalities along the auditory pathway and other abnormalities in the brainstem. Patients who had full neurologic recoveries had BAER measurements that were similar to controls. The BAER measurements for those with poor long-term outcomes were normal after resuscitation but showed significant reduction in wave V amplitudes over the ensuing days post-injury. When compared to controls, patients with a vegetative outcome had abnormally prolonged wave I-V interpeak latencies, diminished wave V amplitudes, and large-wave I/V amplitude ratios following resuscitation.[19] Long-term musculoskeletal impairments secondary to poor neurologic outcome include equinus, contractures of the hip adductors, hamstrings, and quadriceps, hip subluxation or dislocation, and scoliosis.[14] Children with status dystonicus, characterized by frequent and severe episodes of generalized dystonia, tend to have more significant long-term orthopaedic impairments and deformities. Common abnormal movement patterns in the first few months postinjury include decorticate posturing and dystonia with opisthotonos. Torsion spasms (especially those causing painful opisthotonos) may be treated pharmaceutically with muscle relaxants such as tizanidine and baclofen, and/or trazodone and propanolol. The common ADRs that can affect rehabilitation interventions include dizziness, hypotension, somnolence, ataxia, and bradycardia.

Physical Therapy Patient/Client Management

The status of a patient with anoxic brain injury may change rapidly. Sometimes, within the first 2 to 10 days postevent, a regression may occur for reasons as yet unknown. At this stage, the patient may become vegetative or even die. The physical therapist must work closely with the team of physicians, nurses, speech pathologists, occupational therapists, and caregivers to ensure a complete understanding of the patient's condition and to promote the maintenance of functional integrity for the patient. The current patient will not be able to verbally communicate since he is intubated and he may have sustained damage to brain regions critical for receptive and expressive language. Therefore, it is important for every person in the healthcare team and the patient's family members to be cognizant of behavioral and physiological indicators of pain and distress, such as changes in facial expression, muscle tone, vocalizations, atypical behaviors, and increases in heart rate and blood pressure.[20] It is vital that all members of the team are consistent in their communications with the family. This child sustained a severe brain injury and recovery depends on the extent of the injury, his previous function, and the postinjury environment. It is important for the family to understand that children do not just "wake up" from a coma. The family should be educated to look for early responses to sensory stimuli, such as responding to light, focusing on a family member's face, and responding to commands. Providing the family with knowledge of signs of improvement to look for and activities to do with their child helps minimize stress and promote coping.

Examination, Evaluation, and Diagnosis

The examination of the patient begins with a detailed chart review of the patient's history and medical management. Discussion with the nursing staff to assess for immediate risks and cautions is vital to ensure that the patient is stable. The physical therapist must interview family and caregivers regarding the patient's previous level of functioning, growth and developmental milestones, living environment, medical/ surgical history, and likes and dislikes. This time can also be used to discuss the family's perspectives on the injury and their goals. Because a toddler is dependent on the family for care and emotional support, family-centered care must be implemented.[7] If possible, a family member should be present during the examination since the child's anxiety is likely to be decreased when the primary caregiver is present.[21]

The child in this case currently has a PGCS score of 11 and he is still intubated. His eyes are open and he is beginning to focus on people and pull away from tactile input. Potential noxious examination techniques, such as moving the child into different positions or performing ROM on joints that may not have not been moved in several days, should be performed in a proactive manner.[18] Positions of comfort, distractions, procedural preparation, and parent coaching[22,23] should be employed when feasible and necessary. A systems review as outlined in the *Guide to Physical Therapist Practice*[24] should be performed as thoroughly as possible.

Specific deficits following a near-drowning episode that are of particular concern to the physical therapist include: learning, memory, attention, executive functions, visuospatial functions, communication skills, and movement disorders including rigidity, dystonia, chorea, action myoclonus, ataxia, dysarthria, dysphagia, and ocular apraxia.[25-28] Careful documentation of muscle tone and movement patterns is necessary in order to predict the development of postural asymmetry, contractures, deformity, and the potential for skin breakdown. A meticulous examination of skin integrity should be performed. Motor functioning should be assessed using both criterion and norm-referenced assessments, such as the **Gross Motor Function Measure** (GMFM)[29] and the Peabody Scales of Motor Development,[30] respectively. The GMFM has demonstrated responsiveness and validity as an evaluative measure of gross motor function in children with traumatic brain injury.[29] The GMFM is responsive to changes in gross motor function secondary to therapeutic interventions. The five dimensions tested include: (1) lying and rolling; (2) sitting; (3) crawling and kneeling; (4) standing; and (5) walking. The lying and rolling dimension and, possibly the sitting dimension would be most appropriate for the initial evaluation of this child. Functional skills should be assessed using tools such as the Wee-FIM36 or the Pediatric Evaluation of Disability Inventory.[31,32] The developmental age of the child determines the tools that should be used to assess pain. For this patient, behavioral and physiological measures such as the Comfort Behavior Scale or the Non-communicating Children's Pain Checklist are indicated.[33]

The physical therapist synthesizes the information gathered from the examination to determine the patient's diagnosis, prognosis, and plan of care. Anticipated musculoskeletal, neuromuscular, and cardiopulmonary secondary impairments must also be considered during this phase in addition to anatomical changes due to growth and further development. Growing evidence regarding neuroplasticity and recovery of function suggest that premorbid status and the quality of the physical and social environment be considered during prognosis.[34] Caregiver coping and degree of optimism may strongly affect long-term outcomes as well.[35-37]

Plan of Care and Interventions

The general physical therapy plan of care includes preventing the predictable secondary impairments that may occur in any critically ill bed-bound individual (joint contracture, muscle atrophy, skin breakdown) and improving or maintaining ventilation and oxygenation. Passive ROM must include functional ROM of every joint in the extremities. Mandibular, cervical, thoracic and lumbar ranges should be maintained as well. Sensory stimulation may increase the arousal and attention of the patient. Such stimuli may be in the form of visual, olfactory, taste, auditory, touch, movement, or position. Attention must be paid to the patient's reactions to each stimulus to gauge for overstimulation. As the patient is unable to verbally communicate, the physical therapist must monitor nonverbal behaviors (e.g., grimacing, increase in tone) and physiologic responses (blood pressure and heart rate) closely.

To the extent that it is possible, the physical therapist should encourage purposeful developmentally appropriate movement patterns. This could be attempted by using **cognitive-behavioral stimulation**.[4,38] Coma disrupts the arousal mechanisms and interferes with the child's ability to respond to the environment. As perception is linked to action, activities that improve a child's awareness of the environment are paramount. Initially, the child could be presented with structured sensory modalities (vision, hearing, smell, taste, touch, posture, and motion) to increase the level of arousal and environmental awareness. The family could be encouraged to bring in the child's favorite items from home—perhaps a favorite stuffed animal or musical book. The aroma from favorite foods could be used as well. Once arousal and awareness increase, the child could be encouraged to make purposeful movements toward the stimulus, such as reaching out to touch a stuffed bear. Auditory stimulation, such as a favorite song, could be paired with movement. For example, if the child is working on head control in supported sitting, music could be played whenever he holds his head erect and then stopped when he drops his head. Localization of visual, auditory, and tactile inputs can be facilitated as well. For example, every time a caregiver says the child's name, the child could be encouraged, at first passively if need be, to turn his head toward the caregiver. To try to improve cognitive level, multimodal stimuli can be used. If there is a neglected side, the visual layout of the social and physical environment should be construed to facilitate movement on the neglected side. As the child's medical stability allows, the physical therapist addresses functional, gross and fine motor, and visuomotor skills as the child's arousal, attention, and communication progress. A typical 2-year-old child should be able to walk well, run, jump in place or from a small step, walk up and down steps with a hand held, kick a small ball forward, catch a rolled ball, throw a ball for a short distance without accuracy, stack several blocks, scribble on a piece of paper, place a small object in a bottle, and put at least one piece of a three-piece formboard in the proper hole.[30]

It is vital to include caregiver education as an intervention. The benefits of caregiver education are twofold: not only is the patient receiving more consistent stimulation and mobilization, but the caregivers have an opportunity to feel as though they are doing something important to the patient's well-being and potential recovery. The effect of this responsibility cannot be overemphasized. Caregivers should be given instruction regarding positioning and complications that may result from improper positioning (e.g., contractures, pressure ulcers, asymmetries). The therapist can instruct caregivers how to perform passive ROM exercises on the patient, perform skin integrity checks, and stimulation techniques to facilitate cognitive improvement. The child in this case will most likely be discharged to a pediatric rehabilitation hospital. Rehabilitation prognosis is very difficult at this point. If the child is to be discharged home, essential equipment to consider include a rental wheelchair or adapted stroller and a bath seat. Additional equipment can be ordered as necessary, depending on the child's recovery.

Evidence-Based Clinical Recommendations

SORT: Strength of Recommendation Taxonomy

A: Consistent, good-quality patient-oriented evidence
B: Inconsistent or limited-quality patient-oriented evidence
C: Consensus, disease-oriented evidence, usual practice, expert opinion, or case series

1. Brainstem auditory evoked response (BAER) is an indicator of future neurologic recovery in patients with anoxic brain injury. **Grade B**

2. The Gross Motor Function Measure (GMFM) is a responsive and valid assessment of gross motor function in children with traumatic brain injury. **Grade B**

3. Cognitive-behavioral stimulation improves outcomes with regards to consciousness, arm control/hand function, and praxis in individuals status/post near-drowning. **Grade B**

COMPREHENSION QUESTIONS

31.1 A physical therapist in the PICU evaluates a patient 5 days after a near-drowning episode. Which of the following is associated with a better prognosis?

   A. Spontaneous, purposeful movements within 24 hours after the episode
   B. Submersion for less than 5 minutes
   C. Submersion in cold water
   D. All of the above

31.2 A physical therapist has been working with a 6-year-old child who survived a near-drowning episode 15 days ago. Strategies to improve the child's attention and promote age-appropriate movement patterns would include:

   A. Reward head lifting in supported sitting by using a multitude of sensory inputs simultaneously—the more stimulation the better.
   B. Place the child in prone and facilitate head lifting by stroking the neck extensors.
   C. Reward head lifting in supported sitting by playing music such as the child's favorite song.
   D. Place the child on a ball in sitting and facilitate head lifting.

ANSWERS

31.1   **D.** In general, neurons die when there is a lack of oxygen for periods of 5 to 10 minutes (option B). When oxygen shortage is severe and/or prolonged, increasing numbers and types of neurons are affected and the resulting sequelae are more severe.[10] Better outcomes have been reported when near-drowning occurs in cold water (option C).[11] One study has reported that children who were sufficiently awake and had spontaneous, purposeful movements and had normal brainstem function 24 hours after near-drowning had satisfactory recovery (option A).[14]

31.2   **C.** It is important to use *structured* sensory modalities to increase arousal and to pair those modalities with active movement.[4,38] Items which the child previously liked are best. Linking motor behavior to practical consequences helps improve motor learning. Sitting is a more functional and age appropriate position for a 6-year-old than prone (option B). Sitting on a dynamic surface such as a ball to facilitate head lifting would likely be too challenging 15 days after a near-drowning injury (option D).

REFERENCES

1. Casmiro M, Maitan S, De Pasquale F, Cova V, Scarpa E, Vignatelli L; NSE Study Group. Cerebro-spinal fluid and serum neuron-specific enolase concentrations in a normal population. *Eur J Neurol.* 2005;12:369-374.

2. Rech TH, Viera SR, Nagel F, Brauner JS, Scalco R. Serum neuron-specific enolase as early predictor of outcome after in-hospital cardiac arrest: a cohort study. *Crit Care*. 2006;10:R133.

3. Mandel R, Martinot A, Delepoulle F, et al. Prediction of outcome after hypoxic-ischemic encephalopathy: a prospective clinical and electrophysiologic study. *J Pediatr.* 2002;141:45-50.

4. Pierro MM, Bollea L, Di Rosa G, et al. Anoxic brain injury following near-drowning in children. Rehabilitation outcome: three case reports. *Brain Inj.* 2005;19:1147-1155.

5. Lee LK, Mao C, Thompson KM. Demographic factors and their association with outcomes in pediatric submersion injury. *Acad Emerg Med.* 2006;13:308-313.

6. DeBoer S, Scott E. Near drowning: prognosis and prevention. *Australian Emerg Nurs J.* 2004;6:27-38.

7. Barat M, Blanchard JY, Darriet D, Giroire JM, Daverat P, Hazaux JM. Les troubles neuropsychologiques des anoxies cerebrales prolongees. Influence sure le devenir functionnel. *Annales de Readaptation et de Medecine Physique.* 1989;32:657-668.

8. Volpe BT, Hirst W. The characterization of an amnesic syndrome following hypoxic ischemic injury. *Arch Neurol.* 1983;40:436-440.

9. Armengol CG. Acute oxygen deprivation: neuropsychological profiles and implications for rehabilitation. *Brain Inj.* 2000;14:237-250.

10. Beyda DH. Pathophysiology of near-drowning and treatment of the child with a submersion incident. *Crit Care Nurs Clin North Am.* 1991;3:273-280.

11. Lezak MD. *Neuropsychological Assessment.* 3rd ed. New York: Oxford University Press; 1995.

12. Wilson BA. Cognitive functioning of adult survivors of cerebral hypoxia. *Brain Inj.* 1996;10:863-874.

13. Medical aspects of the persistent vegetative state. The Multi-Society Task Force on PVS. *N Engl J Med.* 1994;330:1499-1508.

14. Abrams RA, Mubarak S. Musculoskeletal consequences of near-drowning in children. *J Pediatr Orthop.* 1991;11:168-175.

15. Shaw KN, Briede CA. Submersion injuries: drowning and near-drowning. *Emerg Med Clin North Am*. 1989;7:355-370.

16. Fields AI. Near-drowning in the pediatric population. *Crit Care Clin*. 1992;8:113-129.

17. Bratton SL, Jardine DS, Morray JP. Serial neurologic examinations after near drowning and outcome. *Arch Pediatr Adolesc Med*. 1994;148:167-170.

18. Farah MJ. *Visual Agnosia: Disorders of Object Recognition and What They Tell Us about Normal Vision*. Cambridge, MA: Massachusetts Institute of Technology Press; 1990.

19. Fisher B, Peterson B, Hicks G. Use of brainstem auditory-evoked response testing to assess neurologic outcome following near drowning in children. *Crit Care Med*. 1992;20:578-585.

20. Swiggum M, Hamilton ML, Gleeson P, Roddey T. Pain in children with cerebral palsy: implications for pediatric physical therapy. *Pediatr Phys Ther*. 2010;22:86-92.

21. Piira T, Sugiura T, Champion GD, Donnelly N, Cole AS. The role of parental presence in the context of children's medical procedures: a systematic review. *Child Care Health Dev*. 2005;31:233-243.

22. Stephens BK, Barkey ME, Hall HR. Techniques to comfort children during stressful procedures. *Accid Emerg Nurs*. 1999;7:226-236.

23. Pederson C. Promoting parental use of nonpharmacologic techniques with children during lumbar punctures. *J Pediatr Oncol Nurs*. 1996;13:21-30.

24. American Physical Therapy Association. *Guide to Physical Therapist Practice*. 2nd ed. *Phys Ther*. 2001;81:9-746.

25. Bhatt MH, Obeso JA, Marsden CD. Time course of postanoxic akinetic-rigid and dystonic syndromes. *Neurology*. 1993;43:314-317.

26. Werhahn KJ, Brown P, Thompson PD, Marsden CD. The clinical features and prognosis of chronic posthypoxic myoclonus. *Mov Disord*. 1997;12:216-220.

27. Parkin AJ, Miller J, Vincent R. Multiple neuropsychological deficits due to anoxic encephalopathy: a case study. *Cortex*. 1987;23:655-665.

28. Shah MK, Al-Adawi S, Dorvlo AS, Burke DT. Functional outcomes following anoxic brain injury: a comparison with traumatic brain injury. *Brain Inj*. 2004;18:111-117.

29. Russell DJ, Rosenbaum PJ, Avery L, Lane M. *Gross Motor Function Measure (GMFM-66 and GMFM-88): User's Manual*. London, United Kingdom: MacKeith Press; 2002.

30. Folio MR, Fewell RR. *Peabody Developmental Motor Scales-2*. Austin, TX: PRO-ED; 2000.

31. Haley S, Coster W, Ludlow L, Haltiwanger J, Andrellos P. *Pediatric Evaluation of Disability Inventory (PEDI). Version 1.0*. Boston: New England Medical Center Hospitals; 1992.

32. Msall ME, Braun S, Granger CV. Use of the functional independence measure for children (Wee FIM): an interdisciplinary training tape. *Dev Med Child Neurol*. 1990;32(46):93.

33. O'Rourke D. The measurement of pain in infants, children, and adolescents: from policy to practice. *Phys Ther*. 2004;84:560-570.

34. Shumway-Cook A, Woollacott MH. *Motor Control: Translating Research into Clinical Practice*. 3rd ed. Baltimore, MD: Lippincott Williams & Wilkins Publishing; 2007.

35. Swiggum M. *Prediction of Adaptive Motor Skill Performance in School-Aged Children with Low Birth Weight without Major Neurosensory Impairment*. (dissertation). Houston, TX: School of Physical Therapy, Texas Woman's University; 2010.

36. Allen EC, Manuel JC, Legault C, Naughton MJ, Pivor C, O'Shea TM. Perception of child vulnerability among mothers of former premature infants. *Pediatrics*. 2004;113:267-273.

37. Eiser C, Eiser JR. Mothers' rating of quality of life in childhood cancer: initial optimism predicts improvement over time. *Psych Health*. 2007;22:535-543.

38. Liscio M, Adduci A, Galbiati S, Poggi G, Sacchi D, Strazzer S, Castelli E, Flannery J. Cognitive-behavioural stimulation protocol for severely brain-damaged patients in the post-acute stage in developmental age. *Disabil Rehabil*. 2008;30:275-285.

Listing of Cases

Listing by Case Number

Listing by Health Condition (Alphabetical)

Listing by Case Number

Listing by Health Condition (Alphabetical)

NOTE: Page numbers followed by *f* or *t* indicate figures or tables, respectively.